Infectious Diseases
and Antimicrobial Stewardship
in Critical Care Medicine

Infectious Diseases and Antimicrobial Stewardship in Critical Care Medicine

Fourth Edition

Edited by

Cheston B. Cunha

Medical Director, Antimicrobial Stewardship Program
Rhode Island Hospital and Miriam Hospital
Attending Physician, Division of Infectious Diseases and
Assistant Professor of Medicine
Brown University Alpert School of Medicine
Providence, Rhode Island

Burke A. Cunha

Formerly Chief, Infectious Disease Division
Winthrop-University Hospital
Mineola, New York
Professor of Medicine
State University of New York School of Medicine
Stony Brook, New York

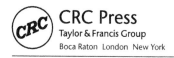

CRC Press
Taylor & Francis Group
Boca Raton London New York

CRC Press is an imprint of the
Taylor & Francis Group, an **informa** business

CRC Press
Taylor & Francis Group
6000 Broken Sound Parkway NW, Suite 300
Boca Raton, FL 33487-2742

First issued in paperback 2022

ISBN-13: 978-1-138-29706-7 (hbk)
ISBN-13: 978-1-03-233603-9 (pbk)
DOI: 10.1201/9781315099538

*For **Marie***

Peerless wife and mother

Provider of domestic peace and tranquility

Paragon of truth and beauty

Paradigm of earthly perfection…

With gratitude for her love and constant support

Burke A. Cunha

Contents

SECTION I Clinical Diagnostic Approach in the Critical Care Unit

SECTION II   Clinical Syndromic Approach in the Critical Care Unit

Foreword

The complexity of patients hospitalized in the United States is clearly increasing, especially in critical care departments. Patients are kept alive and salvaged from devastating illnesses and injuries by new mechanisms of support such as sophisticated mechanical ventilation, extracorporeal membrane oxygenation, renal replacement therapy, and ventricular assist devices. Cancer, autoimmune diseases, and transplant recipients are treated with more potent and more selective biologic agents. More and more solid organ transplants and stem cell transplants are being performed.

With the rising complexity of patients, the complexity of infectious complications is also increasing. As patients live longer with devastating diseases, as patients are immunosuppressed more substantially by their underlying primary process or by the therapies they receive, and as patients are treated with therapeutic and prophylactic antimicrobials for longer periods of time, they are being infected with a broader spectrum of bacterial, fungal, and viral pathogens compared with those seen one or two decades ago.

For healthcare providers, successful management of patients in critical care units requires new skills. The natural history of many diseases is changing due to the support these patients can receive. Thus, providers need to understand the complications that are most likely to occur, so that they can design effective preventive, diagnostic, or therapeutic strategies.

Methods to establish diagnoses of infectious complications are changing. Imaging, interventional radiology, bronchoscopy, and biliary and gastrointestinal endoscopy are some of the many ways that clinicians now obtain specimens for diagnostic analysis. Matrix-assisted laser desorption/ionization-time of flight mass spectrometry and nucleic acid amplification are among the techniques that have revolutionized diagnostic microbiology. However, these new approaches present challenges regarding how to interpret ultrasensitive techniques and how to determine which genes recognized by diagnostic tests are being expressed or might be inducible for future expression.

After years of pleas for new antimicrobials, there is a trickle of new antivirals, antifungals, and antibacterials entering into the antimicrobial armamentarium. Some of these are being used prophylactically, which prevents important clusters of infections but selects previously uncommon and highly resistant pathogens. Others are being used therapeutically, with highly encouraging results. Intensivists must know how to use these drugs, but they must also recognize the consequences of using them on the individual patient as well as on the ecology of the critical care unit (CCU), the hospital, or the global community.

The fourth edition of *Infectious Diseases and Antimicrobial Stewardship in Critical Care Medicine* recognizes that the field of infectious diseases is changing rapidly, especially for patients with the most complex and the most life-threatening illnesses. Indeed, the field is so complex that a new subspecialty is emerging, critical care-infectious diseases, which is attracting expert clinicians to focus specifically on the infectious complications that occur in this patient population. Chet and Burke Cunha have assembled experienced clinicians who focus on providing practical information for providers caring for critically ill patients. They have appropriately focused more attention on antibiotic stewardship.

This book has a unique focus, which expert clinicians will continue to learn from, refer to, and utilize to improve the outcome of individual patients in their CCUs and the long-term performance of their clinical programs.

Henry Mazur
Department of Critical Care Medicine, Clinical Center
National Institutes of Health
Bethesda, Maryland

Preface to the First Edition

Infectious diseases are very important in critical care. In the critical care unit (CCU), infectious diseases are seen in the differential diagnoses of the majority of patients, and maybe, patients acquire infections in the CCU. However, infectious disease is accorded a relatively minor place in most critical care textbooks and does not receive the emphasis it deserves, given its presence in the CCU.

The infectious diseases encountered in the critical care setting are some of the most severe and often difficult to diagnose. This book was developed for critical care practitioners, the majority of whom are not trained in infectious diseases. It is written by clinicians in infectious diseases in critical care and is meant as a handbook to provide valuable information not included in critical care textbooks.

The text is unique in its emphasis and organization. It comprises four main sections: The first section deals with general concepts of infectious diseases in the CCU; the second deals with infectious diseases on the basis of clinical syndromes; the third deals with specific infectious disease problems; and the fourth deals with therapeutic considerations in critical care patients.

One of the unique features of this book is its emphasis on differential diagnosis rather than therapy. The main problem in the CCU is not therapeutic but diagnostic. If the patient's problem can be clearly delineated diagnostically, treatment is a relatively straightforward matter. Therapy cannot be appropriate unless related to the correct diagnosis. *Infectious Diseases in Critical Care Medicine* emphasizes the importance of differential diagnoses in each chapter and includes chapters on various "mimics" of infectious diseases. In fact, it is with the "mimics" of various infectious disorders that clinicians often face the most difficult diagnostic challenges. This book should help CCU clinicians readily discern between infectious diseases and the noninfectious disorders that mimic infection.

This is the first and only book that deals solely with infectious diseases in critical care medicine. It is not meant to be a comprehensive textbook of infectious diseases. Rather, it focuses on the most common infections likely to present diagnostic or therapeutic difficulties in the critical care setting. The authors have approached their subjects from a clinical perspective and have written in a style useful to clinicians. In addition to its usefulness to critical care intensivists, this book should also be helpful to internists and infectious disease clinicians participating in the care of patients in the CCU.

Burke A. Cunha

Preface to the Second Edition

Infectious diseases continue to represent a major diagnostic and therapeutic challenge in the critical care unit (CCU). Infectious diseases maintain their pre-eminence in the CCU setting because of their frequency and importance in the critical unit patient population.

Since the first edition of *Infectious Diseases in Critical Care Medicine*, there have been newly described infectious diseases to be considered in differential diagnosis, and new antimicrobial agents have been added to the therapeutic armamentarium.

The second edition of *Infectious Diseases in Critical Care Medicine* continues the clinical orientation of the first edition. Differential diagnostic considerations in infectious diseases continue to be the central focus of the second edition.

Clinicians caring for acutely ill patients in the CCU are confronted with the common problem of differentiating noninfectious disease mimics from their infectious disease counterparts. For this reason, the differential diagnosis of noninfectious diseases remains an important component of infectious diseases in the second edition. The second edition of *Infectious Diseases in Critical Care Medicine* emphasizes differential clinical features that enable clinicians to sort out complicated diagnostic problems.

Because CCU patients often have complicated/interrelated multisystem disorders, subspecialty expertise is essential for optimal patient care. Early utilization of infectious disease consultation is important to ensure proper application/interpretation of appropriate laboratory tests and for the selection/optimization of antimicrobial therapy.

Selecting the optimal antimicrobial for use in the CCU is vital. The optimization of antimicrobial dosing to take into account the antibiotic's pharmacokinetic and pharmacodynamic attributes is equally important. The infectious disease clinician, in addition to optimizing dosing considerations, is also able to evaluate potential antimicrobial side effects as well as drug-drug interactions, which may affect therapy. Infectious disease consultations can be helpful in differentiating colonization ordinarily not treated from infection that should be treated. Physicians who are not infectious disease clinicians lack the necessary sophistication in clinical infectious disease training, medical microbiology, pharmacokinetics/pharmacodynamics, and diagnostic experience. Physicians in CCUs should rely on infectious disease clinicians as well as other consultants to optimize care for these acutely ill patients.

The second edition of *Infectious Diseases in Critical Care Medicine* has been streamlined, maintaining the clinical focus in a more compact volume. Again, the authors have been selected for their expertise and experience. The contributors to the book are world-class teacher/clinicians who have in their writings imparted wisdom accrued from years of clinical experience for the benefit of the CCU physicians and their patients. The second edition of *Infectious Diseases in Critical Care Medicine* remains the only book dealing with infections in critical care.

Burke A. Cunha

Preface to the Third Edition

Infectious disease aspects of critical care have changed much since the first edition was published in 1998. Infectious diseases are ever present and are becoming important in critical care. *Infectious Diseases in Critical Care Medicine* (third edition) remains the only book exclusively dedicated to infectious diseases in critical care.

Importantly, *Infectious Diseases in Critical Care Medicine* (third edition) is written from the infectious disease perspective by clinicians for clinicians who deal with infectious diseases in critical care. The infectious disease perspective is vital in the clinical diagnostic approach to noninfectious and infectious disease problems encountered in critical care. The third edition of this book is not only completely updated but includes new topics that have become important in infectious diseases in critical care since the publication of the second edition.

The hallmark of clinical excellence in infectious disease consultation is the diagnostic experience and expertise of the infectious disease consultant. The clinical approach should not be to arrive at a diagnosis by ordering a bewildering number of clinically irrelevant tests, hoping for clues from abnormal findings. The optimal differential diagnostic approach depends on the infectious disease consultant carefully analyzing the history, physical findings, and pertinent nonspecific laboratory tests in critically ill patients to focus on diagnostic efforts. Before a definitive diagnosis is made, the infectious disease consultant's role as diagnostician is to correctly interpret and correlate nonspecific laboratory tests in the correct clinical context, which should prompt specific laboratory testing to rule in or rule out the most likely diagnostic possibilities. As subspecialist consultants, infectious disease clinicians are excellent diagnosticians. For this reason, infectious disease consultation is of vital importance for all but the most straightforward infectious disease problems encountered in critical care.

Another distinguishing characteristic of infectious disease clinicians is that they are both diagnostically and therapeutically focused. Many noninfectious disease clinicians often tend to empirically "cover" patients with an excessive number of antibiotics to provide coverage against a wide range of unlikely pathogens. Currently, most of resistance problems in critical care units result from not appreciating the resistance potential of some commonly used antibiotics in many multidrug regimens, such as ciprofloxaxin, imipenem, and ceftazidime. Some contend that this approach is defensible because with antibiotic "de-escalation," the unnecessary antibiotics can be discontinued subsequently. Unfortunately, except for culture results from blood isolates cultures with skin/soft tissue infections, or cerebrospinal fluid with meningitis, usually there are no subsequent microbiologic data upon which to base antibiotic de-escalation, such as nosocomial pneumonia, abscesses, and intra-abdominal/pelvic

infections. The preferred infectious disease approach is to base initial empiric therapy or to cover the most likely pathogens rather than clinically unlikely pathogens. Should diagnostically valid data become available, a change in antimicrobial therapy may or may not be warranted based on new information.

Because infectious disease consultation is so important in the differential diagnostic approach in critical care, this book's emphasis is on differential diagnosis. If the diagnosis is inaccurate/incorrect, empiric therapy will necessarily be incorrect. To assist those taking care of critically ill patients, chapters on physical exam clues and their mimics, ophthalmologic clues and their mimics in infectious disease, and radiologic clues and their mimics in infectious disease have been included in this edition. In addition, several chapters, notably "Clinical Approach to Fever" and "Fever and Rash," also emphasize on physical findings.

Since the last edition, some infectious diseases, such as *Clostridium difficile* diarrhea/colitis, severe acute respiratory syndrome, hantavirus pulmonary syndrome, avian influenza (H5N1), and swine influenza (H1N1), have become important in critical care medicine.

Another important topic has been added on infections related to immunomodulating/immunosuppressive agents. The widespread introduction of immune modulation therapy has resulted in a recrudescence of many infections due to intracellular pathogens, which are important to be recognized in patients receiving these agents. Because miliary tuberculosis is so important and is not an infrequent complication of steroid/immunosuppressive therapy, a chapter on this topic also has been included in the third edition.

As mentioned, antibiotic resistance in the critical care unit is a continuing problem with short- and long-term clinical consequences. Currently, methicillin-resistant *Staphylococcus aureus* and vancomycin-resistant enterococci are the most important gram-positive pathogens in critical care, and a chapter has been added on antibiotic therapy for these pathogens. Among the multidrug-resistant aerobic gram-negative bacilli, *Klebsiella pneumoniae*, *Pseudomonas aeruginosa*, and *Acinetobacter baumannii* continue to pose difficult therapeutic problems, and a chapter has been included on this important topic.

The contributors to the third edition of *Infectious Diseases in Critical Care Medicine* are nationally or internationally acknowledged experts in their respective fields. The authors have been selected for their clinical excellence and experience. They are teacher-clinicians also known for their ability to effectively distill the key points related to their topics.

The third edition is not just a compendium of current guidelines. Guidelines are not definitive and for this reason often change over time. Guideline followers may not agree with this book's clinical approach, which is evidence based but tempered by clinical experience. Especially in critical care, the key determinant of optimal patient care is experienced based clinical judgment, which the clinician contributors have provided.

In summary, this edition is both up-to-date and better than ever. Now in its third edition, *Infectious Diseases in* *Critical Care Medicine*, written by clinicians for clinicians, remains the only major text exclusively dealing with the major infectious disease syndromes encountered in critical care medicine.

Burke A. Cunha

Preface to the Fourth Edition

Infectious Diseases and Antimicrobial Stewardship in Critical Care Medicine (4th edition) maintains its clinical emphasis on practical problem solving of the major infectious disease syndromes encountered daily in the critical care unit (CCU). The first edition of *Infectious Disease in Critical Care Medicine* was published in 1998 and was the first book devoted entirely to infectious disease problems in the CCU. Each subsequent edition has maintained emphasis on the clinical approach. The fourth edition maintains this clinical practical approach to difficult diagnostic and therapeutic problems in the CCU. The main challenge in critical care remains making a time-critical correct clinical syndromic diagnosis, on which correct therapy is based. Diagnosis is still largely based on the history (80%) and physical exam (10%) and is accordingly emphasized throughout the book.

Infectious Diseases and Antimicrobial Stewardship in Critical Care Medicine (fourth edition) consists of four sections, i.e., clinical diagnostic approach, clinical syndromic approach, clinical approach in compromised hosts, and antimicrobial therapy and antibiotic stewardship. The 38 chapter topics were selected because of the clinical relevance. Topics focus on commonest diagnostic and therapeutic problems encountered daily in the CCU. Intentionally, all topics are not covered, and some topics are repeated from a different perspective in different chapters.

The fourth edition of *Infectious Diseases and Antimicrobial Stewardship in Critical Care Medicine* is written with continued emphasis on clinical diagnostic reasoning based on a pertinent history, relevant physical exam, and key related nonspecific test clues to assist the critical care consultant in making an accurate and timely clinical syndromic diagnosis. Overreliance on non-clue-directed testing brings with it a variety of negative consequences for patients. Most of the diagnostic confusion in the CCU results from irrelevant or misleading laboratory tests and imaging. *Infectious Diseases and Antimicrobial Stewardship in Critical Care Medicine* (fourth edition) provides critical care clinicians with a carefully considered clinical approach, assisting clinicians to order key tests and to properly interpret the clinical relevance of test results in the clinical context.

The new final section of *Infectious Diseases and Antimicrobial Stewardship in Critical Care Medicine* of the (fourth edition) is devoted to antimicrobial stewardship. Once the most likely clinical syndromic diagnosis has been established by clinical problem solving, selecting and optimizing antibiotic therapy completes the CCU consultant's role. Antibiotic stewardship programs (ASPs) optimize antimicrobial therapy by utilizing dosing based on pharmacokinetic/pharmacodynamic (PK/PD) considerations, site of infection, antibiotic resistance potential, antibiotic drug-drug interactions, and antibiotic side effects. Each hospital has its own epidemiology, resistance profiles, and medical staff expertise. The ASPs should be tailored to the institution's particular problems, i.e., "one size does not fit all." However, with each ASP, "the devil is in the details." An effective ASP program requires a multidisciplinary approach tailored to each hospital, which includes support from the medical microbiology laboratory, infection control, and the pharmacy under the direction of an infectious disease clinician expert in antimicrobial therapy. This new section recognizes the increasing importance of antibiotic stewardship in the CCU.

The contributors of *Infectious Diseases and Antimicrobial Stewardship in Critical Care Medicine, Fourth Edition* are experienced clinicians who are recognized experts in their fields. We are grateful to the distinguished contributors for sharing their clinical wisdom for the benefit of critical care physicians and their patients.

Cheston B. Cunha

Burke A. Cunha

Editors

Cheston B. Cunha, MD, FACP, is medical director of the Antimicrobial Stewardship Program at Rhode Island Hospital and the Miriam Hospital in Providence, Rhode Island, USA. He is also an attending in adult infectious disease in the Division of Infectious Diseases and assistant professor of medicine at Brown University Alpert School of Medicine. Dr. Cunha has written/co-written 51 articles, 53 book chapters, and 7 books. He has been an editor of *Antibiotic Stewardship, Antibiotic Essentials* (15th and 16th editions), *Clinical Infectious Diseases* (3rd edition), and *Infectious Diseases in Critical Care Medicine and Antibiotic Stewardship* (4th edition). He has been an annual recipient of the Dean's Excellence in Teaching Award from the Alpert Medical School of Brown University.

Burke A. Cunha, MD, MACP, formerly Chief, of the Infectious Disease Division at Winthrop-University Hospital, Mineola, New York, and professor of medicine at State University of New York School of Medicine, Stony Brook, New York. He is one of the world's leading authorities on antimicrobial therapy and clinical infectious diseases. He has written/edited 1355 articles, 221 book chapters, and 36 books. He has received numerous teaching awards, including the Aesculapius Award for teaching excellence and the Spatz Award for clinical excellence. Dr. Cunha is a Master of the American College of Physicians, awarded for lifetime achievement as a Master Clinician and Master Teacher.

Contributors

Müge Ayhan
Atatürk Training and Research Hospital
Ankara, Turkey

Divyansh Bajaj
Department of Medicine
St. Vincent's Medical Center
Bridgeport, Connecticut

David Bernstein
Department of Medicine
Northwell Health
Zucker School of Medicine at Hofstra/Northwell
Manhasset, New York

Emilio Bouza
Clinical Microbiology and Infectious Diseases Department
Hospital General Universitario Gregorio Marañón
and
Department of Medicine
School of Medicine
Universidad Complutense de Madrid
and
Instituto de Investigación Sanitaria
Hospital Gregorio Marañón
and
CIBER Enfermedades Respiratorias-CIBERES
    (CB06/06/0058)
Madrid, Spain

Kristina Bruno
College of Pharmacy and Health Sciences
St. John's University
New York City, New York

John L. Brusch
Division of Infectious Diseases
Cambridge Health Alliance
Cambridge, Massachusetts

Almudena Burillo
Clinical Microbiology and Infectious Diseases Department
Hospital General Universitario Gregorio Marañón
and
Department of Medicine
School of Medicine
Universidad Complutense de Madrid
and
Instituto de Investigación Sanitaria
Hospital Gregorio Marañón
Madrid, Spain

Kevin Cahill
NSLIJ, Lenox Hill Hospital
New York City, New York

Abdullah Chahin
Critical Care and Infectious Diseases
Warren Alpert Medical School of Brown University
Providence, Rhode Island

Burke A. Cunha
Infectious Disease Division
Winthrop-University Hospital
Mineola, New York
and
State University of New York School of Medicine
Stony Brook, New York

Cheston B. Cunha
Infectious Disease Division
Department of Medicine
Rhode Island and Miriam Hospitals
Warren Alpert Medical School of Brown University
Providence, Rhode Island

Lee S. Engel
Department of Medicine
Louisiana State University Health Science Center
New Orleans, Louisiana

Donald E. Fry
Departments of Surgery
Northwestern University Feinberg School of Medicine
Chicago, Illinois
and
The University of New Mexico School of Medicine
Albuquerque, New Mexico

Joseph Metmowlee Garland
Division of Infectious Disease
Department of Medicine
The Miriam Hospital and Rhode Island Hospital
and
Warren Alpert Medical School of Brown University
Providence, Rhode Island

Bronwen Garner
Department of Medicine
Division of Infectious Diseases
The University of Utah
Salt Lake City, Utah

Sonali Gupta
Department of Medicine
St. Vincent's Medical Center
Bridgeport, Connecticut

John J. Halperin
Overlook Medical Center
Atlantic Neuroscience Institute
Summit, New Jersey
and
Department of Neurology and Medicine
Sidney Kimmel Medical College of Thomas Jefferson
    University
Philadelphia, Pennsylvania

Kimberly Hanson
ARUP Laboratories
The University of Utah
Salt Lake City, Utah

John M. Horne
Section of Infectious Diseases
Departments of Medicine
Medical Microbiology and Immunology
Creighton University School of Medicine
and
V.A. Medical Center
Omaha, Nebraska

Sana Idrees
Department of Medicine
St. Vincent's Medical Center
Bridgeport, Connecticut

Douglas S. Katz
Department of Radiology
NYU Winthrop Hospital
Mineola, New York

Elise Kochoumian
Department of Medicine
NSLIJ, Lenox Hill Hospital
New York City, New York

Jason M. Lazar
Department of Medicine
Director of non-invasive Cardiology
State University of New York Downstate Medical Center
Brooklyn, New York

Andrew Levinson
Division of Pulmonary, Critical Care, and Sleep Medicine
and
Department of Medicine
The Miriam Hospital and Rhode Island Hospital
Warren Alpert Medical School of Brown University
Providence, Rhode Island

Huei-Wen Lim
Department of Internal Medicine
Northwell Health
Manhasset, New York

Fred A. Lopez
Department of Medicine
Louisiana State University Health Science Center
New Orleans, Louisiana

Michael Lorenzo
Pharmacy Department
The Miriam Hospital and Rhode Island Hospital
Providence, Rhode Island

Olivier Lortholary
Université Paris Descartes
Centre d'Infectiologie Necker-Pasteur
Hôpital Necker-Enfants Malades
IHU Imagine, APHP
Paris, France

Jocelyn A. Luongo
Department of Radiology
NYU Winthrop Hospital
Mineola, New York

Larry I. Lutwick
Infectious Disease Division
Mayo Clinic Hospital
Eau Claire, Wisconsin

Danielle Maffei
College of Pharmacy and Health Sciences
St. John's University
New York City, New York

Eleni E. Magira
First Department of Critical Care
National and Kapodistrian University of Athens Medical School
Athens, Greece

Thomas J. Marrie
Department of Medicine
Dalhousie University
Halifax, Nova Scotia, Canada

Joseph Mattana
Department of Medicine
St. Vincent's Medical Center
Bridgeport, Connecticut
and
The Frank H. Netter MD School of Medicine
Quinnipiac University
North Haven, Connecticut

Bushra Mina
Pulmonary Medicine
Critical Care Medicine
Lenox Hill Hospital
New York City, New York

Yehia Y. Mishriki
Department of Medicine
Lehigh Valley Health Network
Allentown, Pennsylvania

Jonathon Moore
Pulmonary and Critical Care Department
NSLIJ, Lenox Hill Hospital
New York City, New York

Patricia Muñoz
Clinical Microbiology and Infectious Diseases Department
Hospital General Universitario Gregorio Marañón
and
Department of Medicine
School of Medicine
Universidad Complutense de Madrid
and
Instituto de Investigación Sanitaria
Hospital Gregorio Marañón
and
CIBER Enfermedades Respiratorias-CIBERES (CB06/06/0058)
Madrid, Spain

Steven M. Opal
Infectious Disease Division
Warren Alpert Medical School of Brown University
Providence, Rhode Island
and
Ocean State Clinical Coordinating Center of Rhode Island Hospital
Providence, Rhode Island

Orlando A. Ortiz
Department of Radiology
NYU Winthrop Hospital
Mineola, New York

Diane M. Parente
Pharmacy Department
The Miriam Hospital and Rhode Island Hospital
Providence, Rhode Island

Perrine Parize
Université Paris Descartes
Centre d'Infectiologie Necker-Pasteur
Hôpital Necker-Enfants Malades
IHU Imagine, APHP
Paris, France

Frédéric Pène
Université Paris Descartes
Service de Réanimation, Hôpital Cochin
Paris, France

Anne Pouvaret
Université Paris Descartes
Centre d'Infectiologie Necker-Pasteur
Hôpital Necker-Enfants Malades
IHU Imagine, APHP
Paris, France

Laurel C. Preheim
Section of Infectious Diseases
Departments of Medicine
Medical Microbiology and Immunology
Creighton University School of Medicine
and
V.A. Medical Center
Omaha, Nebraska

Jana Preis
Division of Infectious Diseases
Department of Veterans Affairs
Medical Center Brooklyn
Brooklyn, New York

David A. Quillen
Department of Ophthalmology
George and Barbara Blankenship
College of Medicine
Pennsylvania State University
Hershey, Pennsylvania

Charles V. Sanders
Department of Medicine
Louisiana State University Health Science Center
New Orleans, Louisiana

Edward J. Septimus
Infection Prevention and Epidemiology Clinical Services
    Group
HCA Healthcare System
Texas A&M Health Science Center College of Medicine
    Houston
Houston, Texas

Shabnam Seydafkan
Division of Cardiovascular Medicine
State University of New York Downstate Medical Center
Brooklyn, New York

Boris Shapiro
Department of Radiology
NYU Winthrop Hospital
Mineola, New York

Wendy Sligl
Department of Critical Care Medicine
and
Division of Infectious Diseases
Faculty of Medicine and Dentistry
University of Alberta
Edmonton, Alberta, Canada

Charles W. Stratton
Clinical Microbiology Laboratory
Division of Infectious Diseases
Vanderbilt University Medical Center
Nashville, Tennessee

Praveen Sudhindra
UnityPoint Health
Peoria, Illinois

Damary C. Torres
College of Pharmacy and Health Sciences
St. John's University
New York City, New York
and
Clinical Pharmacist
NYU Winthrop Hospital
Mineola, New York

David Waldner
Division of Infectious Diseases
Faculty of Medicine and Dentistry
University of Alberta
Edmonton, Alberta, Canada

Michael J. Wilkinson
Department of Ophthalmology
College of Medicine
Pennsylvania State University
Hershey, Pennsylvania

Edward Wing
Division of Infectious Disease
Department of Medicine
The Miriam Hospital and Rhode Island Hospital
Warren Alpert Medical School of Brown University
Providence, Rhode Island

Paul-Louis Woerther
Université Paris XII, Service de Microbiologie
Hôpital Henri Mondor
Créteil, France

Gary P. Wormser
Department of Medicine
Division of Infectious Diseases
New York Medical College
Valhalla, New York

Gülden Yilmaz
Department of Infectious Diseases and Clinical
    Microbiology
Gülhane Training and Research Hospital
Ankara, Turkey

Section I

Clinical Diagnostic Approach in the Critical Care Unit

1 Diagnostic Reasoning and Clinical Problem Solving

Burke A. Cunha

CONTENTS

There are only three things that are important in medicine: diagnosis, diagnosis, and diagnosis.

—Charles Bryan

Incorrect diagnoses lead to incorrect treatments.

—William Osler

The value of experience is not in seeing much, but in seeing wisely.

—William Osler

CLINICAL PERSPECTIVE

The diagnostician must recognize and appreciate important aspects of a pertinent history regarding the patient's DDx. Another important factor in DDx considerations is the tempo of the disease process. Disease tempo narrows DDx in acute bacterial meningitis (ABM), acute viral meningitis (AVM), acute viral encephalitis (AVE), and CAPs.

Physical findings are helpful when present, e.g., Horder's spots in psittacosis. Aside from rash and nuchal rigidity in ABM or AVM, the physical examination (PE) in CAP is largely limited to auscultation of the chest. In ABM, if CAP is not present, tenderness over the sinuses or mastoids points to an upper respiratory tract bacterial etiology of the patient's ABM. The PE can be diagnostic in meningococcemia (MC) with ABM. Similarly, in AVM, a vesicular rash points to varicella-zoster virus (VZV) as the cause of the patient's AVM. In AVE, tremor and flaccid paralysis are important

clues to West Nile encephalitis (WNE). Some PE findings in AVE have important Dx value; e.g., *Herpes labialis* in a patient with AVE effectively eliminates herpes simplex virus (HSV) from further Dx consideration. *H. labialis* may precede HSV AVE but does not present at the same time as the AVE. Before proceeding to interpretation of the diagnostic significance of non-specific laboratory tests, the diagnostician should identify/differentiate the characteristic findings from the history, PE, and disease tempo from findings that are only consistent with the DDx. It is as important to identify diagnostic eliminators (DxE) as it is to recognize and appreciate key characteristic diagnostic findings.

Diagnostic eliminators are a powerful Dx tool to rapidly limit the DDx by eliminating some Dx from further consideration. Finding DxE in the history, PE, and non-specific laboratory tests rapidly narrows the DDx. This eliminates unnecessary testing, since some disorders in this DDx have been essentially eliminated from further Dx consideration. The clinical significance of clinical and laboratory test findings lies not in their sensitivity or specificity but rather by the company they keep. For example, in a patient with CAP, the finding of otherwise unexplained of relative bradycardia (RB) is a DxE for all typical and most atypical causes of CAP. In contrast, the DDx of CAP with RB is narrowed to Q fever, psittacosis, and Legionnaire's disease. While RB is not specific for any of these CAP causes, if combined with an elevated ferritin and/or hypophosphatemia, the most probable cause of RB is Legionnaire's disease.

In ABM or AVE, the presence of RBCs in the cerebrospinal fluid (CSF) could represent a traumatic tap or bleed (CVA,

ICH, SAH, etc.). If these causes of the presence of RBCs in the CSF can be eliminated, the DDx is narrowed to *Listeria monocytogenes* or severe HSV AVE. The presence of RBCs in the CSF also acts as a DxE in ruling out other causes of ABM, AVM, and AVE.

The clinical conundrum in the patient with ABM or AVE and otherwise unexplained CSF RBCs is readily resolved by correctly interpreting the CSF lactic acid (LA) level. The CSF glucose is unhelpful in this situation, as it is markedly decreased in ABM and *Listeria monocytogenes* ABM and may be decreased in HSV AVE. The combined Dx difficulty of ABM/AVE with decreased CSF glucose and unexplained RBCs is easily resolved by considering the Dx significance of a highly elevated CSF LA level. In this setting, *L. monocytogenes* ABM may be easily differentiated from AVE (both with a ↓ CSF glucose and CSF RBCs) by CSF LA levels. The CSF LA will be highly elevated in *L. monocytogenes* ABM but not in HSV AVE. Although RBCs may elevate the CSF LA levels somewhat, the CSF LA level is proportional to the number of RBCs present and is easily assessed.

Another important point in increasing the Dx specificity of non-specific findings is by the degree of the elevation. Degree of elevation alone confers Dx specificity to many tests; e.g., relatively few are associated with a very highly elevated ESR, but relatively few if the ESR is very highly elevated. For example, in CAP, an ESR >100 mm/h, just by virtue of the degree of elevation, increases Dx specificity. In the DDx of CAP, DDx is narrowed from more than a dozen entities to only *Streptococcus pneumoniae* or Legionnaire's disease. The ESR should be combined with other characteristic findings associated with *S. pneumoniae* or Legionnaire's disease to increase Dx specificity. Also, before interpreting the Dx significance of a highly elevated ESR in CAP, the clinician must be certain that the ESR elevation is otherwise unexplained by another disorder. Similarly, in ABM, the CSF LA may be elevated due to RBCs in partially treated ABM (PTABM), brain anoxia, hepatic encephalopathy, etc. but is very highly elevated only in ABM.

Combining characteristic clinical and laboratory test findings narrows the DDx and increases the Dx probability of the most likely Dx in the DDx, as the examples in tables show—DxE used in conjunction combined with characteristic findings leads to an accurate clinical syndromic diagnostic clinical syndromic diagnosis (CSD) on which to base specific testing and initial empiric therapy.

TABLE 1.1

Six Steps in Clinical Diagnostic Reasoning to Arrive at a Clinical Syndromic Diagnosis

		Clinical Correlations (see Table 1.2 on CAP)
Step #1	*Localize the main problem to the primary organ system involved.*	Patient presenting *acutely ill with fever and SOB* also has loose stools, HA, and mental confusion. *DDx: Encephalitis? Infectious diarrhea? But most likely it is CAP.*
Step #2	*Factor in the disease tempo* (acute vs. subacute vs. chronic).	*Disease tempo suggests an acute process* arguing against a subacute CNS/GI problem or CAP (due to a less virulent pathogen)
Step #3	From the history and non-specific laboratory tests, search *for characteristic findings[a] for each likely possibility* in the DDx.	*Characteristic finding for CAP would be a pulse-temperature deficit (RB)* with multiple organ system involvement (CNS, GI, etc.).
Step #4	*Take into account any relevant diseases in the PMH* (that could impact disease severity or the clinical presentation).	If this patient had a relevant PMH, e.g., SLE, *SLE with flare could manifest* as SLE cerebritis (with mental confusion) or SLE pneumonitis (mimicking CAP). At this point, R/O SLE flare.
Step #5	Among the narrowed DDx, **search for** DxE (effectively eliminate the diagnosis from further Dx consideration/testing).	The *patient has RB, which may be considered a characteristic finding* in CAPs due to psittacosis, *Q fever, or Legionnaire's disease.* Alternately, *RB is also a DxE in the DDx of CAP, since RB effectively eliminates all typical CAP pathogens* as well as tularemia, M. pneumoniae, and C. pneumoniae (including PCP).
Step #6	From the remaining few diseases in the DDx, (excluding DxE Dx), construct **a Dx point score[b] (to approximate the relative probability of each remaining Dx in the DDx).** • After all DxE have been applied (excluding diagnoses in the DDx eliminated by the DxE), *the remaining diagnoses with + point scores* represent the CSD.	After DxE are removed from the DDx, *remaining point scores for this patient* are as follows: #1: Legionnaire's disease, #2 psittacosis, and #3 Q fever. • *In this clinical vignette, the most likely Dx is Legionnaire's disease.* Psittacosis and Q fever should also be R/O by specific testing.

[a] Characteristic findings are those that are nearly always predictably present. Avoid overinterpreting findings that are only consistent with the diagnosis.

[b] Dx point scores using the presence or absence of characteristic findings: +1 point per characteristic finding; 0 = no DDx value; −1 point per lack of a characteristic finding. Dx point score is an algebraic sum of characteristic findings, e.g., +6−3 = +3.

This chapter is arranged in a tabular format to illustrate these principles (Table 1.1). Acute bacterial meningitis, AVM, and AVE are considered using a diagnostician's problem-solving-based approach by recognizing characteristic clinical and laboratory findings and by combining such findings to increase Dx specificity to quickly narrow the DDx. Lastly, DDx is applied to further limit the Dx and formulate a CSD on which to base antibiotic-stewardship-based empiric antibiotic therapy. Using common CCU, problematic DDx illustrative examples of ABM, AVM, AVE (Table 1.2), and severe CAP (Table 1.3) are presented in a tabular form.

CLINICAL PROBLEM SOLVING COMMENTARY: ACUTE BACTERIAL MENINGITIS (TABLE 1.2)

Clinical Presentation

CC/HPI	PMH
• Elderly 68 y/o male	• CLL (on steroids)
• 3D history of fever, HA, stiff neck	• No recent sick contacts
	• No recent zoonotic contact
	• No recent insect exposure/bites

HISTORY AND EPIDEMIOLOGY

The history may provide some diagnostic clues in an adult presenting with fever and headache ± mental confusion. Fever with chills, headache, a stiff neck, and clear mentation point to likely meningitis. Disease tempo and severity are further useful in differentiating ABM from acute viral (aseptic) meningitis (AVM). Recent sick contact history with someone with meningitis is helpful if the type of meningitis is known. The medical history, if positive for immunosuppressive drugs, or underlying disorders with impaired host defenses can limit the pathogen range in the DDx; e.g., a patient with a past medical history of multiple myeloma is particularly predisposed to infections with encapsulated pathogens (*S. pneumoniae*, *Haemophilus influenzae*, etc.). Such a patient presenting with ABM is most likely to be infected with either of these organisms. Of course, the same patient can have meningococcal (MC) meningitis if there has been recent close contact with a case of MC ABM. Alternatively, multiple myeloma is associated with impaired humoral immunity (↓ B-lymphocyte function), which does not predispose the patient to the various viral causes of AVM.

If the history is predominantly that of fever with mental confusion or obtundation ± mild neck stiffness, then the presumptive diagnosis is AVE. In general, bacterial pathogens cause ABM leptomeningeal infection, but brain parenchyma is unaffected. In contrast, neurotropic viruses cause AVE and primarily involve the brain parenchyma and, unless contiguous, do not affect the leptomeninges. For this reason, there is little or no nuchal rigidity with AVE.

The initial impression, based on history, to be further supported or modified, is limited to ABM vs. AVM or AVE, which most likely directs the focus on diagnostic workup.

A pertinent history can be very useful in limiting the DDx to the likely pathogen. For example, if the patient is elderly or has any sort of malignancy, the most likely pathogen presenting as ABM is *L. monocytogenes*. Since *Listeria* is an intracellular pathogen, defects in cellular immunity (↓ T-lymphocyte function) predispose to ABM in case of this organism. The case vignette is that of an 68-year-old male (elderly with CLL) (↓ CMI), who is on steroids (↓ CMI). Certainly, *Listeria* should be included in DDx. A subacute presentation of AVM should also include aseptic meningitis due to medications, e.g., TMP-SMX. Also, if hamster contact results in a "flu-like illness," which is then followed by AVM presentation, then *lymphocytic choriomeningitis* (LCM) should be strongly considered.

Exposure history is very important in dealing with diagnosis possibilities with AVE. A variety of insect vectors transport a variety of pathogens, e.g., mosquitos and WNE as well as ticks and Lyme neuroborreliosis. The CNS Lyme disease presents as a very mild AVM. In contrast, WNE may present as a fulminant AVE ± tremors or flaccid paralysis. The "great imitator" is HSV, which may present as a mild AVM or as severe acute AVE with obtundation/coma. Important in the history of cases of AVE where HSV is the DDx is a recent past medical history of *H. labialis*. Patients with HSV AVE with a PMH of *H. labialis* may report lip blisters in the preceding 1–3 weeks (gone later when the patient presents). If *H. labialis* is present when the patient with AVE presents, it is not due to HSV. The HSV from *H. labialis* needs time to regress and later invade the brain parenchyma as AVE.

DISEASE TEMPO

Disease tempo is critical in DDx, as all infectious and non-infectious diseases have a characteristic tempo, e.g., MC ABM is fulminant, severe, and acute vs. the subacute course of basilar meningitis due to sarcoidosis, meningeal carcinomatosis, or TB meningitis. The onset of MC ABM is hyperacute. The patient may report symptoms of URI for several days and look well at this time. However, when the infection begins to fully manifest itself, it moves with a frightening speed, which is the basis for the well-known adage "well at noon, dead by three." The prognosis is a function of the number of petechiae. Clinicians should remember there are three clinical MC variants, i.e., meningococcemia without ABM, ABM alone, and ABM with MC.

In general, drug-induced aseptic meningitis and all causes of AVM are less severe and have a slower course than the rapid/severe progression of ABM. Some bacterial pathogens present less acutely with clinical features of ABM and AVE. The classic neuropathogen that displays features of both meningeal inflammation (nuchal rigidity) and mental confusion is *L. monocytogenes* ABM.

PERTINENT PHYSICAL EXAM FINDINGS

Fever is routinely present in ABM, AVM, and AVE. With any of these (and other CNS disorders) a pulse-deficit (RB) is frequent and diagnostically unhelpful. Fever post CVA should not exceed 102°F, but temperatures >102°F are usual after an ICH.

In patients with mental confusion but no fever, the working Dx should be encephalopathy (toxic/metabolic) and not encephalitis. If severe, degree of mental status impairment points to AVE until proven otherwise. There should be no/mild nuchal rigidity with AVE. In contrast, ABM and, to a lesser extent, AVM characteristically have prominent nuchal rigidity. Nuchal rigidity must be differentiated from meningismus or a stiff neck due to cervical spine OA (Kernig/Brudzinski signs are negative).

A maculopapular rash, if present, is a key Dx finding in AVM, particularly when due to an enterovirus. A vesicular rash points to VZV (shingles), with CNS findings manifesting as AVM. Petechial or pustular rash points to MC with ABM. Rhinorrhea, tenderness over the sinuses/mastoids, or typical bacterial CAP indicates that the ABM pathogen is most likely *S. pneumoniae* or less commonly *H. influenzae*.

NON-SPECIFIC LABORATORY TESTS

For ABM, CSF analysis provides Dx clues or the Dx itself. Since ABM involves the leptomeninges, the CSF contains the ASM pathogen and, to a lesser extent, the AVM pathogen. The key CSF test remains the CSF Gram stain, which reveals the interesting intensity of the cellular (WBC) response (pleocytosis) and the morphology of bacterial pathogen. A prominent pleocytosis should be present in the CSF, with a PMN predominance in ABM. In untreated ABM, the PMN predominance should be >90%. Only HSV among the viral causes of AVM may result in this degree of pleocytosis. The Dx of ABM should be questioned if the PMN is <90%. Other key CSF parameters in ABM are the CSF glucose and CSF LA in ABM and some cases of AVM. In ABM, CSF glucose is decreased as a function of ABM severity. Similarly, the CSF

LA is highly elevated (inversely proportional to the CSF glucose) in ABM. Therefore, the usual CSF combination in ABM is markedly decreased CSF glucose, accompanied by a highly elevated CSF LA. The CSF glucose levels are not decreased in AVM/AVE except for HSV, LCM, and in some cases of enterovirus. These two parameters may be also used to assess therapeutic response or as a test of cure if a patient is re-LP.

Excluding a CNS bleed (SAH, CVA, and ICH) or a traumatic tap, RBCs in the CSF (aside from being a DxE) may provide an important Dx clue. The CSF RBCs in ABM point to *L. monocytogenes*, whereas subacute chronic meningitis may suggest meningeal carcinomatosis or TB meningitis. Importantly, RBCs in the CSF are not a feature of sarcoid meningitis. Viral causes of AVE RBCs, if present, point to severe HSV AVE (not mild HSV AVE or HSV AVM). In severe HSV AVE, RBC numbers are reflective of the extent of brain parenchymal damage to the frontoparietal lobe.

Imaging in ABM should follow the LP unless there are reasons to suspect ↑ ICP. Otherwise, LP should precede head CT/MRI, which is unhelpful in ABM but useful to R/O a suspected associated tumor or brain abscess. In HSV AVE, changes on the head CT takes days to occur, and the EEG is the preferred early Dx test, since AVE by definition is an electrical storm in the brain (localized, as in HSV) or diffuse global slowing (as in most other causes of AVE).

The CSF usually is diagnostically unhelpful in AVE, since the disease process is located in the brain parenchyma by definition and not in the leptomeninges/CSF. The CSF in AVE, not infrequently, is entirely normal. Viral PCR of the CSF may be negative in AVE. The CSF viral PCR is most useful when the infective process involves the CSF/leptomeninges, as in AVM. Typically, with AVM, the CSF cellular response is less intense than in ABM, and there is usually a lymphocytic predominance. A PMN predominance is common in many acute CNS infections, but the PMNs should always be <90% (see above for exceptions).

The EEG is the preferred early test to diagnose AVE. In HSV AVE, typically, there is unilateral frontotemporal lobe localization. Other causes of AVE may involve the thalamus, e.g., in WNE. In most cases of AVE, there is diffuse global slowing, which is Dx. The CSF Gram stain may be negative in ABM due to *L. monocytogenes*. Interestingly, even though the Gram stain is negative (~50%), CSF cultures are nearly always positive. Blood cultures may also be positive for *L. monocytogenes*. Most CSF bacterial pathogens may be presumptively identified by their morphology on CSF Gram stain (and definitively identified on CSF culture).

TABLE 1.2
Meningitis: Clinical Diagnostic Problem Solving

Pertinent History/Epidemiology	Disease Tempo	Pertinent PE	Pertinent Laboratory Tests		

Pertinent History/Epidemiology

Clinical Presentation

CC/HPI
- Elderly 68-year-old male
- 3D history of fever, HA, and stiff neck

PMH
- CLL (on steroids)
- No recent sick contacts
- No recent zoonotic contact
- No recent insect exposure/bites

Disease Tempo

Acute
- S. pneumoniae
- MC with ABM

Subacute
- H. influenzae
- Listeria
- LCM
- AVM (EV and HSV)

Chronic
- NA in this case (TB, meningeal Ca, and sarcoidosis)

Pertinent PE

Nuchal Rigidity
- Most prominent with S. pneumoniae and H. influenzae
- Less prominent with AVM, AVE, and Listeria

Rash
- Rash may occur with EV, S. pneumoniae, H. influenzae, and MC with ABM

Respiratory Tract
- No tenderness over sinuses/mastoids
- Chest clear

Pertinent Laboratory Tests

CSF

Gram Stain
- PMNs and organisms usually seen with ABM but may be negative with Listeria and S. pneumoniae

Glucose ↓↓↓
- Typical of ABM, some causes of AVM (EV, LCM), normal with AVE (except with HSV)

LA ↑↑↑
- Highly elevated in ABM but not in AVM or AVE
- Most useful if CSF RBCs present and ↓ CSF glucose to Dx ABM

Serum
- ↑Ferritin useful clue to WNE
- BCs: pending

ASP Empiric Therapy (Based on CSD)
- **PCN Tolerant**
  Ampicillin 2g (IV) q4h +
  Ceftriaxone 2g (IV) q8h
- **PCN Allergic**
  Meropenem 2g (IV) q8h (meningeal dosed)

CSD — ABM Most Likely Due To
- #2 S. pneumoniae
- #3 H. influenzae
- #1 Listeria monocytogenes

Final Dx: Listeria ABM
- CSF cultures + Listeria monocytogenes
- BCs: −

DDx	Pertinent History/Epidemiology	Disease Tempo	Relevant History	Pertinent PE	Relevant Laboratory Tests CSF			Dx Point Scores (Excluding DxE)
					RBCs +	Glucose ↓↓	LA ↑↑	
ABM								
S. pneumoniae	+	+	0	+	−	+	+	5 − 1 = +4
H. influenzae	+	+	0	+	−	+	+	5 − 1 = +4
MC with ABM	+	−	0	−	−	+	+	
L. monocytogenes	+	+	0	+	+	+	+	6 − 0 = +6
AVM								
HSV	+	+	0	+	+	−	−	
EV	+	+	0	+	−	+	−	
LCM	+	+	−	+	−	+	−	
AVE								
HSV	+	+	0	0	+	+	−	
VZV	−	+	−	−	−	−	−	
WNE	−	+	0	−	−	−	−	
ARBOV	−	−	−	−	0	−	−	

Abbreviations: 0, no DDx value; CSD, clinical syndromic diagnosis; ABM, acute bacterial meningitis; AVM, acute viral meningitis; AVE, acute viral encephalitis; LA, CSF lactic acid; DDx, differential diagnosis; VZV, varicella-zoster virus; MC, meningococcemia with ABM; HSV, Herpes simplex; EV, enterovirus; LCM, lymphocytic choriomeningitis; WNE, West Nile encephalitis; ARBOV, arbovirus encephalitis.

SUMMARY

Comparing the disease presentation, disease, history, and epidemiologic features, clinicians can usually differentiate ABM from AVM. AVE is not usually confused with ABM, but often with various causes of aseptic of viral AVM. In ABM or AVM, CSF analysis is a key to the etiologic diagnosis. In contrast, the CSF is often unhelpful or non-diagnostic in AVE. In AVE, the EEG is the most important early Dx test. In ABM, empiric therapy is based on the likely presence or absence of *L. monocytogenes* as the likely pathogen. In AVE, HSV and VZV encephalitis are the only CNS viral infection that are treatable, e.g., with acyclovir (Table 1.2).

Acute Bacterial Meningitis: Pearls and Pitfalls

- *Listeria monocytogenes* is the commonest ABM pathogen in patients with malignancies.
- *Listeria monocytogenes* presents subacutely with some mental confusion and moderate nuchal rigidity.
- CSF clues are a negative Gram stain with elevated LA with *L. monocytogenes*.
- CSF Gram stain + in ~ 50% but culture + in ~ 100% with *L. monocytogenes*.
- ABM usually presents acutely with nuchal rigidity and no/mild mental confusion (encephalitis).
- Mental confusion without fever suggests encephalopathy due to a non-infectious (toxic/metabolic) cause.
- *Neisseria meningitidis* may present as MC alone (petechiae rash) without meningitis or as ABM without MC, or with both.
- Except for HSV, near all viral causes of AVM/AVE have normal CSF glucose (other causes include LCM and enterovirus) and an unelevated CSF LA.
- If there is mental confusion with fever ± nuchal rigidity, the Dx is AVE. The preferred initial test in AVE is an EEG, not a brain CT/MRI.
- In AVE due to HSV, the CSF may have few/no WBCs, since the infection involves the brain parenchyma and not leptomeninges.
- The severity of ABM is reflected by the degree of decreased glucose and elevated CSF LA.
- CSF protein is ~ blood-brain permeability and an indicator of relative CSF antibiotic penetration.
- Commonest causes of ABM (aside from MC are *S. pneumoniae* and *H. influenzae*) may be accompanied by petechiae rash-mimicking MC/ABM.
- No cause of ABM is accompanied by flaccid paralysis, which should suggest WNE or enterovirus D68 or D71.
- *L. monocytogenes* in the CSF may be differentiated rapidly from dipterous by a preparation that demonstrates its diagnostic "tumbling motility."
- In suspected ABM, recent contact with a person with ABM points to an MC etiology. Antecedent history of respiratory tract infection (sinusitis, mastoiditis, and CAP) points to *S. pneumoniae* or *H. influenzae* as likely ABM pathogen.
- In elderly patients with ABM, infection is most likely due to *S. pneumoniae, H. influenzae,* or *L. monocytogenes.*
- In untreated ABM, the CSF pleocytosis is intense. The PMNs are ≥ 90%, which rule out viral AVM/AVE (except for HSV encephalitis).

CLINICAL PROBLEM SOLVING COMMENTARY: SEVERE CAP (TABLE 1.3)

Clinical Presentation

CC/HPI	PMH
• 76-year-old female pet shop owner	• RA (on anti-TNF meds)
• 4-day history of fever, chills, headache, mild myalgias, dry cough, and loose stools	• Recent flight from West Coast 2 weeks ago
	• No recent sick contacts

PERTINENT HISTORY AND EPIDEMIOLOGY

The patient is an elderly woman who presents acutely with a CAP requiring hospitalization. Epidemiologic features include her recent airplane trip and contact with birds and animals (she works in a pet shop). The DDx at this point includes all causes of typical CAP as well as atypical zoonotic and non-zoonotic CAP. Given the possibility of airborne exposure in the airplane, the DDx should include influenza, influenza-like infections (ILIs), and less likely pertussis. She is a compromised host on immunosuppressive medications (anti-TNF immuno-suppression), which may increase the severity of any cause of CAP and particularly predispose to Legionnaire's disease.

DISEASE TEMPO

Rapidity on onset (acuteness) has diagnostic implications. PCP and CMV CAP usually manifest subacutely over a week. In this case, the patient presents acutely with a severe CAP. The acuteness as well as the severity of her CAP may, in part, be due to her immunosuppression.

Acute-onset severe CAPs are most often due to *S. pneumoniae*, influenza, or Legionnaire's disease. ILIs and pertussis are usually less severe. CMV causes CAP in normal hosts but is more common in compromised hosts such as the patient presented here.

PCP progresses gradually over a week, presenting acutely as a severe CAP with severe hypoxemia. Severe influenza CAP is the other common cause of CAP presenting with severe hypoxemia.

PERTINENT PHYSICAL EXAM FINDINGS

The typical CAP, particularly *S. pneumoniae*, presents with fever/chills ± pleuritic chest pain. On chest exam, there are localized rales; one/two lobe cavitation should suggest an alternative etiology, e.g., aspiration during abscess (subacute onset) occurring after 3–5 days. The only cause of rapid cavitation (<72 hours) and acute/severe CAP is MSSA/MRSA CAP only in patients with influenza. If present, CAP with pleural effusion is typically unilateral and most common with *H. influenzae* (RLL). With *S. pneumoniae*, pleural empyema (resembling pleural effusion on CXR) is usual and pleural effusion is uncommon. If present, pleural effusion due to *S. pneumoniae* is small whereas that due to *H. influenzae* is mild to moderate in size. Dullness may also be due to consolidation.

There is a paucity of physical findings in CAP patients. Rash (Horder's spots) occurs on the face in some patients with psittacosis. In a CAP patient, splenomegaly only occurs with psittacosis and Q fever. Before ascribing any findings to any Dx, be sure that it is otherwise unexplained. If there is alternate explanation, the findings cannot be used in DDx reasoning, e.g., CAP with splenomegaly in a patient with regional enteritis (RE) splenomegaly may be due to the RE.

If the host can generate a fever, the only CAP presenting without a fever is pertussis. Pulse-temperature relationships have important Dx implications in CAP as well in many ID DDx problems. Relative bradycardia refers to a slowed pulse relative to the temperature of 103°F (the appropriate pulse rate is 120/min). Excluding other causes of a slowed pulse (pacemaker, β-blockers, verapamil, diltiazem, etc.), RB occurs only with psitticosis, Q fever, and Legionnaire's disease. If not otherwise unexplained, its presence is a DxE and immediately excludes all other causes of typical/atypical CAP.

Otherwise-unexplained loose stools/watery diarrhea essentially narrows Dx possibilities in severe CAP to *Mycoplasma pneumoniae* of Legionnaire's disease. In contrast, if present amid otherwise unexplained, generalized or localized abdominal pain (usually without tenderness/rebound) in a CAP patient limits Dx possibilities to Legionnaire's disease.

Many causes of CAP particularly and ILIs may be accompanied by a generalized headache. Among the non-viral causes of CAP, psittious, Q fever, and Legionnaire's disease are often present with headache in addition to their respiratory symptoms of greater diagnostic significance is the presence of mental confusion (encephalopathy) alone or with headache, mental confusion, otherwise unexplained, with severe CAP limits DDx possibilities to psittacosis influenza, *Mycoplasma pneumoniae* (with very high cold agglutinin titers) and Legionnaire's disease. As with other findings, these findings, if otherwise unexplained, have DDx significance, e.g., cirrhosis with hepatic encephalopathy and *S. pneumoniae* CAP. It makes little sense to ascribe the CAP to psittacosis, influenza, or Legionnaire's disease.

NON-SPECIFIC LABORATORY TESTS

The diagnosis significance of leukocytosis (with or without an L shift) is often given undue Dx significance. At best, in a critically ill patient, leukocytosis is a measure of stress (ill in the CCU) and not infection per se. Of much greater diagnostic significance is leukopenia. If present, otherwise-unexplained leukopenia points to a viral etiology in a CAP patient. Leukopenia can also serve as DxE in some CAP cases, e.g., Legionnaire's disease. Legionnaire's disease is consistently accompanied by a marked leukocytosis. Therefore, the presence of in patient where Legionnaire's disease is in the DDx should eliminate it from further diagnostic consideration. Of more diagnostic usefulness is relative lymphopenia. Once again, this, like all other diagnostic findings, is useful only if otherwise unexplained. In a severe CAP patient, relative lymphopenia points to Legionnaire's disease, CMV, or influenza as the likely cause of CAP.

Of course, any patient on steroids or some immunosuppressants may have drug induced relative lymphopenia unrelated to the cause of the patient's CAP. The platelet count isn't very useful in the setting of acute/severe CAP. Thrombocytosis may occur after 1–2 weeks with Q fever *M. pneumoniae* or *S. pneumoniae*. Importantly, thrombocytosis is not an acute-phase reactant (only increases acutely with a GI bleed). In contrast, thrombocytopenia may be a clue to a viral CAP etiology, e.g., influenza, ILIs, adenovirus, and CMV. Thrombocytopenia is not a characteristic feature of any other typical or atypical CAPs e.g., thrombocytopenia is a DxE for Legionnaire's disease.

The ESR may be elevated in many disorders. Diagnostic specificity of ESR elevations is increased when elevated. An acutely elevated ESR >100 mm/Hg limits Dx possibilities to *S. pneumoniae* or Legionnaire's disease. Unelevated or moderately elevated ESRs may occur with any cause of CAP. Similarly, a very highly elevated CRP (>130) points to Legionnaire's disease, but as an accurate phase reactant, it may be elevated in many acute pulmonary and non-pulmonary disorders.

In CAP patients, otherwise-unexplained mild elevations of the serum transaminases suggest a systemic infection with liver involvement. Therefore, all causes of typical CAPs are effectively ruled out if and or are elevated without explanation. The usual causes of severe CAP with elevated AST/ALT are psittacosis, Q fever, CMV, adenovirus, and Legionnaire's disease.

While hyponatremia is frequent and profound in Legionnaire's disease, it is a non-specific finding that may occur with other CAP causes as well a variety of other pulmonary disorders (due to SIADH). If Legionnaire's disease is suspected, the clinician should look for other Legionnaire's disease clinical/laboratory findings, particularly if more characteristic, e.g., early hypophosphatemia. In contrast to hyponatremia, hypophosphatemia, when present, is only associated with Legionnaire's disease. If present in Legionnaire's disease, it occurs early (usually day #1 in the CCU) and rapidly resolves during the course of Legionnaire's disease. The absence of hypophosphatemia has no exclusionary Dx significance.

In CAP patients, highly increased CPK levels occur only with influenza, ILIs, and Legionnaire's disease. However, the absence of CPK elevations does not rule out these diagnoses. Otherwise-unexplained highly elevated ferritin levels in a severely ill CAP adult should suggest Legionnaire's disease Although mild/transient elevated ferritin levels may occur as an acute-phase reactant, the ferritin levels in Legionnaire's disease are highly elevated and sustained.

Urinalysis with otherwise-unexplained microscopic hematuria points to a Legionnaire's disease etiology in a CAP patient. Since Legionnaire's disease is a systematic infection with a pulmonary component, extrapulmonary manifestations are the rule in all atypical CAPs, including Legionnaire's disease. Renal involvement in Legionnaire's disease and often manifested as mild/reversible acute renal failure (ARF).

TABLE 1.3

Severe CAP: Clinical Diagnostic Problem Solving

Pertinent History/Epidemiology	Disease Tempo	Pertinent PE	Pertinent Laboratory Tests
Clinical Presentation	**Acute**	**Vital Signs**	**Serum Tests**
CC/HPI	• Typical CAP	• T = 103.8°F	**WBC**
• 76-year-old female pet shop owner	• Atypical CAP	• P = 100/min	• 24 K/mm³
• 4-day history of fever, chills, headache, mild myalgias, dry cough, and loose stools	• Influenza	**Skin**	• L = 6% (n <21%)
	• ILIs	• No rash	• Atypical L = 5%
PMH	**Subacute**	**Neuro**	• PLT = N
• RA (on anti-TNF meds)	• PCP	• HA but no mental confusion	**Other**
• Recent flight from West Coast 2 weeks ago	• CMV	**HEENT**	• ESR = ↑↑↑
• No recent sick contacts	**Chronic**	• No pharyngitis	• LDH = ↑
	• Not applicable in this case	• No conjunctival suffusion	• ALT/AST = ↑
		Lungs	• Na⁺ = N
		• R LL rales without dullness	• PO₄ = ↓
		Abdomen	• CPK = ↑↑
		• No organomegaly	• Ferritin = ↑↑↑
		• Mild RLQ tenderness without rebound	• Cold agg = 1:64
			• β 1,3 glucan = N
			CXR
			• Bilateral (R > L) nodular infiltrates (no consolidation, cavitation, or pleural effusion)
			• No hilar or mediastinal adenopathy
			• A-a gradient (room air) = 30

DDx	Pertinent History/ Epidemiology	Disease Tempo	Pertinent PE		Non-Specific Laboratory Tests					Dx Point Scores (excluding DxE)	CSD	ASP Empiric Therapy (Based on CSD)	Final Dx
			RB	Fever ≥ 102°F	Relative Lymphopenia	↑ LFTs	Cold Agg 1:64	↑↑ CPK	CXR (Nodular Infiltrates)				
Typical CAP													
S. pneumoniae	+	+	–	0	–	–	–	–	+				
H. influenzae	+	0	–	0	–	–	–	–	–				
M. catarrhalis	–	–	–	0	–	–	–	–	–				
Pertussis	–	–	–	–	–	–	–	–	–				

(Continued)

TABLE 1.3 (*Continued*)
Severe CAP: Clinical Diagnostic Problem Solving

DDx	Pertinent History/ Epidemiology	Disease Tempo	Pertinent PE		Non-Specific Laboratory Tests					Dx Point Scores (excluding DxE)	CSD	ASP Empiric Therapy (Based on CSD)	Final Dx
			RB	Fever ≥ 102°F	Relative Lymphopenia	↑ LFTs	Cold Agg 1:64	↑↑ CPK	CXR (Nodular Infiltrates)				
Atypical CAP													
Zoonotic													
Psittacosis	+	+	+	0	–	+	–	–	0	+5 – 3 = +2	#3 Psittacosis		
Q fever	+	+	+	0	–	+	–	–	+	+5 – 2 = +3	#2 Q fever		
Tularemia	+	+	–	0	–	–	–	–	–				
Non-zoonotic													
M. pneumoniae	0	+	–	–	–	–	+	–	+				
C. pneumoniae	0	–	–	–	–	–	–	–	–				
Legionnaire's disease	+	+	+	+	+	+	–	+	+	+8 – 1 = +7	#1 Legionnaire's disease	**PCN Tolerant/ Allergic** Levofloxacin 500 mg (IV/ PO) × 2 weeks or doxycycline 200 mg (IV) q12h × 3 days, then 100 mg IV/ PO q12h × 11 days or azithromycin 500 mg (IV/PO) q24h × 2 weeks	Legionnaire's disease • Legionella urinary antigen+ • BCs: negative
Viral CAP													
Influenza	+	–	–	–	+	–	+	+	–				
ILIs[a]	+	–	–	–	0	0	+	0	–				
CMV	–	–	–	–	+	+	+	–	–				
Adenovirus	+	0	–	–	0	0	0	0	+				
Other CAP													
PCP	–	–	–	+	+[a]	0	–	–	–				

Abbreviations: ILIs, influenza-like illnesses; CMV, cytomegalovirus; adenov, adenovirus; PCP, pneumocystis (carinii) jiroveci pneumonia; RA, rheumatoid arthritis; CSD, clinical syndromic diagnosis; RB, relative bradycardia; ASP, antibiotic stewardship program; CXR, chest X-ray; HA, headache.

a Unless due to underlying disorder, e.g., HIV.

SUMMARY

The clinical characteristic features cited previously are the basis of diagnostic reasoning and clinical problem solving in admitted adults with acute onset of severe CAP (see Table 1.3).

Clinicians using this approach will not have to test all CAPs for Legionnaire's disease, but rather test only those patients with a high point score in the CSD. Similarly, there is no need in a CAP patient to "cover atypicals" when there are no clinical findings/features suggesting an atypical CAP, i.e., no extrapulmonary features.

Severe CAP: Pearls and Pitfalls

- Atypical pneumonias are CAPs that are part of a systemic disease, primarily with pneumonia *plus* a variety of *extrapulmonary* laboratory/ clinical manifestations.
- Atypical CAPs may be further classified into two groups based on the presence or absence of zoonotic vector contact, i.e., zoonotic CAPs (psittacosis, Q fever, and tularemia) and atypical non-zoonotic CAP (*M. pneumoniae*, *Chlamydia pneumoniae*, and Legionnaire's disease).
- Bacterial CAPs are usually due to *S. pneumoniae*, *H. influenzae*, *Moraxella catarrhalis*, and, less commonly, pertussis.
- Frequent causes of viral CAPs include influenza and ILIs due to RSV, HPIV-3, and HMPV. However, influenza is most likely to present as severe CAP.
- Another important cause of viral CAPs includes adenovirus, which may mimic a typical bacterial CAP. It is the only viral CAP that may present as a segmental/lobar pneumonia.
- In adults, less common causes of CAP include pertussis. Pertussis presents as a prolonged dry cough with *Mycoplasma*-like illness but without fever/chills. A hallmark of pertussis is intense lymphocytosis (often >60%).
- PCP occurs primarily in immunosuppressed individuals. PCP usually presents with ↑ SOB/DOE over a week. Initial CXR is clear (like early influenza). Later, bilateral fluffy infiltrates occur as the pneumonia progresses and hypoxemia worsens. The A-a gradient is typically >35.
- The most useful non-invasive test for PCP is a highly elevated β1,3 glucan level. An elevated LDH is diagnostically less useful.
- As with influenza, auscultation of the chest with PCP is conspicuous by the absence of rales.
- Psittacosis, transmitted by psittacine birds, presents with fever and headaches (± mental confusion), often with a facial rash (Horder's spots).
- RB is a feature of Q fever, psittacosis, and Legionnaire's disease but is a DxE for other typical/atypical CAP etiologies.
- Mildly increased serum transaminases often accompany Q fever, psittacosis, and Legionnaire's disease but not other causes of CAP.
- The only CAP associated with highly increased ferritin levels or hypophosphatemia is Legionnaire's disease.
- CAP with dry cough and fever suggests a viral ILI, *Mycoplasma pneumoniae* or *C. pneumoniae*, but without fever consider pertussis.
- Legionnaire's disease may be acquired from *Legionella*-containing aerosols and is frequently travel-related, e.g., hotels, fountains, whirlpool baths, humidifiers, showers, and aircraft.
- Some immunosuppressive medications, e.g., anti-TNF inhibitors, predispose to Legionnaire's disease by ↓ CMI.
- Legionnaire's disease is often accompanied by headache and/or mental confusion.
- CAP with splenomegaly limits Dx possibilities to Q fever or psittacosis.
- An ↑ CPK in CAP patients points to influenza or Legionnaire's disease.
- CAP with a very high ESR (>100 mm/h) limits diagnostic possibilities to *S. pneumoniae* and Legionnaire's disease.

(Continued)

- Hyponatremia is not specific for Legionnaire's disease and may occur with any infectious pulmonary disorder.
- Unless highly elevated, an ↑ LDH is not specific and not indicative for PCP.
- CAP with otherwise-unexplained microscopic hematuria or ARF points to a Dx of Legionnaire's disease.
- Legionnaire's disease is mimicked most closely by *S. pneumoniae*, Q fever, and psittacosis.
- Typically, tularemia pneumonia is accompanied by hilar adenopathy and a bloody pleural effusion.
- Clues to severe influenza CAP are acuteness of onset, profound fatigue, and prominent myalgias ± hemoptysis.

SUGGESTED READING

Bean RB, Bean WB. *Osler Aphorisms from His Bedside Teachings in Writings.* Springfield, MO: CC Thomas, 1961.

Bryan CS, Longo LD. Perspective: Teaching and mentoring the history of medicine: An oslerian perspective. *Acad Med* 2013;88:97–101.

Bryan CS. *Osler: Inspirations from a Great Physician.* New York: Oxford University Press, 1997.

Cabot R. *Differential Diagnosis.* Philadelphia, PA: W.B. Saunders, 1911.

Campbell EJM. The diagnosing mind. *Lancet* 1987;11:849–851.

Casscells W, Schoenberger A, Graboys TB. Interpretation by physicians of clinical laboratory results. *NEJM* 1978;299:999–1001.

Crombie DL. Diagnostic process. *J Coll Gen Prac* 1963;54:579–589.

Cunha BA, Cunha CB. Legionnaire's disease and its mimics: A clinical perspective. *Infect Dis Clin North Am* 2017;31:95–109.

Cunha BA. Characteristic predictors that increase the pretest probability of Legionnaires disease: "Don't order a test just because you can" revisited. *South Med J* 2015;108:761.

Cunha BA. Difficulties in teaching diagnostic reasoning in the digital age: The critical role of the teacher-clinician mentor. *Am J Med* 2017;130:517–519.

Cunha BA. How to make a clinical diagnosis in medicine: How Osler connected the diagnostic dots. *Winthrop Univ Hosp Med J* 2013;33:783–774.

Cunha BA. Osler on typhoid fever: Differentiation of typhoid from typhus and malaria. *Inf Dis Clin of North Am* 2004;18:111–126.

Cunha BA. Physician heal thyself, make haste slowly. In: Papadakos PJ, Bertman S eds. *Distracted Doctoring, Make Haste Slowly.* New York: Springer-Verlag, 2017.

Cunha BA. Potential pitfalls of basing specific antibiotic therapy on rapid susceptibility reporting. *Am J Health Syst Pharm* 2014;71:1246–1247.

Cunha BA. Teaching fever aphorisms: Osler revisited. *Eur J Clin Micro Inf Dis* 2007;26:371–373.

Cunha BA. The clinical and laboratory diagnosis of acute meningitis and acute encephalitis. *Expert Opin Med Diagn* 2013;7:343–364.

Cunha BA. The diagnosing mind: The diagnostic significance of non-specific laboratory tests. *Winthrop-University Hosp Med J* 2006;28:489–493.

Cunha CB, Cunha BA. The gram stain re-visited: Importance to antibiotic stewardship programs (ASP). In: Khardori NM ed. *Bench to Bedside: Microbiology for Clinicians.* Boca Raton, FL: CRC Press, 2018.

Cunha BA. The master clinician's approach to diagnostic reasoning. *Am J Med* 2017;130:5–7.

Cunha CB, Cunha BA. Brief history of the clinical diagnosis of malaria: From Hippocrates to Osler. *J Vector Borne Dis* 2008;45:194–199.

Cunha CB, Cunha BA. Legionnaire's disease and its protean clinical manifestations: The ongoing challenges of the most interesting atypical pneumonia. *Infect Dis Clin North Am* 2017;31:13–16.

Harvey AM, Boardly J, Barondess JA. *Differential Diagnosis, The Interpretation of Clinical Evidence* (3rd ed.). Philadelphia, PA: WB Saunders Co, 1979.

Kassirer JP, Kopelman RI. *Learning Clinical Reasoning.* Baltimore, MD: Williams & Wilkins, 1991.

Kirch W, Schafii C. Misdiagnosis at a university hospital in 4 medical eras: Report on 400 cases. *Medicine* 1996;75:29–40.

Orient JM. *Sapira's Art and Science of Bedside Diagnosis* (4th ed.). New York: Lippincott Williams & Wilkins, 2009.

Peterson MC, Holbrook JH, Von Hales D, et al. Contribution of the history, physical examination and laboratory investigation in making medical diagnoses. *West J Med* 1992;156:163–165.

Sackett DL, Rennie D. The science of the art of the clinical examination. *JAMA* 1992;267:2650–2652.

Sandler G. The importance of the history in the medical clinic and the cost of unnecessary tests. *Am Heart J* 1980;100:928–931.

Schattner A, Zimhony O, Avidor B, et al. Asking the right question. *Lancet* 2003;361:1786.

Schattner A. Simple is beautiful, the neglected power of simple tests. *Arch Intern Med* 2014;164:2198–2200.

Tumulty P. What is a clinician and what does he do? *NEJM* 1970;283:120–124.

2 Clinical Approach to Fever in the Critical Care Unit

Burke A. Cunha

CONTENTS

CLINICAL PERSPECTIVE

The approach to fever depends on associated findings related to the fever (height, duration, fever pattern, pulse-temperature relationships, and relative bradycardia) and chills. Nearly always, there are clinical signs pointing to a particular organ/source of the infection.

Clinically, Cunha's "102°F rule" has a great differential diagnosis (DDx) utility in providing a relatively efficient way to differentiate infectious from most non-infectious disorders. In general, <102°F likely indicates a non-infectious etiology.

The relationship of temperature to pulse is next in the diagnostic importance in DDx. The pulse increases 10 beats per minute for every degree Fahrenheit increase in temperature and is the usual pattern with the infectious causes of fever >102°F. However, if there is a pulse-temperature deficit, i.e., relative bradycardia, then the DDx is quickly limited to few possibilities. To use relative bradycardia as a DDx finding, the patient must not be on drugs that decrease the pulse when fever is present, e.g., β-blockers, diltiazem, verapamil, or a pacemaker-induced pulse. Relative tachycardia suggests a non-infectious etiology with the exception of infectious myocarditis. Very high temperature elevations >106°F indicate extreme hyperpyrexia, which is always on a non-infectious basis.

Similarly, single fever spikes (not fevers terminated by antipyretics) are always on a non-infectious basis, usually due to blood/blood products infusion 1–3 days preceding the single fever spike, manipulation/irrigation of colonized/infected mucosa or device related (insertion/removal of urinary catheters, central-venous catheters [CVCs], drainage tubes, tracheostomy, and endotracheal tubes), wound irrigation/debridement. Chills, (frank rigors), not chilliness, suggests bacteremia, fungemia, or viremia unless present following antipyretic medications. A hectic/septic fever curve is often mimicked by antipyretics for fever. For pain, non-antipyretics are preferred since they do not affect temperature.

Antipyretics should only be given in extreme hyperpyrexia (T > 106°F) if the patient has severe cardiopulmonary disease or CNS trauma/hemorrhage. Fever is a critical host defense mechanism and should not be treated unless the fever itself poses a threat to the patient. Not only is fever beneficial, but giving antipyretics results in diagnostic confusion in interpreting fever clues. Decreasing fever eliminates a guide to assessing the efficacy of antimicrobial therapy.

Unless the fever poses specific harm to the patient (*vide supra*), do not give antipyretics, since they complicate the diagnostic and therapeutic significance of fever.

Non-infectious fevers tend to be both low grade (<102°F) and subacute/chronic. In contrast, infective fevers in the critical care unit (CCU) are usually acute in onset.

The clinical diagnostic approach to the CCU febrile patient depends on fever-associated aspects that are clinically correlated with the history physical examination and pertinent non-specific laboratory tests.

Fever is a cardinal sign of disease and may be caused by many infectious and non-infectious disorders. The number of DDx disorders that occur in seriously ill patients in CCU is more limited than in hospital patients. The main clinical DDx problems in the CCU are to differentiate between infectious and non-infectious causes of fever and to try to determine the specific Dx of the patient's fever.

The clinical approach to the DDx of fever in the CCU is based on characteristics of the fever, the fever pattern, the relationship of the pulse to the fever, the acuteness and duration of the fever, and the presence or absence of imaging studies. Characteristics of the patient's fever in the appropriate clinical context to determine DDx possibilities. These findings are the basis of formulating a clinical syndromic diagnosis (narrowed based on Dx probability DDx, not possibility). Then, after narrowing the DDx, it is usually relatively straightforward to order specific tests to arrive at a diagnosis.

Most patients in the CCU have low-grade fevers due to non-infectious causes. Alternately, new or high-grade fevers suggest a possible infectious etiology (Table 2.1) [1–10].

CLINICAL SYNDROMIC DIAGNOSIS OF FEVERS IN THE CCU

NON-INFECTIOUS CAUSES OF FEVER IN THE CCU

Infectious and non-infectious disorders may cause fevers that may be low, i.e., ≤102°F, or high, i.e., ≥102°F. In general, most non-infectious disorders are associated with low-grade fevers of ≤102°F. Exceptions to the "102°F fever rule" include malignant hyperthermia, relative adrenal insufficiency, massive intracranial hemorrhage, central fever, drug fever, systemic lupus erythematosus (SLE) flare, heat stroke, vasculitis, and certain malignancies, e.g., lymphomas. The most common non-infectious disorders in the CCU have low-grade fevers ≤102°F, e.g., acute myocardial infarction, pulmonary embolism/infarct, phlebitis, catheter-associated bacteriuria, acute pancreatitis, acute viral hepatitis, dry gangrene, uncomplicated wound infections, subacute bacterial endocarditis (SBE), cerebrovascular accidents, splenic infarcts, renal infarcts, small/moderate intracerebral hemorrhages, pulmonary hemorrhage, acute respiratory distress syndrome (ARDS), bronchiolitis obliterans organizing pneumonia (BOOP), pleural effusions, pericardial effusion, atelectasis, cholecystitis, non-infectious diarrheas, *Clostridium difficile* diarrhea, ischemic colitis, gas gangrene, surgical toxic shock syndrome (TSS), acute gout flare, small bowel obstruction, and uncomplicated cellulitis/wound infection [1,3,5,11–30].

Extreme hyperpyrexia (temperature ≥106°F) is rarely, if ever, due to an infectious disease. There are relatively few disorders, all non-infectious, which present with extreme hyperpyrexia (Table 2.2) [1,3,5].

TABLE 2.1
Causes of Fever in the CCU

System Etiology	Infectious Etiology	Non-infectious
Central nervous	Meningitis	Cerebral infarction
	Encephalitis	Cerebral hemorrhage
	Brain abscess	Posterior fossa syndrome
		Seizures
		CNS tumors
Cardiovascular	Endocarditis	Myocardial infarction
	IV line sepsis	Postpericardiotomy
	Septic thrombophlebitis	syndrome
	Thrombophlebitis	Dressler's syndrome
	Postperfusion syndrome	Cholesterol emboli syndrome
	(CMV)	Deep vein thrombosis
	Pericarditis	Atrial myomas
	Pacemaker/defibrillator	
	infection	
Pulmonary	Pneumonia	Atelectasis
	Empyema	SLE pneumonitis
	Tracheobronchitis	Pleural effusion
	Lung abscess	Pulmonary emboli/infarction
	Empyema	ARDS
		Pulmonary drug reactions
		BOOP
		Fat emboli
Gastrointestinal	Liver abscess	Gastrointestinal hemorrhage
	Splenic abscess	Acalculous cholecystitis
	Intra-abdominal abscess	Non-viral hepatitis
	Cholecystitis/cholangitis	Pancreatitis
	Viral hepatitis	Inflammatory bowel disease
	Peritonitis	Non-*C. difficile* diarrhea
	Appendicitis	Ischemic/non-*C. difficile*
	Diverticulitis	colitis
	C. difficile diarrhea/colitis	Splenic infarct
Renal	Acute cystitis	Renal infarct
	Acute Pyelonephritis	
	Renal abscess	
Rheumatologic	Osteomyelitis	Acute gout/pseudogout
	Septic arthritis	SLE/RA flare
		Vasculitis
Skin/soft tissue	Cellulitis	Hematoma
	Wound infection	Intramuscular injections
	Decubitus ulcer	Burns
Endocrine/		Acute adrenal insufficiency
metabolic		Hyperthyroidism/thyroiditis
		Alcohol withdrawal/DTs
GU	Prostatic abscess	Hemorrhage into ovarian cyst
	PID	
	Tubo-ovarian abscess	
Other	Transient bacteremias	Drug fever
	Septicemia	Blood/blood products
	Parotitis	transfusion
	Pharyngitis	
	Transient bacteremia	

Abbreviations: PID, pelvic infectious disease syndrome; DTs, delirium tremens; SLE, systemic lupus erythematosus; RA, rheumatoid arthritis; ARDS, acute respiratory distress syndrome; BOOP, bronchiolitis obliterans with organizing pneumonia; CNS, central nervous system.

TABLE 2.2
Clinical Applications of the "102°F Rule" in the CCU

Common Causes of Temperature	Comments ≤102°F
Acute myocardial infarction	H/O chest pain/community-acquired pneumonia EKG/cardiac enzymes
Pulmonary embolism	H/O PE underlying reasons predisposing to pulmonary emboli
	VQ scan positive (pulmonary angiography for large emboli)
	↑ FSPs with multiple small pulmonary emboli
GI bleed	Hyperactive BS, BRB per rectum/melena
	↑ BUN (except in alcoholic liver disease)
	Endoscopy/abdominal CT scan → bleeding source
Acute pancreatitis	Severe abdominal pain: may be associated with ARDS
	↑ amylase and ↑ lipase or pancreatitis on abdominal CT scan
Hematomas	H/O recent surgery/bleeding diathesis
	Visible on skin, e.g., Grey-Turner's/Cullen's sign, or on CT scan
Phlebitis	Local erythema without suppuration/vein tenderness
Catheter-associated bacteriuria	Urine with bacteria and WBCs nearly always represent colonization, not infection
	Bacteremia (urosepsis) does not result from bacteriuria unless pre-existing renal disease, urinary tract obstruction, or patient has SLE, DM, steroids, etc.
Pleural effusions	Bilateral effusions are never due to infection: look for a non-infectious etiology
Uncomplicated wound infections	"Wounds" with temperatures ≥102°F should prompt a search for an underlying abscess
Atelectasis/dehydration	Temperatures usually ≤101°F
	May be confused with pulmonary emboli/early pneumonia
Tracheobronchitis	Purulent endotracheal secretions with negative chest X-ray for pneumonia
	Tracheobronchitis does not → temperatures ≥102°F
Thrombophlebitis	Warm, tender calf/foot veins ± palpable cord
	Thrombophlebitis does not → pulmonary emboli
	Phlebothrombosis → pulmonary emboli
C. difficile	Stools positive for C. difficile toxin
	Fecal WBC positive ~50%. Stools are watery, green, foul smelling
	If temperatures ≥102°F with blood/mucous diarrhea, C. difficle or ischemic colitis is probable
Nosocomial pneumonia/ventilator-associated pneumonia	May have temperatures >102°F also
	Pulmonary infiltrate consistent with a bacterial pneumonia occurring ≥1 week after hospitalization
	Must be differentiated from ARDS, LVF, etc.
	Diagnosis supported by quantitative protected catheter tip culture (PBB/BAL)
	Endotracheal secretions represent upper airway colonization and are not reflective of lower respiratory tract organisms causing VAP pneumonia

(Continued)

TABLE 2.2 (*Continued*)
Clinical Applications of the "102°F Rule" in the CCU

Common Causes of Temperature	Comments >102°F
IV-line infections	Central venous line infections
	Organisms from blood cultures taken from non-involved extremity same as positive semiquantitative catheter culture (≥15 colonies)
	If all other sources of fever are ruled out, consider IV-line infection, especially with overdue lines (even if site not infected visually)
C. difficile	Stools positive for C. difficile toxin
	Bloody diarrhea, temperature ≥102°F
	Abdominal CT scan shows thumb printing/colitis/toxic megacolon
Drug fever	In patients with otherwise unexplained fevers, consider drug fever
	Blood cultures are negative (excluding contaminants)
	Patients with drug fever usually have ≥102°F accompanied by relative bradycardia
	↑ WBC with left shift is common as is ↑ ESR
	Mild-moderate elevations serum transaminases common
	Eosinophils nearly always present but eosinophils less common
	Patient with infection may also have a drug fever
	Commonest causes of drug fever are diuretics, pain/sleep medications, sulfa-containing stool softeners as well as sulfa drugs and β-lactam antibiotics
Blood/blood product transfusion	Single fever spike (1–3 or 5–7 days posttransfusion)
Transient bacteremia due to manipulation of a colonized/infected mucosal surface	Single temperature spike 1–3 days, post-manipulative, that spontaneously resolves without treatment

The clinical diagnostic approach to non-infectious fevers is usually relatively straightforward because of their associated findings of non-infectious disorders causing fevers; it includes features of the history, physical, or routine laboratory/radiology studies. By knowing that most non-infectious disorders are associated with fevers <102°F, the diagnostic approach to fevers >102°F should prompt an alternate explanation (if non-infectious diseases suspected with temperature of >102°F can be eliminated on a clinical basis). The clinical problem arises when a patient has a multiplicity of infectious and non-infectious causes. Fevers are virtually always due to a single, not multiple, casuses (Tables 2.3 and 2.4) [1–6,10].

TABLE 2.3
Causes of Extreme Hyperpyrexia (>106°F)

Hypothalamic dysfunction
Malignant neuroleptic syndrome
Central fevers (hemorrhagic, trauma, malignancy)
Heat stroke
Malignant hyperthermia
Drug fever

TABLE 2.4
Diagnostic Significance of Fever Patterns

Fever Patterns	Usual Causes
Single fever spike	Manipulation of a colonized/infected mucosal surface (not systemic infectious diseases)
	Blood/blood products transfusion
	Infusion-related sepsis (contaminated infusate)
	Temperature error
Intermittent (hectic/septic) fevers	Gram-negative/positive sepsis
	Abscesses (renal, abdominal, pelvic)
	Acute bacterial endocarditis
	Kawasaki's disease
	Malaria
	Miliary tuberculosis
	Peritonitis
	Toxic shock syndrome
	Antipyretics
Remittent fevers	Viral upper respiratory tract infections
	Plasmodium falciparum malaria
	ARF
	Legionella
	Mycoplasma
	Tuberculosis
	SBE (viridans streptococci)
Continuous/sustained fevers	Central fevers
	Roseola infantum (human herpesvirus-6)
	Brucellosis
	Kawasaki's disease
	Psittacosis
	Rocky Mountain spotted fever
	Scarlet fever
	Enterococcal SBE (tularemia)
	Typhoid fever
	Drug fever
Double quotidian fevers	Adult Still's disease (adult-juvenile rheumatoid arthritis)
	Visceral leishmaniasis
	Miliary tuberculosis
	Mixed malarial infections
	Right-sided gonococcal endocarditis
Biphasic (Camelback) fevers	Colorado tick fever
	Dengue fever
	Leptospirosis
	Brucellosis
	Lymphocytic choriomeningitis
	Yellow fever

(Continued)

TABLE 2.4 (*Continued*)
Diagnostic Significance of Fever Patterns

Fever Patterns	Usual Causes
	Poliomyelitis
	Smallpox
	Rate-bite fever (*Spirillum minus*)
	Chikungunya fever
	Rift Valley fever
	African hemorrhagic fevers (Marburg, Ebola, Lassa, etc.)
	Echovirus (Echo 9)
Relapsing fevers	Relapsing fever (*B. recurrentis*)
	Yellow fever
	Smallpox
	Ascending (intermittent) cholangitis
	Brucellosis
	Dengue
	Chronic meningococcemia
	Malaria
	Rate-bit fever (*S. moniliformis*)

DIAGNOSTIC SIGNIFICANCE OF FEVER DEFERVESCENCE PATTERNS

Most of this chapter is concerned with the diagnosis of fever in the CCU. This is done by analyzing the rapidity of onset of the fever, the height of the fever, the relationship of the fever to the pulse, the fever patterns, and the duration of the fever. The characteristics of fever resolution also have diagnostic significance. Fever defervescence patterns may be interpreted in two ways. The rapidity and completeness of the fever patterns resolution attest to the effective treatment or resolution of the non-infectious or infectious process. Fever defervescence patterns are as predictable as fever patterns and are also useful in suspecting complications secondary to the disorder or therapy.

With bacterial meningitis, temperature resolution with appropriate therapy is related to the pathogen causing the meningitis. Meningococcal meningitis defervesces quickly over 1–3 days, whereas *Haemophilus influenzae* meningitis resolves over 3–5 days, and severe pneumococcal meningitis may take a week or longer for the fever to decrease/become afebrile. Viral causes of meningitis or encephalitis defervesce vary slowly over a 7-day period, and by monitoring the fever defervescence pattern, a clinician can easily differentiate viral meningitis/encephalitis from bacterial meningitis. Because fever defervescence patterns may also point to complications, the astute clinician will monitor the fever pattern post-therapy, looking for an unexpected temperature spike after the patient has defervesced.

H. influenzae meningitis, e.g., defervesces after 3–5 days, but if the patient's temperature spikes after 5 days, this would suggest either a complication of the infection, i.e., subdural empyema, or a complication of therapy, i.e., drug fever secondary to antimicrobial therapy [1,2,5].

In patients with endocarditis, the fever defervescence pattern is also pathogen related. Patients with SBE have fevers <102°F, which defervesce after a few days of effective antimicrobial therapy. A subsequent temperature spike after the fever with viridians streptococcal SBE has resolved should suggest either a complication of SBE, i.e., septic emboli/infarcts, or a complication of SBE therapy, i.e., drug fever. With *Staphylococcus aureus* acute bacterial endocarditis (ABE), patients initially have temperatures ≥102°F (excluding SBE in intravenous drug abusers). Patients with *S. aureus* endocarditis defervesce within 3–5 days after initiation of effective anti-*S. aureus* therapy. The persistence of fever in a patient being treated appropriately should suggest the possibility of a paravalvular/mild myocardial abscess. With *S. aureus* ABE, the reappearance of fever after initial defervescence should suggest a septic complication, i.e., septic emboli/infarcts, paravalvular/myocardial abscess, or complication of antimicrobial therapy, e.g., drug fever. Patients with enterococcal endocarditis have a fever defervescence pattern intermediate between viridians streptococcal SBE and ABE. Patients with enterococcal endocarditis usually defervesce slowly over 5 days, and recrudescence of fever in patients with enterococcal endocarditis should suggest a septic complication or drug fever [1,5,20,42].

Fever defervescence patterns are also important in patients with CAP as well as nosocomial pneumonias. In normal hosts with CAP, owing to typical bacterial pathogens, i.e., *Streptococcus pneumoniae*, *Haemophilus influenzae*, or *Moraxella catarrhalis*, fever resolves rapidly over the first few days with effective treatment. *S. pneumoniae* CAP has three possible fever defervescence patterns: The first and most common is a rapid decrease in temperature, similar to that found in *H. influenzae* or *M. catarrhalis* CAP in normal hosts. The second pattern with pneumococcal pneumonia is that of initial defervescence within in 3–5 days, followed by a secondary rise in fever. A secondary fever rise is a normal variant and does not indicate an infectious complication. The third pattern with *S. pneumoniae* is found in patients with impaired humoral immunity, i.e., patients with alcoholic cirrhosis, multiple myeloma, and chronic lymphatic leukemia. In patients with impaired β-lymphocyte function, the fever slowly remits during the first week of therapy. Patients with overwhelming pneumococcal sepsis, with no humoral immunity, i.e., asplenia, remain febrile and critically ill until the infection resolves or there is a fatal outcome.

Patients with nosocomial pneumonias NP/VAP may have temperature elevations that are above or below 102°F, and fever is not a way to rule out the diagnosis of nosocomial pneumonia. The NP/VAP is an imprecise diagnosis and is routinely given to most patients in the CCU who have fever, leukocytosis, and pulmonary infiltrates. Therefore, most patients who have a working diagnosis of NP/VAP in fact do not have NP/VAP but have infiltrates, fever, and leukocytosis due to other causes. Patients should be treated appropriately with monotherapy or combination therapy for NP/VAP defervesce rapidly if the infiltrates do, in fact, represent NP/VAP [5,46–49].

Monotherapy or combination therapy for NP/VAP should be with at least one agent that has a high degree of anti-*Pseudomonas aeruginosa* activity. Patients with *bona fide* NP/VAP defervesce quickly within a week. The persistence of fever, i.e., lack of a fever defervescence pattern in patients with NP/VAP, suggests two possibilities: First, the patient has a non-infectious disorder that is mimicking NP/VAP and, for this reason, is not responding to antimicrobial therapy. Second, the patient could have an infectious disease, a process that is unresponsive to antipseudomonal antimicrobial therapy, i.e., herpes simplex virus 1 (HSV-1) pneumonia. HSV-1 pneumonia is common in the CCU setting and presents as persistent fever and infiltrates unresponsive to antibiotics or as "failure to wean" in ventilated patients. In patients with good pulmonary function prior to admission who present as "failure to wean." Bacterial NP/VAP with empiric treatment should see an improvement/resolution of infiltrates and a defervescence of fever within 2 weeks. Persistence of fever with or without infiltrates after 2 weeks, in the absence of another cause for the fever, should suggest HSV-1 pneumonia, until proven otherwise. HSV-1 pneumonia is easily diagnosed by bronchoscopy, demonstrating cytopathic effects HSV CPEs from cytology specimens, or direct fluorescent antibody test/monoclonal tests of respiratory secretions will be positive for HSV. Importantly, no vesicles are present in the bronchi in bronchoscoped patients with HSV-1 pneumonitis [5,50–52].

The clinical approach to the delayed resolution of fever, persistence of fever, or new appearance of fever is related to a complication of therapy, i.e., drug fever. After initial improvements in temperature/fever, a recrudescence of fever manifested by new fever/fever spikes may be related to the infectious process or to a non-infectious complication unrelated to therapy, i.e., myocardial infarction, gastrointestinal hemorrhage, acute pancreatitis, acute gout, deep vein thrombosis, phlebitis, and pulmonary emboli/infarcts. The time that the fever spike occurs in relation to the initial defervescence, pulse-temperature relationships and other associated findings are the key determinants diagnostically in sorting out the possible explanations for the reappearance of fever in CCU patients with central lines or in patients on prolonged/high-dose steroid or immunosuppressive therapy. Lack of response to antimicrobial therapy suggests inadequate spectrum, suboptimal dosing, or insufficient activity against the pathogen viral or non-infectious disorder [3,5,52].

INFECTIOUS CAUSES OF FEVER IN THE CCU

Most non-toxin–mediated infections elicit a febrile response. While all infectious diseases may not manifest with temperatures >102°F, they have the potential to exceed 102°F; e.g., nosocomial pneumonia may be associated with temperatures <102°F or >102°F. Although all infectious diseases are not associated with temperatures ≥102°F, acute infections usually.

Infectious diseases in the CCU usually associated with high-grade fevers ≥102°F include acute meningitis, acute encephalitis, brain abscess, septic thrombophlebitis, jugular septic vein thrombophlebitis, pelvic septic thrombophlebitis, septic pulmonary emboli, pericarditis, acute bacterial endocarditis, perivalvular/myocardial abscess, community-acquired pneumonia, pleural empyema, lung abscess, postoperative abscesses cholangitis, intrarenal/perinephric abscess, prostatic abscess, urosepsis, CVC infections, contaminated infusates, pylephlebitis, liver abscess, *Clostridioides (Clostridium) difficile* colitis, complicated skin and soft tissue infections/abscesses, AV graft infections, foreign body–associated infections (pacemakers/AICDs, CVCs, Hickman/Broviac catheters), and septic arthritis. Infectious diseases likely in the CCU setting with low-grade fevers <102°F include chronic sacral osteomyelitis, decubitus ulcers, uncomplicated wound infections, and cellulitis [5,18,20,22].

The clinical diagnostic approach analyzes the fever in the patient's clinical context, i.e., correlates these clinical findings with other aspects of the patient's condition to arrive at a likely clinical syndromic diagnosis for the cause of the fever. The clinical approach utilizes the height of the fever, abruptness of onset, pulse-temperature relationships (relative bradycardia), response to antibiotic therapy, duration of fever, and the defervescence pattern, all of which have diagnostic importance (Table 2.5) [5].

TABLE 2.5
Fevers Prone to Relapse

Infectious Causes

Relapsing fever (*Borrelia recurrentis*)	Colorado tick fever
Trench fever (*Rochalimaea quintana*)	Dengue fever
Q fever	Leptospirosis
Typhoid fever	Brucellosis
Vibrio fetus	Bartonellosis (Oroyo fever)
Syphilis	Acute rheumatic fever
Tuberculosis	Rate-bite fever (*Spirillum minus*)
Histoplasmosis	Visceral leishmaniasis
Coccidioidomycosis	Lyme disease
Blastomycosis	Malaria
Pseudomonas pseudomallei (meliodosis)	Non-influenza respiratory viruses
Lymphocytic choriomeningitis	Babesiosis
Dengue fever	Epstein–Barr virus
Yellow fever	Cytomegalovirus
Chronic meningococcemia	

Non-infectious Causes

Bechet's disease	Familial Mediterranean fever
Crohn's disease	Fever, adenitis, pharyngitis, aphthous ulcer syndrome
Weber-Christian disease (panniculitis)	Systemic lupus erythematosus
Leukocytoclastic angiitis	Hyper IgD syndrome
Sweet's syndrome	

SINGLE FEVER SPIKES >102°F

Patients in the CCU who have been afebrile or had low-grade fevers, i.e., ≤102°F, may suddenly develop a single fever spike >102°F. Single fever spikes are never infectious in origin. The causes of single fever spikes include insertion/removal of a urinary catheter, insertion/removal of a venous catheter, suctioning/manipulation of an endotracheal tube, wound packing/lavage, wound irrigation, etc. Any procedure that involves a manipulation of a colonized/infected surface can induce a transient bacteremia. Such transient bacteremias are unsustained and do not result in infection or spread to other organs and for this reason should not be treated. The cause of single fever spikes is a diagnostic, not a therapeutic, problem.

The other common causes of single fever spikes are blood/blood product transfusions. Most febrile reactions occur within the first 72 hours after the blood/blood product transfusion, and most of these occur in the first 24–48 hours. There are few reactions after 72 hours, but some occur 5–7 days after the blood transfusion.

In patients with a single fever spike due to transient bacteremias following manipulation of a colonize/infected mucosal surface or secondary to blood product/blood transfusion, may be inferred by the temporal relationship of the causative event and the appearance of the fever. The characteristic fever curve, i.e., a single isolated temperature spike resolves spontaneously without treatment [1,5,11,31].

DDx OF LOW-GRADE FEVERS (<102°F) IN THE CCU

Most of the acute, non-infectious disorders that occur in the CCU are accompanied by low-grade fevers, i.e. <102°F. Fevers <102°F secondary to acute myocardial infarction, pulmonary embolus, and acute pancreatitis, are associated with fevers of relatively short duration. Other conditions that commonly present as with low-grade fevers include dehydration, atelectasis, wound inflammation, hematoma, seromas, ARDS, BOOP, deep vein thrombosis, pleural effusions, tracheobronchitis, decubitus ulcers, cellulitis, phlebitis, etc. Prolonged low-grade fevers (<102°F) are, in the main, not infectious. Try to identify the non-infectious disorder, so that undue resources will not be wasted looking for an unlikely infectious disease explanation for the fever [1,10,17–23].

There are relatively few prolonged fevers in the CCU that last for over a week. Such low-grade (<102°F) prolonged fevers lasting over a week are usually due to non-infectious disorders, e.g., central fever, drug fever, post-perfusion syndrome, atelectasis, dehydration, undrained seromas, and tracheobronchitis. Prolonged high-grade fevers may be due to an undrained abscess. Nosocomial sinusitis from prolonged nasotracheal intubation may also cause prolonged fever in the CCU [2,5,6,35–39].

CLINICAL SYNDROMIC DIAGNOSIS

COMMON DIAGNOSTIC PROBLEMS IN THE CCU

Drug Fever

Drug fevers are common in the CCU setting due to the multiplicity of medications. Physicians should always be suspicious of the possibility of drug fever when other diagnostic possibilities have been exhausted. Drug fever may occur in individuals who have just recently been started on the sensitizing medication but more commonly in those who have been on a sensitizing medication for a long period of time, without previous problems. Patients with drug fever do not necessarily have multiple allergies to medications and are not usually atopic. However, the likelihood of drug fever is more likely in patients who are atopic and have multiple drug allergies (Table 2.6).

Patients with drug fever, i.e., hypersensitivity reaction without rash, may present with any degree of fever, but most commonly, drug fevers are in the 102°F–104°F range. Patients with drug fever look "inappropriately well" for the degree of fever, which is different from that of the toxemic patient with a bacterial systemic infection. Relative bradycardia is invariably present (excluding patients on β-blocker therapy, those with arrhythmias, heart block, or pacemaker-induced rhythms) [1,5,40,41]. Laboratory tests include an increase in the WBC count, with a shift to the left. Eosinophils are often present in the differential count, but patients less commonly have eosinophilia. The ESR is elevated with drug fever, but this may be compounded by other causes of increased ESR with the multitude of disorders in CCU patients. Serum transaminases are also mildly/transiently elevated in drug fever. Often, such mild increases in the serum transaminases are overlooked by clinicians. Drug fever is a diagnosis of exclusion, but in patients with an obscure, otherwise-unexplained fever, the constellation of non-specific findings, including relative bradycardia, mildly increased serum transaminases, and eosinophils in the differential count, is sufficient to make a presumptive diagnosis of drug fever (Tables 2.7 and 2.8) [1–5,8,29–34].

It is a popular misconception that antibiotics are the most common cause of drug fever. Among the antibiotics, β-lactams and sulfonamides are the most common causes of drug fever. More common causes of drug fever in the CCU setting are antiarrhythmics; antiseizure medications; sulfa-containing diuretics, e.g., furosemide, tranquilizers, sedatives, sleep medications, and antihypertensive medications; sulfa-containing stool softeners, e.g., Colace; and, to a lesser extent, β-blockers. Since CCU patients are usually receiving multiple medications, it is not always possible to discontinue the one agent likely to be the cause of the drug fever. Often, two or three agents must be discontinued simultaneously. The clinician should discontinue the most likely agent that is not life supporting first, in order to properly interpret the decrease in temperature, if, indeed, that was the sensitizing agent responsible for the drug fever. If the agent that is likely

TABLE 2.6
Causes of Relative Bradycardia

Infectious	Non-infectious
Legionella	Beta blockers
Psittacosis	CNS lesions
Q fever	Lymphomas
Typhoid fever	Factitious fever
Typhus	Drug fever
Babesiosis	
Malaria	
Leptospirosis	
Yellow fever	
Dengue fever	
Viral hemorrhagic fevers	
Rocky Mountain spotted fever	

Determination of Relative Bradycardia

Inclusive criteria

1. Patient must be an adult, i.e., ≥13 years
2. Temperature ≥102°F
3. Pulse must be taken simultaneously with the temperature elevation

Exclusive criteria

1. Patient has NSR without arrhythmia, second-/third-degree heart block or pacemaker-induced rhythm
2. Patient must not be on β-blocker medication

Appropriate Temperature-Pulse Relationships

Pulse (beats/min)	Temperature
150	41.1°C (106°F)
140	40.6°C (105°F)
130	40.7°C (104°F)
120	39.4°C (103°F)
110	38.9°C (102°F)

Source: Cunha, B.A., *Clin. Microbiol. Infect.*, 6, 633–634, 2000.

Note: Relative bradycardia refers to heart rates that are inappropriately slow relative to body temperature (pulse must be taken simultaneously with temperature elevation). Applies to adult patients with temperature ≥ 102°F; does not apply to patients with second-/third-degree heart block, pacemaker-induced rhythms, or those taking beta-blockers.

to cause the drug fever cannot be discontinued, an attempt should be made to find an equivalent non-allergic substitute, i.e., ethacrynic acid in place of furosemide and a carbapenem in place of a β-lactam. If the agent responsible for the drug fever is discontinued, temperatures will decrease to near normal/normal within 72 hours. If no decrease in temperature within 72 hours, consider an alternate diagnosis. Resolution of drug fever returns temperature to normal, the leukocytosis decreases, and the eosinophils disappear (Tables 2.7 and 2.8) [5,32,34]. If the patient has a drug rash and fever, the diagnosis is drug rash. Fever is associated with drug rash and may take days to weeks to resolve after the sensitizing drug is discontinued (Tables 2.7 and 2.8) [5,26,40–42].

TABLE 2.7
Clinical Features of Drug Fever

History
    Many individuals are atopic
    "Sensitizing medication" taken for days or years
Physical Examination
    Look "inappropriately well" for degree of fever
    Low to high-grade fevers (102°F ≥ 106°F)
    Relative bradycardia (with temperature ≥102°F if not on β-blockers, etc.)
    No rash[a]
Laboratory Tests
    ↑ WBC count (often with left shift)
    Eosinophils usually present in peripheral smear (often missed with
        automated counters)
    Eosinophilia is uncommon
    ↑ ESR in most (may reach ≥100 mm/h)
    Mild/transient ↑ of serum transaminases (early)

[a]   If present, diagnosis is drug rash with fever.

TABLE 2.8
Drug Fever (2° Sensitizing Medications)

Common Causes	Rare Causes
Antibiotics	Digoxin
β-lactams	Steroids
Sleep medications	Diphenhydramine (Benadryl)
Antiseizure medications	Aspirin
Sulfa-containing drugs	Vitamins
Stool softeners (Colace)	Tetracyclines
Diuretics (Lasix)	Erythromycins
Antimicrobials	Ketolides
(TMP-SMX,	Clindamycin
pentamidine)	Aminoglycosides
Antidepressants/	Chloramphenicol
tranquilizers	Vancomycin
Antiarrhythmics	Teicoplanin
β-blockers	Aztreonam
ACE inhibitors	Carbapenems
	Quinolones
	Quinupristin/dalfopristin
	Daptomycin
	Tigecycline
	TMP
	Anti-virals
	Anti-fungals

DIAGNOSTIC SIGNIFICANCE OF RELATIVE BRADYCARDIA

Relative bradycardia combined in a patient with an obscure fever is an extremely useful diagnostic sign. Fever plus relative bradycardia immediately limits diagnostic possibilities to central fevers, drug fevers, and lymphomas, among the non-infectious disorders commonly causing fever in the CCU. Among the infectious causes of fever in the CCU, relative bradycardia in patients with pneumonia narrows diagnostic possibilities to *Legionella*, (psitticosis or Q fever). Patients without pneumonia, but with fever and relative bradycardia in the CCU limit diagnostic possibilities to a variety of arthropod-borne infections, i.e., RMSF, typhus, and typhoid fever, and arthropod-borne hemorrhagic fevers, i.e., yellow fever, Ebola, and dengue fever. Relative bradycardia, like other signs, should be interpreted in concert with other clinical findings to prompt further diagnostic testing for specific infectious diseases and to eliminate the non-infectious disorders associated with relative bradycardia from further consideration (Tables 2.9 and 2.10) [5,40,41].

TABLE 2.9
Persistent Fever in the CCU

Antibiotic-Related Problems
    Inadequate coverage/spectrum
    Inadequate antibiotic blood levels
    Inadequate antibiotic tissue levels
        Undrained abscess
        Foreign body-related infection
        Protected focus
            Abscess
            Foreign body
            Chronic osteomyelitis, etc.
        Organ hypoperfusion/diminished local blood supply
    In vitro susceptibility but inactive *in vivo*
    Antibiotic "tolerance" (gram-positive cocci)
    Drug-induced interactions
        Antibiotic inactivation
        Antibiotic antagonism

Non-antibiotic-Related Problems
    Treating colonization
    Non-infectious diseases mimics
        SLE
        Drug fever
        Atelectasis
        Pleural effusions
        Seroma
        Dehydration
        Acute pancreatitis
        Pulmonary emboli/infarction
        Acute myocardial infarction
        Central nervous system hemorrhage/cerebrovascular accident
    Antibiotic-unresponsive infectious diseases
        Viral infection

TABLE 2.10

Clinical Syndromic Approach to Fever in the CCU

System	Community-Acquired	Nosocomial	Either	Usual Maximum Temp at Presentation	
				≥102°F	≤102°F
Central nervous system	Meningitis			+	+
	Encephalitis				
	Brain abscess				+
		Neurosurgical shunt infection		+	
		Posterior fossa syndrome			+
			Central fevers	+	
			Cerebrovascular accident		+
			Massive intraventricular hemorrhage	+	
			Seizures		+
Cardiovascular	Subacute bacterial endocarditis				+
					+
			Acute bacterial endocarditis	+	
			Myocardial infarction		+
		Temporary IV/central line/ infected pacemaker		+	
	Permanent IV/central line/infected pacemaker			+	
		Postpericardiotomy syndrome			+
	Viral pericarditis		Myocardial/perivalvular abscess	+	
	Postperfusion syndrome				+
		Balloon pump fever		+	
		Sternal osteomyelitis			+
Pulmonary	CAP			+	
	Lung abscess			+	
		VAP		+	
			Pulmonary emboli/infarction		−
			ARDS		−
	Empyema			+	
			Pleural effusion		−
			Atelectasis/dehydration		+
	Systemic lupus erythematosus Pneumonitis			+	
			Tracheobronchitis		+
	BOOP				+
	Broncogenic carcinomas (without postobstructive pneumonia)				+
	Pulmonary cytotoxic drug reactions		Mediastinitis	+	
Gastrointestinal	Cholecystitis				
			Intra-abdominal abscess	+	
			Cholangitis	+	
			Viral hepatitis		+
			Acalculous cholecystitis	+	
			Peritonitis	+	
			Pancreatitis		+

(Continued)

TABLE 2.10 (*Continued*)

Clinical Syndromic Approach to Fever in the CCU

System	Community-Acquired	Nosocomial	Either	Usual Maximum Temp at Presentation	
				≥102°F	≤102°F
	Ischemic colitis				+
			Gastrointestinal hemorrhage		+
			Antibiotic-associated diarrhea (*C. difficile*)	+	
			Antibiotic-associated colitis (*C. difficile*)	+	
Urinary tract			Urosepsis	+	
		Catheter-associated bacteremia		+	
	Pyelonephritis			+	
	Cystitis				+
Skin/soft tissue	Cellulitis			+	
			Uncomplicated wound infection		+
	Gas gangrene				+
	Mixed soft tissue infection with gas			+	
Bone/joint			Decubitus ulcer		+
			Chronic osteomyelitis		+
	Acute osteomyelitis			+	
			Septic arthritis	+	
			Acute gout	+	
			RA joint flare		+
Other		Fat emboli		+	
			Adrenal insufficiency	+	
			Hematomas		
		Transient bacteremia		+	
		Blood/blood product transfusion		+	
		Sinusitis			+
	Alcohol withdrawal syndrome			+	+
	Delirium tremens			+	
	SLE flare				

CLINICAL APPROACH TO FEVER IN THE CCU

Problems that occur in the CCU that are related to new problems, complications of the original/new problems, and the effect of multiple medications make the diagnostic possibilities of explaining fever in the CCU complex. The cause of fever may be suggested by epidemiologic factors as well as the history, physical, laboratory, and radiology tests. If the main thrust of the diagnostic approach is to identify reversible/curable causes of fever, analysis of the fever characteristics is the best way to sort out DDx possibilities in the CCU. Careful attention should be given to whether the fever spike is isolated or sustained, whether the fever is greater than or less than 102°F, the duration of the fever, and the relationship of the temperature with the pulse. Careful review of all the medications is essential not only to recognize drug side effects/interactions but also to entertain the possibility of drug fever if other diagnoses are unlikely. Clinicians should also be familiar with the fever defervescence patterns of infectious and non-infectious disorders. Most situations are fairly straightforward, e.g., a steroid-dependent patient with SLE and flare who is in the CCU for the management of renal insufficiency and develops a fever >102°F without relative bradycardia, which is sustained. While there are many possibilities to explain fevers, i.e., superimposed cytomegalovirus (CMV) or bacterial infections, the most important correctable factor to identify as the cause of the fever is inadequate steroid dosage. Patients on chronic corticosteroids when admitted to the CCU require stress doses of corticosteroids. Without increasing the corticosteroid daily dose, patients develop a fever from a flare of their SLE/relative bradycardia and adrenal insufficiency, which presents as otherwise-unexplained fever in such patients (Table 2.11) [1,5,6,8,53].

TABLE 2.11
Clinical Diagnostic Approach to Fever in CCU

Early infectious disease consultation
- All febrile CCU patients should have an infectious disease consultation
- Infectious disease consultation to evaluate mimics of infections (pseudosepsis) and microbiologic data

Persistent low grade fevers (≤102°F)
- Non-infectious medical diseases most likely
- Infectious disease causes also important

Acute high, spiking fevers (≥102°F)
- Infectious disease etiology most likely
- Medical disorders excluded by fevers ≥102°F:

MI/LVF	Thrombophlebitis
PE	*C. difficile* diarrhea
Acute pancreatitis	GI hemorrhage
ARDS	Cholecystitis
Atelectasis/dehydration	Uncomplicated wound infection
Hematomas	

- Only non-infectious diseases with temperatures ≥102°F in CCU
  Drug fevers
  Malignant neuroleptic syndrome
  Central fevers
  Fevers 2° to blood/blood product transfusion
  Transient bacteremias 2° to manipulation of a colonized/infected mucosa

TABLE 2.12
Therapeutic Approach to Fever in the CCU

Microbiologic data evaluation
- Critical to differentiate colonization from infection
  Respiratory secretion isolates
  Urinary isolates
  Analysis of origin of blood culture isolates
- Rule out pseudoinfections

Common causes of fevers
- Nosocomial pneumonia/VAP
  Chest X-ray
  - If negative, no nosocomial pneumonia/VAP
  - If positive, rule out LVF, ARDS, etc.
  Perform semiquantitative PBB/BAL to confirm diagnosis
- Check central IV lines
  Duration of insertion
  - The longer the IV line is overdue, the more likely the fever is due to IV-line infection
  - Otherwise-unexplained fevers in a patient with overdue IV lines should be regarded as IV line infection until proven otherwise
  Evidence of infections at local site
  - If IV shows sign of infection, remove IV line immediately, send tip for semiquantitative culture, and obtain blood cultures from peripheral vein
  - If IV site non-erythematous, IV line infection not ruled out; remove/replace IV line and send removed catheter tip for semiquantitative culture
- If nosocomial pneumonia and IV-line infection eliminated from diagnostic consideration, consider drug fever

Early empiric therapy
- Coverage based on site/organism correlations: colonization should not be treated
- Infectious disease consultant recommendations should be followed

If an infectious etiology is suspected/diagnosed, empiric coverage should be based on site/pathogen associations. Specific therapy, if different from empiric therapy, may be used if empiric therapy is ineffective. Duration of therapy is a function of the type/site of infection and the status of the host defenses (Tables 2.12 and 2.13) [54–56].

Non-infectious causes of relapsing fevers in the CCU include Crohn's disease, leukoclastic angiitis, Sweet's syndrome, and SLE. The infectious causes of fevers that are prone to relapse include viral infections, i.e., CMV, Epstein–Barr virus, lymphocytic choriomeningitis, dengue, yellow fever, and Colorado tick fever. Zoonotic bacterial infections, i.e., leptospirosis, bartonellosis, brucellosis, malaria, babesiosis, ehrlichiosis/Q fever, anaplasmosis, and typhoid fever [1,5].

TABLE 2.13
Sepsis/Septic Shock

Subset	Usual Pathogens	Preferred IV Therapy	Alternate IV Therapy	IV-to-PO Switch
Unknown source	*Enterobacteriaceae* *B. fragilis*	Meropenem 1 g (IV) q8h × 2 weeks or piperacillin/tazobactam 4.5 g (IV) q8h × 2 weeks or imipenem 500 mg (IV) q6h × 2 weeks or ertapenem 1 g (IV) q24h × 2 weeks or combination therapy with ceftriaxone 1 g (IV) q24h × 2 weeks plus metronidazole 1 g (IV) q24h × 2 weeks	Quinolone[a] (IV) × 2 weeks plus either metronidazole 1 g (IV) q24h × 2 weeks or clindamycin 600 mg (IV) q8h × 2 weeks	Moxifloxacin 400 mg (PO) q24h × 2 weeks or combination therapy with clindamycin 300 mg (PO) q8h × 2 weeks plus either ciprofloxacin 500 mg (PO) q12h × 2 weeks or gatifloxacin 400 mg (PO) q24h × 2 weeks or levofloxacin 500 mg (PO) q24h × 2 weeks
	Group D streptococci[b] *E. faecalis*	Meropenem 1 g (IV) q8h × 2 weeks or piperacillin/tazobactam 4.5 g (IV) q8h × 2 weeks	Ampicillin/sulbactam 3 g (IV) q6h × 2 weeks or quinolone[c] (IV) × 2 weeks	Quinolone[c] (PO) × 2 weeks
	E. faecium (VRE)	Linezolid 600 mg (IV) q12h × 2 weeks or quinupristin/dalfopristin 7.5 mg/kg (IV) q8h × 2 weeks	Chloramphenicol 500 mg (IV) q6h × 2 weeks or doxycycline 200 mg (IV) q12h × 3 days, then 100 mg (IV) q12h × 11 days	Linezolid 600 mg (PO) q12h × 2 weeks or doxycycline 100 mg (PO) q12h × 2 weeks
Lung source	*S. pneumoniae* *H. influenzae* *K. pneumoniae*	Ceftriaxone 1 g (IV) q24h × 2 weeks or cefepime 2 g (IV) q12h × 2 weeks	Quinolone[c] (IV) q24h × 2 weeks or Any second-generation cephalosporin (IV) × 2 weeks	Quinolone[c] (PO) q24h × 2 weeks or doxycycline 200 mg (PO) q12h × 3 days, then 100 mg (PO) q12h × 11 days
IV-line sepsis, bacterial (Treat initially for MSSA; if later identified as MRSA, treat accordingly)	*S. epidermidis* *S. aureus* (MSSA) *Klebsiella* *Enterobacter* *Serratia* *S. aureus* (MRSA)	Meropenem 1 g (IV) q8h × 2 weeks or cefepime 2 g (IV) q12h × 2 weeks Vancomycin 1 g (IV) q12h × 2 weeks or linezolid 600 mg (IV) q12h × 2 weeks or quinupristin/dalfopristin 7.5 mg/kg (IV) q8h × 2 weeks	Ceftriaxone 1 g (IV) q24h × 2 weeks or quinolone[d] (IV) q24h × 2 weeks Vancomycin 1 g (IV) q12h × 2 weeks or linezolid 600 mg (IV) q12h × 2 weeks or quinupristin/dalfopristin 7.5 mg/kg (IV) q8h × 2 weeks	Quinolone[d] (PO) q24h × 2 weeks or cephalexin 500 mg (PO) q6h × 2 weeks Linezolid 600 mg (PO) q12h × 2 weeks or minocycline 100 mg (PO) q12h × 2 weeks

(Continued)

TABLE 2.13 (*Continued*)
Sepsis/Septic Shock

Subset	Usual Pathogens	Preferred IV Therapy	Alternate IV Therapy	IV-to-PO Switch
IV-line sepsis, fungal (Treat initially for non-albicans Candida; if later identified as *C. albicans*, treat accordingly)	*Candida albicans*	*Preferred IV therapy:* fluconazole 800 mg (IV) × 1, then 400 mg (IV) q24h × 2 weeks *Alternate IV therapy:* caspofungin 70 mg (IV) × 1 dose, then 50 mg (IV) q24h × 2 weeks or lipid-associated formulation of amphotericin B (p. 369) (IV) q24h × 2 weeks or amphotericin B deoxycholate 0.7 mg/kg (IV) q24h × 2 weeks or voriconazole (see "usual dose," p. 480) or itraconazole 200 mg (IV) q12h × 2 days, then 200 mg (IV) q24h × 2 weeks	*Preferred IV therapy:* fluconazole 800 mg (IV) × 1, then 400 mg (IV) q24h × 2 weeks *Alternate IV therapy:* caspofungin 70 mg (IV) × 1 dose, then 50 mg (IV) q24h × 2 weeks or Lipid-associated formulation of amphotericin B (p. 369) (IV) q24h × 2 weeks or amphotericin B deoxycholate 0.7 mg/kg (IV) q24h × 2 weeks or voriconazole (see "usual dose," p. 480) or itraconazole 200 mg (IV) q12h × 2 days, then 200 mg (IV) q24h × 2 weeks	Fluconazole 400 mg (PO) q24h × 2 weeks or voriconazole (see "usual dose," p. 480) or itraconazole 200 mg (PO) solution q12h × 2 weeks
	Non-albicans *Candida*[e]	Caspofungin or lipid amphotericin B or amphotericin B deoxycholate (see *C. albicans*, above) × 2 weeks	Fluconazole or itraconazole (see *C. albicans*, above) or voriconazole (see "usual dose," p. 480) × 2 weeks	Fluconazole (see *C. albicans*, above) or itraconazole 200 mg (PO) solution q24h or voriconazole (see "usual dose," p. 480) × 2 weeks[e]
	Aspergillus	Voriconazole (see "usual dose," p. 480) × 2 weeks or caspofungin 70 mg (IV) × 1 dose, then 50 mg (IV) q24h × 2 weeks or itraconazole 200 mg (IV) q12h × 2 days, then 200 mg (IV) q24h × 2 weeks	Lipid-associated formulation of amphotericin B (p. 369) (IV) q24h × 2 weeks or amphotericin B deoxycholate 1–1.5 mg/kg (IV) q24h × 2 weeks	Voriconazole (see "usual dose," p. 480) × 2 weeks or itraconazole 200 mg (PO) solution q12h × 2 days, then 200 mg (PO) solution q24h × 2 weeks
Intra-abdominal/pelvic source	Enterobacteriaceae *B. fragilis*	Meropenem 1 g (IV) q8h × 2 weeks or piperacillin/tazobactam 4.5 g therapy with (IV) q8h × 2 weeks or imipenem 500 mg (IV) q6h × 2 weeks or combination therapy with ceftriaxone 1 g (IV) q24h × 2 weeks plus metronidazole 1 g (IV) q24h × 2 weeks	Quinolone[a] (IV) × 2 weeks plus either metronidazole 1 g (IV) q24h × 2 weeks or clindamycin 600 mg (IV) q8h × 2 weeks	Moxifloxacin 400 mg (PO) q24h × 2 weeks or combination therapy with clindamycin 300 mg (PO) q8h × 2 weeks plus either ciprofloxacin 500 mg (PO) q12h × 2 weeks or gatifloxacin 400 mg (PO) q24h × 2 weeks or levofloxacin 500 mg (PO) q24h × 2 weeks

(Continued)

TABLE 2.13 (*Continued*)
Sepsis/Septic Shock

Subset	Usual Pathogens	Preferred IV Therapy	Alternate IV Therapy	IV-to-PO Switch
Urosepsis gram (−) bacilli	Enterobacteriaceae	Ceftriaxone 1 g (IV) q24h × 1–2 weeks	Aztreonam 2 g (IV) q8h × 1–2 weeks or any aminoglycoside (IV) × 1–2 weeks	Quinolone (PO)[a] × 1–2 weeks
Gram + streptococci (treat initially for *E. faecalis*; if later identified as VRE, treat accordingly)	Group B streptococci *E. faecalis*	Quinolone (IV)[a] × 1–2 weeks	Ampicillin 1–2 g (IV) q4h × 1–2 weeks or vancomycin 1 g (IV) q12h × 1–2 weeks	Amoxicillin 1 g (PO) q8h × 1–2 weeks or quinolone (PO)[a] × 1–2 weeks
Urosepsis gram (+) streptococci Treat initially for *E. faecalis*; if later identified as VRE, treat accordingly)	*E. faecium* (VRE*)*	Linezolid 600 mg (IV) q12h × 1–2 weeks or Quinupristin/dalfopristin 7.5 mg/kg (IV) q8h × 1–2 weeks	Linezolid 600 mg (IV) q12h × 1–2 weeks or Quinupristin/dalfopristin 7.5 mg/kg (IV) q8h × 1–2 weeks	Linezolid 600 mg (PO) q12h × 1–2 weeks or doxycycline 200 mg (PO) q12h
Organism not known	Enterobacteriaceae Group B, D streptococci	Quinolone (IV)[a] × 2 weeks	Piperacillin/tazobactam 4.5 g (IV) q8h × 1–2 weeks	Quinolone (PO)[a] × 2 weeks
Asplenia or hyposplenia	*S. pneumoniae* *H. influenzae* *N. meningitidis*	Ceftriaxone 2 g (IV) q24h × 2 weeks or quinolone[d] (IV) Q24h × 2 weeks	Cefepime 2 g (IV) q12h × 2 weeks or cefotaxime 2 g (IV) q6h × 2 weeks	Quinolone[d] (PO) Q24h × 2 weeks
Steroids (high chronic dose)	*Candida* *Aspergillus*	Treat the same as for fungal infection	Treat the same as for fungal infection	Treat the same as for fungal infection
Miliary TB	*M. tuberculosis*	Treat the same as pulmonary TB (p. 47) plus steroids × 1–2 weeks	Treat the same as pulmonary TB (p. 47) plus steroids × 1–2 weeks	Treat the same as pulmonary TB (p. 47) plus steroids × 1–2 weeks
Miliary BCG (disseminated)	Bacillus Calmette-Guerin (BCG)	Treat with four anti-TB drugs (NIH, rifampin, ethambutol, and cycloserine) q24h × 6–12 months plus steroids (e.g., prednisone 40 mg q24h) × 1–2 weeks	Treat with four anti-TB drugs (NIH, rifampin, ethambutol, and cycloserine) q24h × 6–12 months plus steroids (e.g., prednisone 40 mg q24h) × 1–2 weeks	Treat with four anti-TB drugs (NIH, rifampin, ethambutol, and cycloserine) q24h × 6–12 months plus steroids (e.g., prednisone 40 mg q24h) × 1–2 weeks
Severe sepsis	Gram-negative or gram-positive bacteria	Appropriate antimicrobial therapy plus surgical decompression/drainage if needed plus drotrecogin alpha (Xigris) 24 µg/kg/h (IV) × 96 hours	Appropriate antimicrobial therapy plus surgical decompression/drainage if needed plus drotrecogin alpha (Xigris) 24 µg/kg/h	Appropriate antimicrobial therapy plus surgical decompression/drainage if needed plus drotrecogin alpha (Xigris) 24 µg/kg/h

Abbreviations: MSSA/MRSA, methicillin-sensitive/-resistant *S. aureus*.

Notes: Duration of therapy represents total time IV or IV + PO. Most patients on IV therapy able to take PO meds should be switched to PO therapy after clinical improvement. Duration of therapy represents total time IV or IV + PO.

[a] Ciprofloxacin 400 mg (IV) or 500 mg (PO) q12h or gatifloxacin 400 mg (IV or PO) q24h or levofloxacin 500 mg (IV or PO) q24h.

[b] Treat initially for *E. faecalis*; if later identified as *E. faecium* (VRE), treat accordingly.

[c] Ciprofloxacin 400 mg (IV) or 500 mg (PO) q12h or gatifloxacin 400 mg (IV or PO) q24h or levofloxacin 500 mg (IV or PO) q24h or moxifloxacin 400 mg (IV or PO) q24h.

[d] Gatifloxacin 400 mg or levofloxacin 500 mg or moxifloxacin 400 mg.

[e] Best agent depends on infecting species. Fluconazole susceptibility varies predictably by species. *C. glabrata* (usually) and *C. krusei* (almost always) are resistant to fluconazole. *C. lusitaniae* is often resistant to amphotericin B (deoxycholate and lipid-associated formulations). Others are generally susceptible to all agents.

TABLE 2.14

Treatment of Fever in the CCU

Obligatory reduction in temperatures >106°F
- Heat stroke
- Malignant hyperthermia
- Malignant neoplastic syndrome
- Central fevers
- Drug fever

Obligatory reduction in temperatures >102°F[a]
- Acute myocardial infarction
- Borderline pulmonary function
- Central nervous system trauma

Optional reduction in temperatures >102°F[a]
- Blood/blood product transfusion reactions
- Post-diagnosis of infectious/non-infectious diseases febrile disorders

[a] Temperatures should be lowered to <102°F.

TREATMENT OF FEVER

Fever is an important clinical sign indicating a non-infectious or infectious disorder. The presence of fever should prompt the clinician to analyze its height, frequency, pattern, and associated history, physical findings, and laboratory tests to determine the cause of fever and initiate appropriate treatment [1,4,5,26,41–45,52]. Fever, per se, should not be treated unless the fever itself is a threat to the patient, i.e., extreme hyperpyrexia could result with CNS damage. Temperatures >102°F in patients with severe cardiac/pulmonary diseases could precipitate acute myocardial infarction or respiratory failure [5,57]. Fever is also an important host defense mechanism that should not be suppressed without a compelling clinical rationale (Table 2.14) [57–59].

REFERENCES

1. Cunha BA. Clinical approach to fever in the CCU. *Crit Care Clin* 1998;8:1–14.
2. Cunha BA. Fever in the intensive care unit. *Intensive Care* 1999;25:648–651.
3. Cunha BA, Shea KW. Fever in the intensive care unit. *Infect Dis Clin North Am* 1996;10:185–209.
4. Fry DE. Postoperative fever. In: Mackowiak PA ed. *Fever: Basic Mechanisms and Management*. New York: New York Press, 1991:293–254.
5. Cunha BA. Approach to fever. In: Gorbach SL, Bartlett JB, Blacklow NR eds. *Infectious Diseases in Medicine and Surgery* (4th ed.). Baltimore, MD: Lippincott Williams & Wilkins, 2005:54–63.
6. McGowan JE, Rose RC, Jacobs NF, et al. Fever in hospitalized patients. *Am J Med* 1987;82:580–586.
7. Ryan M, Levy MM. Clinical review: Fever in intensive care unit patients. *Crit Care* 2003;7:221–225.
8. Stumacher RJ. Fever in the ICU. *Infect Dis Pract* 1996;20:89–92.
9. Tu RP, Cunha BA. Significance of fever in the neurosurgical intensive care unit. *Heart Lung* 1998;17:608–611.
10. Petersen PE. Fever in the ICU. *Chest* 2000;117:855–869.
11. Cunha BA. Bacteremia and septicemia. In: Rakel RE, Bope ET eds. *Conn's Current Therapy—2003* (55th ed.). Philadelphia, PA: WB Saunders, 2004:113–118.
12. Gabby DS, Cunha BA. Pseudosepsis secondary to bilateral adrenal hemorrhage. *Heart Lung* 1998; 27:348–351.
13. Lai KK, Melvin ZS, Menard MJ, et al. Clostridium difficile-associated diarrhea: Epidemiology, risk factors, and infection control. *Infect Cont Hosp Epidemiol* 1997;18:628–632.
14. Boulant JA. The preoptic-anterior hypothalamus in thermo-regulation and fever. *Clin Infect Dis* 2000;31:S157–S161.
15. Cunha BA. Fever in malignant disorders. *Infect Dis Pract* 2004;28:335–336.
16. Engoren M. Lack of association between atelectasis and fever. *Chest* 1995;107:81–84.
17. Garibaldi RA, Brodine S, Matsumiya S, et al. Evidence for the non-infectious etiology of early postoperative fever. *Infect Cont* 1985;6:273–277.
18. Paradisi F, Corti G, Mangani V. Urosepsis in the critical care unit. *Crit Care Clin* 1998;114:165–180.
19. Warren JW. Catheter-associated urinary tract infections. *Infect Dis Clin North Am* 1997;11:609–619.
20. Cunha BA, Gill MV, Lazar J. Acute infective endocarditis. *Infect Dis Clin North Am* 1996;10:811–834.
21. Marx N, Neumann FJ, Ott I, et al. Induction of cytokine expression in leukocytes in acute myocardial infarction. *J Am Coll Cardiol* 1997;30:165–170.
22. Caines C, Gill MV, Cunha BA. Non-Clostridium difficile nosocomial diarrhea in the intensive care unit. *Heart Lung* 1997;26:83–84.
23. Barton JC. Nonhemolytic, noninfectious transfusion reactions. *Semin Hematol* 1981;18:95–121.
24. Ferrara JL. The febrile platelet transfusion reaction: A cytokine shower. *Transfusion* 1995;35:89–90.
25. Fenwick JC, Cameron M, Naiman SC, et al. Blood transfusion as a cause of leucocytosis in critically ill patients. *Lancet* 1994;344:855–856.
26. Cunha BA. The diagnostic approach to rash and fever in the CCU. *Crit Care Clinics* 1998;8:35–54.
27. Petersen SR, Sheldon GF. Acute acalculous cholecystitis: A complication of hyperalimentation. *Am J Surg* 1979;138:814–817.
28. Marik PE, Andrews L, Maini B. The incidence of deep venous thrombosis in ICU patients. *Chest* 1997;111:661–664.
29. Hamid N, Spadafora P, Khalife ME, Cunha BA. Pseudosepsis: Rectus sheath hematoma mimicking septic shock. *Heart Lung* 2006;35:434–437.
30. Mieszczanska H, Lazar J, Cunha BA. Cardiovascular manifestations of sepsis. *Infect Dis Pract* 2003;27:183–186.
31. Wormser GP, Ororato IM, Preminger TJ, et al. Sensitivity and specificity of blood cultures obtained through intravascular catheters. *Crit Care Med* 1990;18:152–156.
32. Johnson DH, Cunha BA. Drug fever. *Infect Dis Clin North Am* 1996;10:85–91.

33. Mackowiak PA, LeMaistre CF. Drug fever: A critical appraisal of conventional concepts. *Ann Intern Med* 1987;106:728–733.

34. Mackowiak PA. Drug fever: Mechanisms, maxims and misconceptions. *Am J Med Sci* 1987;294:275–286.

35. Fernandez-hidalgo N, Almirante B, Tornos P, et al. Contemporary epidemiology and prognosis of health care-associated infective endocarditis. *Clin Infect Dis* 2008;47:1287–1296.

36. Bartlett JG, Gerding DN. Clinical recognition and diagnosis of clostridium difficile infection. *Clin Infect Dis* 2008;46:12–18.

37. Maki DG. Pathogenesis, prevention, and management of infections due to intravascular devices used for infusion therapy. In. Bisno A, Waldvogel F, eds. *Infections Associated with Indwelling Medical Devices.* Washington, DC: American Society for Microbiology, 1989:161–177.

38. Williams JF, Seneff MG, Friedman BC, et al. Use of femoral venous catheters in critically ill adults: Prospective study. *Crit Care Med* 1991;19:550–553.

39. Rouby JJ, Laurent P, Gosnach M, et al. Risk factors and clinical relevance of nosocomial maxillary sinusitis in the critically ill. *Am J Respir Crit Care Med* 1994;150:776–783.

40. Cunha BA. Diagnostic significance of relative bradycardia. *Infect Dis Pract* 1997;21:38–40.

41. Cunha BA. The diagnostic significance of relative bradycardia in infectious disease. *Clin Microbiol Infect* 2000;6:633–634.

42. Cunha BA. Rash and fever in the intensive care unit. In: Abraham E, Vincent JL, Kochanek P, eds. *Textbook of Critical Care Medicine* (5th ed.). Philadelphia, PA: Elsevier, 2005:113–119.

43. Cunha BA. The diagnostic significance of fever curves. *Infect Dis Clin North Am* 1996;10:33–44.

44. Musher DM, Fainstein V, Young EJ, et al. Fever patterns: Their lack of clinical significance. *Arch Intern Med* 1979;139:1225–1228.

45. Sideridis K, Canario D, Cunha BA. Dengue fever, the diagnostic importance of a camelback fever pattern. *Heart Lung* 2003; 32:414–418.

46. Meduri GU, Mauldin GI, Wunderink RG, et al. Causes of fever and pulmonary densities in patients with clinical manifestations of ventilator-associated pneumonia. *Chest* 1994;106:221–235.

47. Timsit JF, Misset B, Goldstein FW, et al. Reappraisal of distal diagnostic testing in the diagnosis of ICU-acquired pneumonia. *Chest* 1995;108:1632–1639.

48. Meduri GU. Diagnosis and differential diagnosis of ventilator-associated pneumonia. *Clin Chest Med* 1995;16:61–93.

49. Cunha BA. Ventilator associated pneumonia: Monotherapy is optimal if chosen wisely. *Crit Care Med* 2006;10:e141–e142.

50. Chastre J, Fagon JY, Trouillet JL. Diagnosis and treatment of nosocomial pneumonia in patients in intensive care units. *Clin Infect Dis* 1995;21(suppl 3):S226–S237.

51. Eisenstein I, Cunha BA. Herpes simplex virus type I (HSV-I) pneumonia presenting as failure to wean. *Heart Lung* 2003;32:65–66.

52. Cunha BA. Nosocomial fever of unknown origin (FUO). *Infect Dis Pract* 2005;29:282–287.

53. Laupland KB, Shahpori R, Kirkpatrick AW, et al. Occurrence and outcome of fever in critically ill adults. *Crit Care Med* 2008;36:1531–1535.

54. Cunha BA. Factors in antibiotic selection for the seriously ill hospitalized patients. *Antibiot Clin* 2003;7(S2):19–24.

55. Cunha BA. *S. aureus* bacteremia: Clinical treatment guideline. *Antibiot Clin* 2006;10:365–367.

56. Cunha BA. *Antibiotic Essentials* (8th ed.). Sudbury, MA: Jones & Bartlett, 2009.

57. Mackowiak PA. Physiological rationale for suppression of fever. *Clin Infect Dis* 2000;31(suppl 5):S185–S189.

58. Kluger MJ, Ringler DH, Anver MR. Fever and survival. *Science* 1975;188:166–168.

59. Kluger MJ, Kozak W, Conn CA, et al. The adaptive value of fever. *Infect Dis Clin North Am* 1996;10:1–20.

3 Physical Exam Clues and Their Mimics in Infectious Diseases in the Critical Care Unit

Yehia Y. Mishriki

Non semper ea sunt quae videntur. (Things are not always what they seem.)

—Phaedrus

Under the best of circumstances, the physical examination (PE) of an CCU patient is quite challenging. To make matters more difficult, many physical findings are neither specific nor sensitive. What have been touted as "pathognomonic" findings are rarely, if ever, so. The astute physician must always consider that a given PE finding may be due to more than one disease entity. Premature closure and availability bias can further trip up the unwary clinician. As with various clinical syndromes, PE findings in infected patients can be mimicked by a variety of non-infectious diseases. The table that follows lists many of the PE findings one may encounter in the infected CCU patient, along with their non-infectious mimics and hints to help distinguish them apart.

System	ID Exam Finding	Non-infectious Mimics	Diagnostic Features
Fever	Usually the *sine qua non* of infection	Drug or drug withdrawal Cotton fever Central fever/subarachnoid hemorrhage Periodic fevers Sarcoidosis Neoplasms (esp. lymphoma and renal cell cancer) Autoimmune diseases (SLE, adult Still's disease, PMR) Neuroleptic malignant syndrome Malignant hyperthermia Serotonin syndrome Sympathomimetic toxidrome Immune reconstitution inflammatory syndrome Reaction to blood products Jarish-Herxheimer reaction Tumor lysis syndrome Pancreatitis Organ transplant rejection Acute gout Stroke (esp. intracerebral bleed) Myocardial infarction (STEMI) Adrenal insufficiency Acalculous cholecystitis Postoperative (first 24 hours) Pulmonary aspiration Pulmonary embolism Atrial myxoma	Non-infectious causes of fever must always be considered in patients with fever and no obvious source of infection, especially in the setting of relative bradycardia or extreme elevations of temperature (i.e., >106°F). Rash and/or eosinophilia suggest a drug fever, as does a high fever in an asymptomatic patient. The clinical setting, timing, and associated findings can suggest a non-infectious cause of fever (i.e., rigidity in neuroleptic malignant syndrome, recent institution of HAART in IRIS, use of serotonergic medications, etc.). Relative bradycardia may be present in non-infectious fever but may also occur in certain infections such as typhoid, Legionnaire's disease, dengue, malaria, babesiosis, and others.
Extreme hyper pyrexia (>106°F)	Gram-negative bacteremia (rare)	Malignant hyperthermia Neuroleptic malignant syndrome Central fever including post craniotomy Drug fever Heatstroke Thyrotoxicosis crisis Cocaine/phencyclidine	Fever >106°F is almost never due to an infection. Suppressed TSH with elevated free T4 and free T3 is seen in thyrotoxicosis. Muscle rigidity and increased creatine kinase in neuroleptic malignant syndrome.

(Continued)

System	ID Exam Finding	Non-infectious Mimics	Diagnostic Features
Sustained fever	Gram-negative pneumonia Typhoid Typhus Bacterial endocarditis Lobar pneumonia Tuberculosis Fungal disease	Central fever Autoimmune disorders Neoplasms	Blood cultures/chest X-ray in pneumonia and endocarditis. There may be relative bradycardia in central fever and also in typhoid. Serologic testing for autoimmune disorders.
Double quotidian fever	Gonococcal endocarditis Mixed malarial infection Visceral leishmaniasis	Adult onset Still's disease Juvenile rheumatoid arthritis	Blood culture positive in gonococcal endocarditis. Blood smear positive in malaria. Biopsy of bone marrow, liver, lymph node, or spleen in leishmaniasis. Clinical criteria and markedly elevated ferritin to diagnose AOSD and JRA.
Hypothermia	Overwhelming sepsis	Exposure/immersion Drugs (ethanol, phenothiazines, sedatives/hypnotics) Metabolic (hypothyroidism, hypoadrenalism, hyper-pituitarism, hypoglycemia) Acute spinal cord transection Burns/exfoliative dermatitis Aggressive fluid resuscitation	Clinical setting. Glucose, TSH, cortisol level, or cosyntropin stimulation test in suspected metabolic causes.
Relative bradycardia (Faget sign, pulse-temperature dissociation)	Legionellosis Psittacosis Q fever Typhoid fever Typhus Babesiosis Malaria Leptospirosis Yellow fever Dengue fever Viral hemorrhagic fevers Rocky Mountain spotted fever	β-blockers CNS lesions Lymphomas Factitious fever Drug fever Intrinsic heart disease	A pneumonic process and relative bradycardia suggest legionellosis, Q fever, and psittacosis. Hemolytic anemia suggests malaria or babesiosis. Leukopenia suggests typhoid fever. Capillary leak syndrome suggests viral hemorrhagic fever.
Orthopnea	Biapical pneumonia Tuberculous pericardial effusion	Left-sided CHF Diffuse interstitial lung disease Intrathoracic anterior mediastinal mass (goiter, thymoma, lymphoma, teratoma) Bilateral diaphragmatic paralysis Pulmonary veno-occlusive disease	Fever, crackles, and signs of consolidation in the upper lung fields in pneumonia. Increase JVP, edema, and S3 gallop in CHF. Immobility of the diaphragms on percussion of the lungs during deep inspiration. Imaging to detect mediastinal masses. Pulmonary hypertension on echocardiography or right-sided cardiac catheterization with a normal PCWP suggests pulmonary veno-occlusive disease.
Platypnea	Bibasilar pneumonia	Cirrhosis Bilateral pulmonary emboli Severe emphysema Bilateral pleural effusions	Fever suggests pneumonia. Imaging (X-ray, CT) for other pulmonary disorders. Stigmata of chronic liver disease in cirrhosis.
Trepopnea	Infectious pleuritis (affected side down)	Left-sided CHF Unilateral extensive lung disease or post-pneumonectomy Swyer-James syndrome Endobronchial mass with ball-valve effect	Fever in infective pleuritis. Elevated JVP, S3 gallop, basilar crackles, and edema in CHF. X-ray or CT scan of the chest for pulmonary disorders.

(Continued)

System	ID Exam Finding	Non-infectious Mimics	Diagnostic Features
Cellulitis	Bacterial	Allergic contact dermatitis erythema nodosum Insect bite–induced hypersensitivity (papular urticaria) Stasis dermatitis lipodermatosclerosis	Fever and leukocytosis favor infection. Clinical context and exam findings for other diagnoses.
Subcutaneous nodules	Acute rheumatic fever Nocardiosis Sporotrichosis Atypical mycobacterial infections *Rochalimaea henselae* *Dirofilaria immitis* Cutaneous leishmaniasis Onchocerciasis	Rheumatoid arthritis SLE Tophaceous gout Sarcoidosis Granuloma annulare	Jones' criteria in ARF. Fever >102°F suggestive of, but not diagnostic of, infection. Appropriate cultures and serological tests. Synovitis and joint changes in RA. Biopsy for others.
Tender violaceous acral papules	Infectious endocarditis Typhoid Gonococcemia	Cholesterol emboli Chilblains Vasculitis Cryoglobulinemia SLE Non-bacterial thrombotic endocarditis	Fever favors infection. Murmur and positive blood cultures in endocarditis. Livedo reticularis in cholesterol emboli. Echocardiography for NBTE.
Painful unilateral eye proptosis	Orbital cellulitis Septic cavernous sinus thrombosis Sino-orbital aspergillosis Mucormycosis	Graves' disease Orbital pseudotumor Orbital myositis Lymphoma Metastatic cancer Primary tumors of the orbit Tolosa-Hunt syndrome Retro-orbital hemorrhage Leukemia	Fever favors infection. Immunosuppression present in aspergillosis and mucormycosis. Cranial nerve III, IV, V, and VI involvement in septic cavernous sinus thrombosis.
Ptosis, miosis, possible anhidrosis (Horner's syndrome)	Chronicle apical pneumonia (staphylococcal, fungal, *Aspergillus*, *Pasteurella*) Tuberculosis Hydatid cyst of the thoracic outlet Mycotic thoracic aortic aneurysm Basilar meningitis	Central lesions: Wallenberg syndrome, TIA/stroke, brain tumors, MS Preganglionic lesions: thoracic tumors, phrenic nerve syndrome, thyroid enlargement, DISH, neck trauma, carotid dissection, Arnold-Chiari malformation, syringomyelia Postganglionic lesions: skull fracture, cluster headaches, migraines, middle-ear infections	Fever suggests infection. Blood cultures/serologic testing. Imaging (chest X-ray/CT/MRI). MRI brain/spinal cord.
Optic head swelling/inflammation (papillitis)	Bacterial: esp. brucellosis, endocarditis, leptospirosis, Lyme disease, *Mycoplasma pneumoniae*, syphilis, tuberculosis Fungal: candidiasis, coccidioidomycosis, mucormycosis, cryptococcosis Viral: AIDS; VZV; equine encephalitis; hepatitides A, B, C; EBV; influenza; measles; mumps; poliomyelitis; yellow fever; West Nile virus Protozoan: malaria, toxoplasmosis, trypanosomiasis Rickettsial: typhus, Q fever, Rocky Mountain spotted fever Helminths: *Acanthamoeba*, echinococcosis, onchocerciasis, toxocariasis, trichinellosis	Idiopathic Non-arteritic anterior ischemic optic neuropathy Demyelinating/degenerative diseases: adrenoleukodystrophy, hereditary ataxia, MS, neuromyelitis optica Drugs/vaccines/toxins Inflammatory/autoimmune: Henoch-Schönlein purpura, polyarteritis nodosa, sarcoidosis, granulomatosis with polyangiitis, Behçet's disease, progressive systemic sclerosis, RA, SLE, giant cell arteritis, Takayasu arteritis, thromboangiitis obliterans Multiple myeloma	Distinguished by CSF findings, including culture and serology. MRI and CT scanning for demyelinating and degenerative CNS disorders. Clinical criteria and serologic testing for autoimmune disorders.

(Continued)

System	ID Exam Finding	Non-infectious Mimics	Diagnostic Features
Sudden sensorineural hearing loss (i.e., negative ipsilateral Rinne test and/or contralateral localization on the Weber test)	Viral cochlear or vestibular labyrinthitis Viral auditory nerve neuritis Meningoencephalitis Specific viruses (mumps, CMV, EBV, rubella, rubeola, VZV, HSV, parainfluenza, Lassa fever, HIV) Syphilis Scrub typhus Leptospirosis Psittacosis Typhoid fever	High viscosity syndromes: macroglobulinemia, P vera Small vessel obstruction: sickle cell anemia, microemboli, Caisson disease Thromboangiitis obliterans Hypercoagulable states Autoimmune disorders: inner ear autoimmune disease, relapsing polychondritis, SLE, polyarteritis nodosa, Cogan's syndrome Neurologic disorders: MS, migraine Ototoxic drugs	Historical context. Fever suggests an infection. Autoimmune disorders diagnosed by criteria and serology. Culture and/or serologic testing will identify most, but not all, of the infectious etiologies.
Parotid enlargement and tenderness	Viral parotitis (mumps, parainfluenza, influenza, Coxsackievirus, CMV) Bacterial parotitis	Bulimia Drug-induced/iodide parotitis Sialolithiasis Parotid neoplasms	Fever suggests infection. Pus emanating from Stenson's duct in bacterial parotitis.
Erythema/edema external auditory canal	Acute otitis externa (esp. pseudomonal) Eczema herpeticum	Acute contact dermatitis Eczematous dermatitis Psoriasis SLE	Fever favors infection. HSV culture or DFA. Historical context.
Inflamed pinna	Bacterial perichondritis Chronic granulomatous infectious process (TB, fungal, syphilis, leprosy)	Relapsing polychondritis Frostbite Irritant contact dermatitis Trauma	Distinguished based on the history. Fever favors an infectious process. Culture and/or biopsy, if indicated.
Clear nasal discharge	CSF rhinorrhea in a patient with meningitis and a basal skull/cribriform plate fracture	Vasomotor rhinitis Allergic rhinitis Viral rhinitis	Beta-2 transferrin level is elevated in CSF rhinorrhea and not in other causes of rhinorrhea.
Saddle nose deformity	Syphilis Leprosy	Relapsing polychondritis Trauma, including post rhinoplasty Granulomatosis and polyangiitis	Distinguished based on history, serologic testing, and/or biopsy.
Intranasal eschar	Rhinocerebral mucormycosis Phaeohyphomycosis in allergic fungal sinusitis Rhinocerebral aspergillosis	Granulomatosis and polyangiitis Cocaine abuse	Culture first, then biopsy and/or serologic testing if necessary.
Nasal septal perforation	Syphilis Tuberculosis	Cocaine/oxymetazoline abuse Granulomatosis and polyangiitis Midline granuloma SLE Mixed cryoglobulinemia Rheumatoid arthritis Mixed connective tissue disease	Culture/biopsy. Serologic testing.
Swelling of the cheek	Buccal space infection	Angioedema	Fever and tenderness in infection.
Tongue ulcer	*Histoplasma capsulatum* Herpes viruses CMV Tuberculosis Syphilis *Leishmania donovani* *Blastomyces dermatitis*	Oral lichen planus Behçet's disease Granulomatosis and polyangiitis Amyloidosis Crohn's disease Carcinoma TUGSE	Distinguished by culture, serology and/or biopsy. Wickham's striae are seen in lichen planus. Macroglossia in amyloidosis.
Palatal ulcer	Mucormycosis Other fungal infection (e.g., phaeohyphomycosis) Syphilis	Drug-induced (esp. methotrexate) Cancer/lymphoma Granulomatosis and Polyangiitis Crohn's disease Midline granuloma Major aphthous ulcer Sweet's syndrome	Distinguished by culture, serology (if necessary), and/or biopsy.

(Continued)

System	ID Exam Finding	Non-infectious Mimics	Diagnostic Features
Palatal purpura	Early KS	Trauma Coagulopathy	KS will progress over time, whereas true purpura will resolve. Biopsy definitive in KS.
Uvular edema/ inflammation	Uvulitis: bacterial (esp. streptococcal, *Haemophilus influenzae*), viral Tuberculosis	Angioedema, hereditary or acquired Allergic Myxedematous changes of hypothyroidism Inhalation injury *Ecballium elaterium* topical use Cocaine or marijuana smoking Sauna exposure Trauma Postanesthesia and deep sedation (with or without endotracheal intubation) Obstructive sleep apnea Heavy-chain disease	Fever favors an infectious process. Acute infectious uvulitis may be associated with epiglottitis. Appropriate history. Culture in streptococcal disease. TSH in thyroid disease.
Tonsillar inflammation/ enlargement	Tonsillar abscess Syphilis	Cancer Amyloidosis Lymphoma Sarcoidosis	Culture and/or biopsy.
Gingival edema, inflammation, ulceration	Acute necrotizing ulcerative gingivitis (Vincent's angina) Herpangina	Leukemic gingivitis Scurvy Agranulocytosis Cyclic neutropenia Acatalasia	Leukopenia suggests agranulocytosis or cyclic neutropenia. Follicular hyperkeratosis, purpura, and corkscrew hairs are seen in scurvy. Premature WBCs form on peripheral smear in leukemia.
Smooth erythematous tongue	Infectious glossitis due to type b *H. influenzae* Atrophic thrush	Vitamin B complex deficiency Non-tropical sprue Pernicious anemia Iron deficiency Alcoholism Amyloidosis Crohn's disease	Culture will be positive in bacterial/fungal glossitis.
Blanching of half of the tongue	Bacterial endocarditis embolism	Giant cell arteritis Air embolism (Liebermeister sign)	Fever >102°F favors endocarditis. Air embolism with petechial rash, tachypnea, and confusion.
Buccal/gingival violaceous papule/ nodule	KS Bacillary angiomatosis	Venous lake or varicosity Pyogenic granuloma Scurvy Hemangioma	Biopsy will distinguish the entities.
Pre-auricular lymphadenopathy/ mass	Parinaud's oculoglandular syndrome (TB, cat scratch disease, syphilis, tularemia, *Chlamydia trachomatis*, adenovirus, *Bartonella*) Toxoplasmosis Acute parotitis Actinomycosis Infection of the scalp, face, ear Orbital adnexal infection	Metastatic cancer Branchial cleft cyst Pre-auricular sinus Parotid tumor Lymphoma	Culture/serology/biopsy. CT scanning, if needed.
Submental/ submandibular lymphadenopathy	Oral, buccal, dental infections (sialadenitis, diphtheria, primary HSV gingivostomatitis, gonorrhea, syphilis, etc.) Parinaud's oculoglandular conjunctivitis	Metastatic cancer Lymphoma	Culture or biopsy. CT scanning, if needed.
Anterior cervical lymphadenopathy	Oropharyngeal infections Toxoplasmosis Mycobacterial infections HIV	Metastatic cancer Kikuchi-Fujimoto disease Sarcoidosis Lymphoma	Culture/serology/ biopsy. CT scan, if needed.

(Continued)

System	ID Exam Finding	Non-infectious Mimics	Diagnostic Features
Posterior cervical lymphadenopathy	Infectious mononucleosis Rubella HIV Scalp infection Toxoplasmosis Trypanosomiasis *Neorickettsia sennetsu*	Castleman's disease Kikuchi-Fujimoto disease Lymphoma Metastatic cancer Tornwaldt's disease	Culture/serology/ biopsy. CT scanning, if needed.
Occipital lymphadenopathy	Rubella Scalp infection Toxoplasmosis Cat scratch disease Pediculosis Tinea capitis Tularemia	Seborrheic dermatitis	Culture and/or serology in infectious causes. Scaling, greasy, and erythematous rash in seborrhea.
Supraclavicular lymphadenopathy	Thoracic bacterial or fungal infections Parinaud's oculoglandular syndrome	Metastatic cancer (GI, lung, ovarian, GU) Lymphoma	Culture, imaging, and biopsy.
Axillary lymphadenopathy, unilateral	Upper extremity infection Mastitis Cat scratch disease Sporotrichosis Tuberculosis Brucellosis Chickenpox Herpes zoster HIV	Lymphoma Cancer-breast, lung, melanoma Reactive lymphadenitis (i.e., vaccination, allergic reaction) Silicone breast implant	Culture, serology, and biopsy.
Axillary lymphadenopathy, bilateral	Infectious mononucleosis Cat scratch disease	Autoimmune diseases: RA, scleroderma, SLE, dermatomyositis, Sjögren's Lymphoma/leukemia Metastatic cancer Diabetic mastopathy IRIS Granulomatous diseases: sarcoidosis, tuberculosis, silicone breast implants Kikuchi-Fujimoto disease	Culture, serology, and biopsy, as indicated. Clinical history/setting.
Bicipital/ epitrochlear lymphadenopathy	Upper extremity infection Cat scratch disease Tularemia Secondary syphilis EBV Sporotrichosis Leprosy Leishmaniosis tuberculosis Filariasis Infectious mononucleosis	Lymphoma Sarcoidosis SLE	Clinical setting. Culture, serology, and biopsy.
Inguinal lymphadenopathy	Infection of the foot/leg STDs (syphilis, chancroid, LGV, genital herpes, granuloma inguinale) Plague Filariasis Onchocerciasis Rectal infections (CMV, mycobacteria) Cat scratch disease EBV Orchitis Pediculosis Intersphincteric abscess Mayora virus infection	Metastatic cancer (urogenital tract) Lymphoma Rosai-Dorfman disease	Clinical setting. Culture, serology, and biopsy.

(Continued)

System	ID Exam Finding	Non-infectious Mimics	Diagnostic Features
Generalized lymphadenopathy	EBV CMV Rubella Tuberculosis Secondary syphilis Lyme disease Hepatitis A and B Typhoid fever Brucellosis Leptospirosis Histoplasmosis HIV HTLV-1 infection Bartonellosis Mycoplasma Toxoplasmosis Cryptococcosis West Nile virus Measles Scarlet fever Rickettsia (scrub typhus, rickettsial pox) Dengue Leishmaniasis Lassa fever Monkeypox Chagas disease Trypanosomiasis Penicilliosis Melioidosis Glanders	Lymphoma Leukemia Rheumatoid arthritis SLE Drug reaction (phenytoin, sulfonamides, others) Adult-onset Still's disease Multicentric Castleman's disease Kikuchi-Fujimoto disease Storage diseases (glycogen, lipid, lysosomal) X-linked lymphoproliferative disease Serum sickness	Clinical history and setting. Culture, serology, and biopsy. Evanescent salmon rash, and elevated ferritin in Still's disease.
Tender thyroid	Acute suppurative thyroiditis Infection of a thyroid nodule	Subacute (de Quervain) thyroiditis Thyroid amyloidosis	Fever >102°F suggests infection. Scanning/biopsy for others.
Hemoptysis	Lung abscess Pneumonia Tuberculosis Mycetoma ("fungus ball") Invasive pulmonary aspergillosis Infectious tracheobronchitis Bronchiectasis Paragonimiasis	Pulmonary neoplasm (malignant or benign) Pulmonary embolus/infarction Goodpasture's syndrome Idiopathic pulmonary hemosiderosis Granulomatosis and polyangiitis Henoch-Schönlein purpura Antiphospholipid antibody syndrome Behçet's disease Lupus pneumonitis Lung trauma/contusion Foreign body Diffuse alveolar damage Lymphangioleiomyomatosis Arteriovenous malformation Mitral stenosis Veno-occlusive disease Pseudohemoptysis	Imaging, serologic tests (ANA, anti-GBM antibodies, and cANCA), and sputum Gram stain/AFB stain. Bronchoscopy.
Inspiratory stridor	Epiglottitis Peritonsillar abscess Laryngeal TB	Upper-airway foreign body Upper-airway tumor Vocal cord dysfunction Postextubation laryngeal edema Vocal cord edema or paralysis Tracheomalacia Inhalational injury	Endoscopy, sputum AFB.

(Continued)

System	ID Exam Finding	Non-infectious Mimics	Diagnostic Features
Tracheal deviation (with the patient sitting up)	Toward the lung with a lobar pneumonia	Toward the lung with significant atelectasis Large goiter Away from a pleural effusion	Fever favors infection. Dullness, decreased tactile fremitus with effusion. Imaging.
Unilateral or focal loss of inspiratory intercostal retractions	Lobar pneumonia	Pleural effusion Tension pneumothorax Unilateral diaphragmatic paralysis	Fever, increased tactile fremitus, and egophony in pneumonia. Hyperresonance in pneumothorax.
Chest wall tenderness	Epidemic pleurodynia Septic arthritis of the sternoclavicular, sternomanubrial, or costoclavicular joint	Tietze syndrome Chest trauma Intercostal/mammary thrombophlebitis (Mondor disease) SAPHO syndrome Relapsing polychondritis	Fever favors infection. Tender chest wall thrombosed vein in Mondor disease. Imaging in SAPHO.
Chest wall mass	"Pointing" empyema TB of a rib Actinomycosis Nocardiosis Aspergillosis	Neoplasm, malignant or benign	The skin over a "pointing" empyema is warm. Chest X-ray, culture, and biopsy.
Chest dullness to percussion	Lobar pneumonia with or without empyema	Atelectasis Pleural effusion Pleural thickening	Fever favors infection. Chest X-ray.
Wheezing	Lower respiratory tract infection (esp. with RSV, human metapneumovirus) Chronic pneumonia PIE (*Strongyloides stercoralis*, hookworm, *Ascaris lumbricoides*, *Schistosoma japonicum*) Tropical pulmonary eosinophilia Allergic bronchopulmonary aspergillosis	Asthma/COPD CHF Endobronchial tumors Sarcoidosis Cystic fibrosis Pulmonary embolism Lymphangioleiomyomatosis Acute chest syndrome in sickle-cell disease Drug-induced bronchospasm Bronchiectasis Bronchiolitis obliterans Hypersensitivity pneumonitis	Culture and serology for infections. Imaging (X-ray and CT scan). Peripheral smear in SS disease. Occasionally, biopsy (bronchiolitis and hypersensitivity pneumonitis). Serology.
Late inspiratory crackles (rales)	Pneumonia	Atelectasis CHF Pulmonary fibrosis Collagen vascular disorders (SLE, granulomatosis with polyangiitis, scleroderma, others)	Culture, sputum Gram stain, and serologic testing (ANA, cANCA, and Scl-70). Rarely, lung biopsy. Elevated JVP, S3 gallop, and peripheral edema in CHF.
Pleural friction rub	Viral pleurisy Pneumonia Tuberculous pleuritis	Pulmonary embolism/infarction Sickle-cell chest syndrome Asbestosis/mesothelioma Postpericardiotomy SLE Post-thoracotomy Drug-induced pleuritis	Imaging (X-ray and CT scan). Sputum culture/Gram stain. Peripheral smear in SS disease. Pleural biopsy for tuberculosis.
Amphoric breath sounds	Lungs abscess Tubercular cavity Fungal pulmonary cavity	Cyst, bleb, or bulla of any etiology communicating with a bronchus (e.g., COPD, cavitary cancer, etc.) Open pneumothorax	Imaging (X-ray and CT). Sputum culture for TB and fungal. Bronchoscopy with biopsy and culture.
Tender, inflamed superficial vein	Septic thrombophlebitis	Trousseau syndrome Thromboangiitis obliterans Chemical phlebitis	Fever >102°F and positive blood cultures in septic thrombophlebitis.
Palpable arterial aneurysm	Mycotic aneurysm	Polyarteritis nodosa Traumatic aneurysm Neurofibromatosis Pseudoaneurysm	Fever and positive blood cultures in mycotic aneurysm. Multi-organ involvement and ANCA positivity in PAN. Cutaneous neurofibromas in NF.

(Continued)

System	ID Exam Finding	Non-infectious Mimics	Diagnostic Features
Right sternal or supra-sternal pulsation	Mycotic or luetic ascending aortic aneurysm	Non-infectious ascending aortic aneurysm Tortuous carotid artery Dissecting aneurysm of the ascending aorta Right-sided aortic arch	Fever and positive blood cultures in mycotic aneurysm. RPR in luetic aneurysm. Echocardiography in other diagnoses.
Pericardial friction rub	Acute viral or bacterial pericarditis	Collagen vascular diseases (esp. SLE) Postpericardiotomy/MI syndrome Uremia Pericardial metastases	Clinical context for postpericardiotomy syndrome. Serologic testing, BUN/creatinine, and echocardiography.
Apical pansystolic murmur	Mitral regurgitation in acute rheumatic fever Mitral regurgitation in bacterial endocarditis	Mitral regurgitation due to other causes: mitral valve prolapse, papillary muscle dysfunction/rupture, ischemia, severe LV dilation	Jones' criteria in ARF. Echocardiography, blood cultures, and Duke criteria in other diagnoses.
Apical diastolic rumbling murmur	Relative mitral stenosis in ARF (Carey Coombs murmur)	Mitral stenosis: late effect of rheumatic fever or degenerative valvular disease Austin Flint murmur	Jones' criteria in ARF. Echocardiography in other diagnoses.
Basilar diastolic blowing murmur left sternal border	Aortic regurgitation in endocarditis Syphilis	Aortic regurgitation due to hypertension, rheumatic heart disease, aortoannular ectasia, aortic dissection Pulmonary insufficiency	Blood cultures and peripheral stigmata for IE. Echocardiography for other diagnoses.
Pansystolic murmur left lower sternal border	Tricuspid regurgitation in endocarditis Tricuspid regurgitation in rheumatic fever	Tricuspid regurgitation in Epstein anomaly, prolapse, carcinoid, papillary muscle dysfunction, connective tissue disorders (e.g., Marfan), RA, radiation injury	Blood cultures and IE stigmata for IE. Jones' criteria for ARF. Echocardiography for other diagnoses.
Jaundice	Viral hepatitides (A, B, E, EBV, CMV) Ascending cholangitis Sepsis-associated cholestasis Leptospirosis Malaria Hemorrhagic fevers Relapsing fever Tuberculosis *Coxiella burnetti* *Histoplasma capsulatum* Schistosomiasis Brucellosis	Alcoholic liver disease Biliary tract obstruction (stone, tumor, stricture) Drug-induced Hemolytic anemia Cancer (primary or metastatic to the liver) Hepatic vein thrombosis Ischemic hepatitis	Clinical context. Serologic testing for viral hepatitides. Blood culture. Peripheral smear for hemolytic anemia and malaria. US for CBD obstruction and tumors/hepatic vein thrombosis.
Doughy abdomen	Tubercular peritonitis	Peritoneal metastases Peritoneal mesothelioma Recent significant weight loss	Imaging (CT and US). Peritoneal/ascites culture and/or biopsy.
Right lower quadrant tenderness	Acute salpingitis Tubo-ovarian abscess Bacterial ileocecitis (*Yersinia enterocolitica, Campylobacter jejuni, Salmonella enteritidis*) Amoebic colitis Tuberculous colitis Actinomycosis *Mycobacterium avium intracellulare* (in AIDS) *Angiostrongylus costaricensis* *Balantidium coli* Ascariasis	Acute appendicitis Cecitis/typhlitis Crohn's disease Diverticulitis Epiploic appendagitis Impaction of a stone in the right ureter Meckel's diverticulitis Ovarian cyst Ectopic pregnancy Cecal adenocarcinoma Carcinoid	Stool culture and specific serology in enteric infections. CT scanning/US for non-infectious etiologies.

(Continued)

System	ID Exam Finding	Non-infectious Mimics	Diagnostic Features
Obturator sign	Pelvic abscess	Appendicitis Pelvic fracture Obturator muscle spasm/dysfunction/ hematoma	Fever and leukocytosis in appendicitis/ pelvic abscess.
Psoas sign	Psoas abscess	Acute appendicitis Psoas hematoma Iliopsoas bursitis	Fever and leukocytosis in appendicitis/ psoas abscess. CT scanning in psoas hematoma.

Tender hepatomegaly	Acute viral hepatitis
	Hepatic abscess (pyogenic, amoebic,
	  toxoplasma)
	Typhoid
	Disseminated candidiasis
	Echinococcosis
	Acute schistosomiasis
	Fascioliasis
	Clonorchiasis
	Hepatic capillariasis
		Acute alcoholic hepatitis
		Drug-induced hepatitis
		Right-sided heart failure/constricted
		  pericarditis
		Hepatic sickle-cell crisis
		Budd-Chiari syndrome
			Clinical context. There may be a friction
			rub over a hepatic abscess. Serology, US,
			and culture to distinguish the various
			ideologies.

Splenomegaly	Acute infections (e.g., EBV, CMV,
	  hepatitis, SBE, psittacosis, cat scratch
	  disease)
	Chronic infections (e.g., miliary TB,
	  malaria, schistosomiasis, AIDS,
	  brucellosis, visceral leishmaniasis,
	  syphilis, toxoplasmosis)
		Congestive: cirrhosis, portal hypertension,
		  CHF, compression or thrombosis of the
		  portal or splenic veins
		Neoplasms: lymphoproliferative disorders,
		  myeloproliferative disorders
		Inflammatory: sarcoidosis, amyloidosis
		Connective tissue diseases: SLE, RA
		Hemolytic anemias
		Storage diseases: Gaucher, Niemann-Pick,
		  etc.
			Based on the clinical context. Blood and
			other appropriate cultures. Serological
			testing.
			Review of peripheral smear.
			Rarely splenic biopsy.

Prostatic nodule	Tuberculosis Prostatic abscess	Cancer Leiomyoma	Fever and toxic state in prostatic abscess. In TB, the seminal vesicles and vas deferens are also involved.
Carpometacarpal ulnar deviation	Jaccoud's arthritis in rheumatic fever	Rheumatoid arthritis SLE Ulnar impaction syndrome Chronic hemiplegia	Initially, the deviation in Jaccoud's arthritis is passively reproducible. MCP synovitis, Swan neck, and boutonniere deformities in RA. Imaging.
Charcot joint	Syphilis Leprosy	Diabetes Alcoholism Trauma Amyloidosis Pernicious anemia Syringomyelia, spina bifida, myelomeningocele MS Charcot-Marie-Tooth disease Connective disorders (RA, scleroderma) Cauda equina lesions	Clinical context. Serology, imaging, and biopsy/culture.

Mono- or pauci-articular arthritis	Bacterial septic arthritis
	Lyme disease
	Viruses (parvovirus B19, hepatitis B,
	  rubella, mumps, adenovirus,
	  Coxsackievirus, retroviruses, EBV,
	  chikungunya)
		Gout
		Pseudogout
		Other crystalline arthritides
		Löfgren's syndrome
		Plant thorn arthritis
		Synovial metastases
		Charcot joint
			Arthrocentesis with microscopy (including
			polarized lens) and culture. Serology and
			imaging.

Sternoclavicular inflammation/ tenderness	Septic arthritis	Trauma/fracture Inflammatory arthritis (e.g., RA, ankylosing spondylitis, psoriatic) Gout SAPHO Friedrich's syndrome	Blood and joint fluid culture and microscopy. Imaging.

(Continued)

System	ID Exam Finding	Non-infectious Mimics	Diagnostic Features
Sacroiliac tenderness	Septic arthritis or osteomyelitis Brucella arthritis Tubercular arthritis	Trauma/fracture Reactive arthritis Crystalline arthritides Spondyloarthropathies (e.g., ankylosing spondylitis, inflammatory bowel disease, psoriatic arthritis)	Blood and joint fluid culture and microscopy. Serology. Imaging.
Tenderness/ inflammation symphysis pubis	Osteomyelitis	Osteitis pubis (sterile) CPPD disease	Blood/bone culture. Imaging.
Muscle swelling/ tenderness	Pyomyositis Necrotizing fasciitis Trichinosis Infected hematoma	Bland hematoma Muscle infarction	Culture and imaging. Occasional muscle biopsy (trichinosis).
Penile ulcer	Syphilis Herpes simplex Chancroid Lymphogranuloma venereum Donovanosis Histoplasma Tularemia Leishmaniasis Amebiasis	Behçet's disease Crohn's disease Lichen planus Cancer Fixed drug eruption	Extreme tenderness and multiple ulcers suggest herpes. A single very tender ulcer in chancroid. Groove sign in LGV. Bilateral lymphadenopathy in syphilis and herpes. Culture, serology, and/or biopsy.
Perineal/scrotal purpura	Early Fournier's gangrene	Retroperitoneal hemorrhage (blue scrotum sign of Bryant)	Recent GU surgery/manipulation, fever, and prostration suggest Fournier's gangrene.
Scrotal swelling/ tenderness	Epididymo-orchitis Pyocele	Testicular cancer Testicular torsion Polyarteritis nodosa	Color Doppler US shows impaired blood flow in torsion and an inhomogeneous collection in a pyocele.
Epididymal beading	Genitourinary tuberculosis	Epididymal cysts in polycystic kidney disease Young's syndrome	Upper and lower GU tract scarring in TB. Imaging.
Nuchal rigidity, meningismus	Infections meningitis (bacterial, viral)	Non-infectious meningitis (drug-induced, SLE, Behçet's syndrome, Sjogren's syndrome, sarcoidosis) Subarachnoid hemorrhage Leptomeningeal metastases Primary CNS angiitis Degenerative cervical spine disease Diffuse idiopathic skeletal hyperostosis	Fever >102°F suggest infection. CSF culture/serology. Imaging.
Chorea	Acute rheumatic fever (Sydenham's chorea) HIV Creutzfeldt-Jakob disease	CNS ischemia/hemorrhage Neurologic disorders (Huntington's chorea, neuroacanthocytosis) SLE Drugs (L-dopa, lithium, methadone, lamotrigine) Toxins Paraneoplastic Antiphospholipid antibody syndrome Metabolic: hyperthyroidism, hypoglycemia, hypocalcemia Other: P vera, basal ganglia calcification, senile	Fever suggests infection but does not exclude CNS lesions such as SLE and hyperthyroidism. Jones' criteria for ARF. Serology, blood work, and imaging for other possibilities.

(Continued)

System	ID Exam Finding	Non-infectious Mimics	Diagnostic Features
Cranial nerve palsies (isolated or in various combinations)	Suppurative intracranial thrombophlebitis: CN II, IV, V, VI, VII Acute bacterial meningitis: III, IV, VI, VII Rhinocerebral mucormycosis: II through VII, IX, X Lyme disease: primarily CN VII, less commonly II, III, the sensory portion of V, VI, and the acoustic portion of VIII Acute HIV meningitis: V, VII, and VIII Malignant otitis externa: VII, less commonly X, XI, XII Orbital cellulitis: III, IV, VI Septic cavernous sinus thrombosis: III, IV, V, VI Cryptococcal meningitis Herpes meningoencephalitis CMV Syphilis: VII and VIII followed by II, III, IV, VI, V Acute botulism: III, IV, VI, IX, X, XI, XII (with fixed dilated pupils) Tuberculous meningitis: VI, VII, VIII Primary amoebic meningoencephalitis Mumps Eastern equine encephalitis: VI, VII, XII Bulbar poliomyelitis: IX, X Diphtheria: III, VI, VII, IX, and X Tick-borne encephalitis: III, VII, IX, X, XI Progressive multifocal leukoencephalopathy Listerial brainstem encephalitis St. Louis encephalitis Japanese encephalitis Cerebral cysticercosis Subacute progressive disseminated histoplasmosis Cephalic tetanus (following a head wound) Relapsing fever Q fever Psittacosis Eosinophilic meningitis (*Angiostrongylus cantonensis*): IV–VI Melioidosis: VII	Nerve infarction (i.e., diabetic) Supratentorial mass with herniation Migraine CNS aneurysm Subarachnoid hemorrhage Sarcoidosis Meningeal carcinomatosis/lymphoma Tolosa-Hunt syndrome Neurologic syndromes (e.g. Weber's, Benedikt's, Nothnagel's) Neoplasms (pituitary, meningioma) Trauma Pseudotumor cerebri Multiple sclerosis Ciguatera fish poisoning	Clinical setting. Culture, serology, and imaging to distinguish the various possibilities.
Peripheral neuropathy (stocking sensory deficit with or without weakness)	HIV Leprosy CMV *M. pneumoniae* Lyme disease Hepatitis B, C VZV Parvovirus Neuroborreliosis Neurosyphilis Trypanosomiasis Botulism Diphtheria *Tropheryma whipplei*	Diabetes mellitus Alcohol abuse Drugs Vasculitis Myxedema Renal failure Rheumatoid arthritis Sarcoidosis Amyloidosis Acromegaly Multifocal CIDP Porphyria Hereditary (e.g., Charcot-Marie-Tooth) Vitamin D deficiency Heavy-metal poisoning	Clinical setting. Culture, serology, and imaging to distinguish the various possibilities.

(Continued)

System	ID Exam Finding	Non-infectious Mimics	Diagnostic Features
Flaccid paralysis, acute	West Nile virus Eastern equine virus Diphtheria Lyme disease Enteroviruses Poliomyelitis Botulism	Guillain-Barré syndrome Acute axonal neuropathy Demyelinating diseases (e.g., multiple sclerosis, transverse myelitis, acute disseminated encephalomyelitis) Myasthenia gravis Acute toxic neuropathies (e.g., heavy metals, organophosphate poisoning) Tick bite paralysis Snakebite Acute porphyria Critical illness neuropathy Cord compression Spinal cord ischemia	
Brachial plexopathy	Parvovirus B19 EBV mononucleosis HIV Lyme disease	Pancoast tumor Trauma/compression Parsonage-Turner syndrome Post irradiation Tumor infiltration Paraneoplastic	Clinical setting. Culture, serology, and imaging to distinguish the various possibilities.
Lumbosacral plexopathy (a) T12–L4: decreased flexion, adduction, and eversion of the thigh; absent patellar reflex (b) L5–S3: sensory loss in L5–S3 distribution; hip extension and abduction, knee flexion, plantar and dorsiflexion of the foot are weak; the Achilles reflex absent with preserved patellar reflex (c) Entire plexus: variable weakness of the hip girdle, thigh, and foot muscles	CMV (in AIDS) Herpes zoster *C. pneumoniae* Tuberculosis	Trauma/parturition Retroperitoneal hemorrhage Neoplastic Diabetic Vasculitis (RA, SLE, PAN)	Clinical setting. Culture, serology, and imaging to distinguish the various possibilities.
Paraplegia/paresis with a sensory level	Spinal epidural abscess Tuberculous adhesive arachnoiditis Transverse myelitis (mycoplasma, TB, Lyme disease, syphilis, viral, HTLV-1)	Arachnoiditis due to epidural drug injection, hemorrhage, or postsurgical Arachnoiditis due to seeding of a CNS or metastatic cancer Transverse myelitis (MS, autoimmune/vasculitis, drugs, neuromyelitis optica)	Significant spinal pain and fever suggest an epidural abscess. Blood and CSF culture/serology. Imaging and serologic testing for vasculitis.

(Continued)

System	ID Exam Finding	Non-infectious Mimics	Diagnostic Features
Cerebellar ataxia	Lyme disease Brain abscess Toxoplasma encephalitis *Listeria monocytogenes* CNS syphilis Tick-borne encephalitis Viral encephalitis (Japanese, St. Louis, West Nile, enterovirus, varicella, Venezuelan equine, CMV) Rickettsia (*Rickettsia rickettsii, Coxiella burnetti*) JC virus (including PML) Cerebral malaria Subacute progressive disseminated histoplasmosis West African trypanosomiasis Whipple's disease Primary amoebic meningoencephalitis Hendra virus *Francisella tularensis*	CNS tumors Drugs Multiple sclerosis Miller-Fisher syndrome Ataxia-telangiectasia syndrome Friedrich's ataxia Celiac disease Posterior circulation ischemia/stroke Alcoholic cerebellar disease Idiopathic cerebellar degeneration MELAS Vitamin E deficiency Periodic ataxia Olivopontocerebellar atrophy Paraneoplastic Exposure to toxins (lead, anticonvulsants, salicylates, aminoglycosides, sedatives) Autoimmune disorders (SLE, Sjogren's) Neurotoxic shellfish poisoning	Fever favors an infectious etiology. Chronicity suggests hereditary syndromes. Culture (including CSF), serology, and imaging to distinguish the other etiologies.
Descending paralysis with absent MSRs	Botulism Bulbar poliomyelitis	Miller Fisher syndrome	Fever and asymmetry suggest polio. Anti-GQ1b antibody titers in Miller Fisher syndrome. Normal CSF in botulism.

Abbreviations: AIDS, acquired immune deficiency syndrome; AFB, acid fast bacillus; ANA, antinuclear antibody; cANCA, antineutrophil cytoplasmic antibody; AOSD, adult-onset Still's disease; ARF, acute rheumatic fever; CBD, common bile duct; CHF, congestive heart failure; CIDP, chronic inflammatory demyelinating polyneuropathy; CMV, cytomegalovirus; CN, cranial nerve; CNS, central nervous system; COPD, chronic obstructive pulmonary disease; CPPD, calcium pyrophosphate dihydrate; CSF, cerebrospinal fluid; DFA, direct fluorescent antibody; DISH, diffuse idiopathic skeletal hyperostosis; EBV, Epstein–Barr virus; GI, gastrointestinal; GU, genitourinary; HAART, highly active anti-retroviral therapy; HIV, human immunodeficiency virus; HSV, herpes simplex virus; HTLV-1, human T-cell lymphotropic virus 1; IE, infectious endocarditis; IRIS, immune reconstitution inflammatory syndrome; IVDA, intravenous drug abuse; JRA, juvenile rheumatoid arthritis; JVP, jugular venous pressure; KS, Kaposi sarcoma; LGV, lymphogranuloma venereum; LV, left ventricle; MCP, metacarpophalangeal; MELAS, mitochondrial encephalomyopathy, lactic acidosis and stroke-like episodes; MI, myocardial infarction; MS, multiple sclerosis; NBTE, non-bacterial thrombotic endocarditis; NF, neurofibromatosis; PAN, polyarteritis nodosa; PIE, pulmonary infiltrates with eosinophilia; PMR, polymyalgia rheumatica; P vera, polycythemia vera; RA, rheumatoid arthritis; RPR, rapid plasma reagin; SAPHO, synovitis, acne, pustulosis, hyperostosis, osteitis; STD, sexually transmitted disease; STEMI, ST elevation myocardial infarction; TB, tuberculosis; TSH, thyroid-stimulating hormone; TIA, transient ischemic attack; TSH, thyroid-stimulating hormone; TUGSE, traumatic ulcerative granuloma with stromal eosinophilia; US, ultrasound; VZV, varicella-zoster virus.

BIBLIOGRAPHY

Acevedo F, Baudrand R, Letelier LM, Gaete P. Actinomycosis: A great pretender. Case reports of unusual presentations and a review of the literature. *Int J Infect Dis* 2008;12(4):358–362.

Bruce AJ, Rogers III RS. Acute oral ulcers. *Dermatol Clin* 2003;21(1):1–5.

Carsons SE. Fever in rheumatic and autoimmune disease. *Infect Dis Clin* 1996;10(1):67–84.

Chalifoux JR, Vachha B, Moonis G. Imaging of head and neck infections: Diagnostic considerations, potential mimics, and clinical management. In: *Seminars in Roentgenology* 2017;52(1):10–16, WB Saunders.

Cunha BA, Shea KW. Fever in the intensive care unit. *Infect Dis Clin* 1996;10(1):185–209.

Cunha BA. Pneumonia in the elderly. *Clin Microbiol Infect* 2001;7(11):581–588.

Cunha BA. The clinical significance of fever patterns. *Infect Dis Clin.* 1996;10(1):33–44.

Cunha BA. The mimics of endocarditis. In: Brusch J, Jassal D, Kradin R eds. *Infective Endocarditis.* Boca Raton, FL: CRC Press, 2007, Chapter 17, pp. 345–353.

Gayle A, Ringdahl E. Tick-borne diseases. *Am Fam Physician* 2001;64(3):461–466.

Goetz CG, ed. *Textbook of Clinical Neurology.* 3rd ed. Philadelphia: Saunders/Elsevier, 2007.

Goldman, L Ausiello, D. Cecil Medicine. 23rd ed. Philadelphia: Elsevier health Sciences, 2008.

Habermann TM, Steensma DP. Lymphadenopathy. *Mayo Clin Proc* 2000 (Vol. 75, No. 7, pp. 723–732).

Hahn BH, Tsao B, Firestein GS, Budd RC, Harris ED, McInnes IB, Ruddy S, Sergent JS. Kelley's textbook of rheumatology. et al. Eds. Pathogenesis of systemic lupus erythematosus. 2009:1174–1200.

Hoffman R, Benz Jr EJ, Heslop H, Weitz J, Silberstein LE, Anastasi J. Hematology: Basic principles and practice. 6th ed. Philadelphia: Elsevier Health Sciences, 2013.

Johnson DH, Cunha BA. Drug fever. *Infect Dis Clin* 1996;10(1):85–91.

Karnath BM. Approach to the Patient with Lymphadenopathy. *Hosp Physician* 2005;41(7):29.

Larici AR, Franchi P, Occhipinti M, Contegiacomo A, del Ciello A, Calandriello L, Storto ML, Marano R, Bonomo L. Diagnosis and management of hemoptysis. *Diagn Interv Radiol* 2014;20(4):299.

LeBlond RF, DeGowin RL, Brown DD. *DeGowin's Diagnostic Examination*. 9th ed. New York: McGraw-Hill Medical, 2009.

Lio PA. The many faces of cellulitis. *Arch Dis Child Educ Pract* 2009;94(2):50–54.

Mandell GL, Bennett JE, Mandell DR. Douglas, and Bennett's principles and practice of infectious diseases. 2010, 2.

Mann D, Zipes D, Libby P, Bonow R. Braunwald's Heart Disease: A Textbook of Cardiovascular Medicine. 10th ed. Philadelphia: Elsevier, 2014.

Marik PE. Fever in the ICU. *Chest J* 2000;117(3):855–869.

Mason RJ, Broaddus VC, Martin TR, King TE, Schraufnagel D, Murray JF. Murray and Nadel's textbook of respiratory medicine. 5th ed. Philadelphia: Saunders/Elsevier, 2010.

Orient JM, Sapira JD. *Sapira's Art & Science of Bedside Diagnosis*. 3rd ed. Philadelphia: Lippincott Williams & Wilkins, 2010.

Østergaard L, Huniche B, Andersen PL. Relative bradycardia in infectious diseases. *J Infect* 1996;33(3):185–191.

Powers JH, Scheld WM. Fever in neurologic diseases. *Infect Dis Clin* 1996;10(1):45–66.

Ramik D, Mishriki YY. The other "Cotton Fever". *Infect Dis Clin Pract* 2008;16(3):192–193.

dos Santos JW, Torres A, Michel GT, de Figueiredo CW, Mileto JN, Foletto VG, de Nóbrega Cavalcanti MA. Non-infectious and unusual infectious mimics of community-acquired pneumonia. *Respir Med* 2004;98(6):488–494.

Siva C, Velazquez C, Mody A, Brasington R. Diagnosing acute monoarthritis in adults: A practical approach for the family physician. *Am Fam Physician* 2003;68(1):83–92.

Talwani R, Gilliam BL, Howell C. Infectious diseases and the liver. *Clin Liver Dis* 2011;15(1):111–130.

Vichinsky EP, Styles LA, Colangelo LH, Wright EC, Castro O, Nickerson B, Cooperative Study of Sickle Cell Disease. Acute chest syndrome in sickle cell disease: Clinical presentation and course. *Blood* 1997;89(5):1787–1792.

Wein A, Kavoussi L, Campbell M. Campbell-Walsh Urology. 10th ed. Philadelphia: Elsevier/Saunders, 2012.

4 Ophthalmologic Clues to Infectious Diseases and Their Mimics in the Critical Care Unit

Cheston B. Cunha, Michael J. Wilkinson, and David A. Quillen

CONTENTS

The eyes, like a sentinel, occupy the highest place in the body.

—Marcus Tulius Cicero

Eye examination is one element of a physical examination that is frequently overlooked by clinicians, despite its ability to provide key diagnostic clues. Often, an eye examination is deferred because of a lack of comfort or familiarity with funduscopic and, to a lesser degree, external ocular examinations. However, clinicians should take time to carefully inspect the internal and external anatomy of the eye in search of a physical finding that may tip the scales toward one diagnosis over another.

This is the most common case in critically ill patients, who are often unable to provide historical clues as to the nature of their condition. We should, therefore, not relegate this examination solely to the purview of ophthalmologists but rather add it to our armamentarium of diagnostic tools.

This chapter, presented in a tabular form, contains a collection of both internal and external eye findings in conditions that may be seen in an intensive care setting. This is designed to act as a guide to supplement the internists' ocular examination of critically ill patients and is to be used for initial evaluation of a patient or when an ophthalmologist is not readily available. These findings, in concert with the history, physical, and laboratory analyses, may help to identify the etiology of the patient's illness [1–4].

Note that physical findings that are visible on slit lamp examination are found under "SL:" in the table. All other findings are visible on general examination of the eye.

INFECTIOUS DISEASES

Disease	External Eye Findings	Fundoscopic Findings
Mycobacterium tuberculosis (TB)	• Chronic conjunctivitis (often unilateral) • Conjunctival granulomas • Phlyctenulosis (focal translucent nodules along the limbus of the eye) • Ulcerative/interstitial keratitis • Scleritis • Orbital tuberculoma	• Tuberculoma of the choroid (usually unilateral, but diffuse choroidal granulomas may be seen in miliary TB)

(Continued)

Disease	External Eye Findings	Fundoscopic Findings

SL:
- Chronic granulomatous iritis
- Panuveitis
- Interstitial keratitis
- Keratic precipitates

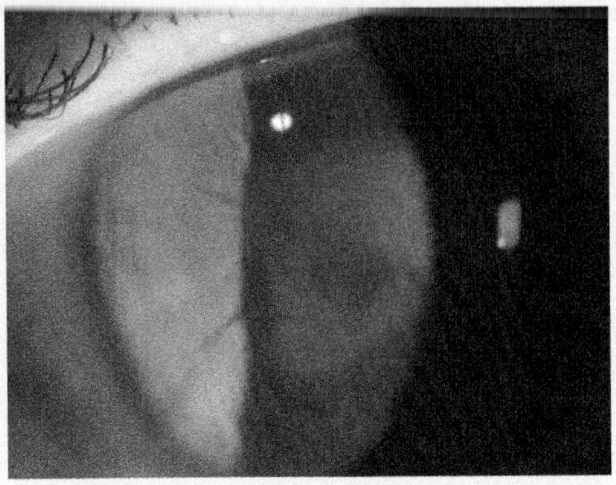

FIGURE 4.1 Interstitial keratitis.

Adenovirus
- Follicular conjunctivitis with watery/mucoid discharge (often begins with unilateral involvement and later spreads to contralateral eye)
- Subepithelial corneal infiltrates
- Eyelid edema
- Subconjunctival hemorrhage
- Ciliary flush
- Corneal haziness
- Preauricular lymph node enlargement

- None

Toxic shock syndrome
- Conjunctival suffusion
- Anterior scleritis
- Scleral ectasia

SL:
- Uveitis
- Keratic precipitates
- Vitreous opacities
- Choroiditis

- Retinal detachments
- Cystoid macular edema

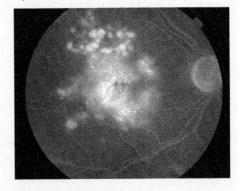

FIGURE 4.2 Cystoid macular edema.

Leptospirosis (Weil's syndrome)
- Conjunctival suffusion (often dramatic hemorrhagic)
- Conjunctival discharge
- Subconjunctival hemorrhage
- Hypopyon (a small hypopyon may require SL evaluation)
- Scleral icterus +/−

SL:
- Mutton fat keratic precipitates
- Uveitis (anterior or posterior)

- Retinal hemorrhage
- Retinal exudates
- Optic neuritis

(Continued)

Disease	External Eye Findings	Fundoscopic Findings
Rocky mountain spotted fever	• Conjunctivitis with papillae • Conjunctival petechiae • Subconjunctival hemorrhage • Corneal ulceration SL: • Panuveitis • Iritis	• Retinal hemorrhage • Retinal exudates • Optic nerve pallor • Roth spots
Tularemia (oculoglandular)	• Conjunctivitis with purulent discharge • Conjunctival nodules (1–5 mm) • Chemosis • Eyelid edema • Necrosis of conjunctivae • Eyelid edema • Eyelid ulceration SL: • Corneal edema • Peripheral corneal infiltrates (relatively rare but have a very high specificity when present) • Nodules along the limbus	• Optic neuritis  FIGURE 4.3 Optic neuritis. • None
Hantavirus pulmonary syndrome	• Conjunctival suffusion SL: • None	
Bacterial endocarditis	• Conjunctival hemorrhage • Subconjunctival hemorrhage SL: • None	• Roth spots • Cotton-wool spots • Retinal hemorrhages • Branch/central retinal artery occlusion 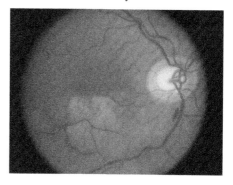 FIGURE 4.4 Branch retinal artery occlusion. (*Continued*)

Disease	External Eye Findings	Fundoscopic Findings
Cytomegalovirus Ocular cytomegalovirus seen in HIV-infected patients with CD4 <50 cells/mm³	• Often has no remarkable external ocular manifestations SL: • Fine keratic precipitates • Anterior uveitis +/–	• Granular yellow-white opacities with irregular borders (lesions usually originate on the periphery and spread centrally) • Retinal hemorrhage "Cheese Pizza" appearance • "Frosted branch angiitis" (vascular sheathing)

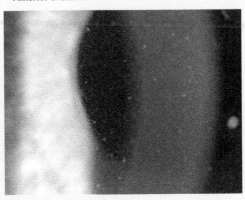

FIGURE 4.5 Keratic precipitates.

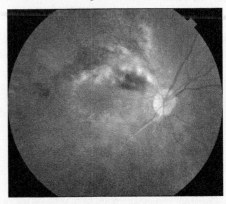

FIGURE 4.6 CMV retinitis.

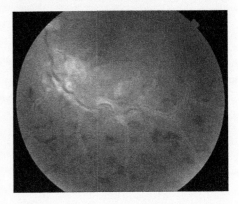

FIGURE 4.7 Frosted branch angiitis.

Toxoplasmosis	• Nystagmus SL: • Granulomatous iridocyclitis	• "Headlight in the fog" (focal necrotizing retinitis with overlying vitritis) • Chorioretinitis • Papilledema • Retinal hemorrhage • Retinal vasculitis • Retinal vein/artery occlusion

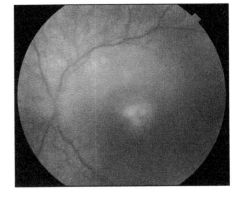

FIGURE 4.8 Headlight in the fog.

(Continued)

Disease	External Eye Findings	Fundoscopic Findings
Meningococcemia	• Severe bilateral eyelid edema (this is a relatively common, but overlooked, early sign of meningococcal meningitis as well as disseminated disease) • Purulent, bilateral conjunctivitis (this may be the presenting feature of meningococcal infection) • Chemosis • Petechiae on the eyelids • Subconjunctival hemorrhage SL: • Anterior uveitis	• Retinal detachment • Retinal vein occlusion 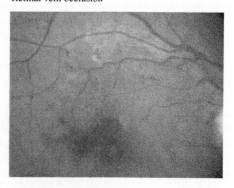 FIGURE 4.9 Branch retinal vein occlusion.
Cat scratch disease	• Unilateral conjunctivitis with papillae (Parinaud's oculoglandular syndrome) • Bacillary angiomatosis (relatively uncommon) SL: • Intermediate uveitis	• Optic nerve edema with "macular star" (typically unilateral) • Cotton-wool spots 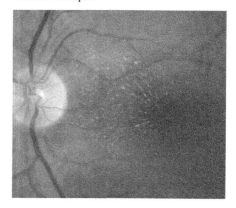 FIGURE 4.10 Macular star.
Invasive fungal infection (disseminated histoplasmosis and candidiasis)	• Conjunctival suffusion • Strabismus • Corneal infiltrates • Dacryocystitis • Proptosis • CN palsies SL: • Anterior uveitis (+/− hypopyon)	• Chorioretinitis • Roth spots • Vitreous opacities ("string of pearls" appearance) • Candida endophthalmitis

(Continued)

Disease	External Eye Findings	Fundoscopic Findings
Herpes zoster virus	• Unilateral conjunctivitis • Blepharitis • Scleritis • Hutchinson's sign SL: • Pseudodendritic keratitis • Interstitial keratitis • Uveitis • Iritis	• Retinitis

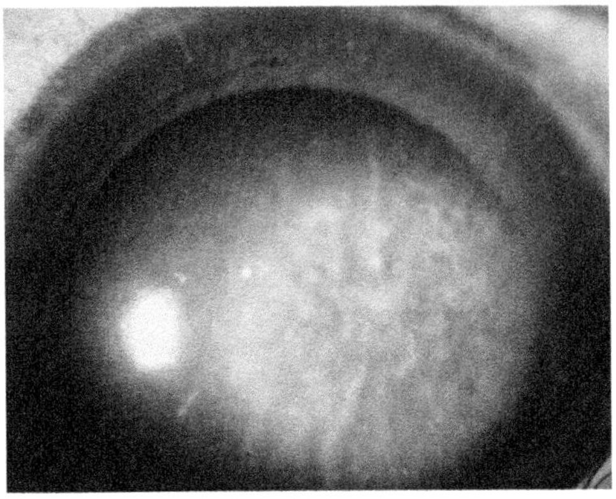

FIGURE 4.11   Pseudodendritic keratitis.

Lyme disease	• Scleritis • Proptosis • Follicular conjunctivitis • Keratitis • CN palsies (CN III, VI, VII) • Eyelid edema SL: • Uveitis • Iritis	• Papilledema • Retinal detachment • Optic neuritis • Choroiditis • Retinal vasculitis
Primary and secondary syphilis	• Lid ulcer (chancre) • Conjunctivitis • Eyebrow loss/thinning SL: • Uveitis • Interstitial keratitis • Scleritis	• None • Optic neuritis • Chorioretinitis • Retinal vasculitis
Tertiary syphilis	• Argyll Robertson pupil • Conjunctival gumma SL: • Interstitial keratitis	• Optic atrophy • Retinal scarring

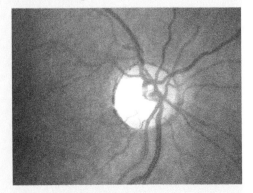

FIGURE 4.12   Optic atrophy.

NON-INFECTIOUS DISEASES

Disease	External Eye Findings	Fundoscopic Findings
Sarcoidosis	• Conjunctival granuloma • Eyelid nodules • Painless dacryoadenitis • Argyll Robertson or Adie's pupil anomalies • CN palsies (CN III, IV, VI, VII) • Proptosis • Scleritis SL: • Mutton fat keratic precipitates • Band keratopathy • Keratoconjunctivitis sicca • Anterior uveitis • Koeppe nodules (pupil margin) • Busacca nodules (stromal) • Cataracts	• Candle wax drippings • Retinal granuloma • Retinal neovascularization • Optic disk edema • Optic neuritis • Optic atrophy • Retinal venous sheathing • Branch retinal vein occlusion • Chorioretinitis • Retinal hemorrhage • Cystoid macular edema

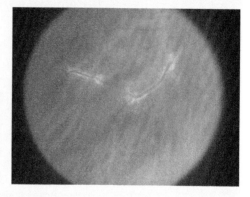

FIGURE 4.15   Candle wax drippings.

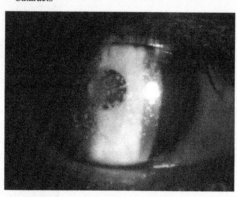

FIGURE 4.13   Keratic precipitates.

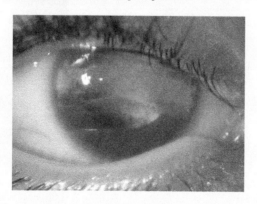

FIGURE 4.14   Band keratopathy.

(Continued)

Disease	External Eye Findings	Fundoscopic Findings
Systemic lupus erythematosus	• Eyelid nodules • Conjunctivitis • Scleritis • Internuclear ophthalmoplegia • One-and-a-half syndrome (a conjugate horizontal gaze palsy in one direction and an internuclear ophthalmoplegia in the other) SL: • Keratoconjunctivitis sicca • Uveitis	• Cotton-wool spots • Roth spots • Hard exudates • Macular ischemia • Retinal neovascularization • Papillitis • Chorioretinitis 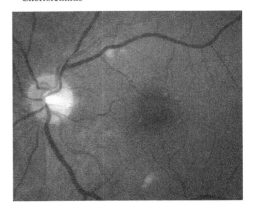 **FIGURE 4.16** Cotton-wool spots.
Wegener's granulomatosis	• Conjunctival suffusion • Bilateral eyelid edema • Eyelid nodules • Painful ptosis • Necrotizing sclerokeratitis (corneal ulceration) occlusion • Proptosis • Orbital cellulitis • Orbital pseudotumor • Painful dacryoadenitis/dacryocystitis • CN palsies (can involve any, but most common are CN II, VI, VII) SL: • Posterior uveitis	• Cotton-wool spots • Retinal hemorrhages • Retinal vasculitis (perivascular sheathing) • Central retinal artery occlusion • Central/branch retinal vein occlusion 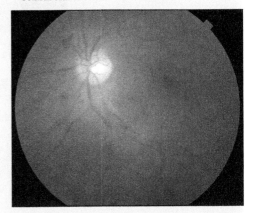 **FIGURE 4.17** Retinal vasculitis.
Temporal arteritis/giant cell arteritis	• Decreased visual acuity • Amaurosis fugax • Relative afferent pupillary defect • Horner's syndrome • Scleritis SL: • Marginal corneal ulceration	• Cotton-wool spots • Central retinal artery occlusion • Chorioretinal scarring (secondary to choroidal infarctions)

(*Continued*)

Disease	External Eye Findings	Fundoscopic Findings
Cholesterol emboli syndrome	• Amaurosis fugax SL: • None	• Hollenhorst plaques • Retinal infarction 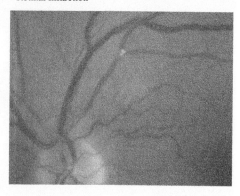 FIGURE 4.18 Hollenhorst plaque.
Stevens–Johnson syndrome	• Bilateral hemorrhagic conjunctivitis • Ulcerative keratitis • Symblepharon • Entropion • Trichiasis SL: • Stromal opacification	• None

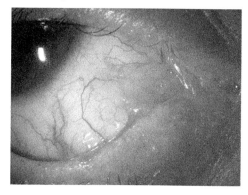

FIGURE 4.19 Symblepharon.

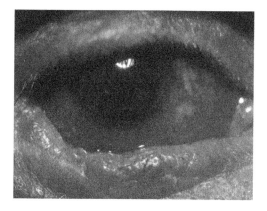

FIGURE 4.20 Hemorrhagic conjunctivitis.

(Continued)

Disease	External Eye Findings	Fundoscopic Findings
Acute pancreatitis	• Xanthelasma (seen in hypertriglyceridemia-related pancreatitis) • Corneal arcus (seen in hypertriglyceridemia-related pancreatitis) SL: • None	• Lipemia retinalis (seen in hypertriglyceridemia-related pancreatitis) • Purtscher-like retinopathy (seen in alcoholic pancreatitis)

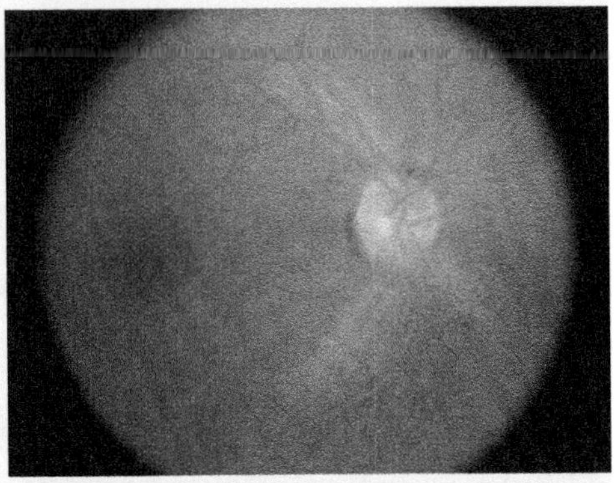

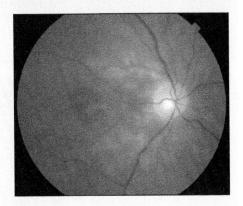

FIGURE 4.21 Lipemia retinalis.

FIGURE 4.22 Purtscher-like retinopathy.

Disease	External Eye Findings	Fundoscopic Findings
Kawasaki's disease	• Bilateral nonexudative bulbar conjunctivitis (limbal sparing) • Subconjunctival hemorrhage SL: • Anterior uveitis • Superficial keratic precipitates	• Papilledema

ACKNOWLEDGMENTS

Unless otherwise noted, all photographs in this chapter are reproduced with permission from Penn State Department of Ophthalmology. Digital image reproduction courtesy of ophthalmic photographers Timothy Bennett, CRA, FOPS, and James D. Strong, BS, CRA.

REFERENCES

1. Gold DH, Weingeist TA. *Color Atlas of the Eye in Systemic Disease*. Philadelphia, PA: Lippincott Williams & Wilkins, 2001.
2. Kanski JJ. *Clinical Ophthalmology*. London, UK: Butterworth Heinemann Publishing, 1994.
3. Tasman W, Jaeger EA. *The Wills Eye Hospital Atlas of Clinical Ophthalmology*. Philadelphia, PA: Lippincott-Raven Publishers, 1996.
4. Quillen DA, Blodi BA, eds. *Clinical Retina*. Chicago, IL: AMA Press, 2002.

5 Radiology of Infectious Diseases and Their Potential Mimics in the Critical Care Unit

Jocelyn A. Luongo, Boris Shapiro, Orlando A. Ortiz, and Douglas S. Katz

CONTENTS

CLINICAL PERSPECTIVE

Radiologic diagnosis of infection in the critically ill population can be challenging. Various imaging modalities are usually needed in the workup of infection in these patients to exclude or diagnose alternate disorders, including malignancy and autoimmune disease. In this chapter, the radiologic presentation of various abdominal, neurologic, and thoracic infections, as well as the findings in other diseases that may mimic infection on imaging, are discussed, as are potentially helpful differentiating factors.

ABDOMINAL AND PELVIC INFECTIOUS PROCESSES AND THEIR MIMICS

CLINICAL AND RADIOLOGIC DIAGNOSIS OF ACUTE PYELONEPHRITIS

Acute pyelonephritis is a bacterial infection involving the renal pelvis, tubules, and interstitium. The most common pathogen is *Escherichia coli*. Infection occurs primarily via ascending spread of a urinary tract infection (UTI), although hematogenous spread can occur less frequently. Uncomplicated disease is rarely, if ever, fatal. However, complications such as emphysematous pyelonephritis in diabetics, abscess formation, or sepsis increase the morbidity and mortality substantially. Risk factors for the development of complications include age greater than 65 years, bedridden status, immunosuppression, diabetes, and a long-term indwelling urinary tract catheter [1].

The diagnosis of acute pyelonephritis is usually made via history and physical examination in conjunction with positive urinalysis, and imaging is not generally needed, except in patients with an atypical presentation or a suspected complication. IV contrast-enhanced CT is the imaging method of choice in adult patients. The classic findings of acute pyelonephritis on CT are wedge-shaped and striated areas of decreased enhancement. There is also usually stranding of the

perinephric fat and thickening of Gerota's fascia. The kidney involved may also be enlarged or demonstrate areas of focal swelling in the acute setting, and then may become scarred and contracted if the infection progresses to a chronic state. The imaging abnormalities, however, usually resolve over 1–5 months. Persistent pyuria after appropriate antibiotic treatment correlates with residual inflammation that may still be detected with imaging. However, in most patients, clinical signs such as fever abate within 24–48 hours after appropriate antibiotic therapy, and patients are considered clinically cured within 4–5 days [2].

Ultrasound may be used for screening, although it is not as sensitive or specific as CT. Findings include a normal or enlarged kidney with decreased echogenicity and wedge-shaped zones of hypoechogenicity (hyperechogenic foci, which are less likely, usually indicate a hemorrhagic component). There is also blurring of the corticomedullary junction. Anechoic regions are indicative of abscess formation. Ultrasound is also used in neonates and young children with a febrile UTI to detect urinary tract anomalies associated with hydronephrosis or ureterocele. A voiding cystourethrogram (VCUG) is indicated if there is an abnormal ultrasound or a repeat episode of febrile UTI. VCUG entails catheterization of the urethra and bladder under fluoroscopy, and it is used for evaluation of vesicoureteral reflux and/or posterior urethral valves, which puts the child at risk for repeat episodes of pyelonephritis and renal failure [1–4].

MIMICS OF ACUTE PYELONEPHRITIS

Xanthogranulomatous pyelonephritis (XGPN) is a relatively rare form of pyelonephritis, which is associated with a chronically obstructed kidney, usually in conjunction with a staghorn calculus. The disorder results in destruction of the renal parenchyma and a non-functioning kidney. Unlike conventional bacterial pyelonephritis, which is usually treated medically, the treatment for XGPN is usually nephrectomy,

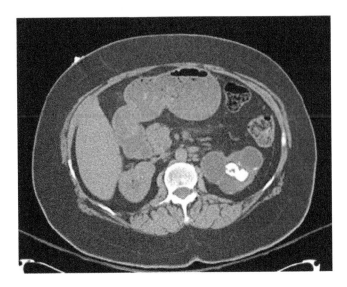

FIGURE 5.1 Non-contrast axial CT image of the abdomen in a 53-year-old woman demonstrates a large obstructing staghorn calculus in the pelvis of the left kidney with diffuse calyceal dilatation and diffuse cortical thinning. These findings are diagnostic of XGPN, when combined with a history of recurrent urinary tract infection. *Abbreviation*: XGPN, xanthogranulomatous pyelonephritis.

or partial nephrectomy if only a portion of the kidney is involved. XGPN is most frequently seen in diabetic or immunocompromised patients [1,2].

The CT findings of XGPN include low-attenuation collections in the kidney involved, which represent dilated calyces filled with pus and debris, as well as a dilated renal pelvis (Figure 5.1). There is prominent IV contrast enhancement of the rims of the collections secondary to inflammation and formation of granulation tissue. There is also little to no excretion of IV contrast into the collecting system, as the kidney is non-functioning. As in conventional pyelonephritis, there is inflammatory change of the perinephric fat, but in contrast, there is much more frequent involvement of adjacent structures, particularly of the ipsilateral psoas muscle, with rare involvement of other structures such as the colon. Unlike in conventional pyelonephritis, as noted, a staghorn calculus is usually present. Gas within the kidney may rarely be seen [1–3].

Renal infarction is another entity that may present clinically similar to acute pyelonephritis. It commonly presents with flank pain, fever, microscopic hematuria, and elevated inflammatory markers, with lactate dehydrogenase being the most specific for renal infarction. The most common cause of renal infarction is atrial fibrillation, but other causes include endocarditis, atherosclerosis, angiocatheterization, aortic stent placement, vasculitis, medical-renal disease, and coagulopathy. Renal infarcts are commonly associated with concomitant splenic infarcts on CT, which may be bland if due to non-septic emboli, or alternatively may be related to septic emboli (e.g., from atrial fibrillation in the former or from endocarditis in the latter). The most common finding on IV contrast-enhanced CT is one or more wedge-shaped hypodensities within an otherwise-normal-appearing kidney, which

are similar to the CT findings in pyelonephritis. As with acute pyelonephritis, these hypodensities may become hyperdense if additional CT images are obtained after a 1- to 6-hour delay. This phenomenon is called a persistent nephrogram or flip-flop enhancement. This pattern may represent multiple renal infarcts, but pyelonephritis may look the same. In a large renal infarct, a thin cortical rim sign may appear, which is capsular enhancement due to collateral blood supply to the outer renal cortex; this differentiates it from an inflammatory/infectious process. Absence of perinephric fat stranding on CT is also relatively common in renal infarcts [5–9].

CLINICAL AND RADIOLOGIC DIAGNOSIS OF RENAL ABSCESS

Focal or multifocal bacterial infection can result in the formation of a renal abscess. The location of the abscess may indicate its etiology. Cortical abscesses can result from hematogenous spread of infection, with *Staphylococcus aureus* being the most common pathogen. Much more commonly, in contrast, corticomedullary abscesses result from ascending spread of infection from organisms in the urine. The latter type of abscess is more likely to extend to the renal capsule and perforate, resulting in perinephric abscess formation (Figure 5.2). Corticomedullary abscesses are uncommon complications of UTIs; risk factors for their development include recurrent infections, untreated or ineffectively treated infections, renal calculi, instrumentation, vesicoureteral reflux, and diabetes mellitus [10].

There are multiple options for imaging a patient with a suspected renal abscess, with IV contrast-enhanced CT considered the method of choice. Radiographs may show radiopaque calculi or intraparenchymal gas in patients with emphysematous pyelonephritis, but are generally not helpful for the identification of an abscess alone. Ultrasound findings include an ill-defined mass, which is either hyperechoic or hypoechoic, with low-level internal echoes and disruption of the corticomedullary junction. The "comet sign," consisting of internal

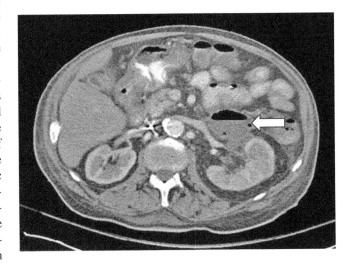

FIGURE 5.2 IV contrast-enhanced axial CT image of the abdomen in a 72-year-old man demonstrates an abscess in the left anterior pararenal space, containing gas and fluid (*arrow*).

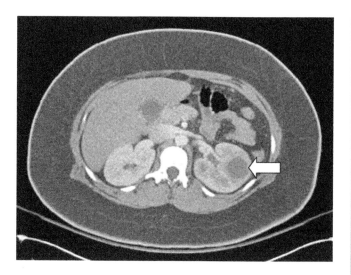

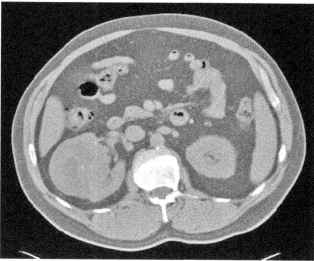

FIGURE 5.3 IV contrast-enhanced axial CT image of the abdomen in a 15-year-old female demonstrates an abscess in the interpolar region of the left kidney (*arrow*), with rim enhancement and adjacent diffuse low density and left renal swelling, representing associated pyelonephritis.

FIGURE 5.4 Non-enhanced axial CT image of the abdomen in a 47-year-old man who presented with left flank pain, demonstrates a large mixed solid and cystic/necrotic tumor in the upper pole of the right kidney, containing internal foci of calcification, which subsequently proved to be renal cell carcinoma.

echogenic foci, indicates the presence of gas. IV contrast-enhanced CT demonstrates a round, well-marginated, low-attenuation mass with wall enhancement (Figure 5.3). Gas may or may not be present, and there is no enhancement centrally. Perinephric inflammatory change is also often seen. A nuclear white blood cell scan may also be helpful for diagnosis. Uptake of indium-111-labeled leukocytes within the abscess can be seen, although false-negative results may occur if the patient has already been on antibiotic therapy, if the abscess is walled off, or if there is a poor inflammatory response [3,10].

MIMIC OF RENAL ABSCESS

Renal cell carcinoma may mimic renal abscess on imaging examinations. Both form focal masses within the kidney; however, unlike renal abscess, which does not enhance centrally, renal cell carcinoma typically demonstrates heterogeneous enhancement. Internal calcifications may or may not be present (Figure 5.4). For this reason, the recommendation for known or suspected renal masses that could be cancers rather than abscesses includes short-term interval imaging follow-up with non-enhanced CT, followed by multi-phasic contrast-enhanced CT performed at the same sitting [3,11].

CLINICAL AND RADIOLOGIC DIAGNOSIS OF PSOAS ABSCESS

The iliopsoas compartment is located between the spine and the retroperitoneal organs and constitutes an important anatomic conduit of disease from the thorax to the pelvis and proximal femur. Diseases of the psoas often present with vague abdominal complaints, with painful hip flexion deformity present in less than half of patients. Psoas abscess is defined as primary when there is no local cause identified,

and it is then usually attributed to hematogenous spread of a distant, and sometimes occult, infectious process. It is associated with immunosuppression, diabetes, and/or drug abuse. The most common causative pathogen is *S. aureus.* Secondary psoas abscess is more common in immunocompetent patients and is due to local infectious spread from the intestines, kidneys, or bone. It is usually polymicrobial. Fistulizing Crohn disease is reportedly the most common cause. Iatrogenic causes of psoas abscess include urologic surgeries and surgeries on the lumbar or hip areas. Underlying retroperitoneal space malignancy is a very rare cause of secondary psoas abscess [16,17].

Signs/symptoms are, as noted, often non-specific, and unanticipated iliopsoas abscess may be identified on CT. The CT findings of psoas abscess include enlargement of the muscle by a low-attenuation mass, which displays rim enhancement after IV contrast administration. Other findings include obliteration of normal fat planes, as well as adjacent bone destruction and gas formation. Gas within a psoas abscess may also be related to an underlying bowel fistula, such as in Crohn disease or diverticulitis. MRI is the most sensitive modality to look for infectious/inflammatory changes in the adjacent bone and cartilage, and is particularly helpful if there is concern for associated discitis, osteomyelitis, or sacroiliitis. Increased signal on fluid-sensitive sequences within muscle, however, is not specific for a psoas abscess, and may be due to a primary pathologic process in the spine causing muscle edema. Abnormal uptake on a Ga-67 scan may also be used for diagnosis, although other entities, such as lymphoma, also show increased uptake; this finding is therefore not specific. CT-guided percutaneous drainage is the primary treatment of choice for iliopsoas abscesses, and it also helps to exclude alternative diagnoses and to guide targeted antibiotic therapy [12–21].

Mimic of Psoas Abscess

Differentiation from tumor, such as lymphoma, can be difficult with imaging alone, as both can present as low-attenuation masses on CT, although the presence of gas makes the diagnosis of abscess far more likely. Adjacent structures should be examined to determine if there is a source of secondary infection. In the case of lymphoma originating from para-aortic lymph nodes, a potential helpful differentiating feature is that there may be medial or lateral displacement of the muscle by tumor, rather than extension into the muscle, as would be seen in an abscess [22,23]. Positron emission tomography (PET)-CT is an imaging modality that can be used to depict skeletal muscle metastases, manifesting as increased metabolic activity within the muscle. However, an abscess has a similar increased metabolic uptake, and therefore, PET-CT is more useful for staging and monitoring response to treatment in known malignancies [24,25].

Retroperitoneal hemorrhage can present as a clinically occult, yet important cause of blood loss, and when subacute to chronic, can also mimic a psoas abscess. Common causes include anticoagulation medications, bleeding diathesis, surgical procedures, trauma, and ruptured aortic aneurysm. Hematomas cause diffuse enlargement of the involved muscle(s) and/or mass-like infiltration of the retroperitoneal spaces. Fresh blood has high attenuation (up to 80 HU) on non-contrast CT, and appears hyperdense compared with soft tissue and normal muscle. Subsequently, IV contrast-enhanced CT is sometimes obtained, and if there is contrast extravastation, this indicates the specific site of active bleeding. Fluid-fluid levels can be seen immediately in anticoagulated patients on CT, also known as a "hematocrit effect," due to the impaired clotting cascade in this patient population. Retroperitoneal hemorrhage caused by a ruptured aortic aneurysm may involve the iliopsoas compartment, but can be distinguished from hematomas caused by coagulopathy due to the presence of hemorrhage in the periaortic space and the absence of the "hematocrit effect." Chronic hematomas eventually become hypodense, potentially mimicking the appearance of abscesses or tumors, and hence, correlation with clinical history is necessary. Complicating things further, a psoas hematoma can become infected and develop into an abscess [17,26].

Clinical and Radiologic Diagnosis of Prostate Abscess

Prostatic abscess occurs as a complication of acute bacterial prostatitis. The most common organism is *E. coli*. Diabetic and immunocompromised patients are especially prone to this complication. The symptoms are similar to acute bacterial prostatitis, including fever, chills, and urinary frequency, with focal prostatic tenderness on physical examination [26].

Both CT and ultrasound are used for diagnosis, with ultrasound also having therapeutic utility in transrectal drainage. Abscesses can occur anywhere in the prostate, although they are usually centered away from the midline. Findings on transabdominal and/or transrectal ultrasound include focal hypoechoic or anechoic masses, with thickened or irregular walls, septations, and internal echoes. On CT, findings include an enlarged gland containing multiple well-demarcated, non-enhancing fluid collections within the gland and/or periprostatic tissues. These collections may be multi-septated or demonstrate enhancing rims [3,27,28,31].

Mimic of Prostate Abscess

A potential mimicker of prostate abscess is prostate carcinoma. Prostate cancer is the most common non-cutaneous cancer in American men, and the second most common cause of male cancer deaths after lung cancer. Unlike prostate abscess, which can occur anywhere in the gland, prostate cancer occurs mainly in the peripheral zones. Diagnosis is made via a combination of digital rectal examination findings, elevated PSA level, transrectal ultrasound, and MR, with a definitive diagnosis established by biopsy [3,29].

Ultrasound findings are somewhat similar to abscess in that carcinoma appears as an anechoic to hypoechoic mass. The contour is classically asymmetric or triangular with the base close to the capsule, and extending centrally into the gland based on the pattern of tumor growth. While CT is an excellent means for diagnosing and following treatment of prostatic abscess, it has limited use in the diagnosis of carcinoma due to relatively poor sensitivity and specificity for detection of cancer within the gland compared with MRI. CT findings may include an enlarged gland with evidence of extracapsular extension in more advanced tumors (obliterated periprostatic fat plane, invasion of adjacent bladder or rectum) and pelvic lymphadenopathy (Figure 5.5). T2-weighted MRI demonstrates prostate cancer as a relatively low-intensity area within the gland, whereas abscess should demonstrate areas of central high signal intensity related to the fluid content [29,30]. Chronic prostatitis, which may also

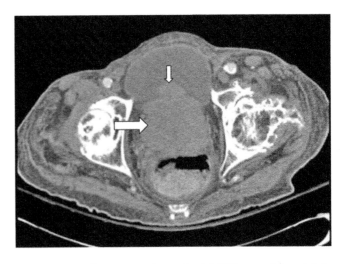

FIGURE 5.5 IV contrast-enhanced axial CT image of the pelvis in a 91-year-old man with known prostate cancer demonstrates a large, slightly heterogeneous prostate (*large arrow*) protruding into the bladder base (*small arrow*).

present with elevated PSA and non-specific urinary symptoms, is much more difficult to distinguish from prostate cancer, but it usually has a different, less defined, pattern of T2 hypointensity, and only a subtly pathologic pattern of restricted diffusion on magnetic resonance imaging (MR), as compared to prostate cancer [32,33].

CLINICAL AND RADIOLOGIC DIAGNOSIS OF LIVER ABSCESS

There are three main types of liver abscess: pyogenic, amebic, and fungal. Pyogenic abscesses occur most often in the United States. Pyogenic liver abscesses occur by direct extension from infected adjacent structures or by hematogenous spread via the portal vein or hepatic artery. *Klebsiella pneumoniae* is more often "cryptogenic," is thought to be caused by hematogenous spread, and is associated with a higher rate of septic hematogenous complications. Polymicrobial pyogenic abscesses are most often associated with adjacent biliary tract obstruction, intra-abdominal infection, or malignancy. The risk of abscess is increased in patients with diabetes, prior bilioenteric anastomosis, or an incompetent sphincter of Oddi. Clinical presentation may be insidious, with fever and right upper quadrant pain being the most common presenting complaints. The right lobe of the liver is more often affected secondary to bacterial seeding via the blood supply from both the superior mesenteric and portal veins. Untreated, the disease is usually fatal, but with prompt abscess identification and then antibiotic administration and drainage, mortality is significantly decreased, now reported to be in the range of 2%–10% [34,38–40].

Both CT and ultrasound can be used for diagnosis and follow-up of liver abscess, as well as for guiding percutaneous drainage. The CT appearance of a liver abscess is a round, well-defined hypodense mass that may contain gas centrally (Figure 5.6). A commonly seen finding is the "cluster sign" representing a conglomerate of small abscesses

coalescing into a single large cavitating mass. Abscesses caused by *Klebsiella* are more likely to be solid, that is, higher in attenuation than fluid, have thin (<2 mm) abscess walls, and necrotic debris within the cavity similar to the aforementioned "cluster sign." They are also associated with a higher rate of hepatic vein thrombophlebitis, which is seen as linear areas of hypoattenuation corresponding to the hepatic veins [39,40]. Arterial-phase CT may show increased attenuation of adjacent liver parenchyma, which is caused by reduced portal venous flow due to inflammation/stenosis and compensatory increased hepatic arterial flow [38]. Secondary findings include right pleural effusion and right lower lobe atelectasis. On ultrasound, the abscess is usually spherical or ovoid with hypoechoic, irregular walls. Centrally, the abscess may be anechoic or less often hyperechoic or hypoechoic, depending on the presence of septa, debris, or necrosis [3].

MIMIC OF LIVER ABSCESS

A non-liquefied abscess (particularly from *Klebsiella* species) can sometimes be confused with hepatic tumor, including hepatocellular carcinoma (HCC) and metastatic disease from gastrointestinal primary tumors, or vice versa (Figure 5.7), particularly when solitary. As with abscesses, these also appear more often on the right side of the liver when solitary. A helpful differentiating factor is that most patients with HCC have underlying cirrhosis [3,37].

On ultrasound, the mass appears mixed in echogenicity and demonstrates increased vascularity on color Doppler. The appearance on portal-venous phase (i.e., routine delay following IV contrast) CT is usually that of a hypodense mass with or without necrosis. The tumor may have a capsule, which enhances after IV contrast administration. Portal vein thrombosis occurring in conjunction with liver abscess is clinically and radiologically difficult to differentiate from tumor thrombus in HCC. HCC demonstrates characteristic

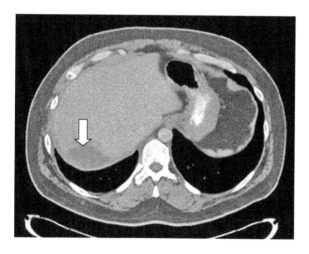

FIGURE 5.6 Axial CT image of the abdomen with oral contrast only, demonstrating an abscess in the right hepatic lobe (*arrow*) in a 36-year-old man with fever and abdominal pain following recent laparoscopic appendectomy for perforated appendicitis.

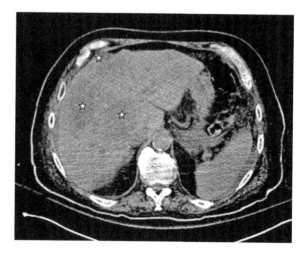

FIGURE 5.7 Non-enhanced axial CT image of the abdomen in a 77-year-old man with colon cancer demonstrating multiple large, relatively low-density masses throughout the liver (*stars*), representing metastases.

enhancement patterns on multi-phasic CT scans performed, with at least both arterial and portal venous phases, which aid in diagnosis and differentiation from other entities. The tumor is heterogeneous on arterial-phase CT (or MR) imaging, intermixed with areas of hypoperfusion from portal vein occlusion by tumor thrombus. There is then washout of contrast on the portal venous phase, as the tumor is supplied almost exclusively by the hepatic artery [3,34,35].

MR can also be used, although it is mostly reserved for those patients whose findings on CT are indeterminate or when there is a contraindication to iodinated contrast for CT and when IV gadolinium can be administered for MR. On T1-weighted imaging, HCC is typically hypointense, whereas on T2-weighted images, it is usually somewhat hyperintense. With IV gadolinium administration, the enhancement pattern varies from central to peripheral, and from homogeneous to rim enhancing. Also, on T2-weighted imaging, the hyperintensity surrounding an abscess is typically much greater than what would be seen for HCC [3,35,36].

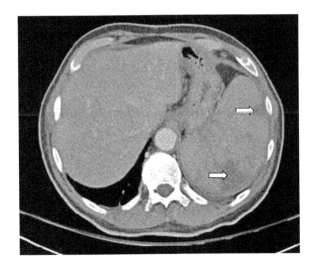

FIGURE 5.8   IV contrast-enhanced axial CT image of the abdomen in an 82-year-old man demonstrating multiple peripheral, wedge-shaped, low-density areas in a mildly enlarged spleen (*arrows*), which are acute and subacute infarcts.

CLINICAL AND RADIOLOGIC DIAGNOSIS OF SPLENIC ABSCESS

Splenic abscess is a relatively rare entity with a high mortality rate. The most common etiology is hematogenous spread of infection from elsewhere in the body. Alcoholics, diabetics, and immunocompromised patients are most susceptible. There is a diverse array of pathogens, including bacteria (both aerobic and anaerobic) and fungi [41].

Diagnosis cannot be made solely through history and physical examination. CT is the standard imaging modality for diagnosis and therapeutic drainage planning. CT findings include a low-attenuation, ill-defined mass or masses within the splenic parenchyma. As with abscesses elsewhere in the abdomen and pelvis, there may be gas or a gas-fluid level. There is no enhancement of the central portion after IV contrast administration, although as with hepatic abscesses, there is often peri-abscess enhancement as well as surrounding edema. There may be inflammatory stranding of the perisplenic fat. Ultrasound demonstrates a hypoechoic mass, which may contain internal septations and low-level internal echoes, representing either debris or hemorrhage. There is no blood flow within the central areas on Doppler imaging [3,42].

MIMIC OF SPLENIC ABSCESS

Splenic infarcts may have a similar clinical presentation, including fever, chills, and left upper quadrant pain. Differentiating the two entities is important, as an infarct can be managed conservatively, whereas an abscess requires antibiotic therapy and possibly drainage. On CT, a splenic infarct is classically a peripheral, wedge-shaped low-attenuation region after IV contrast administration (Figure 5.8). However, infarcts may be rounded, similar to an abscess, or irregular in shape. Lack of mass effect on the splenic capsule may be a helpful differentiating factor from abscess. Further complicating matters, as noted earlier regarding renal infarcts in patients with septic emboli (e.g., from endocarditis), the CT findings

may be identical to those of bland infarction (e.g., from atrial fibrillation), and differentiating between these two entities is difficult to impossible without clinical correlation [3,42].

Unlike in splenic abscess, on follow-up cross-sectional imaging an infarct should become better demarcated and eventually resolve, leaving an area of fibrotic contraction and volume loss. A deviation from this expected course suggests a complication such as hemorrhage or superimposed infection [42].

CLINICAL AND RADIOLOGIC DIAGNOSIS OF CHOLANGITIS/CALCULOUS CHOLECYSTITIS

Acute infection of the biliary system is most often caused by biliary obstruction from gallbladder calculi. A dislodged calculus from the gallbladder may pass into the intestines without causing any symptoms, or it may lodge at various points along the biliary tract, which is termed choledocholithiasis. Acute calculous cholecystitis is caused by an impacted calculus with resultant obstruction at the level of the cystic duct and gallbladder wall inflammation. It presents with persistent right upper quadrant tenderness and elevated inflammatory markers. Ten to 20% of people with symptomatic gallbladder calculi also have choledocholithiasis, which puts them at risk for gallstone pancreatitis and for cholangitis, even after cholecystectomy [38,43,51].

Acute cholangitis is most commonly caused by an impacted calculus in the common bile duct, leading to bile stasis and infection. Through a similar mechanism, it may be caused by a benign or malignant stricture. Increased intrabiliary pressure is a key factor in the breakdown of biliary defenses and overgrowth with intestinal bacteria. Procedures such as bilioenteric anastomosis or insertion of biliary stents also put individuals at risk for cholangitis due to the now easy pathway for enteric contents to migrate retrograde into the biliary system. The most common pathogens are *E. coli* and *Enterococci*. Cholangitis classically presents as Charcot's triad of fever, jaundice, and

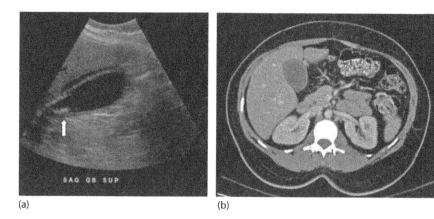

(a) (b)

FIGURE 5.9 (a) Ultrasound examination demonstrates a thickened gallbladder wall, pericholecystic fluid, and gallstones (*arrow*). Correlating with a positive sonographic Murphy's sign, these findings were diagnostic of acute cholecystitis in this patient. (b) IV contrast-enhanced axial CT image of the abdomen in the same patient demonstrates thickening and increased enhancement of the gallbladder wall, but the gallstones are not identifiable.

right upper quadrant pain. However, elderly patients and smokers are more likely to face a severe form of cholangitis, even in the absence of some of these clinical findings [49–55].

On ultrasound, cholangitis appears as thickened walls of the bile ducts, which may be dilated and contain pus or debris. Visualization of an obstructing calculus increases diagnostic certainty, although MR cholangiography (see below) is more accurate for identification of such calculi. The ultrasound criteria for acute cholecystitis include cholelithiasis and a sonographic Murphy's sign, considered the most sensitive findings, with additional findings of a thickened gallbladder wall (>3 mm) and pericholecystic fluid (Figure 5.9a) [3,43,44].

Nuclear scintigraphic examinations are useful in confirming cholecystitis and for differentiating between acute and chronic forms in selected patients. 99m-Tc iminodiacetic acid derivatives (i.e., hepatobiliary iminodiacetic acid [HIDA] and its derivatives) are injected intravenously, are taken up by hepatocytes, and are then transported into the biliary system in a fashion similar to bilirubin. Non-visualization of the gallbladder at four hours has a 99% specificity for diagnosing cholecystitis. Intravenous morphine may be administered if initial images do not demonstrate the gallbladder, to cause sphincter of Oddi spasm, increasing biliary pressure and forcing radiotracer into a chronically inflamed gallbladder, but not in acute gallbladder inflammation [3].

CT is nearly as sensitive as ultrasound or HIDA when evaluating for cholecystitis, and is often the first imaging examination obtained, because patients may have non-specific and non-localizing symptoms, and many other inflammatory conditions of the abdomen can mimic cholecystitis clinically [38]. CT findings in cholecystitis include a distended gallbladder, gallbladder wall thickening, pericholecystic fat stranding, and calcified gallstones, when present. There is also mural enhancement with IV contrast administration (Figure 5.9b). Complications include gangrenous changes in the wall, with heterogeneity of enhancement, and pericholecystic abscesses, which are also identifiable on CT [3,38,44]. Arterial-phase CT is relatively sensitive and specific for the diagnosis of acute cholangitis. CT may show

enhancement of bile ducts, with patchy inhomogeneous areas of liver enhancement, which are reversible with treatment. This is thought to be due to increased arterial flow to compensate for the decreased portal venous flow in the setting of biliary stasis. The extent of these compensatory hepatic attenuation differences is even greater in the setting of infection. Dilated bile ducts and an obstructing process, most commonly a calculus, may also be identified on CT as the cause of cholangitis [38,55,56].

MRI findings of acute cholecystitis include a distended gallbladder with calculi, gallbladder wall thickening and edema, and increased signal in the pericholecystic fat on T2-weighted images. MR cholangiopancreatography (MRCP, i.e., multi-planar heavily T2-weighted images) can be used to visualize obstructing calculi within the biliary tract with a high degree of accuracy in patients with suspected cholecystitis and/or cholangitis, which are seen as filling defects and/or a cutoff of the common duct [3]. Identification of a calculus in a dilated (>10 mm) common bile duct may be an indication for urgent endoscopic drainage, even in the absence of clinical symptoms, due to an increased risk of developing severe cholangitis. On the other hand, MRCP is a reliable way to exclude clinically significant choledocholithiasis and thus prevent unnecessary invasive procedures [55,57].

MIMIC OF CALCULOUS CHOLECYSTITIS

Approximately 90% of patients with cholecystitis are associated with calculi, but 10% occur without them, i.e., acalculous cholecystitis (AC). The precise etiology of AC is still not fully understood. Existing theories propose the noxious effect of superconcentrated bile due to prolonged fasting and the lack of cholecystokinin-stimulated emptying of the gallbladder. Gallbladder wall ischemia from low-flow states in patients with fever, dehydration, or heart failure has also been proposed. The disease occurs in very ill patients, such as those on mechanical ventilation or those having experienced severe trauma or burns. Mortality is much higher with AC, as the entity is much more prone to gangrene and perforation [43,45,46].

AC has proven to be an elusive diagnosis to correctly establish, both clinically and radiologically. In the appropriate clinical context, in any patient with presumed cholecystitis without demonstration of calculi on ultrasound, CT, or MR, AC should be the leading diagnosis. Prior studies have shown decreased sensitivity for both ultrasound and nuclear medicine examinations for the detection of AC. Sonographic findings include an enlarged gallbladder, diffuse or focal wall thickening with focal hypoechoic regions, pericholecystic fluid, and diffuse homogeneous echogenicity (possibly from debris) in the gallbladder lumen without identifiable calculi. Visualization of the gallbladder on HIDA scans is possible in some patients with AC due to a patent cystic duct, leading to false negatives. False positives on HIDA scans may also occur since parenteral alimentation, prolonged fasting, and hepatocellular dysfunction, all of which can be seen in the critically ill, are the same factors that cause non-visualization of the gallbladder despite the absence of acute or chronic inflammatory gallbladder disease [46,47,58].

CLINICAL AND RADIOLOGIC DIAGNOSIS OF EMPHYSEMATOUS CHOLECYSTITIS

Emphysematous cholecystitis is a form of cholecystitis caused by gas-forming organisms, most commonly *E. coli, Clostridium perfringens,* and *Bacilis fragilis.* Gallstones are often present, although there are also affected patients without calculi. Those most prone to infection are diabetics and the elderly. It carries a five-times greater risk of perforation than uncomplicated acute cholecystitis [38,44,48].

Gas within the gallbladder wall may be identified on radiographs. The most sensitive and specific imaging examination is CT, which not only demonstrates gas in the gallbladder wall, but also may show spread of inflammation and, in some patients, gas extending into surrounding tissues and into the rest of the biliary system [38,44,48].

MIMIC OF EMPHYSEMATOUS CHOLECYSTITIS

Aside from calculous and AC, gas in the biliary system from a biliary-enteric fistula (spontaneous or iatrogenic) is a differential consideration in the diagnosis of emphysematous cholecystitis, although relatively rare (Figure 5.10). Specific considerations include gallstone ileus (i.e., chronic cholecystitis with fistula to the adjacent small bowel) and malignancy. Extension of inflammation into the pericholecystic tissues and extrahepatic ducts may be a helpful differentiating feature, as this is considered more specific for emphysematous cholecystitis [48].

CLINICAL AND RADIOLOGIC DIAGNOSIS OF PANCOLITIS

Colonic infection results from bacterial, viral, fungal, or parasitic infections. An increasingly prevalent agent in both hospitalized and non-hospitalized patients is *Clostridium difficile.* It is associated with recent use of antibiotics, and often presents with watery diarrhea, fever, and leukocytosis. Symptoms vary, however, from mild to severe.

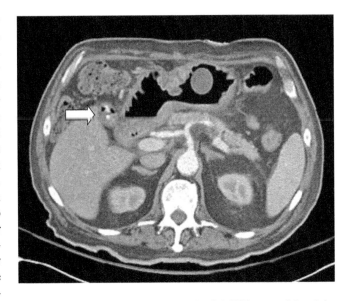

FIGURE 5.10 IV contrast-enhanced axial CT image of the abdomen demonstrates air in the gallbladder (which also contains calculi [*arrow*]), secondary to erosion of the stomach into the biliary system, in a 71-year-old man with metastatic gastric cancer. This is a gastrocholedochal fistula. A gastrostomy tube is also present.

Radiographic findings of *C. difficile* colitis include polypoid mucosal thickening, severe haustral fold thickening or "thumbprinting" represented by widened opaque transverse bands, and gaseous distention of the colon. On CT, the colonic wall is thickened and low in attenuation, secondary to edema (Figure 5.11). Wall thickening may be circumferential, eccentric, smooth, irregular, or polypoid, and ranges from 3 to 32 mm. There is mucosal and serosal enhancement. Inflammation of the pericolonic fat and ascites may be present. The "target sign" on CT consists of two to three concentric

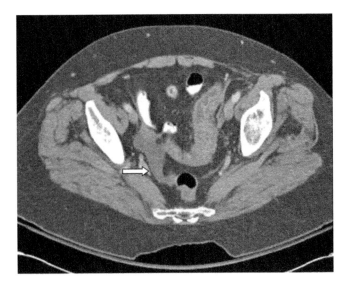

FIGURE 5.11 IV contrast-enhanced axial CT image of the pelvis demonstrates wall thickening of the sigmoid colon with intramural low density, representing submucosal edema. Mild pericolonic inflammation is noted. These findings represent colitis. A small amount of right pelvic ascites is also present (*arrow*).

rings of different attenuation within the colonic wall, and represents mucosal hyperemia and submucosal edema or inflammation. This sign is helpful, but not very specific, as it is also seen in inflammatory bowel disease, including ulcerative colitis (UC), among other disorders. The "accordion sign" is due to trapping of oral contrast between markedly thickened haustral folds, resulting in alternating bands of high and low attenuation, oral contrast, and edematous bowel wall, respectively. Pericolonic fat stranding, while often present, is generally mild in comparison with the degree of bowel wall thickening, which may be helpful in differentiating *C. difficile* from inflammatory colitis [3,59].

MIMIC OF PANCOLITIS

Ulcerative Colitis

UC is an inflammatory bowel disorder, with a variable disease course, which primarily involves the colorectal mucosa and submucosa. The wall thickening in UC is characteristically diffuse and symmetric. CT findings are typically of a non-specific, contiguous colitis involving a portion of the distal colon or the entire colon, without skip areas, which is in and of itself difficult if not impossible to differentiate from infection at initial presentation. CT is used to determine extent/severity of colitis and any complications (obstruction, perforation, etc.) [3,60].

Ischemic Colitis

Ischemic colitis results from compromise to the colonic blood supply, either by global changes in circulation or by local changes in mesenteric vasculature. As such, findings occur in a territorial distribution, typically in watershed areas, particularly the splenic flexure (superior mesenteric artery/inferior mesenteric artery junction) and the rectosigmoid junction (inferior mesenteric artery/hypogastric artery junction). It is the most common form of gastrointestinal ischemia, is usually transient and self-limited, and the cause is often somewhat elusive and multifactorial. Most of the patients affected are elderly, with non-specific abdominal pain, and occasionally bloody diarrhea. It is associated with cardiovascular disease, numerous medications, coagulopathic states, and hypovolemia. Again, bowel wall thickening, mucosal irregularity, and pericolic inflammatory changes may be seen on CT. Specific, but uncommon, findings for bowel ischemia include pneumatosis (in the correct clinical context), which may be difficult to distinguish from intraluminal gas in some patients, and the absence of submucosal enhancement in the region of infarction [3,61].

CNS INFECTIONS AND THEIR MIMICS

CLINICAL AND RADIOLOGIC DIAGNOSIS OF BRAIN ABSCESS

Focal infection in the brain is most often bacterial, although fungal and parasitic infections also occur. Pathogens can be introduced into the brain via direct extension (such as from sinus or dental infection), hematogenous spread, or after penetrating injury or brain surgery. There is a substantially increased incidence of CNS infection in immunocompromised patients. There are four stages of infection: Early and late cerebritis, and early and late abscess capsule formation. Capsule formation typically occurs over a period of 2–4 weeks [62,63].

CT and MRI are both utilized in diagnosis. The appearance of the abscess on either depends on the stage of infection. Classically, a brain abscess appears as a smooth, ring-enhancing mass; gas-containing abscesses are rarely seen. Early cerebritis is more readily detected on MR than CT. CT during this stage may demonstrate a poorly defined, low-attenuation subcortical mass with mass effect, or may alternatively be normal. On MR, an ill-defined, heterogeneous mass is seen, hypointense to isointense on T1-weighted images, and hyperintense on T2-weighted images. During the late cerebritis stage, a rim appears on MR, high intensity on T1-weighted images (Figure 5.12) and low intensity on T2-weighted images, as well as increasing mass effect and vasogenic edema on both CT and MR. The early capsule on CT appears as a thin, enhancing rim, with low attenuation in the center of the mass (Figure 5.13a and b). On MR, the rim becomes increasingly well defined, and the center of the mass demonstrates increased signal relative to cerebrospinal fluid (CSF) on T1-weighted images. The rim is typically thickest on the cortical aspect and thinnest in its deep aspect, which is a phenomenon believed to be related to the higher oxygenation of blood flow closer to the gray matter. A feature that can be used to differentiate late cerebritis from the early capsular stage, as both demonstrate rim formation, is the phenomenon of "filling in," in which a 20- to 40-minute delay on a contrast-enhanced MR will show enhancement in the central

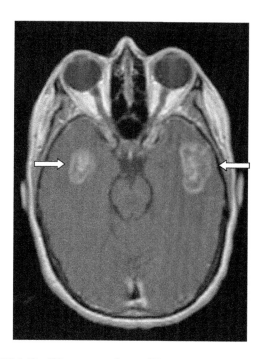

FIGURE 5.12 IV contrast-enhanced T1-weighted axial MR image of the brain demonstrates two ring-enhancing masses in the temporal lobes (*arrows*) in a 52-year-old woman with *Nocardia* cerebritis.

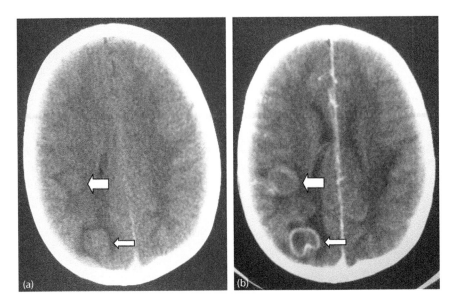

FIGURE 5.13 (a) Axial CT image of the brain in a 3-year-old boy with congenital heart disease demonstrates two subcortical, low-attenuation masses in the right cerebral hemisphere (*arrows*). (b) After IV contrast administration, both masses demonstrate thin, peripheral enhancement (*arrows*) with central low density, which is highly consistent with brain abscesses.

portion of the abscess during late cerebritis but not once the actual capsule has formed [62,64]. A recently described "dual rim" sign, which depicts an inner hyperintense and an outer hypointense ring on magnetic-susceptibility MR imaging, has been shown to be highly specific for a pyogenic abscess. The hyperintense ring is thought to represent the low magnetic-susceptibility granulation tissue, which is located between the abscess cavity and the free-radical rich fibro-collagenous abscess capsule. The center of the abscess also demonstrates high signal on diffusion-weighted MR imaging, presumably due to the elevated viscosity of the necrotic material. Resolution of the restricted diffusion in response to treatment precedes the reduction in size of the abscess. On the other hand, persistent high signal on diffusion-weighted imaging indicates failed treatment, and extension of restricted diffusion into the ventricle is diagnostic for intra-ventricular rupture of the abscess [71,72,76].

CLINICAL AND RADIOLOGIC DIAGNOSIS OF CNS TUBERCULOSIS

While isolated involvement of the central nervous system in tuberculosis (TB) is rare, CNS involvement is seen in approximately 5% of patients with TB, with increased prevalence in immunocompromised individuals. Infection mostly occurs via hematogenous spread. Various forms of cerebral involvement can occur, including tuberculous meningitis, cerebritis, tuberculoma, abscess, or miliary TB. Tuberculoma (or tuberculous granuloma) is the most common CNS parenchymal manifestation of TB. These may be solitary or multiple, and can occur anywhere in the brain, although there is a predilection for the frontal and parietal lobes [65,66].

On CT, tuberculomas may be round or lobulated, high or low in attenuation, and enhancement patterns vary from homogeneous to ring enhancing (Figure 5.14a and b). The tuberculomas may also have irregular walls of varying thickness. When chronic, they are associated with mass effect, surrounding edema, and calcification. The "target sign," consisting of central calcification, surrounding edema, and peripheral enhancement, is suggestive of, but not entirely diagnostic for, tuberculoma. On MR, tuberculomas are initially hypointense on T1-weighted and T2-weighted images, and homogeneously enhance. When it undergoes caseous necrosis, the typical tuberculoma is hypointense on T1- and T2-weighted images, but it also demonstrates a peripheral rim of enhancement. If a tuberculoma undergoes liquefactive necrosis, it becomes hyperintense on T2-weighted images, and also acquires restricted diffusion, similar to a pyogenic abscess [62,66,73].

CLINICAL AND RADIOLOGIC DIAGNOSIS OF TOXOPLASMOSIS

In immunocompetent individuals, toxoplasmosis causes a self-limited flu-like illness. However, in the immunocompromised patient, there can be fulminant infection with significant morbidity and mortality. Toxoplasmosis is the most common focal neurologic abnormality in the brain in the AIDS population. Multiple ring-enhancing masses are the most common imaging finding (Figure 5.15a–c). The masses vary in size, and demonstrate surrounding edema, and are hypodense to isodense on non-enhanced CT. With IV contrast administration, rim enhancement is present, and can be either thin and smooth, or solid and nodular. The masses are hypointense on non-enhanced T1-weighted imaging and are typically hyperintense on T2-weighted imaging, although this is variable [62,67].

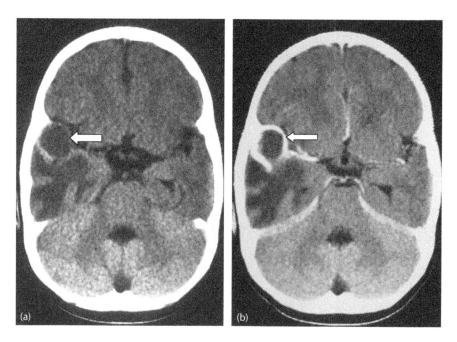

FIGURE 5.14   (a) Axial CT image of the brain in a male patient demonstrates a round, low-attenuation mass in the right temporal lobe (*arrow*), with surrounding vasogenic edema. (b) After IV contrast administration, this mass demonstrates thick peripheral enhancement, which subsequently proved to be a tuberculoma.

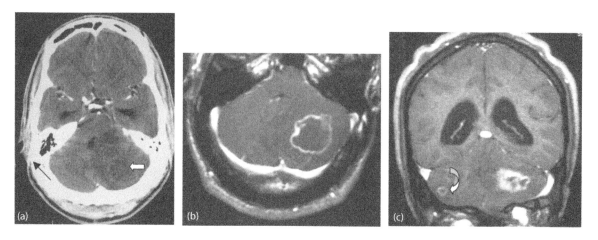

FIGURE 5.15   (a) Axial CT image of the brain in a 34-year-old immunocompromised man demonstrates a 3-cm area of low attenuation in the left cerebellar hemisphere (*arrow*), with associated mass effect on the fourth ventricle and acute hydrocephalus. (b) Axial T1-weighted MR image with gadolinium demonstrates peripheral ring enhancement. (c) Coronal T1-weighted IV gadolinium-enhanced MR image from the same patient demonstrates a second mass in the right cerebellar hemisphere (*curved arrow*); these findings proved to be toxoplasmosis.

MIMICS OF BRAIN ABSCESS, CNS TUBERCULOSIS, AND TOXOPLASMOSIS

BRAIN TUMOR

Necrotic brain tumors, both primary and metastatic, may also present as ring-enhancing parenchymal masses. Unlike an abscess, which typically has smooth margins, a tumor classically demonstrates thick, nodular rim enhancement. The mass(es) may be multi-loculated and complex. The entities can further be differentiated via diffusion-weighted MR imaging, in which the tumor will usually be low in signal, consistent with lack of restricted diffusion, whereas an abscess

usually does exhibit increased intensity due to restricted diffusion. The enhancement pattern is also different, as residual foci of viable tumor within a necrotic center will continue to enhance, resulting in a heterogeneous enhancement pattern. The center of an abscess does not enhance [62,64]. MR perfusion imaging is another technique that helps differentiate a tumor from a benign process. The rim of a pyogenic abscess is less vascular than the capsule of a tumor, and will show decreased relative cerebral blood volume (rCBV) compared with normal white matter, in contrast to a tumor [71].

Differentiation of tuberculoma from tumor can be difficult. Imaging characteristics on MRI can be nearly indistinguishable.

In addition, a tuberculoma may have similar increased peripheral rCBV as a tumor. MR spectroscopy (MRS) has been utilized to successfully differentiate an unusual presentation of an extra-axial tuberculoma from a meningioma. The high lipid and lactate peaks and lack of amino acid resonances may prove useful for distinguishing tuberculoma from other entities in the correct clinical context, potentially sparing unnecessary biopsy [68].

CNS Lymphoma

Primary CNS lymphoma is a B-cell lymphoma that originates from and generally remains within the brain, spinal cord, optic tract, or leptomeninges. It is highly associated with immunodeficiency, and carries a poor prognosis relative to non-CNS lymphomas. The disease incidence in immunocompromised patients peaked in the 1990s due to the AIDS epidemic. Disease incidence is now very low in the immunocompetent population, but it is on the rise among patients 75 years of age or older [74]. Differential diagnoses differ between immune competent and compromised patients, with primary or metastatic tumor considered for the former, and opportunistic infection, such as toxoplasmosis, for the latter. The enhancement pattern of lymphoma is usually heterogeneous on both CT and MR. However, in the immunocompromised population, enhancement can be heterogeneous or ring enhancing (Figure 5.16a and b). Masses are isointense to hypointense on T1-weighted images, and hyperintense on T2-weighted images. There is often leptomeningeal or periventricular/intraventricular extension [62,64].

Toxoplasmosis is difficult to differentiate from primary CNS lymphoma. Both affect gray and white matter, particularly the basal ganglia, and affect immunocompromised patients. Multiplicity can be observed in both conditions. Lymphoma may demonstrate ependymal spread, which is not characteristic of toxoplasmosis. PET findings do differ, as toxoplasmosis is usually hypometabolic, whereas CNS lymphoma is usually hypermetabolic [62].

Clinical and Radiologic Features of Cerebritis

Cerebritis is a term used to describe an acute inflammatory reaction in the brain, with altered permeability of blood vessels, but not angiogenesis. Cerebritis is the earliest form of brain infection that may then progress to abscess formation, as previously noted. Cerebritis alone can be managed nonsurgically with antibiotics [64].

The appearance of early cerebritis on T1-weighted MR imaging is a hypointense or isointense area with minimal mass effect, and little to no enhancement after IV contrast administration. The affected area is hyperintense on T2-weighted and fluid-attenuated inversion recovery (FLAIR) images. It may demonstrate restricted diffusion on diffusion-weighted imaging, which has been attributed to increased cellularity (from infiltrating neutrophils), ischemia, and cytotoxic edema [62].

Mimic of Cerebritis

As opposed to infectious cerebritis, autoimmune cerebritis occurs with systemic lupus erythematosus (SLE). CNS involvement in SLE typically occurs within 3 years of diagnosis and may even precipitate a full-blown SLE presentation. On CT, there is cerebral atrophy and possible focal infarcts or calcification, as well as extensive, potentially reversible white matter changes [28].

MRI is superior for demonstrating active abnormalities that appear as hyperintense white matter foci on FLAIR imaging, with restricted diffusion and IV contrast enhancement. Differentiating old abnormalities from infectious cerebritis may be difficult, as both are bright on T2-weighted imaging, and neither entity enhances with IV contrast administration. MRS and MR perfusion imaging can be utilized to further evaluate for

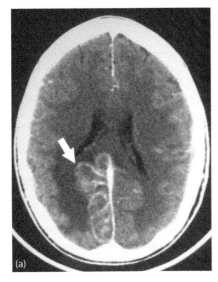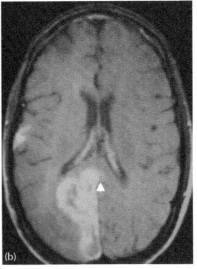

FIGURE 5.16 (a) IV contrast-enhanced axial CT image of the brain in an HIV-positive man demonstrates a gyriform enhancing mass in the right occipital lobe associated with vasogenic edema (*arrow*). (b) IV contrast-enhanced T1-weighted axial MR image demonstrates intense right occipital lobe enhancement as well as a second small right frontal cortical focus of enhancement in this patient with lymphoma.

suspected lupus cerebritis, if necessary. MRS findings, though non-specific, include a decreased *N*-acetyl aspartate peak, and increased choline and lactate peaks. MR perfusion imaging demonstrates decreased cerebral blood flow and volume in the regions of chronic abnormalities caused by autoimmune cerebritis, relative to the normal white matter [62,75].

CLINICAL AND RADIOLOGIC DIAGNOSIS OF MENINGITIS

Meningitis is an inflammatory infiltration of the pia mater, the arachnoid, and the CSF. The disease can have an infectious or non-infectious etiology. Early in the course of disease, the initial diagnosis is made on clinical evaluation, including lumbar puncture, as imaging findings are often normal. On CT, there may be hydrocephalus with enlargement of the subarachnoid space and effacement of the basal cisterns. There is enhancement within the sulci and cisterns after IV contrast administration, secondary to breakdown in the blood–brain barrier, as well as areas of low attenuation from altered perfusion patterns. On MR, exudate in the subarachnoid space is isointense on T1-weighted images and hyperintense on T2-weighted images. Again, there is leptomeningeal enhancement after IV contrast administration, which is typically smooth and linear (Figure 5.17). Diffusion-weighted imaging findings depend on altered perfusion and the presence of vascular complications, including arterial occlusion [62,64].

MIMIC OF MENINGITIS

Carcinomatous meningitis occurs from both secondary and primary brain tumors. The most common distant primary tumors include breast and lung cancer. Glioblastoma multiforme, pineal tumors, and choroid plexus tumors can also

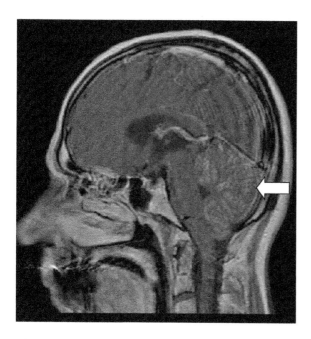

FIGURE 5.17 IV contrast-enhanced sagittal MR image of the brain demonstrates mild leptomeningeal enhancement, most pronounced in the posterior fossa (*arrow*), in a 53-year-old man with cryptococcal meningitis on CSF analysis.

extend along the leptomeninges. The enhancement pattern of carcinomatous meningitis is often thicker and irregular compared with the one that is seen with infectious meningitis, although thin and linear enhancement can also occur. In such patients, clinical information, including the presence of a primary malignancy, and CSF analysis may be needed to definitively differentiate between the two entities [62,64].

CLINICAL AND RADIOLOGIC DIAGNOSIS OF ENCEPHALITIS

Encephalitis is an inflammation of the brain parenchyma that may be focal or diffuse, and is most commonly associated with viral infection (rather than cerebritis, which is associated with bacterial infection). Potential agents include eastern and western equine, herpes simplex, Epstein–Barr, and varicella viruses, as well as cytomegalovirus (CMV). Herpes encephalitis, to which the elderly are particularly vulnerable, is a dangerous form of the disease with high mortality rates if therapy is not promptly initiated.

CT is often negative in these patients. Abnormal findings on MR and nuclear imaging examinations depend on the specific virus. Herpes typically involves the medial temporal and inferior frontal lobes (Figure 5.18a), whereas Japanese encephalitis affects the thalami, brain stem, cerebellum, spinal cord, and cerebral cortex. Abnormal high-intensity abnormalities can be demonstrated on T2-weighted and FLAIR sequences (Figure 5.18b). Contrast enhancement may range from none to intense [62,64,69,76].

MIMIC OF ENCEPHALITIS

Restricted diffusion may be present, which, depending on clinical presentation, may rarely lead to confusion of the entity with acute infarction. In such patients, MRS and nuclear medicine imaging may be helpful. Tc-99m hexamethylpropyleneamine oxime (HMPAO) single-photon emission CT has shown utility for the detection of both herpes encephalitis and Japanese encephalitis [70].

CLINICAL AND RADIOLOGIC DIAGNOSIS OF HIV ENCEPHALOPATHY/ENCEPHALITIS

HIV encephalopathy/encephalitis (HIVE) is a syndrome of cognitive, behavioral, and motor abnormalities attributed to the effect of HIV infection on the brain in the absence of other opportunistic infection. HIVE is the most common neurologic manifestation of HIV. Diffuse cortical atrophy is the most common finding on both CT and MR. White matter disease is also present, and the areas most affected are the periventricular regions and centrum semiovale, the basal ganglia, cerebellum, and the brainstem. On T2-weighted MR images, white matter signal changes may be focal or diffuse, and the distribution and extent of the abnormalities do not necessarily correlate with clinical presentation. FLAIR sequences may demonstrate focal abnormalities not revealed on T2-weighted images, particularly those smaller than 2 cm. Foci of HIVE do not enhance on MR examination after IV gadolinium administration, a characteristic feature [62,76].

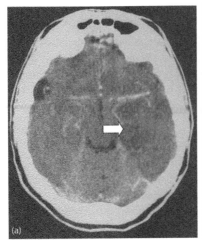
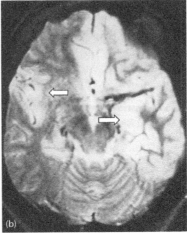

FIGURE 5.18   (a) IV contrast-enhanced axial CT image of the brain in a patient with herpes encephalitis demonstrates low attenuation in the left temporal lobe (*arrow*). (b) A corresponding T2-weighted axial MR image from the same patient demonstrates high signal intensity in both medial temporal lobes (*arrows*), consistent with the diagnosis of herpes encephalitis.

MIMIC OF HIVE

The differential for white matter abnormalities is broad, encompassing infectious, inflammatory, and autoimmune causes. In multiple sclerosis (MS), the abnormalities are usually focal, although with severe illness, they can become confluent (Figure 5.19a–c). Unlike in HIV, active MS foci do enhance. They are isointense to hypointense on T1-weighted imaging, whereas such foci are not visualized on T1-weighted images in HIVE [62,76].

Acute disseminated encephalomyelitis is a condition whereby multifocal white matter and basal ganglia abnormalities occur, typically 10–14 days after infection or vaccination. They involve both the brain and spinal cord. CT is initially negative but with time demonstrates low-density, flocculent, and asymmetric abnormalities, which are better

visualized on FLAIR MR sequences. IV contrast enhancement may be punctate or ring-like (complete or incomplete). Again, IV contrast enhancement is one helpful differentiating feature from HIVE [62,76].

THORACIC INFECTIONS AND THEIR MIMICS

CLINICAL AND RADIOLOGIC DIAGNOSIS OF BACTERIAL PNEUMONIA

Bacterial pneumonia presents with fever, cough, dyspnea, and can be divided into three main radiologic patterns. The causative organism generally determines what type of pneumonia results. However, the host immune response and various other undetermined factors also play a role in the clinical and radiologic manifestations of pneumonia.

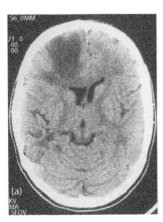
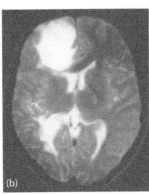
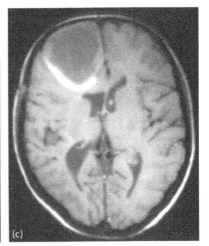

FIGURE 5.19   (a) Axial CT image of the brain in a 15-year-old female with known multiple sclerosis demonstrates a low-attenuation "mass" in the right frontal lobe, with little mass effect relative to its size. (b) T2-weighted axial MR image demonstrates high signal intensity within the mass. (c) IV gadolinium-enhanced T1-weighted axial MR image demonstrates partial rim enhancement in this patient, with tumefactive multiple sclerosis.

Lobar, or focal pneumonia, is the most common type and is associated with community-acquired pneumonia (CAP). The most common pathogen is *Streptococcus pneumoniae.* The main risk factor in the healthy adult population is smoking. Special populations, such as children younger than 2 years and patients with asplenia, immunodeficiency, or sickle cell disease, are susceptible to this pathogen due to inability to neutralize encapsulated bacteria. The infection starts in the distal air-spaces, in the periphery of the lobe, and leads to homogenous opacification of a part or of an entire lobe. The airways remain patent, therefore air bronchograms are present, and lobar volume is preserved or even enlarged due to infiltrative process. *Klebsiella* is another important cause of CAP, and also usually presents with a focal consolidation. It is associated with chronic alcoholism, and has a higher rate of complications, including lung necrosis and cavitations [88,89].

Lobular, multifocal, or bronchopneumonia, is the main pattern associated with hospital-acquired pneumonia. It is caused by aspiration of colonized tracheal secretions, and the most common pathogen is *Pseudomonas*, followed by *S. aureus.* The classic appearance on chest radiography and CT is a "patchwork-quilt" pattern of air-space opacification, reflecting diseased and adjacent non-diseased pulmonary lobules. Air bronchograms are uncommon due to inflammatory exudates filling the distal airways, but are present if the airways remain patent (Figure 5.20a and b) [77,78]. Pulmonary infection is the most common cause of death in patients with hematologic malignancies, and the most common bacterial pathogen is *Pseudomonas* [94].

Interstitial pneumonia is characterized by cellular inflammation in the walls of the bronchioles and alveolar septa, and by inflammatory exudate or mucus partially filling the bronchiolar lumen. It commonly presents with atypical "walking" pneumonia symptoms, and reticulonodular opacities on imaging. The most common bacterial pathogen is *Mycoplasma pneumoniae*, but viruses, *Legionella*, and *Pneumocystis* are other common causes of interstitial pneumonia. Serology and risk factors such as immunodeficiency are sometimes the best clue to the diagnosis. *Mycoplasma* pneumonia has variable appearance on imaging, with bronchial wall thickening the most common feature on CT. While not specific to *Mycoplasma*, centrilobular or branching tree-in-bud patterns of nodules strongly suggest an acute infectious process in the distal airways on CT, as opposed to non-infectious causes of interstitial lung disease (ILD). Radiologic resolution of pneumonia often lags behind clinical improvement, and may take up to 12–14 weeks [88,89].

MIMICS OF BACTERIAL PNEUMONIA

Pulmonary Embolus

Although many chest radiographs in patients with pulmonary embolus (PE) are not entirely normal, the findings are usually not specific for PE, and confirmation or exclusion with additional imaging, particularly with pulmonary CT angiography (the current imaging reference standard), ventilation/

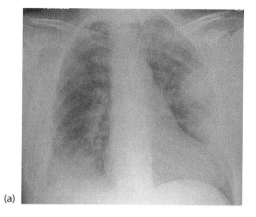

(a)

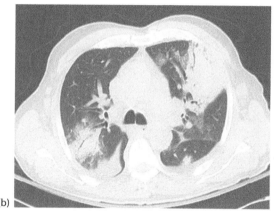

(b)

FIGURE 5.20 (a) Chest radiograph demonstrates dense opacification in the left upper lobe and at the right lung base in an adult patient with multi-lobar pneumonia. (b) Axial CT image of the chest in the same patient demonstrates consolidation in the left lower and right upper lobes containing air bronchograms, again consistent with multi-focal pneumonia. Bilateral pleural effusions are also present posteriorly.

perfusion (V/Q) scan, and lower extremity venous Doppler, are required for diagnosis. Radiographic findings include right heart enlargement, central pulmonary artery enlargement (usually when chronic, but occasionally when acute with a large clot burden), localized peripheral oligemia with or without distention of more proximal vessels ("Westermark sign"), and peripheral air-space opacification due to localized pulmonary hemorrhage. When lung infarction occurs, in a minority of patients, a pleural-based, wedge-shaped opacity can be identified, the "Hampton's hump." Lung infarction can have a similar appearance to segmental pneumonia, and correlation with CT angiography is usually needed to differentiate the two entities (Figure 5.21a and b). The utility of chest radiography is more for identifying between alternate diagnoses and for interpretation of V/Q scans, to correlate with abnormal areas of perfusion or ventilation [77].

Neoplasm

Invasive mucinous adenocarcinoma usually presents as a spiculated nodule or a lobulated lung mass, but it may also present as a focal consolidation at the periphery of a lobe. The patient

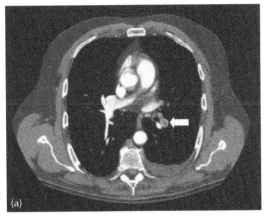

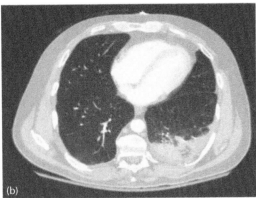

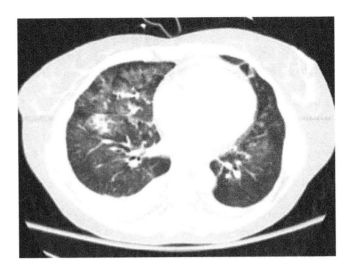

FIGURE 5.22 Axial CT image of the mid-chest demonstrates bilateral alveolar and ground-glass opacities as well as interlobular septal thickening in a 38-year-old woman with lupus. These findings were not present on a CT performed 4 days earlier (not shown), and are compatible with lupus pneumonitis and/or hemorrhage. Bilateral pleural effusions as well as a pericardial effusion are also present.

FIGURE 5.21 (a) IV contrast-enhanced axial CT image of the mid-chest demonstrates an embolus in the central left lower lobe pulmonary artery (*arrow*), as well as a small left pleural effusion. (b) An area of consolidation in the left lower lobe posteriorly represents pulmonary infarction. Although the appearance may be similar to pneumonia in some patients, the presence of embolus and absence of other clinical signs of infection in this patient establish the diagnosis of pulmonary infarction with certainty.

is usually not acutely ill as compared with a patient with focal pneumonia. Findings suspicious for cancer include narrowed air bronchograms within the consolidation, and bubble-like low attenuation areas on CT. This process may look similar to the "Swiss-cheese" appearance of focal pneumonia in the setting of underlying emphysema. Thickening of surrounding vessels is also concerning for lung adenocarcinoma, or less likely primary lung lymphoma. Bronchial wall thickening proximal to a consolidation, on the other hand, supports the diagnosis of infectious pneumonia. Ipsilateral pleural thickening is also more common in an infectious process, unless the tumor has invaded the pleura [91,92].

Lupus Pneumonitis (SLE)

Pulmonary manifestations of SLE include acute lupus pneumonitis and chronic interstitial disease. The former is rapid in onset and may mimic a focal or multi-focal pneumonia, with CT findings of ground-glass attenuation and patchy consolidation that then coalesces (Figure 5.22). Additional radiographic findings include elevated hemidiaphragms due to myopathy and resultant low lung volumes with linear bibasilar atelectasis. The opacities will respond to steroids, unlike most

pneumonia and chronic interstitial disease. Lupus patients are also at increased risk for pulmonary emboli, pulmonary hemorrhage, and infectious pneumonia [77,79].

Congestive Heart Failure

Congestive heart failure (CHF) is usually bilateral and symmetric with pulmonary findings of interstitial edema, which may mimic interstitial pneumonia. Unilateral disease can also occur much less commonly. A specific condition associated with pulmonary edema isolated to the right upper lobe is mitral regurgitation. The radiographic findings may easily be confused with pneumonia. As in the case of diffuse CHF changes, initiation of therapy should rapidly reverse the findings, unlike in pneumonia [80].

CLINICAL AND RADIOLOGIC DIAGNOSIS OF CAVITARY PNEUMONIA

The term "cavity" with respect to the lung is used to describe an air-containing nodule with a thick wall (>4 mm) or within a surrounding area of pneumonia or an associated mass. Cavitary lung nodules and masses result from neoplastic, autoimmune, and infectious processes. Cavities with a wall thickness >15 mm are most likely malignant. Squamous cell cancer of the lung is the most common malignancy to cavitate. There may relatively rarely be co-existence of pulmonary infection and malignancy in a cavitary nodule or mass [93].

The common bacterial pneumonias that may progress to cavitation include *S. aureus*, *Klebsiella*, and *P. aeruginosa* [81]. Hospitalized, debilitated patients are most susceptible to these pathogens. They typically present with lobar consolidation in the case of *Klebsiella*, or multifocal opacities in the case of *S. aureus* or *Pseudomonas*, as described previously. Sputum culture is essential in diagnosis, and it may occasionally reveal anaerobic oropharyngeal pathogens, such as *Bacteroides, Fusobacterium,* or *Actinomyces* [88]. Exudative pleural effusion is a common complication associated with these pneumonias. This may progress to an empyema, which is an infected fluid collection that may demonstrate locules of gas within a fluid density, surrounded by thickened parietal and visceral pleura. Abscess formation occurs late in the infection, and is demonstrated by increasing demarcation of an initially ill-defined opacity with evolution into a round cavity with an irregular thick wall and possibly an air-fluid level [77,88]. Lung abscess tends to make an acute angle with the pleura, in contrast to the obtuse angle of an empyema [89].

MIMICS OF CAVITARY PNEUMONIA

Septic Emboli

Venous thromboembolism is a common cause of initially aseptic cavitary nodules or masses, which form as a result of pulmonary infarcts, within two months of the initial embolic event. A minority of these aseptic cavities can become superinfected, most commonly with *Clostridium* species. More commonly, infected cavities form from an infectious embolic source. The most common cause of septic emboli is prosthetic intravascular devices such as central venous catheters. Other special populations include children with *S. aureus* osteomyelitis, young adults with oropharyngeal infections leading to Lemierre syndrome, IV drug abusers with *S. aureus* bacteremia, and immunocompromised patients who are at risk for *Salmonella* bacteremia [93]. Cavitations caused by septic emboli may be thick or thin-walled on chest radiographs and CT. On CT, these are peripherally distributed and frequently have associated feeding vessels (Figure 5.23). They may be at different stages of development and healing [81].

Aspergillosis

Aspergillus mold causes several distinct forms of pulmonary disease, ranging in severity from allergic reaction to angioinvasive pulmonary infection. This may present as fever in a neutropenic patient, not responsive to antibiotics. Invasive pulmonary aspergillosis frequently results in focal lung infarctions and cavitary transformation. The organism invades small blood vessels in the lung, the early appearance of which is relatively small pulmonary nodules with surrounding hemorrhage seen as ground-glass opacity secondary to hemorrhagic infarction, the "CT halo" sign (Figure 5.24). The vessel(s) involved can sometimes be identified ("feeding vessel" sign). The classic "air crescent" sign appears during the healing process, and is due to separation of infected necrotic lung from normal lung parenchyma or an aspergilloma that develops within a pre-existent cavity (Figure 5.25). Aspergillomas, which are not frankly angioinvasive in contrast to invasive aspergillosis but which may cause hemoptysis or may be asymptomatic, move freely within the cavity, and thus should change position between prone and supine imaging, a highly helpful identifying feature [77,78,94].

Tuberculosis

Tuberculous cavitations occur mainly in post-primary TB and have a preponderance for the upper lobes. The inner wall of a tuberculous focus can be either smooth or irregular in appearance. Post-primary TB is also associated with characteristic dense tree-in-bud opacities, which are indicative of endobronchial spread of the disease (Figure 5.26) [82,88,91].

CLINICAL AND RADIOLOGIC DIAGNOSIS OF VIRAL PNEUMONIA

Diffuse, or interstitial, pneumonias are often viral in etiology, as described previously. The infections can be divided

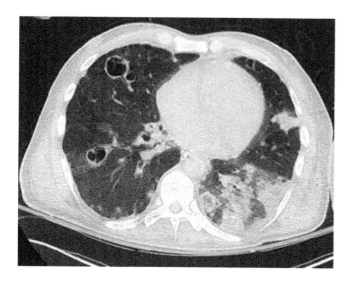

FIGURE 5.23 Non-contrast axial CT image of the mid-chest in a 30-year-old man with endocarditis demonstrates multiple nodules throughout both lungs, some of which are cavitating, as well as left and right lower lobe pneumonia. The nodules are septic pulmonary emboli.

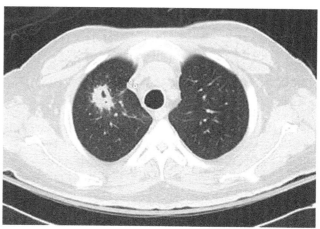

FIGURE 5.24 Non-contrast axial CT image of the upper chest in an immunocompromised 29-year-old man demonstrates a thick-walled spiculated cavitary mass in the right lung apex. Additional nodules with surrounding ground-glass opacity, some of which were cavitating, were also seen throughout both lungs. The findings combined with the clinical information are compatible with invasive aspergillosis.

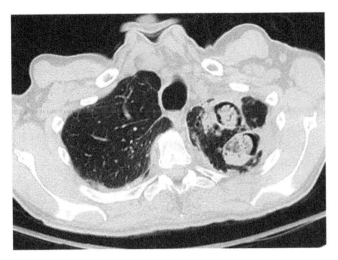

FIGURE 5.25 Non-contrast axial CT image of the upper chest demonstrates two cavitary masses in the left lung apex, containing soft-tissue material, with lucent areas and surrounding crescents of air ("air crescent" sign), representing aspergillomas. There is also tracheal dilatation and pre-existent bronchiectasis, as well as architectural distortion of the upper lobes.

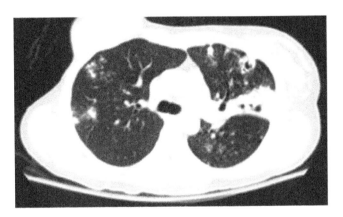

FIGURE 5.26 Axial CT image of the chest in a 39-year-old woman with pulmonary tuberculosis demonstrates left upper lobe consolidation along the left major fissure with areas of cavitation. Additional nodular opacities of varying size are seen diffusely in both lungs, some of which demonstrate a "tree-in-bud" configuration.

into two broad categories: Those in immunocompetent hosts, most often influenza A and B, and those in immunocompromised hosts, such as CMV, herpes simplex virus (HSV), and the *Pneumocystis* pneumonia (PCP) [77]. Viral pneumonias make up approximately 10% of CAP in immunocompetent population, and patients with CHF are also at increased risk of developing viral pneumonia [90].

Nodules ranging in size from 1 to 20 mm, best depicted on CT, are a common feature in all forms of viral pneumonia [89]. Influenza pneumonia in a normal, healthy host usually has a mild course. In the elderly or debilitated patient, infection can be fulminant and potentially fatal within a matter of days. Influenza pneumonia initially appears on chest CT as diffuse bilateral reticulonodular areas, 1–2 cm

in diameter, and patchy ground-glass opacities. There may be small centrilobular nodules representing alveolar hemorrhage. Over the course of days to weeks, depending on the condition of the patient, diffuse consolidation may develop. Pleural effusions rarely occur. In a healthy host, the findings should resolve within approximately three weeks [77,83].

HSV pneumonia is a rare entity, occurring primarily in the immunocompromised or those with airway trauma, such as the chronically intubated. Infection occurs either via aspiration, via extension from oropharyngeal infection, or hematogenously in patients with sepsis.

On radiographs, the most common findings are patchy segmental or subsegmental areas of air-space disease. CT demonstrates multifocal segmental and subsegmental areas of ground-glass opacity with smaller areas of focal consolidation. Pleural effusion is commonly present with herpes pneumonia [83].

CMV is the most common viral cause of pneumonia in transplant patients as well as in AIDS patients. On CT, the appearance may vary. Mixed alveolar and interstitial abnormalities; consolidation, small, ill-defined centrilobular nodules, bronchial dilatation, and thickened interlobular septa, are all potential findings [83,84].

Unlike the typical viral diffuse pneumonias, PCP is caused by the fungus *P. jirovecii*, a common organism found in otherwise normal human lungs, but which in the immunocompromised host may cause pneumonia. The radiographic appearance of PCP varies widely. Chest radiographs are often completely normal early in the infection. Fine reticular or ground-glass opacities, predominantly in the hilar regions, may be seen on CT (Figure 5.27). Progressive disease results in formation of confluent areas of air-space opacification. Asymmetric or focal areas of interstitial disease are also highly suggestive of *Pneumocystis* pneumonia in the correct clinical context. Significant adenopathy and pleural effusions are highly unusual, and their presence usually indicates an

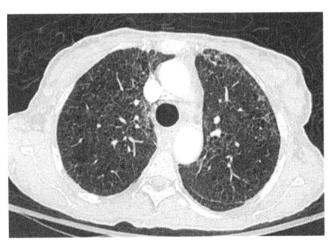

FIGURE 5.27 Non-contrast axial CT image of the chest demonstrates emphysematous change with superimposed diffuse ground-glass opacity in a 58-year-old immunocompromised woman with *Pneumocystis* pneumonia.

alternate diagnosis. Thin-walled cysts or pneumatoceles can also be seen with PCP, as can pneumothorax [78,83].

COVID-19 pneumonia is caused by an apparently new, highly contagious coronavirus (SARS-CoV-2) of unclear origination, which led the World Health Organization to declare a global pandemic on March 11, 2020. Viral nucleic acid testing is the reference standard for diagnosis, and it may also be used to detect asymptomatic carriers of the virus. Symptomatic patients typically present to the emergency department with fever, dyspnea, dry cough, and lymphopenia, and may occasionally have gastrointestinal signs and symptoms. Although a spectrum of disease, the condition of some patients may rapidly deteriorate, which then prompts evaluation with chest radiography as well as, if needed, chest CT evaluation. Initial CT of the chest typically shows bilateral patchy but relatively well-defined and/or nodular ground-glass opacities in a peripheral and lower lobe predominant distribution [95–97]. The opacities tend to solidify and become more confluent and diffuse in the later stage of the disease (Figure 5.28). Additional

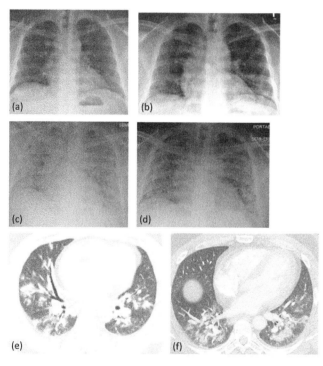

later imaging findings may include interseptal thickening and bronchus deformation. Pleural effusion, pericardial effusion, and lymphadenopathy are characteristically very uncommon [96], but we have anecdotally and very recently seen patients with associated adenopathy on chest CT, as well as patients who have presented with predominantly abdominal complaints where findings were then identified on chest radiography and/or in the lower thorax on abdominal CT.

MIMICS OF DIFFUSE BILATERAL PNEUMONIA

Congestive Heart Failure

Congestive changes occur in two phases: interstitial edema and alveolar flooding or edema. With increased transmural arterial pressure, the earliest findings are loss of definition of subsegmental and segmental vessels, enlargement of peribronchovascular spaces, and the appearance of Kerley A, B, and C lines, reflecting fluid in the central connective septa, peripheral septa, and interlobular septa, respectively. If allowed to progress, increasing accumulation of fluid results in spillage into the alveolar spaces, which is exhibited by confluent opacities primarily in the mid and lower lungs. A "bat's wing" or "butterfly" appearance is classic for CHF, although this is relatively rarely seen. A potentially helpful differentiating feature from other causes of diffuse bilateral air-space opacities is the rapid time frame in which these changes occur. CT findings can also be helpful for demonstrating thickening of subpleural, septal, and bronchovascular structures, along with ground-glass opacities with a gravitational anterior–posterior gradient. Common associated findings are cardiomegaly, pulmonary venous distention, and pleural effusions [77,85].

Pulmonary Hemorrhage

Pulmonary hemorrhage may result from trauma, bleeding diathesis, infection, and autoimmune causes. It is also the most common non-infectious pulmonary complication of acute leukemia, in which case hemoptysis is uncommon. Radiographic findings include bilateral coalescent air-space opacities, which develop rapidly and commonly improve rapidly with a time course of hours, as opposed to days or weeks, such as with most patients with pneumonia [77,94].

Pulmonary Leukostasis

This is one of the most common non-infectious complications of patients with hematologic malignancies, especially in those with a white blood cell count of >100,000. It presents with non-specific symptoms, including cough, fever, and dyspnea. Radiographs may be normal, even in the setting of severe symptoms; however, characteristic findings include bilateral smooth interstitial thickening and pleural effusions, mimicking cardiogenic pulmonary edema or fluid overload. Non-segmental ground-glass opacities seen on CT are caused by leukemic infiltrates in the alveolar spaces, with hemorrhage and edema from diffuse alveolar damage [94].

FIGURE 5.28 43-year-old man with insulin-dependent diabetes, who is a hospital employee with six days of intermittent fever and dry cough, who presented to the Emergency Department with an SpO2 of 93% on room air, and lymphopenia. The patient recovered without intubation/mechanical ventilation, and was discharged from the hospital 17 days later. Initial frontal (PA) chest radiograph on admission (a) shows mildly increased central interstitial markings. There is middle cardiomegaly and tortuosity of the thoracic aorta, more evident on the subsequent AP chest radiographs (b–d). Chest radiograph (b) at day 3 shows patchy nodular mid to lower lung opacities, better demonstrated on axial CT images of the chest performed with IV contrast (e,f). CT also shows mild lower right hilar adenopathy, and subcarinal adenopathy (calipers, e). Chest radiograph at day 8 (c) shows diffuse pulmonary opacification, which is improved on day 12 (d).

Adult Respiratory Distress Syndrome

Adult respiratory distress syndrome (ARDS) occurs as a response to a variety of insults, including trauma, sepsis, pancreatitis, and drug overdose. Leakage of protein-rich fluid from damaged capillary membranes into the interstitial and alveolar spaces leads to decreased inflated lung volumes and decreased lung compliance [77].

On chest radiographs, there are diffuse bilateral opacities located more peripherally due to predominance of capillaries in the periphery of the lung. Presumably, proteinaceous fluid remains in the periphery rather than migrating centrally due to poor diffusion, and there is decreased clearance of the material leading to persistence of the opacities for days to weeks with little change in appearance. CT findings include bilateral ground-glass opacities, consolidation, or a combination of both. Opacities are most often most severe in dependent portions of the lung [84,86].

Interstitial Lung Disease

ILDs are, in general, chronic inflammatory processes that may result in fibrotic change. There are many classifications of the disease, describing both etiology and pattern of pulmonary change. Usual interstitial pneumonia, the most common form of ILD, is initially seen on chest radiography as bibasilar fine reticular opacities progressing to a coarse reticular or reticulonodular pattern, and eventual honeycombing and loss of lung volume. On CT, areas of ground-glass opacity are seen with irregular septal and subpleural thickening, and eventual honeycombing and traction bronchiectasis. Pulmonary fibrosis, while not always seen in ILD, is a helpful feature in differentiating it from pneumonia (Figure 5.29). The time course is also more likely to be chronic, based on months to years, rather than acute or subacute, as with pneumonia [77].

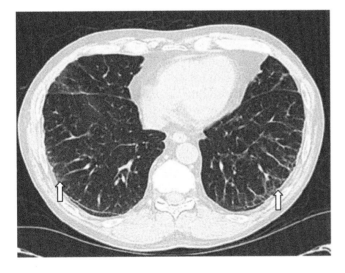

FIGURE 5.29 Axial CT image of the chest in a woman with rheumatoid arthritis demonstrates peripheral fibrotic changes (*arrows*) compatible with rheumatoid arthritis (RA)-associated interstitial lung disease.

Bilateral Massive Aspiration

Aspirated material may include food, water, or sand (as in near drowning) or other foreign objects such as dental material. On chest radiographs, the characteristic appearance is of dependent pulmonary opacities, which then typically coalesce. In healthy individuals, the opacities should resolve rapidly because of mucociliary clearance. There are other specific findings on both radiographs and CT depending on the material aspirated. A specific foreign body may be identified within a bronchus. Legumes, such as lentils, are known to cause a granulomatous pneumonitis. Also, sand or gravel particles may become lodged in small airways, leading to the diagnostic appearance of sand or gravel bronchograms [77,87]. This should not be confused with aspiration pneumonia caused by repetitive inhalation of oropharyngeal bacteria or gastric acid in the setting of impaired swallowing mechanism or reflux esophagitis. Patients with impaired consciousness, alcoholism, tracheostomy, or gastrostomy tubes are at risk for bronchopneumonia via this mechanism. Patients with reflux esophagitis may present with symptoms of CAP, and diffuse centrilobular nodules and bronchiectasis on imaging, due to repetitive aspiration of gastric contents [88,91].

CONCLUSIONS

In conclusion, imaging is extremely helpful and often necessary in the diagnosis of infection in a critically ill patient. However, neoplastic, immunologic, and inflammatory processes can have very similar appearances on imaging, including on radiographs and on CT scans of various parts of the body. Subtle findings are often relied upon to separate these entities, and in many patients, diagnostic certainty is not achieved solely through imaging, but in combination with pertinent clinical and laboratory information and, where necessary, with more invasive procedures, including imaging-guided aspiration and biopsy.

REFERENCES

1. Fulop T. Pyelonephritis, acute. In: eMedicine 2017. Available at: http://www.emedicine.com/Med/topic2843.htm. Accessed on January 5, 2018.
2. Craig WD, Wagner BJ, Travis MD. Pyelonephritis: Radiologic-pathologic review. *Radiographics* 2008;28:255–276.
3. Federle MP, Jeffrey RB, Desser TS, et al. *Diagnostic Imaging: Abdomen* (1st ed.). Salt Lake City, UT: Amirsys, 2005.
4. Karmazyn B, Alazraki A, Anupindi S, et al. American College of Radiology ACR Appropriateness Criteria® Urinary Tract Infection–Child. Revised—2016. Available at: https://acsearch.acr.org/docs/69444/Narrative/. Accessed on December 15, 2017.
5. Piccoli GB, Priola AM, Vigotti FN, et al. Renal infarction versus pyelonephritis in a woman presenting with fever and flank pain. *Am J Kidney Dis* 2014;64(2):311–314.
6. Wolin EA, Hartman DS, Olson JR. Nephrographic and pyelographic analysis of CT urography: Differential diagnosis. *Am J Roentgenol* 2013;200(6):1197–1203.

7. Antopolsky M, Simanovsky N, Stalnikowicz R, et al. Renal infarction in the ED: 10-year experience and review of the literature. *Am J Emerg Med* 2012;30(7):1055–1060.

8. Suzer O, Shirkhoda A, Jafri SZ, et al. CT features of renal infarction. *Eur J Radiol* 2002;44(1):59–64.

9. Kawashima A, Sandler CM, Ernst RD, et al. CT evaluation of renovascular disease. *Radiographics* 2000;20(5): 1321–1340.

10. Benson A, Tarter TH, Teague JL, et al. Renal corticomedullary abscess. In: eMedicine 2015. Available at: http://www. emedicine.com/med/topic2848.htm. Accessed on January 5, 2018.

11. Sheth S, Scatarige JC, Horton KM, et al. Current concepts in the diagnosis and management of renal cell carcinoma: role of multidetector CT and three-dimensional CT. *Radiographics* 2001;21:S237–S254.

12. Muttarak M, Peh WCG. CT of unusual iliopsoas compartment lesions. *Radiographics* 2000;20:S53–S66.

13. Riyad MNYM, Sallam MA, Nur A. Pyogenic psoas abscess: Discussion of its epidemiology, etiology, bacteriology, diagnosis, treatment and prognosis—Case report. *Kuwait Med J* 2003;35:44–47.

14. Torres GM, Cernigliaro JG, Abbitt PL, et al. Iliopsoas compartment: Normal anatomy and pathologic processes. *Radiographics* 1995;15:1285–1297.

15. Shifrin A, Lu Q, Lev MH, Meehan TM, et al. Paraspinal edema is the most sensitive feature of lumbar spinal epidural abscess on unenhanced MRI. *Am J Roentgenol* 2017;209(1):176–181.

16. Dieker CA, De Las Casas LE, Davis BR. Retroperitoneal metastatic germ cell tumor presenting as a psoas abscess: A diagnostic pitfall. *Am J Med Sci* 2013;346(1):70–72.

17. Tonolini M, Campari A, Bianco R. Common and unusual diseases involving the iliopsoas muscle compartment: Spectrum of cross-sectional imaging findings. *Abdom Imaging* 2012;37(1):118–139.

18. Tonolini M, Ravelli A, Campari A, et al. Comprehensive MRI diagnosis of sacral osteomyelitis and multiple muscle abscesses as a rare complication of fistulizing Crohn's disease. *J Crohns Colitis* 2011;5(5):473–476.

19. Cronin CG, Gervais DA, Hahn PF, et al. Treatment of deep intramuscular and musculoskeletal abscess: Experience with 99 CT-guided percutaneous catheter drainage procedures. *Am J Roentgenol* 2011;196(5):1182–1188.

20. Cronin CG, Gervais DA, Hahn PF, et al. Anatomy, pathology, imaging and intervention of the iliopsoas muscle revisited. *Emerg Radiol* 2008;15(5):295–310.

21. Doita M, Yoshiya S, Nabeshima Y, et al. Acute pyogenic sacroiliitis without predisposing conditions. *Spine* (Phila Pa 1976) 2003;28(18):E384–E389.

22. Cortes-Blanco A, Martinez-Lazaro R. Lymphoma mimicking a psoas abscess on Ga-67 scintigraphy. *Clin Nucl Med* 2000;25:567–568.

23. Hopkins TJ, Raducan V, Sioutos N, et al. Lumbar lymphoma presenting as psoas abscess/epidural mass with acute cauda equina syndrome. *Spine* 1993;18:774–778.

24. Bocchino M, Valente T, Somma F, et al. Detection of skeletal muscle metastases on initial staging of lung cancer: A retrospective case series. *Jpn J Radiol* 2014;32(3):164–171.

25. Basu S, Mahajan A. Psoas muscle metastasis from cervical carcinoma: Correlation and comparison of diagnostic features on FDG-PET/CT and diffusion-weighted MRI. *World J Radiol* 2014;6(4):125–129.

26. Federle MP, Pan KT, Pealer KM. CT criteria for differentiating abdominal hemorrhage: Anticoagulation or aortic aneurysm rupture? *Am J Roentgenol* 2007;188:1324–1330.

27. Deem SG, Rhee JJ, Piesman M, et al. Acute bacterial prostatitis and prostatic abscess. In: eMedicine 2017. Available at: http://www.emedicine.com/med/topic2845.htm. Accessed on January 5, 2018.

28. Nghiem HT, Kellman GM, Sandberg SA, et al. Cystic lesions of the prostate. *Radiographics* 1990;10:635–650.

29. Lee F, Littrup PJ, Kumasaka GH, et al. The use of transrectal ultrasound in the diagnosis, guided biopsy, staging and screening of prostate cancer. *Radiographics* 1987;7:627–644.

30. Lawton CA, Grignon D, Newhouse JH, et al. Prostate carcinoma. *Radiographics* 1999;19:185–203.

31. Lee DS, Choe HS, Kim HY, et al. Acute bacterial prostatitis and abscess formation. *BMC Urol* 2016;16(1):38(1–8).

32. Schull A, Monzani Q, Bour L, et al. Imaging in lower urinary tract infections. *Diagn Interv Imaging* 2012;93(6):500–508.

33. Meier-Schroers M, Kukuk G, Wolter K, et al. Differentiation of prostatitis and prostate cancer using the Prostate Imaging-Reporting and Data System (PI-RADS). *Eur J Radiol* 2016;85(7):1304–1311.

34. Peralta R, Lisgaris MV, Salata RA, et al. Liver abscess. In: eMedicine 2017. Available at: http://www.emedicine.com/ MED/topic1316.htm. Accessed on January 5, 2018.

35. Brown KT, Gandhi RT, Covey AM, et al. Pylephlebitis and liver abscess mimicking hepatocellular carcinoma. *Hepatobil Pancreat Dis Int* 2003;2:221–225.

36. Lee KHY, O'Malley ME, Kachura JR, et al. Hepatocellular carcinoma: Imaging and imaging-guided intervention. *Am J Roentgenol* 2003;180:1015–1022.

37. Santosh D, Low G. Pylophlebitis with liver abscess secondary to chronic appendicitis: A radiological conundrum. *J Clin Imaging Sci* 2016;6:37.

38. Patel NB, Oto A, Thomas S. Multidetector CT of emergent biliary pathologic conditions. *Radiographics* 2013;33(7): 1867–1888.

39. Alsaif HS, Venkatesh SK, Chan DS, et al. CT appearance of pyogenic liver abscesses caused by Klebsiella pneumoniae. *Radiology* 2011;260(1):129–138.

40. Lee NK, Kim S, Lee JW, et al. CT differentiation of pyogenic liver abscesses caused by Klebsiella pneumoniae vs non-Klebsiella pneumoniae. *Br J Radiol* 2011; 84(1002):518–525.

41. Losanoff JE, Basson MD. Splenic abscess. In: eMedicine 2016. Available at: http://www.emedicine.com/Med/topic2791.htm. Accessed on January 6, 2018.

42. Rabushka LS, Kawashima A, Fishman EK. Imaging of the spleen: CT with supplemental MR examination. *Radiographics* 1994;14:307–332.

43. Bloom, AA. Cholecystitis. In: eMedicine 2017. Available at: http://www.emedicine.com/MED/topic346.htm. Accessed on January 6, 2018.

44. Hanbidge AE, Buckler PM, O'Malley ME, et al. Imaging evaluation for acute pain in the right upper quadrant. *Radiographics* 2004;24:1117–1135.

45. Shojamanesh H, Roy PK. Acalculous cholecystitis. In: eMedicine 2017. Available at: http://www.emedicine.com/Med/topic3526.htm. Accessed on January 6, 2018.

46. Shuman WP, Rogers JV, Rudd TG, et al. Low sensitivity of sonography and cholescintigraphy in acalculous cholecystitis. *Am J Roentgenol* 1984;142:531–534.

47. Mirvis SE, Vainright JR, Nelson AW, et al. The diagnosis of acalculous cholecystitis: A comparison of sonography, scintigraphy and CT. *Am J Roentgenol* 1986;147:1171–1175.

48. Bloom AA, Remy P. Emphysematous cholecystitis. In: eMedicine 2015. Available at: http://www.emedicine.com/med/TOPIC655.HTM. Accessed on January 6, 2018.

49. Shibata T, Yamamoto Y, Yamamoto N, et al. Cholangitis and liver abscess after percutaneous ablation therapy for liver tumors: Incidence and risk factors. *J Vasc Interv Radiol* 2003;14(12):1535–1542.

50. Marangoni G, Ali A, Faraj W, et al. Clinical features and treatment of sump syndrome following hepaticojejunostomy. *Hepatobiliary Pancreat Dis Int* 2011;10(3):261–264.

51. Sung JY, Costerton JW, Shaffer EA. Defense system in the biliary tract against bacterial infection. *Dig Dis Sci* 1992;37(5):689–696.

52. Elmunzer BJ, Noureldin M, Morgan KA, et al. The impact of cholecystectomy after endoscopic sphincterotomy for complicated gallstone disease. *Am J Gastroenterol* 2017;112(10):1596–1602.

53. Lee JG. Diagnosis and management of acute cholangitis. *Nat Rev Gastroenterol Hepatol* 2009;6(9):533–541.

54. Yeom DH, Oh HJ, Son YW, et al. What are the risk factors for acute suppurative cholangitis caused by common bile duct stones? *Gut Liver* 2010;4(3):363–367.

55. Yamashita Y, Ueda K, Abe H, et al. Common bile duct dilatation with stones indicates requirement for early drainage in patients with or without cholangitis. *Gastroenterology Res* 2013;6(6):219–226.

56. Kim SW, Shin HC, Kim HC, et al. Diagnostic performance of multidetector CT for acute cholangitis: Evaluation of a CT scoring method. *Br J Radiol* 2012;85(1014):770–777.

57. Hjartarson JH, Hannesson P, Sverrisson I, et al. The value of magnetic resonance cholangiopancreatography for the exclusion of choledocholithiasis. *Scand J Gastroenterol* 2016;51(10):1249–256.

58. Wang AJ, Wang TE, Lin CC, et al. Clinical predictors of severe gallbladder complications in acute acalculous cholecystitis. *World J Gastroenterol* 2003;9(12):2821–2823.

59. Kawamoto S, Horton KM, Fishman EK. Pseudomembranous colitis: Spectrum of imaging findings with clinical and pathologic correlation. *Radiographics* 1999;19:887–897.

60. Buck JL, Dachman AH, Sobin LH. Polypoid and pseudopolypoid manifestations of inflammatory bowel disease. *Radiographics* 1991;11:293–304.

61. Theodoropoulou A, Koutroubakis IE. Ischemic colitis: clinical practice in diagnosis and treatment. *World J Gastroenterol* 2008;14(48):7302–7308.

62. Osborn AG, Blaser SI, Salzman KL, et al. *Diagnostic Imaging: Brain* (1st ed.). Salt Lake City, UT: Amirsys, 2004.

63. George N, Siket MS. Brain abscess. In: eMedicine 2017. Available at: http://www.emedicine.com/EMERG/topic67.htm. Accessed on January 6, 2018.

64. Smirniotopoulos JG, Murphy FM, Rushing EJ, et al. Patterns of contrast enhancement in the brain and meninges. *Radiographics* 2007;27:525–551.

65. Corr PD. Tuberculosis, CNS. In: eMedicine. 2015. Available at: http://www.emedicine.com/radio/TOPIC720.HTM. Accessed on January 6, 2018.

66. Engin G, Acunas B, Acunas G, et al. Imaging of extrapulmonary tuberculosis. *Radiographics* 2000;20:471–488.

67. Hokelek M. Toxoplasmosis. In: eMedicine 2017. Available at: http://www.emedicine.com/EMERG/topic601.htm. Accessed on January 6, 2018.

68. Khanna PC, Godinho S, Patkar DP, et al. MR spectroscopy-aided differentiation: "Giant" extra-axial tuberuloma masquerading as meningioma. *Am J Neuroradiol* 2006;27:1438–1440.

69. Howes DS, Lazoff M. Encephalitis. In: eMedicine 2017. Available at: http://www.emedicine.com/emerg/topic163.htm. Accessed on January 2018.

70. Kimura K, Dosaka A, Hashimoto Y, et al. Single-photon emission CT findings in acute Japanese encephalitis. *Am J Neuroradiol* 1997;18:465–469.

71. Muccio CF, Caranci F, D'Arco F, et al. Magnetic resonance features of pyogenic brain abscesses and differential diagnosis using morphological and functional imaging studies: A pictorial essay. *J Neuroradiol* 2014;41(3):153–167.

72. Toh CH, Wei KC, Chang CN, et al. Differentiation of pyogenic brain abscesses from necrotic glioblastomas with use of susceptibility-weighted imaging. *Am J Neuroradiol* 2012;33(8):1534–1538.

73. Patkar D, Narang J, Yanamandala R, et al. Central nervous system tuberculosis: Pathophysiology and imaging findings. *Neuroimaging Clin N Am* 2012;22(4):677–705.

74. Villano JL, Koshy M, Shaikh H, et al. Age, gender, and racial differences in incidence and survival in primary CNS lymphoma. *Br J Cancer* 2011;105(9):1414–1418.

75. Gasparovic CM, Roldan CA, Sibbitt WL Jr, et al. Elevated cerebral blood flow and volume in systemic lupus measured by dynamic susceptibility contrast magnetic resonance imaging. *J Rheumatol* 2010;37(9):1834–1843.

76. Rath TJ, Hughes M, Arabi M, et al. Imaging of cerebritis, encephalitis, and brain abscess. *Neuroimaging Clin N Am* 2012;22(4):585–607.

77. Brant WE, Helms CA. *Fundamentals of Diagnostic Radiology* (3rd ed.). Philadephia, PA: Lippincott Williams & Wilkins, 2007.

78. Kuhlman JE, Reyes BL, Hruban RH, et al. Abnormal air-filled spaces in the lung. *Radiographics* 1993;13:47–75.

79. Lalani TA, Kanne JP, Hatfield GA, et al. Imaging findings in systemic lupus erythematosus. *Radiographics* 2004;24:1069–1086.

80. Schnyder PA, Sarraj AM, Duvoisin BE, et al. Pulmonary edema associated with mitral regurgitation: Prevalence of predominant involvement of the right upper lobe. *Am J Roentgenol* 1993;161:33–36.

81. Ryu JH, Swensen SJ. Cystic and cavitary lung diseases: Focal and diffuse. *Mayo Clin Proc* 2003;78:744–752.

82. Harisinghani MG, McLoud TC, Shepard JO, et al. Tuberculosis from head to toe. *Radiographics* 2000;20:449–470.

83. Kim EA, Lee KS, Primack SL, et al. Viral pneumonias in adults: Radiologic and pathologic findings. *Radiographics* 2002;22:S137–S149.

84. Collins J, Stern EJ. Ground-glass opacity at CT: The ABCs. *Am J Roentgenol* 1997;169:355–367.

85. Gluecker T, Capasso P, Schnyder P, et al. Clinical and radiologic features of pulmonary edema. *Radiographics* 1999;19:1507–1531.

86. Milne ENC, Pistolesi M, Miniati M, et al. The radiologic distinction of cardiogenic and noncardiogenic edema. *Am J Roentgenol* 1985;144:879–894.

87. Marom EM, McAdams HP, Erasmus JJ, et al. The many faces of pulmonary aspiration. *Am J Roentgenol* 1999;172:121–128.

88. Gharib AM, Stern EJ. Radiology of pneumonia. *Med Clin North Am* 2001;85(6):1461–1491.

89. Reynolds JH, McDonald G, Alton H, et al. Pneumonia in the immunocompetent patient. *Br J Radiology* 2010;83(996):998–1009.

90. De Roux A, Marcos MA, Garcia E, et al. Viral community-acquired pneumonia in nonimmunocompromised adults. *Chest* 2004;125(4):1343–1351.

91. Nambu A, Ozawa K, Kobayashi N, et al. Imaging of community-acquired pneumonia: Roles of imaging examinations, imaging diagnosis of specific pathogens and discrimination from non-infectious diseases. *World J Radiol* 2014;6(10):779–793.

92. Kim TH, Kim SJ, Ryu YH, et al. Differential CT features of infectious pneumonia versus bronchioloalveolar carcinoma(BAC) mimicking pneumonia. *Eur Radiol* 2006;16(8):1763–1768.

93. Gadkowski B, Stout, J. Cavitary pulmonary disease. *Clin Microbiol Rev* 2008;21(2):305–333.

94. Choi MH, Jung JI, Chung WD, et al. Acute pulmonary complications in patients with hematologic malignancies. *Radiographics* 2014;34(6):1755–1768.

95. Zhou Y, Wang TZ, Liming X. CT features of coronavirus disease 2019 (COVID-19) pneumonia in 62 patients in Wuhan, China. *Am J Roentgenol* 1–8. doi:10.2214/AJR.20.22975.

96. Yan L, Liming X. Coronavirus disease 2019 (COVID-19): Role of chest CT in diagnosis and management. *Am J Roentgenol* 1–7. doi:10.2214/AJR.20.22954.

97. Rui H, Lu H, Hong J, et al. Early clinical and CT manifestations of coronavirus disease 2019 (COVID-19) pneumonia. *Am J Roentgenol* 1–6. doi:10.2214/AJR.20.22961.

6 Non-specific Laboratory Tests in the Critical Care Unit

Charles W. Stratton

CONTENTS

CLINICAL PERSPECTIVE

The terms critical care unit (CCU) and intensive care unit (ICU) are used interchangeably and have been defined as "an organized system for the provision of care to critically ill patients that provides intensive and specialized medical and nursing care, an enhanced capacity for monitoring, and multiple modalities of physiologic organ support to sustain life during a period of life-threatening organ system insufficiency" [1]. Infections on admission to the CCU or acquired while in the CCU are recognized as a major determinant of mortality [2]. In particular, sepsis and septic shock [3] are associated with a high mortality rate for patients admitted to or in the CCU [4,5]. Indeed, septic shock has been defined as "a subset of sepsis in which underlying circulatory, cellular, and metabolic abnormalities are associated with a greater risk of mortality than sepsis alone" [3]. The rapid diagnosis of sepsis and septic shock, combined with appropriate therapy, is a key factor for reducing the morbidity and mortality in this process [6,7]. This chapter will focus primarily on non-specific laboratory tests commonly used in the CCU and their value for the diagnosis of infection as well as for the rapid diagnosis of sepsis and septic shock. Specific laboratory tests such as blood cultures as well as specific therapy for sepsis and septic shock such as fluid resuscitation will be covered in separate chapters.

NON-SPECIFIC SCREENING TESTS IN THE CCU

Fever is a common symptom/sign in patients admitted to the CCU, or new fever may occur in patents already admitted to the CCU; such fevers may involve infectious or non-infectious causes [8–11]. Fever in emergency department (ED) patients and/or CCU patients has been used to predict bacteremia as well as survival. For example, fever seen in the ED patients with sepsis and septic shock has been noted to predict the survival of such patients admitted to the CCU [12]. In the late-twentieth century, fever was often combined with non-specific laboratory tests such as white blood cell (WBC) count and erythrocyte sedimentation rate (ESR) to better predict bacteremia and/or sepsis and septic shock [13–16]. In the first part of the twenty-first century, other clinical signs, comorbid conditions, and additional non-specific laboratory tests were added to better stratify patients in the ED, in order to predict which patients needed to be admitted to the hospital [17,18]. These screening indexes have also been used in CCU patients who already have fever or develop new fever while in the CCU [13–16]. These non-specific laboratory tests used in such screening indexes will be reviewed in this Chapter. This review will be in the order in which these tests have been historically used for evaluating the febrile CCU patient. Both well-established non-specific laboratory screening tests and emerging non-specific laboratory screening tests will be discussed.

WELL-ESTABLISHED NON-SPECIFIC LABORATORY SCREENING TESTS

WHITE BLOOD CELL COUNT WITH LEUKOCYTE DIFFERENTIAL COUNT

An elevated WBC count as well as an increase in the number of immature polymorphonuclear cells (i.e., bands) in the leukocyte differential count have long been considered as markers for infection in a febrile CCU patient [19–21]; however, the band neutrophilia contributes relatively little new information beyond that provided by an elevated WBC. Inflammation due to non-infectious causes as well as due to other factors such as young age [22] and demargination of WBCs after steroid use [23,24] was also recognized to contribute to leukocytosis, which made the use of this marker somewhat controversial [25]. Moreover, the clinical use of the WBC count and the leukocyte differential count as markers for bacterial infection was interrupted in the 1990s by the introduction of fully automated hematology analyzers [26–31]. Evaluation of these automated hematology analyzers found that in normal patients and in patients with reactive disorders, the analyzers' automated differential provides true and accurate results. The diagnostic value of the elevated WBC and the neutrophil left shift in predicting inflammatory and infectious processes has continued to be evaluated using automated hematology analyzers [32–39]. A number of conclusions have been made from these studies. The first, and most important, is that an elevated WBC count has many potential etiologies. A repeat complete blood count with peripheral smear often provides helpful information, with the findings of immature granulocytes (i.e., bands) and toxic granulation suggesting infection. Stressors capable of producing an increase in WBCs include surgery, exercise, trauma, and emotional stress [38]. Leukocytosis is a common finding in infection, and an elevated WBC with immature granulocytes and toxic granulation should prompt clinicians to look for other signs and symptoms of infection.

Erythrocyte Sedimentation Rate

The ESR (or sed rate) reflects plasma viscosity by measuring the distance in millimeters at which red blood cells in a blood plasma fall in a vertical tube during 1 hour [40]. The ESR is not a highly reproducible test, because it is largely determined by acute-phase proteins in the plasma [41]. Acute-phase proteins are proteins that are produced by hepatocytes in response to cytokines; these cytokines are a result of the acute-phase response that is seen with tissue injury, hypoxia, infection, or inflammation [42–44]. An acute-phase protein has been defined as a protein whose plasma concentration increases (positive acute phase protein) or decreases (negative acute phase protein) by at least 25% during an inflammatory process [45]. Such acute-phase proteins are termed either positive or negative acute-phase reactants. Positive acute-phase reactants include a wide variety of proteins such as C-reactive protein (CRP), procalcitonin (PCT), presepsin, apolipoproteins (e.g., serum amyloid A), haptoglobin, alpha-1 antitrypsin, alpha-1-antichymotrypsin, hepcidin, ferritin, fibrinogen, and others. Negative acute-phase reactants primarily include albumin, transferrin, and transthyretin. Acute-phase proteins have variable half-lives and are also influenced by estrogens, end-stage renal disease, obesity (interleukin 6 [IL-6] secretion by adipose tissue), and genetic variants, all of which can thus impact the ESR [46]. In general, the ESR reflects chronic inflammation, whereas other acute-phase proteins such as CRP, PCT, and presepsin reflect acute inflammation [42–45]. Other causes of abnormal elevations of plasma proteins (e.g., immunoglobulins), such as that seen with multiple myeloma [47] or macroglobulinemia [48], may result in an elevated ESR in the absence of a significant acute-phase response. In addition, the ESR is markedly influenced by the morphology and number of erythrocytes; anemia is known to increase the ESR. Increases in the levels of acute-phase proteins per se are generally due to an increased production by hepatocytes, which, in turn, is driven by cytokines produced by macrophages, monocytes, and other cells during the inflammatory process [42–46]. Interleukin 6 is the major inducer of acute-phase proteins [49]. A markedly elevated ESR often has been associated with infection; however, malignancy, renal disease, tissue injury (e.g., ischemia and trauma), and inflammatory connective tissue disorders also are known to cause an elevated ESR [50,51]. The single most common infection causing a markedly elevated ESR is pyelonephritis [51]. Most patients with malignancies with an ESR greater that 100 mm/h have metastases. The ESR is not per se a particularly useful screening test for afebrile CCU patients; however, when seen in febrile CCU patients, the astute clinician will not ignore this result. When used selectively and interpreted with caution, the EST remains a clinically useful test [52–55].

C-Reactive Protein

The CRP was first recognized in 1930 and was isolated in the serum of patients with pneumococcal pneumonia; it was initially named for its capacity to precipitate polysaccharide-F of *Streptococcus pneumoniae* [56]. The CRP was the first acute-phase protein to be recognized as a biomarker for systemic inflammation and tissue damage [57–59]. It is composed of five identical, non-covalently associated subunits arranged in cyclical symmetry around a central pore [60]. This structure is similar to that reported for the C1t subcomponent of the human complement component C1 as well as the amyloid P-component [60,61]. This structural relationship suggests similar functions; the term pentraxin has been proposed to describe these homologous symmetrical proteins [60–62]. The CRP and serum amyloid P are classic "short" pentraxins produced by hepatocytes in response to IL-6 [63], whereas "long" pentraxins are larger proteins in which only the C-terminal halves display the characteristic features of the pentraxin family [64,65]. Long pentraxins are produced by both somatic and immune cells in response to proinflammatory signals other than IL-6 and by engagement of toll-like receptors. The ability of pentraxins to interact with a wide variety of ligands (e.g., microorganisms, the complement system, dead cells, modified plasma proteins, cellular receptors, extracellular matrix components, and growth factors) allows their involvement in many biological functions involving pattern recognition and places them at the interface of innate immunity and inflammation [64–67]. A major function of CRP is its ability to bind phosphocholine [68,69], thus allowing the recognition of pathogens that display this moiety [70] as well as the recognition of the phospholipid of damaged cells [71–73]. The proinflammatory effects of CRP involve the activation of the complement system [74–76] as well as the induction of inflammatory cytokines and tissue factor in monocytes [76–78]. Proinflammatory effects of CRP can be seen when pentameric CRP interacts with phospholipid ligands or when there is a dissociation of pentameric CRP to monomeric CRP [71–73]. In particular, dissociation of pentameric CRP to modified/monomeric CRP can occur within the inflammatory microenvironment, and newly formed monomeric CRP can subsequently exert potent proinflammatory effects on endothelial cells, leukocytes, and platelets [79,80]. In general, CRP concentrations >1 mg/dL indicate clinically significant inflammation, whereas concentrations between 0.3 mg/dL and 1 mg/dL are thought to indicate low-grade inflammation. Such low-grade inflammation is seen with many conditions, including obesity (IL-6 secretion by adipose tissue) and insulin resistance. Conversely, acute inflammation seen with infection and tissue injury results in markedly elevated CRP levels. For the CCU patient, the CRP is more useful than the ESR [81,82]; however, other biomarkers such as immature granulocytes [83] appear to be equally useful. There are other biomarkers such as PCT [84] that are more sensitive (0.91 versus 0.81) but slightly less specific (0.75 versus 0.77) for predicting infection in CCU patients in comparison with the CRP.

PROCALCITONIN

A calcitonin gene-related 32-amino-acid peptide was first described in 1982 [85]; it was soon recognized that this endogenous vasoactive neuropeptide resided in nerve cells distributed throughout the cardiovascular system and was present in all parenchymal tissues [86]. Moreover, this neuropeptide was noted to be elevated in animal models with sepsis as well as in human patients with sepsis [86–88]. A monoclonal immunoradiometric assay was developed for the detection of calcitonin precursors, which identified a 116-amino-acid precursor (i.e., procalcitonin [PCT]). This precursor was initially studied in children with severe infections [89] and then compared with CRP and leucocyte counts in both infants and children [90]. Serum concentrations of PCT in these infected children were noted to correlate with the severity of microbial invasion, to decrease rapidly during antimicrobial therapy, and to provide a better biomarker of bacterial infection than did the CRP and/or leukocyte count [89,90]. Declining PCT levels generally reflect resolution of the infection. Moreover, the measurement of PCT concentrations during multiple organ dysfunctions syndrome (MODS) has been shown to provide more information about the severity and course of MODS than does the measurement of the CRP [91]. The PCT levels between 0.5 and 2 ng/mL imply a moderate risk for progression to systemic inflammation, while the PCT levels greater than 10 ng/mL are associated with a high probability of developing sepsis and septic shock [89–91]. This can be

best appreciated by a review of the kinetic profiles of different biomarkers of bacterial infection; PCT is detectable in serum within 4 hours, with peak levels seen at 12–36 hours [91]. Current data suggest that PCT levels are rarely elevated in viral infections; the reason is thought to be that viral infections stimulate macrophages to synthesize alpha interferon, which, in turn, inhibits the synthesis of tumor necrosis factor (TNF) [89–91]. Tumor necrosis factor must be present in order for tissues to synthesize PCT [89–91]. The PCT also has been widely studied in adult patients [92–94], in particular, in CCU patients [95–101]. One of the issues in evaluating these studies is to decide what parameters should be used. There is generally a trade-off between sensitivity and specificity in a test of diagnostic accuracy. This means that when there is an increase in sensitivity (i.e., the true positive rate), there is usually a reduction in specificity (i.e., the true negative rate). Therefore, sensitivity and specificity may not be the best measures of diagnostic accuracy. Additional ways to evaluate the diagnostic accuracy is to graphically look at the summary receiver-operating characteristic (SROC) of the test or to look at the area under the curve (AUC) for the SROC [101]. The AUC should range from 0.5 to 1 and is a well-established index for estimating the overall diagnostic accuracy. In several of these studies [92,100,101], the area under the SROC for PCT has been calculated for groups of patients. In one of these studies [100], the highest area under the SROC curve (AUC) was found in intensive-care patients; this AUC index for the PCT was 0.88. Low PCT levels (<0.5 ng/mL) have been shown to be useful to rule out the presence of bacteremia; however, levels as low as 0.1 mg/mL did not achieve a 25% reduction in the duration of antimicrobial therapy [98]. In yet another study [97], AUCs were used to predict bacteremia; the AUC for PCT was 0.843 (95% CI 0.796–0.890; p = 0.0001), which was markedly better than the AUCs for CRP, ESR, and WBC count. The PCT has also been used in hematopoietic stem cell transplants (HSCTs) in order to distinguish complications of infectious diseases from complications of non-infectious diseases. The AUC for PCT in this group of HSCT patients was 0.82 versus 0.76 for CRP [102]. In multivariate analysis, the maximum PCT level during a whole course of HSCT ≥2 ng/mL was independently associated with worse overall survival as post-transplant predictor (adjusted hazard ratio 6.42, p = 0.035) [102]. Finally, in patients with suspected bacteremia, the diagnostic accuracy of an elevated PCT was high, with negative predictive values greater than 98% [103]. Although the clinical utility of the PCT continues to evolve [104], there are a number of conclusions and recommendations that can be made at this time. The first is that the evolution of automated assays for PCT detection has greatly increased the sensitivity of PCT testing while decreasing its turnaround time; many of the earlier studies most likely will need to be re-evaluated using these newer highly sensitive assays, as the threshold levels are likely to have changed [105–107]. In healthy adults, PCT levels are usually below 0.05 ng/mL and rapidly increase within 4–6 hours with systemic bacterial infections, with levels of 0.5 to >2 ng/mL suggesting sepsis [91,104,106]. The PCT levels can be high in non-infectious inflammatory conditions such as trauma, surgery, burns, hyperthermia, and neoplasms [91,104,106]. The PCT levels remain high until resolution of the inflammatory event; declining PCT levels with antimicrobial therapy suggest an infectious source [91,104,106]. High PCT levels can also be seen in neonates shortly after birth, but these usually return to normal levels within 48 hours [91,104,106]. Finally, initial data suggest that PCT levels are not affected by the patient's use of non-steroidal anti-inflammatory agents or glucocorticoids [108,109].

EMERGING NON-SPECIFIC LABORATORY SCREENING TESTS

SERUM LACTATE

Until recently, septic shock has been defined as including three components: (1) Systemic arterial hypotension, (2) tissue hypoperfusion associated with organ dysfunction, and (3) hyperlactatemia [110]. A recent revision of the definition of septic shock now includes only two components: (1) Persistent hypotension after fluid resuscitation that requires vasopressors to maintain mean arterial pressure >65 mmHg, and (2) serum lactate level >2 mmol/L [3]. The clinical implication of this recent definition of septic shock is that an increased serum lactate level >2 mmol/L indicates tissue hypoperfusion associated with signs of organ dysfunction in critically ill patients. The serum lactate level as a clinical indicator was first described over 50 years ago by Broder and Weil [111]. At that time, a serum lactate level >4 mmol/L was considered an indicator of shock. Lactic acidosis is frequently encountered in CCU patients and has been recognized as an indicator of both sepsis and increased mortality [112–115]. Initially, it was thought that impaired tissue oxygenations (i.e., oxygen debt) was the main cause of lactic acidosis [116,117]. Although oxygen debt may play an important role in hemorrhagic/post-traumatic shock [117], lactic acidosis during sepsis was noted to be due to excess pyruvate and lactate production, not deficits in tissue oxygen availability [118,119]. More recent studies have demonstrated that early lactate clearance is associated with improved outcome in sepsis and septic shock [120–122]. Importantly, multiple investigators have demonstrated that the serum lactate level at 24 hours (i.e., serum lactate clearance over the first 24 hours of goal-directed therapy) is the best predictor of death [123–127]. Other investigators have suggested that the serum lactate level at 6 hours is the best predictor of death [121,128]. Improvements of the instrumentation for measuring serum lactate levels have been made [129,130], and the serum lactate level that is now considered to be an indicator of shock has been lowered to >2 mmol/L [3]. Regardless of whether serum lactate levels should be measured at 6 hours versus 24 hours, the preponderance of evidence suggests that lactate kinetics in sepsis and septic shock is useful for both children and adults; moreover, further research is justified [115,120–128,131–137].

PRESEPSIN

Presepsin is soluble CD14 (sCD14) [138–140] and is a new biomarker for sepsis [138–142] that performs similarly to PCT [140,143–146]. Importantly, initial levels of presepsin in CCU patients with sepsis have been shown to be a predictive of outcome in a number of comparative studies with PCT [144,147–150]. The story of presepsin begins with the original model for sepsis, which involved the immune response to endotoxin [151]. Innate immune cells are WBCs that mediate innate immunity; these cells include basophils, dendritic cells, eosinophils, Langerhans cells, mast cells, monocytes, macrophages, neutrophils, and natural killer cells [152]. Innate immune cells possess a variety of surface receptors that recognize pathogen-associated molecular patterns (PAMPs); PAMPs may be sugars, peptides, nucleic acids, or anionic polymers [153]. The most important PAMP receptors are toll-like receptors, which are a family of pattern recognition receptors that induce overlapping yet distinct patterns of gene expression that contribute to the inflammatory response [154]. When these toll-like receptors are engaged by a PAMP, innate immune cells such as macrophages produce proinflammatory cytokines [155]. However, macrophage toll-like receptors require CD14 to recognize certain PAMPs such as lipopolysaccharide (LPS) [157,160]. CD14 is a homodimer of a horseshoe-shaped protein, with a pocket for phospholipid; it is a key component of the innate immune response to LPS [156–160]. Moreover, CD14 has the ability to recognize other types of ligands, including peptidoglycan and muramyl dipeptide as well as other surface structures in both gram-positive and gram-negative bacteria [161–164]. After binding of ligands, CD14 expression on the cell surface membrane decreases owing to the cleavage of soluble types of CD14 [165,166]. It is one of these soluble types of CD14 (sCD14-ST) that is presepsin [138,142]. Presepsin is a 64-amino-acid structure that is now considered a regulatory factor and interacts directly with T and B cells [167–169]. Because presepsin is an emerging biomarker for sepsis, evaluations are ongoing. Initial results have been promising [150], and newer studies continue to support the potential value of presepsin as a biomarker for sepsis [170–173]. Several points should be made in terms of the use of such biomarkers. One is that, to date, there is not an ideal biomarker for identifying sepsis in the first few hours [174]; however, currently, presepsin appears to be the most promising biomarker for sepsis. Multimarker approaches that include multiple biomarkers have been used and appear to be promising [175–177]. Only one of these multimarker studies includes presepsin [177]. Finally, continued comparisons of biomarkers are needed as additional studies are published; such steps are being taken [178].

FUTURE BIOMARKERS FOR SCREENING TESTS IN THE CCU

Biomarkers for the assessment of microbial infections in CCU patients have evolved from a simple clinical index [13–16] to the use of proinflammatory cytokines/chemokines [141,179] to the recent use of microRNA (miRNA) molecules [180–183], the last of which have the greatest potential for predicting sepsis due to infection. The miRNAs are evolutionary conserved, small non-coding endogenous RNA molecules with sizes ranging from 19 to 24 nucleotides; miRNAs regulate gene expression at the post-transcriptional level, either through translation repression or by mRNA degradation [181,182]. Because of this basic regulatory role of miRNAs in a wide variety of biological processes, the differential expression of miRNA could theoretically be used as a novel biomarker for specific pathological processes such as sepsis [182,184–186]. For example, multiple miRNAs have been shown to regulate the toll-like receptor pathway in the human innate immune response [187–190]. Importantly, miRNAs are found in blood serum and plasma, where they exhibit marked stability even after repeated cycles of freeze-thawing and long-term storage of frozen samples [191–193]. However, the choice of the starting material can markedly impact the expression profiles of miRNAs that are generated, as different biofluids (e.g., serum versus plasma) can be enriched for a distinct set of miRNAs [191,194,195]. Moreover, there are a variety of expression profiling methods for detecting miRNAs [196,197]. Currently, reverse transcription quantitative real-time polymerase chain reaction (RT-qPCR) is the most commonly used method for miRNA profiling [198–200]. Finally, because transcriptomics experiments are characteristically "noisy," appropriate normalization must be done to minimize technical variation that might otherwise compromise the interpretation of results. Currently, there is a lack of consensus as to an optimal normalization strategy [201,202].

POTENTIAL ROLE OF MICRORNAS AS BIOMARKERS FOR SEPSIS

The use of WBCs to assess bacterial infection and sepsis is still considered useful in the CCU [34–39]. Thus, it is not surprising that initial work focused on miRNA associated with peripheral blood leukocytes [203]. This initial study identified a decreased level of miR-150 in leukocytes and plasma as an early prognostic marker in patients with sepsis [203]. A subsequent study reported that reduced miR-150 serum levels were associated with an unfavorable outcome in patients with critical illnesses, regardless of the presence of sepsis [204]. These studies suggest that circulating miR-150 may be a prognostic marker rather than a diagnostic marker in critically ill patients [203,204]. Other microRNAs have been evaluated as biomarkers for sepsis. For example, miR-15a, miR-15b, miR-16, and miR-122 have been evaluated in several studies [205–207] and are thought to have potential value to distinguish sepsis from systemic inflammatory response syndrome (SIRS). Of note, miR-122 has been recognized as a biomarker of liver injury and liver cell death [208,209] and is upregulated with liver malperfusion as well as with coagulation disorders [210]. In fact, a number of these biomarkers have proven to be more useful for predicting outcome [207,211] than for distinguishing sepsis from SIRS. Additional miRNAs that have been evaluated as biomarkers for sepsis include miR-146a, miR-223, miR-574-5p, and miR-146a [212–215].

Of these, miR-146a and miR-223 appear to be useful in pediatric patients with sepsis [216]. Clearly, the use of miRNAs as biomarkers for sepsis is rapidly evolving and promises to be a useful diagnostic and prognostic tool [217,218]. Importantly, miRNAs regulate the expression of sepsis-related genes, such as IL-6 and TNF, which in turn are regulated by their own expression of these factors [217,219]. A recent proof-of-principle study [220] illustrates the potential usefulness of miRNAs for the differentiation of human sepsis and SIRS. In this study, the levels of circulating miRNAs were noted to be inversely correlated with the levels of circulating inflammatory cytokines. In severe inflammatory disease, the levels of circulating miRNAs changed in the opposite direction to the levels of proinflammatory mediators [220]. In patients with severe sepsis, circulating miRNA levels were lower than in patients with comparably severe non-infectious SIRS [220]. Moreover, six circulating miRNAs (miR-30d-5p, miR-30a-5p, miR-192-5p, miR-26a-5p, miR-23a-5p, and miRNA-191-5p) were noted to be markedly reduced in sepsis compared with non-infectious SIRS; these miRNAs performed well as individual biomarkers of these conditions [220]. Combined together, these six miRNAs were more discriminatory than traditional biomarkers of sepsis such as CRP and PCT and also outperformed any single miRNA [220]. The AUC for the receiver operating characteristic (ROC) curve of these six miRNAs combined was 0.89 after multivariable correction analysis [220]. The number of patients in this study was small and needs to be increased; nonetheless, this study is very promising [220]. Commercialization of this panel of six miRNAs as well as larger studies are needed before this method is routinely used in the CCU. Finally, circulating miRNAs promise to be specific than currently utilized biomarkers for sepsis. In an experimental animal model for sepsis using cecal ligation and puncture [221], Wu et al. demonstrated that the serum levels of seven miRNAs (miR-133a, miR-133b, miR-122, miR-205, miR-1899, miR714, and miR291b) were specifically regulated in gram-positive infection caused by *Staphylococcus aureus*, whereas the serum levels of eight other miRNAs (miR-16, miR-17, miR-20a, miR-26a, miR-26b, miR-106a, miR-106b, and miR-451) were selectively higher in gram-negative sepsis with *Escherichia coli*. Some issues remain to be resolved, such as interstudy variances, standardization of sample collection, data normalization, and analysis; however, currently, miRNAs appear to have the greatest potential as biomarkers for sepsis.

REFERENCES

1. Marshall JC, Bosco L, Adhikari NK, et al. What is an intensive care unit? A report of the task force of the World Federation of Societies of Intensive and Critical Care Medicine. *J Crit Care* 2017;37:270–276.
2. Goncalves-Pereira J, Pereira JM, Ribeiro O, et al. Impact of infection on admission and of the process of care on mortality of patients admitted to the Intensive Care Unit: The INFAUCI study. *Clin Microbiol Infect* 2014;20:1308–1315.
3. Shankar-Hari M, Phillips GS, Levy ML, et al. Developing a new definition and assessing new clinical criteria for septic shock: For the Third International Consensus Definitions for Sepsis and Septic Shock (Sepsis-3). *JAMA* 2016;315:775–787.

4. Honselmann KC, Buthut F, Heuwer B, et al. Long-term mortality and quality of live in intensive care patients treated for pneumonia and/or sepsis: Predictors of mortality and live in patients with sepsis/pneumonia. *J Crit Care* 2015;30:721–726.

5. Damiani E, Donati A, Serafini G, et al. Effect of performance improvement programs on compliance with sepsis bundles and mortality: A systematic review and meta-analysis of observational studies. *PLOS ONE* 2015;10:e0125827.

6. Bloos F, Reinhart K. Rapid diagnosis of sepsis. *Virulence* 2014;1:154–160.

7. Gotts JE, Matthay MA. Sepsis: Pathophysiology and clinical management. *BMJ* 2016;353:i1585.

8. Cunha BA. Fever in the critical care unit. *Crit Care Clin* 1998;14:1–14.

9. O'Grady NP, Barie PS, Bartlett JG, et al. Practice guidelines for evaluating new fever in critically ill adult patients. Task Force of the Society of Critical Care Medicine and the Infectious Diseases Society of America. *Clin Infect Dis* 1998;26:1042–1059.

10. O'Grady NP, Barie PS, Bartlett JG, et al. Guidelines for evaluation of new fever in critically ill adult patients: 2008 update from the American College of Critical Care Medicine and the Infectious Diseases Society of America. *Crit Care Med* 2008;36:1330–1349.

11. Oncu S. A clinical outline to fever in intensive care patients. *Minerva Anesthesiol* 2013;79:408–418.

12. Sunden-Cullberg J, Rylance R, Svefors J, et al. Fever in the emergency department predicts survival of patients with severe sepsis and septic shock admitted to the ICU. *Crit Care Med* 2017;45:591–599.

13. Mellors JW, Horwitz RI, Harvey MR, Horwitz SM. A simple index to identify occult bacterial infection in adults with acute unexplained fever. *Arch Intern Med* 1987;147:666–671.

14. Mellors JW, Kelly JJ, Gusberg RJ, et al. A simple index to estimate the likelihood of bacterial infection in patients developing fever after abdominal surgery. *Am Surg* 1988;54:558–564.

15. Leibovici L, Cohen O, Wysenbeek AJ. Occult bacterial infection in adults with unexplained fever. Validation of a diagnostic index. *Arch Intern Med* 1990;150:1270–1272.

16. Midha NK, Stratton CW. Laboratory tests in critical care. *Crit Care Clin* 1998;14:15–34.

17. Falguera M, Trujillano J, Caro S, et al. A prediction rule for estimating the risk of bacteremia in patients with community-acquired pneumonia. *Clin Infect Dis* 2009;49:409–416.

18. Lee J, Hwang SS, Kim K, et al. Bacteremia prediction model using a common clinical test in patients with community-acquired pneumonia. *Am J Emerg Med* 2014;32:700–704.

19. Weitzman M. Diagnostic utility of white blood cell count and differential cell counts. *Am J Dis Child* 1975;129:1183–1189.

20. Werman HA, Brown CG. White blood cell count and differential count. *Emerg Med Clin North Am* 1986;4:41–58.

21. Shapira MR, Greenfield S. The complete blood count and leukocyte differential count. *Ann Intern Med* 1987;106:65–74.

22. Luszczak M. Evaluation and management of infants and young children with fever. *Am Fam Physician* 2001;64:1219–1226.

23. Dale DC, Fauci AS, Guerry D IV, Wolff SM. Comparison of agents producing a neutrophilic leukocytosis in man. Hydrocortisone, prednisone, endotoxin, and etiocholanolone. *J Clin Infect* 1975;56:808–813.

24. Shoenfeld Y, Gurewich Y, Gallant LA, Pinkhas J. Prednisone-induced leukocytosis. Influence of dosage, method and duration of administration on the degree of leukocytosis. *Am J Med* 1981;71:773–778.

25. Kuppermann N, Walton EA. Immature neutrophils in the blood smears of young febrile children. *Arch Pediatr Adolesc Med* 1999;153:261–266.

26. Hyun BH, Gulati GL, Ashton JK. Differential leukocyte count: Manual or automated, what should it be? *Yonsei Med J* 1991;32:283–291.

27. Hallawell R, O'Malley C, Hussein S, et al. An evaluation of the sysmex NE-8000 hematology analyzer. *Am J Clin Pathol* 1991;96:594–601.

28. Thalhammer-Scherrer R, Knobl P, Korninger L, Schwarzinger I. Automated five-part white blood cell differential counts. Efficiency of software-generated white blood cell suspect flags of the hematology analyzers sysmex SE-9000, sysmex NE-8000, and Coulter STKS. *Arch Pathol Lab Med* 1997;121:573–577.

29. Korninger L, Mustafa G, Schwarzinger I. The haematology analyser SF-3000: Performance of the automated white blood cell differential count in comparison to the haematology analyser NE-1500. *Clin Lab Haematol* 1998;20:81–86.

30. Siekmeier R, Bierlich A, Jaross W. The white blood cell differential: Three methods compared. *Clin Chem Lab Med* 2001;39:432–445.

31. White blood cell counts: Reference methodology. *Clin Lab Med* 2015;35:11–24.

32. Seebach JD, Morant R, Ruegg R, et al. The diagnostic value of the neutrophil left shift in predicting inflammatory and infectious disease. *Am J Clin Pathol* 1997;107:582–591.

33. Cornbleet PJ. Clinical utility of the band count. *Clin Lab Med* 2002;22:101–136.

34. Ishimine N, Honda T, Yoshizawa A, et al. Combination of white blood cell count and left shift level real-timely reflects a course of bacterial infection. *J Clin Lab Anal* 2013;27:407–411.

35. Nierhaus A, Klatte S, Linssen J, et al. Revisiting the white blood cell count: Immature granulocytes count as a diagnostic marker to discriminate between SIRS and sepsis—A prospective, observational study. *BMC Immunol* 2013;14:8.

36. De S, Williams GJ, Hayen A, et al. Value of white blood cell count in prediction serious bacterial infection in febrile children under 5 years of age. *Arch Dis Child* 2014;99:493–499.

37. De S, Williams GJ, Hayen A, et al. Republished: Value of white cell count in predicting serious bacterial infection in febrile children under 5 years of age. *Postgrad Med J* 2015;91:493–499.

38. Riley LK, Rupert J. Evaluation of patients with leukocytosis. *Am Fam Physician* 2015;92:1004–1011.

39. Honda T, Uehara T, Matsumoto G, et al. Neutrophil left shift and white blood cell count as markers of bacterial infection. *Clin Chim Acta* 2016;457:46–53.

40. Wintrobe MM, Landsberg JW. A standardized technique for the blood sedimentation test. *Am J Med Sci* 2013;346(1935):148–153.

41. Bedell SE, Bush BT. Erythrocyte sedimentation rate. From folklore to facts. *Am J Med* 1985;78:1001–1009.

42. Moshage H. Cytokines and the hepatic acute phase response. *J Pathol* 1997;181:257–266.

43. Gabay C, Kushner I. Acute-phase proteins and other systemic responses to inflammation. *N Engl J Med* 1999;340:448–454.

44. Ray S, Patel SK, Kumar V, et al. Differential expression of serum/plasma proteins in various infectious diseases: Specific or nonspecific signatures. *Proteomics Clin Appl* 2014;8:53–72.

45. Kushner I. The phenomenon of the acute phase response. *Ann NY Acad Sci* 1982;389:39–48.

46. Calvin J, Neale G, Fotherby KJ, Price CP. The relative merits of acute phase proteins in the recognition of inflammatory conditions. *Ann Clin Biochem* 1988;25:60–66.
47. Alexandrakis MG, Passam FH, Ganotakis ES, et al. The clinical and prognostic significance of erthryocyte sedimentation rate (ESR), serum interleukin-6 (IL-6) and acute phase protein levels in multiple myeloma. *Clin Lab Haematol* 2003;25:41–46.
48. Ballas SK. The erythrocyte sedimentation rate, rouleaux formation and hyperviscosity syndrome. Theory and fact. *Am J Clin Pathol* 1975;63:45–48.
49. Gauldie J Richards C, Harnish D, et al. Interferon beta 2/B-cell stimulatory factor type 2 shares identity with monocyte-derived hepatocyte-stimulating factor and regulates the major acute phase protein response in liver cells. *Proc Natl Acad Sci USA* 1987;84:7251–7255.
50. Wyler DJ. Diagnostic implications of markedly elevated erythrocyte sedimentation rate: A reevaluation. *South Med J* 1977;70:1428–1430.
51. Fincher RM, Page MI. Clinical significance of extreme elevation of the erythrocyte sedimentation rate. *Arch Intern Med* 1986;146:1581–1583.
52. Sox HC Jr, Liang MH. The erythrocyte sedimentation rate. Guidelines for rational use. *Ann Intern Med* 1986 104:515–523.
53. Brigden M. The erythrocyte sedimentation rate. Still a helpful test when used judiciously. *Postgrad Med* 1998;103:257–262.
54. Brigden ML. Clinical utility of the erythrocyte sedimentation rate. *Am Fam Physician* 1999;60:1443–1450.
55. Litao MK, Kamat D. Erythrocyte sedimentation rate and C-reactive protein: How best to use them in clinical practice. *Pediatr Ann* 2014;43:417–420.
56. Tillett WS, Francis T. Serological reactions in pneumonia with a non-protein somatic fraction of pneumococcus. *J Exp Med* 1930;52:561–571.
57. Morley JJ, Kushner I. Serum C-reactive protein levels in disease. *Ann NY Acad Sci* 1982;389:406–418.
58. Pepys MB, Baltz ML. Acute phase proteins with special reference to C-reactive protein and related proteins (pentaxins) and serum amyloid A protein. *Adv Immunol* 1983;34:141–212.
59. Pepys MB, Hirschfeld GM. C-reactive protein: A critical update. *J Clin Invest* 2003;111:1805–1812.
60. Osmand AP, Friedenson B, Gewurz H, et al. Characterization of C-reactive protein and the complement subcomponent C1t as homologous proteins displaying cyclic pentameric symmetry (pentraxins). *Proc Natl Acad Sci USA* 1977;74:739–743.
61. Emsley J, White HE, O'Hara BP, et al. Structure of pentameric human serum amyloid P component. *Nature* 1994;367:338–345.
62. Gewurz H, Zhang XH, Lint TF. Structure and function of the pentraxins. *Curr Opin Immunol* 1995;7:54–64.
63. Goodman AR, Cardozo T, Abagyan R, et al. Long pentraxins: An emerging group of proteins with diverse functions. *Cytokine Growth Factor Rev* 1996;7:191–202.
64. Deban L, Bottazzi B, Garlanda C, et al. Pentraxins: Multifunctional proteins at the interface of innate immunity and inflammation. *Biofactors* 2009;35:138–145.
65. Inforzato A, Bottazzi B, Garlanda C, et al. Pentraxins in humoral immunity. *Adv Exp Med Biol* 2012;946:1–20.
66. Vilahur G, Badimon L. Biological actions of pentraxins. *Vascul Pharmacol* 2015;73:38–44.
67. Daigo K, Inorzato A, Barajon I, et al. Pentrazins in the activation and regulation of innate immunity. *Immunol Rev* 2016;274:202–217.
68. Thompson D, Pepys MB, Wood SP. The physiological structure of human C-reactive protein and its complex with phosphocholine. *Structure* 1999;7:169–177.
69. Volanakis JE. Human C-reactive protein: Expression, structure, and function. *Mol Immunol* 2001;38:189–197.
70. Clark SE, Weiser JN. Microbial modulation of host immunity with the small molecule phosphorylcholine. *Infect Immun* 2013;81:392–401.
71. Marnell L, Mold C, Du Clos TW. C-reactive protein: Ligands, receptors and role in inflammation. *Clin Immunol* 2005;117:104–111.
72. Bochkov VN. Inflammatory profile of oxidized phospholipids. *Throm Haemost* 2007;97:348–354.
73. Leitinger N. The role of phospholipid oxidation products in inflammatory and autoimmune diseases: Evidence from animal models and in humans. *Subcell Biochem* 2008;49:325–350.
74. Biro A, Rovo Z, Papp D, et al. Studies on the interactions between C-reactive protein and complement proteins. *Immunology* 2007;121:40–50.
75. Klegeris A, Singh EA, McGeer PL. Effects of C-reactive protein and pentosan polysulphate on human complement activation. *Immunology* 2002;106:381–388.
76. Salazar J, Martinez MS, Chavez-Castillo M, et al. C-reactive protein: An in-depth look into structure, function, and regulation. *Int Sch Res Notices* 2014;653045.
77. Cermak J, Key NS, Bach RR, et al. C-reactive protein induces human peripheral blood monocytes to synthesize tissue factor. *Blood* 1993;82:513–520.
78. Egorina EM, Sovershaev MA, Hansen JB. The role of tissue factor in systemic inflammatory response syndrome. *Blood Coagul Fibrin* 2011;22:451–456.
79. Wu Y, Potempa LA, El Kebir D, Filep JG. C-reative protein and inflammation: Conformational changes affect function. *Biol Chem* 2015;396:1181–1197.
80. Trial J, Potempa LA, Entman ML. The role of C-reactive protein in innate and acquired inflammation: New perspectives. *Inflamm Cell Signal* 2016;3:e1409.
81. Vincent JL, Donadello K, Schmit X. Biomarkers in the critically ill patient: C-reactive protein. *Crit Care Clin* 2011;27:241–251.
82. Lelubre C, Anselin S, Zouaoui Boudjeltia K, et al. Interpretation of C-reactive protein concentrations in critically ill patients. *Biomed Res Int* 2013;124021.
83. Van der Geest PJ, Mohseni M, Brouwer R, et al. Immature granulocytes predict microbial infection and its adverse sequelae in the intensive care unit. *J Crit Care* 29:523–527.
84. Wu JY, Lee SH, Shen CJ, et al. Use of serum procalcitonin to detect bacterial infection in patients with autoimmune diseases: A systematic review and meta-analysis. *Arthrit Rheum* 2012;64:3034–3042.
85. Amara SG, Jonas V, Rosenfeld MG, et al. Alternative RNA processing in calcitonin gene expression generates mRNAs encoding different polypeptide products. *Nature* 1982;298:240–244.
86. Russell FA, King R, Smillie SJ, et al. Calcitonin gene-related peptide: Physiology and pathophysiology. *Physiol Rev* 2014;94:1099–1142.
87. Joyce CD, Fiscus RR, Wang X, et al. Calcitonin gene-related peptide levels are elevated in patients with sepsis. *Surgery* 1990;108:1097–1101.
88. Arnalich F, Sanchez JF, Martinez M, et al. Changes in plasma concentrations of vasoactive neuropeptides in patients with sepsis and shock. *Life Sci* 1995;56:75–81.

89. Assicot M, Gendrel D, Carsin H, et al. High serum procalcitonin concentrations in patients with sepsis and infection. *Lancet* 1993;341:515–518.

90. Hatherill M, Tibby SM, Sykes K, et al. Diagnostic markers of infection: Comparison of procalcitonin with C reactive protein and leucocyte count. *Arch Dis Child* 1999;81:417–421.e.

91. Meisner M. Update on procalcitonin measurements. *Ann Lab Med* 2014;34:263–273.

92. Riedel S, Melendez JS, An AT, et al. Procalcitonin as a marker for the detection of bacteremia and sepsis in the emergency department. *Am J Clin Pathol* 2011;135:182–189.

93. Mitsuma SF, Mansour MK, Dekker JP, et al. Promising new assays and technologies for the diagnosis and management of infectious diseases. *Clin Infect Dis* 2013;56:996–1002.

94. Sridharan P, Chamberlain RS. The efficacy of procalcitonin as a biomarker in the management of sepsis: Slaying dragons or tilting at windmills? *Surg Infect (Larchmt)* 2013;14:489–511.

95. Prkno A, Wacker C, Brunkhorst FM, Schlattmann P. Procalcitonin-guided therapy in intensive care unit patients with severe sepsis and septic shock—A systematic review and meta-analysis. *Crit Care* 2013;17:R291.

96. Schuetz P, Raad I, Amin DN. Using procalcitonin-guided algorithms to improve antimicrobial therapy in ICU patients with respiratory infections and sepsis. *Curr Opin Crit Care* 2013;19:453–460.

97. Leli C, Cardaccia A, Ferranti M, et al. Procalcitonin better that C-reactive protein, erythrocyte sedimentation rate, and white blood cell count in predicting DNAemia in patients with sepsis. *Scand J Infect Dis* 2014;46:745–752.

98. Shehabi Y, Sterba M, Garrett PM, et al. Procalcitonin algorithm in critically ill adults with undifferentiated infection or suspected sepsis. A randomized controlled trial. *Am J Respir Crit Care Med* 2014;190:1102–1110.

99. Davies J. Procalcitonin. *J Clin Pathol* 2015;68:675–679.

100. Hoeboer SH, van der Geest PJ, Nieboer D, Groeneveld AB. The diagnostic accuracy of procalcitonin for bacteraemia: A systematic review and meta-analysis. *Clin Microb Infect* 2015;21:474–481.

101. van der Geest PJ, Mohseni M, Linssen J, et al. The intensive care infection score—A novel marker for the prediction of infection and its severity. *Crit Care* 2016;20:180.

102. Koya J, Nannya Y, Ichikawa M, Kurokawa M. The clinical role of procalcitonin in hematopoietic SCT. *Bone Marrow Transplant* 2012;47:1326–1331.

103. Oussalah A, Ferrand J, Fihine-Tresarrieu P, et al. Diagnostic accuracy of procalcitonin for predicting blood culture results in patients with suspected bloodstream infection: An observational study of 35,343 consecutive patients (A STROBE-Compliant Article). *Medicine* 2015;94:e1774.

104. Gilbert DN. Use of plasma procalcitonin levels as an adjunct to clinical microbiology. *J Clin Microbiol* 2010;48:2325–2329.

105. Dipalo M, Guido L, Micca G, et al. Multicenter comparison of automated procalcitonin immunoassays. *Pract Lab Med* 2015;2:22–28.

106. Fortunato A. A new sensitive automated assay for procalcitonin detection: LIASON® Brahms PCT® II GEN. *Pract Lab Med* 2016;6:1–7.

107. Ceriotti F, Marino I, Motta A, Carobene A. Analytical evaluation of the performance of Diazyme and BRAHMS procalcitonin applied to Roche Cobas in comparison with BRAHMS PCT-sensitive Kryptor. *Clin Chem Lab Med* 2017;56:162–169.

108. Preas HL II, Nylen ES, Snider RH, et al. Effects of anti-inflammatory agents on serum levels of calcitonin precursors during experimental endotoxemia. *J Infect Dis* 2001;184:373–376.

109. Perren A, Derutii B, Lepori M, et al. Influence of steroids on procalcitonin and C-reactive protein in patients with COPD and community-acquired pneumonia. *Infection* 2008;36:163–166.

110. Dellinger RP, Levy MM, Rhodes A, et al. Surviving sepsis campaign: International guidelines for management of severe sepsis and septic shock, 2012. *Crit Care Med* 2013;41:580–637.

111. Broder G, Weil MH. Excess lactate: An index of reversibility of shock in human patients. *Science* 1964;143:1457–1459.

112. Mizock BA, Falk JL. Lactic acidosis in critical illness. *Crit Care Med* 1992;20:80–93.

113. Gutierrez G, Wulf ME. Lactic acidosis in sepsis: A commentary. *Intensive Care Med* 1996;22:6–16.

114. Fall PJ, Szerlip HM. Lactic acidosis: From sour milk to septic shock. *J Intensive Care Med* 2005;20:255–271.

115. Mikkelsen ME, Miltiades AN, Gaieski DR, et al. Serum lactate is associated with mortality in severe sepsis independent of organ failure and shock. *Crit Care Med* 2009;37:1670–1677.

116. Dunham CM, Siegel JH, Weireter L, et al. Oxygen debt and metabolic academia as quantitative predictors of mortality and the severity of the ischemic insult in hemorrhagic shock. *Crit Care Med* 1991;19:231–243.

117. Rixen D, Siegel JH. Bench-to-bedside review: Oxygen debt and its metabolic correlates as quantifiers of the severity of hemorrhagic and post-traumatic shock. *Crit Care* 2005;9:441–453.

118. Gore DC, Jahoor F, Hibbert JM, DeMaria EJ. Lactic acidosis during sepsis is related to increased pyruvate production, not deficits in tissue oxygen availability. *Ann Surg* 1996;224:97–102.

119. Hunt TK. Excess pyruvate and lactate production occurs in sepsis and is not caused by anaerobic glycolysis. *Ann Surg* 1997;226:108–109.

120. Leevraut J, Ciebiera JP, Chave S, et al. Mild hyperlactatemia in stable septic patients is due to impaired lactate clearance rather than overproduction. *Am J Respir Crit Care Med* 1998;157:1021–1026.

121. Nguyen HB, Rivers EP, Knoblich BP. Early lactate clearance is associated with improved outcome in severe sepsis and septic shock. *Crit Care Med* 2004;32:1637–1642.

122. Trzeciak S, Dellinger RP, Chansky ME, et al. Serum lactate as a predictor of mortality in patients with infection. *Intensive Care Med* 2007;33:970–977.

123. Friedman G, Berlot G, Kahn RJ, Vincent JL. Combined measurement of blood lactate concentrations and gastric intramucosal pH in patients with severe sepsis. *Crit Care Med* 1995;23:1184–1193.

124. Bakker J, Gris P, Coffermils M, et al. Serial blood lactate levels can predict the development of multiple organ failure following septic shock. *Am J Surg* 1996;171:221–226.

125. McNeilis J, Marini CP, Jurkiewicz A, et al. Prolonged lactate clearance is associated with increased mortality in the surgical intensive care unit. *Am J Surg* 2001;182:481–485.

126. Husain FA, Martin MJ, Mullenix PS, et al. Serum lactate and base deficit as predictors of mortality and morbidity. *Am J Surg* 2003;185:485–491.

127. Marty P, Roquilly A, Vallee F, et al. Lactate clearance for death prediction in severe sepsis or septic shock patients during the first 24 hours in intensive care unit: An observational study. *Ann Intensive Care* 2013;3:3.

128. Lee YK, Hwang SY, Shin TG, et al. Prognostic value of lactate and central venous oxygen saturation after early resuscitation in sepsis patients. *PLOS ONE* 2016;11:e0153305.

129. Nielsen C, Pedersen LT, Lindholt JS et al. An automated plasma D-lactate assay with a new sample preparation method to prevent interference from L-lactate and L-lactate dehydrogenase. *Scand J Clin Lab Infest* 2011;71:507–514.

130. Pundir CS, Narwal V, Batra B. Determination of lactic acid with special emphasis on biosensing methods: A review. *Biosens Bioelectron* 2016;86:777–790.

131. Dettmer M, Holthaus CV, Fuller BM. The impact of serial lactate monitoring on emergency department resuscitation interventions and clinical outcomes in severe sepsis and septic shock: An observational cohort study. *Shock* 2015;43:55–61.

132. Gu WJ, Zhang Z, Bakker J. Early lactate clearance-guided therapy in patients with sepsis: A meta-analysis with trial sequential analysis of randomized controlled trials. *Intensive Care Med* 2015;41:1862–1863.

133. Scott HF, Brou L, Deakyne SJ, et al. Lactate clearance and normalization and prolonged organ dysfunction in pediatric sepsis. *J Pediatr* 2016;170:149–155.

134. Lee SM, An WS. New clinical criteria for septic shock: Serum lactate level as new emerging vital sign. *J Thorac Dis* 2016;8:1388–1390.

135. Javed A, Guirgis FW, Sterling SA, et al. Clinical predictors of early death from sepsis. *J Crit Care* 2017;42:30–34.

136. Bou Chebl R, El Khuri C, Shami A, et al. Serum lactate is an independent predictor of hospital mortality in critically ill patients in the emergency department: A retrospective study. *Scand J Trauma Resusc Emerg Med* 2017;25:69.

137. Scott HF, Brou L, Deakyne SJ, et al. Association between early lactate levels and 30-day mortality in clinically suspected sepsis in children. *JAMA Pediatr* 2017;171:249–255.

138. Yaegashi Y, Shirakawa K, Sato N, et al. Evaluation of a newly identified soluble CD14 subtype as a marker for sepsis. *J Infect Chemother* 2005;11:234–238.

139. Okamura Y, Yokoi H. Development of a point-of-care assay system for measurement of presepsin (sCD14-ST). *Clin Chim Acta* 2011;412:2157–2161.

140. Shozushima T, Takahashi G, Matsumoto N, et al. Usefulness of presepsin (sCD14-ST) measurements as a marker for the diagnosis and severity of sepsis that satisfied diagnostic criteria of systemic inflammatory response syndrome. *J Infect Chemother* 2011;17:764–769.

141. Faix JD. Biomarkers of sepsis. *Crit Rev Clin Lab Sci* 2013;50:23–36.

142. Faix JD. Presepsin—The new kid on the sepsis block. *Clin Biochem* 2014;47:503–504.

143. Ulla M, Pizzolota E, Lucchiari M, et al. Diagnostic and prognostic value of presepsin in the management of sepsis in the emergency department: A multicenter prospective study. *Crit Care* 2013;17:R168.

144. Masson S, Caironi P, Spanuth E, et al. Presepsin (soluble CD14 subtype) and procalcitonin levels for mortality prediction in sepsis: Data from the Albumin Italian Outcome Sepsis trial. *Crit Care* 2014;18:R6.

145. Masson S, Caironi P, Fanizza C, et al. Circulating presepsin (soluble CD14 subtype) as a marker of host response in patients with severe sepsis or septic shock: Data from the multicenter, randomized ALBIOS trail. *Intensive Care Med* 2015;41:12–20.

146. Behnes M, Bertsch T, Lepiorz D, et al. Diagnostic and prognostic utility of soluble CD 14 subtype (presepsin) for severe sepsis and septic shock during the first week of intensive care treatment. *Crit Care* 2014;18:507.

147. Enguix-Armada A, Escobar-Conesa R, Garcia-De La Torre A, De La Torre-Prados MV. Usefulness of several biomarkers in the management of septic patients: C-reactive protein, procalcitonin, presepsin and mid-regional pro-adrenomedullin. *Clin Chem Lab Med* 2016;54:163–168.

148. Leli C, Ferranti M, Marrano U, et al. Diagnostic accuracy of presepsin (sCD14-ST) and procalcitonin for prediction of bacteraemia and bacterial DNAaemia in pateints with suspected sepsis. *J Med Microbiol* 2016;65:713–719.

149. Tsujimoto K, Hata A, Fujita M, et al. Presepsin and procalcitonin as biomarkers of systemic bacterial infection in patients with rheumatoid arthritis. *Int J Rheum Dis* 2016;21:1406–1413.

150. Wu CC, Lan HM, Han ST, et al. Comparison of diagnostic accuracy in sepsis between presepsin, procalcitonin, and C-reactive protein: A systematic review and meta-analysis. *Ann Intensive Care* 2017;7:91.

151. Heumann D, Roger T. Initial responses to endotoxins and Gram-negative bacteria. *Clin Chim Acta* 2002;323:59–72.

152. Brubaker SW, Bonham KS, Zanoni I, Kagan JC. Innate immune pattern recognition: A cell biological perspective. *Annu Rev Immunol* 2015;33:257–290.

153. Akira S, Uematsu S, Takeuchi O. Pathogen recognition and innate immunity. *Cell* 2006;124:783–801.

154. Takeda K, Akira S. Toll-like receptors. *Curr Protoc Immunol* 2015;109:1–10.

155. Janssens S, Beyaert R. Role of Toll-like receptors in pathogen recognition. *Clin Microbiol Rev* 2003;16:637–646.

156. Di Gioia M, Zanoni I. Toll-like receptor co-receptors as master regulators of the immune response. *Mol Immunol* 2015;63:143–152.

157. Triantafilou M, Triantafilou K. Lipopolysaccharide recognition: CD14, TLRs and the LPS activation cluster. *Trends Immunol* 2002;23:301–304.

158. Schumann RR. Function of lipopolysaccharide (LPS)-binding protein (LBP) and CD14, the receptor of LPS/LBP complexes: A short review. *Res Immunol* 1992;143:11–15.

159. Ziegler-Heitbrock HW, Ulevitch RJ. CD14: Cell surface receptor and differentiation marker. *Immunol Today* 1003;14:121–125.

160. Schumann RR, Rietschel ET, Loppnow H. The role of CD14 and lipopolysaccharide-binding protein (LBP) in the activation of different cell types by endotoxin. *Med Microbiol Immunol* 1994;183:279–297.

161. Weidemann B, Schletter J, Dziarski R, et al. Specific binding of soluble peptidoglycan and muramyl dipeptide to CD14 on human monocytes. *Infect Immun* 1997;65:858–864.

162. Rietschel ET, Schletter J, Weidermann B, et al. Lipopolysaccharide and peptidoglycan: CD14-dependent bacterial inducers of inflammation. *Microb Drug Resist* 1998;4:37–44.

163. Muhvic D, El-Samalouti V, Flad HD, et al. The involvement of CD14 in the activation of human monocytes by peptidoglycan monomers. *Mediatorfs Inflamm* 2001;10:155–162.

164. De Marzi MC, Todone M, Ganem MB, et al. Peptidoglycan recognition protein-peptidoglycan complexes increase monocyte/macrophage activation and enhance the inflammatory response. *Immunology* 2015;145:429–442.

165. Pedron T, Girard R, Chaby R. Variation of LPS-binding capacitiy, epitope expression, and shedding of membrane-bound CD14 during differentiation of human monocytes. *J Immunol* 1995;155:1460–1471.

166. Le-Barillec K, Si-Tahar M, Balloy V, Chignard M. Proteolysis of monocyte CD14 by human leukocyte elastase inhibits lipopolysaccharide-mediated cell activation. *J Clin Infects* 1999;103:1039–1046.

167. Mussap M, Noto A, Fravega M, Fanos V. Soluble CD14 subtype presepsin (sCD14-ST) and lipopolysaccharide binding protein (LBP) in neonatal sepsis: New clinical and analytical perspectives for two old biomarkers. *J Matern Fetal Neonatal Med* 2011;24(Suppl 2):12–14.

168. Rey Nores JE, Bensussan A, Vita N, et al. Soluble CD14 acts as a negative regulator of human T cell activation and function. *Eur J Immunol* 1999;29:256–275.

169. Arias MA, Rey Nores JE, Vita N, et al. Cutting edge: Human B cell function is regulated by interaction with soluble CD14: Opposite effects on IgG1 and IgE production. *J Immunol* 2000;164:3480–3486.

170. Montaldo P, Rosso R, Santantonio A, et al. Presepsin for the detection of early-onset sepsis in preterm newborns. *Pediatr Res* 2017;81:329–334.

171. Stoma I, Karpov I, Uss A, et al. Diagnostic value of sepsis biomarkers in hematopoietic stem cell transplant recipients in a condition of high prevalence of gram-negative pathogens. *Hematol Oncol Stem Cell Ther* 2017;10:15–21.

172. Yu H, Qi Z, Hang C, et al. Evaluating the value of dynamic procalcitonin and presepsin measurements for patients with severe sepsis. *Am J Emerg Med* 2017;35:835–841.

173. Matera G, Quirino A, Peronace C, et al. Soluble CD14 Subtype—A new biomarker in predicting the outcome of critically ill septic patients. *Am J Med Sci* 2017;353:543–551.

174. Rogic D, Juros GF, Petrik J, Vrancic AL. Advances and pitfalls in using laboratory biomarkers for the diagnosis and management of sepsis. *EJIFCC* 2017;28:114–121.

175. Han JH, Nachamkin I, Coffin SE, et al. Use of a combination biomarker algorithm to identify medical intensive care unit patients with suspected sepsis at very low likelihood of bacterial infection. *Antimicrob Agents Chemother* 2015;59:6494–6500.

176. Kelly BJ, Lautenbach E, Nachamkin I, et al. Combined biomarkers discriminate a low likelihood of bacterial infection among surgical intensive care unit patients with suspected sepsis. *Diagn Microbiol Infect Dis* 2016;85:109–115.

177. Kim H, Hur M, Moon HW, et al. Multi-marker approach using procalcitonin, presepsin, galectin-3, and soluble suppression of tumorigenicity 2 for the prediction of mortality in sepsis. *Ann Intensive Care* 2017;7:27.

178. Hayashida K, Kondo Y, Hara Y, et al. Head-to-head comparison of procalcitonin and presepsin for the diagnosis of sepsis in critically ill adult patients: A protocol for a systematic review and meta-analysis. *BMJ Open* 2017;7:e014305.

179. Parlato M, Cavaillon JM. Host response biomarkers in the diagnosis of sepsis: A general overview. *Methods Mol Biol* 2015;1237:149–211.

180. Etheridge A, Lee I, Hood L, et al. Extracellular microRNA: A new source of biomarkers. *Mutat Res* 2011;717:85–90.

181. Verma P, Pandey RK, Prajapati P, Prajapati VK. Circulating microRNAs: Potential and emerging biomarkers for diagnosis of human infectious diseases. *Front Microbiol* 2016;7:1274.

182. Correia CN, Nalpas NC, McLoughlin KE, et al. Circulating microRNAs as potential biomarkers of infectious diseases. *Front Immunol* 2017;8:118.

183. Baldassarre A, Felli C, Prantera G, Masotti A. Circulating microRNAs and bioinformatics tools to discover novel diagnostic biomarkers of pediatric diseases. *Genes* 2017;8:E234.

184. O'Connell RM, Rao DS, Baltimore D. MicroRNA regulation of inflammatory responses. *Annu Rev Immunol* 2012;30:295–312.

185. Chen CZ, Schaffert S, Fragoso R, Loh C. Regulation of immune responses and tolerance: The microRNA perspective. *Immunol Rev* 2013;253:112–128.

186. Zhu S, Pan W, Qian Y. MicroRNA in immunity and autoimmunity. *J Mol Med (Berl)* 2013;91:1039–1050.

187. O'Neill LA, Sheedy FY, McCoy CE. MicroRNAs: The fine-tuners of toll-like receptor signaling. *Nat Rev Immunol* 2011;11:163–175.

188. Fabbri M, Paone A, Calore F, et al. MicroRNAs bind to toll-like receptors to induce prometastatic inflammatory response. *Proc Natl Acad Sci USA* 2012;109:E2110–E2116.

189. Fabbri M, Paaone A, Calore F, et al. A new role for microRNAs, as ligands of toll-like receptors. *RNA Biol* 2013;10:169–174.

190. He X, Jing Z, Cheng G. MicroRNAs: New regulators of toll-like receptor signaling pathways. *Biomed Res Int* 2014;2014:945169.

191. Blondal T, Jensby Nielson S, Baker A, et al. Assessing samples and miRNA profile quality in serum and plasma. *Methods* 2013;59:S1–S6.

192. Koberle V, Pleli T, Schmithals C, et al. Differential stability of cell-free circulating microRNAs: Implications for their utilization as biomarkers. *PLOS ONE* 2013;8:e75184.

193. Chevillet JR, Lee I, Briggs HA, et al. Issues and prospects of microRNA-based biomarkers in blood and other body fluids. *Molecules* 2014;19:6080–6105.

194. McDonald JS, Milosevic D, Reddi HV, et al. Analysis of circulating microRNA: Preanalytical and analytical challenges. *Clin Chem* 2011;57:833–840.

195. Brunet-Vega A, Pericay C, Quilez ME, et al. Variability in microRNA recovery from plasma: Comparison of five commercial kits. *Anal Biochem* 2015;488:28–35.

196. Tian T, Wang J, Zhou X. A review: MicroRNA detection methods. *Org Biomol Chem* 2015;13:2226–2238.

197. Hunt EA, Broyles D, Head T, Deo SK. MicroRNA detection: Current technology and research strategies. *Annu Rev Anal Chem (Palo Alto Calif)* 2015;8:217–237.

198. Kroh EM, Parkn RK, Mitchell PS, Tewari M. Analysis of circulating microRNA biomarkers in plasma and serum using quantitative reverse transcription-PCR (qRT-PCR). *Methods* 2010;50:298–301.

199. Costa MC, Leitao AL, Enguita FJ. MicroRNA profiling in plasma or serum using quantitative RT-PCR. *Methods Mol Biol* 2014;1182:121–129.

200. Thorsen M, Bondal T, Mouritzen P. Quantitative RT-PCR for microRNAs in biofluids. *Methods Mol Biol* 2017;1641:379–398.

201. Schwarzenbach H, da Silva AM, Calin G, Pantel K. Data normalization strategies for microRNA quantification. *Clin Chem* 2015;61:1333–1342.

202. Marabita F, de Canddia P, Torri A, et al. Normalization of circulating microRNA expression data obtained by quantitative real-time RT-PCR. *Brief Bioinform* 2016;17:204–212.

203. Vasilescu C, Rossi S, Shimizu M, et al. MicroRNA fingerprints identify miR-150 as a plasma prognostic marker in patients with sepsis. *PLOS ONE* 2009;4:e7405.

204. Roderburg C, Luedde M, Vargas Cardenas D, et al. Circulating microRNA-150 serum levels predict survival in patients with critical illness and sepsis. *PLOS ONE* 2013;8:e54612.

205. Wang H, Zhang P, Chen W, et al. Evidence for serum miR-15a and miR-16 levels as biomarkers that distinguish sepsis from systemic inflammatory response syndrome in human subjects. *Clin Chem Lab Med* 2012;50:1423–1428.

206. Wang HJ, Zhang PJ, Chen WJ, et al. Four serum microRNAs identified as diagnostic biomarkers of sepsis. *J Trauma Acute Care Surg* 2012;73:850–854.

207. Wang H, Zhang P, Chen W, et al. Serum microRNA signatures identified by solexa sequencing predict sepsis patients' mortality: A prospective observational study. *PLOS ONE* 2012;7:e38885.

208. Bihrer V, Friedrich-Rust M, Kronenberger B, et al. Serum miR-122 as a biomarker of necroinflammation in patients with chronic hepatitis C infection. *Am J Gastroenterol* 2011;106:1663–1669.

209. Roderburg C, Benz F, Vargas Cardenas D, et al. Elevated miR-122 serum levels are an independent marker of liver injury in inflammatory diseases. *Liver Int* 2015;35:1172–1184.

210. Wang HJ, Deng J, Wang JY, et al. Serum miR-122 levels are related to coagulation disorders in septic patients. *Clin Chem Lab Med* 2014;52:927–933.

211. Wang HJ, Zhang PJ, Chen WJ, et al. Characterization and identification of novel serum microRNAs in sepsis patients with different outcomes. *Shock* 2013;39:480–487.

212. Wang JF, Yu ML, Yu G, et al. Serum miR-146a and miR-223 as potential new biomarkers for sepsis. *Biochem Biophys Res Commun* 2010;394:184–188.

213. Wang H, Meng K, Chen WJ, et al. Serum miR-574-5p: A prognostic predictor of sepsis patients. *Shock* 2012;37:263–267.

214. Wang L, Wang HC, Chen C, et al. Differential expression of plasma miR-146a in sepsis patients compared with non-sepsis-SIRS patients. *Exp Ther Med* 2013;5:1101–1104.

215. Tacke F, Roderburg C, Benz F, et al. Levels of circulating miR-133a are elevated in sepsis and predict mortality in critically ill patients. *Crit Care Med* 2014;42:1096–1104.

216. Wu Y, Li C, He Y, et al. Relationship between expression of microRNA and inflammatory cytokines plasma level in pediatric patients with sepsis. *Zhonghua Er Ke Za Zhi* 2014;52:28–33.

217. Huang J, Sun Z, Yan W, et al. Identification of microRNA as sepsis biomarkers based on miRNAs regulatory network analysis. *Biomed Res Int* 2014;2014:594350.

218. Dumache R, Rogobete AF, Bedreag OH, et al. Use of miRNAs as biomarkers in sepsis. *Anal Cell Pathol* 2015;2015:186716.

219. Benz F, Roy S, Trautwein C, et al. Circulating microRNAs as biomarkers for sepsis. *Int J Mol Sci* 2016;17:pii:e78.

220. Caserta S, Kern F, Cohen J, et al. Circulating plasma microRNAs can differentiate human sepsis and systemic inflammatory response syndrome (SIRS). *Sci Rep* 2016;6:28006.

221. Wu SC, Yang JC, Rau CS, et al. Profiling circulating microRNA expression in experimental sepsis using cecal ligation and puncture. *PLOS ONE* 2013;8:e77936.

7 Infections and Their Mimics in Returning Travelers in the Critical Care Unit

Elise Kochoumian, Jonathon Moore, Bushra Mina, and Kevin Cahill

CONTENTS

CLINICAL PERSPECTIVE

Global health is defined as "the area of study, research and practice that places a priority on improving health and achieving equity in health for all people worldwide" [1]. Global medicine extends beyond our borders and involves working with international travelers, immigrants and refugees, dealing with educational marginalization and health illiteracy, and addressing issues of maldistribution and access common in urban and rural areas alike [1,2].

Neglected tropical diseases (NTDs) are a diverse group of communicable diseases that prevail in tropical and subtropical conditions in 149 countries. This group of diseases largely affects low-income and politically marginalized people living in rural and urban areas, predominantly in Africa, Asia, and Latin America. Populations mostly at risk are living in poverty, without adequate sanitation, and in close contact with infectious vectors: domestic animals and livestock. Among the 17 NTDs are trachoma, leprosy, dengue, rabies, Chagas, and schistosomiasis. More than 1 billion people were treated for at least one NTD in 2015 [4]. The Global Burden of Disease Study concluded that NTDs comprehensively contributed to approximately 26.06 million disability-adjusted life years in 2010, as well as significant deleterious economic effects [5].

Tropical diseases can be complicated by critical illness with multiple organ involvement. Critically ill patients with tropical diseases have high morbidity and mortality rates, especially among low-income countries (LIC) with insufficient critical care medicine resources. In 2004, an estimated 15 million people died from tropical infectious and parasitic diseases. Among those, mortality rates of 30%–80% were seen in patients in LIC compared with fewer than 20% in those coming from developed countries. The incidence of hospital-acquired infections complicating the course of illness among those patients in LIC is high, resulting in the prevalence of increased drug resistance and higher mortality. Other factors that affect mortality are the lack of infrastructure for transportation, emergency medical services, and proper triage of patient on arrival to the local hospitals. Those factors result in the delivery of suboptimal care to the critically ill patients suffering from tropical disease and their illness-related complications. Supportive care of vital organs, maintaining adequate hemodynamics and tissue perfusions, and treatment of the specific tropical disease are the main measures in the treatment of critically ill patients. Improving critical care in LIC requires a focus on hospital design, training, triage, monitoring, and treatment modifications; the basic principles of critical care; hygiene; and the involvement of multidisciplinary teams [6].

There is a lack of data about critical care units (CCUs) capacity in underdeveloped countries, including resources such as monitoring devices, equipment, and supportive multidisciplinary services. The Task Force of the World Federation of Societies of Intensive and Critical Care Medicine categorized CCU care into three levels. A level 1 CCU can provide oxygen, non-invasive monitoring, and more intensive nursing care than on a ward. A level 2 CCU can provide invasive monitoring and basic life support for a short period. A level 3 CCU provides a full spectrum of monitoring and life support technologies, serves as a regional resource for the care of critically ill patients, and may play an active role in developing the specialty of intensive care through research and education [7].

Delivering efficient critical care services is dependent on essential factors such as the availability of critical care trained physicians and nurses, availability of supportive services such as blood bank, epidemiology, infectious control, medical technicians and ancillary personnel, closed CCUs, designed critical care units that fulfill measures to decrease decontamination based on the international guidelines, adequate workload, availability of adequate isolation measures to decrease contamination, resources to follow international guidelines and customize protocols to meet regional and local requirements, and adequate equipment (such as invasive and non-invasive ventilation, dialysis units, and oxygen supplementation using high-flow nasal cannula [HFNC]) and drugs [6].

Hospital design is essential in supporting critical care patients and proper triage to the necessary required level of care and in delivering required resuscitation measures in a timely manner. Sepsis guidelines improved mortality by implementing sepsis protocol at time zero of presentation in emergency departments. Rapid response teams also improved patient care and triage.

Baker et al. emphasized the importance of certain elements to deliver critical care for patients with tropical illness in LIC. Elements include hospital design, triaging, training of healthcare providers and ancillary personnel, monitoring and treatment modification, airway-breathing-circulation care, hygiene, and multidisciplinary approach, all which are needed requirements [6].

Major shortages of physicians and nurses/midwives are a matter of concern in most countries in the WHO African Region, WHO South-East Asia Region, and WHO Eastern Mediterranean Region. It has been estimated that there was a deficit of approximately 17.4 million health workers in 2013, of which almost 2.6 million were physicians and over 9 million were nurses and midwives. Regionally, the largest deficit of health workers was in Southeast Asia (6.9 million), followed by Africa (4.2 million) [8].

Political and financial factors also influence the delivery of critical care in the tropics. The Universal Health Coverage (UHC) index values based on national coverage levels show substantial differences across WHO regions. Health financing systems in LIC and lower-middle-income countries rely heavily on out-of-pocket payments, owing to the lack of UHC, implying that households are the major contributors to the health financing system (42.3% and 40.6% in 2013, respectively). Such countries face particular challenges, as they have inadequate service delivery systems and additionally struggle to raise domestic revenues to pay for such services [8].

The risk of acquiring infectious diseases varies greatly, depending on socioeconomic determinants such as poverty and housing conditions, sex, and environmental conditions. Lack of safe water, sanitation, and hand hygiene increases mortality. In 2012, an estimated 871,000 deaths (mostly from infectious diseases) were caused by the contamination of drinking water, bodies of water (such as rivers and reservoirs), and soil, and by inadequate hand-washing facilities and practices resulting from inadequate or inappropriate services. Almost half (45%) of these deaths occurred in the WHO African Region [8].

Improvement in critical care delivery in LIC can be accomplished by undertaking certain initiatives, including the adjustment of critical care infrastructure and the availability of health resources, improvement of training levels, adherence to and ensuring the implementation of the international guidelines while adjusting them to meet local and cultural differences, collaboration with global critical care societies and their activities such as the Fundamental Critical Care Support and the Fundamental Disaster Management sponsored by the Society of Critical Care Medicine (USA) [8].

Increased survival and better quality of life for critical care patients suffering from tropical diseases in LIC can be accomplished by participating in global health and WHO initiatives.

MALARIA

EPIDEMIOLOGY

Malaria is a preventable, treatable, and curable mosquito-borne infectious disease caused by the parasites of the genus *Plasmodium*. Malaria is endemic in the tropics but is not limited by borders because of the extensive global tourist travel and expanding business cartels and is considered a global health hazard. Malaria remains one of the top three infectious diseases, with high mortality after HIV and tuberculosis (TB).

According to the latest *World Malaria Report*, released in November 2018, there were 219 million cases of malaria in 2017, up from 217 million cases in 2016. The estimated number of malaria deaths stood at 435,000 in 2017 [3].

In 2017, five countries accounted for nearly half of all malaria cases worldwide: Nigeria (25%), the Democratic Republic of the Congo (11%), Mozambique (5%), India (4%), and Uganda (4%). The WHO African Region continues to carry a disproportionately high share of the global malaria burden. In 2017, the region was home to 92% of malaria cases and 93% of malaria deaths. In areas with high transmission of malaria, children under 5 years of age are particularly susceptible to infection, illness, and death; more than two thirds (70%) of all malaria deaths occur in this age group. The number of under-5 malaria deaths has declined from 440,000 in 2010 to 285,000 in 2016. However, malaria remains a major killer of children under 5 years old, taking the life of a child every 2 minutes (Figure 7.1) [3].

About 1700 cases of malaria are diagnosed in the United States each year. The vast majority of cases in the United States are in travelers and immigrants returning from countries where malaria transmission occurs, many from sub-Saharan Africa and South Asia. The number of malaria cases diagnosed in the United States has been increasing since the mid-1970s. The Institute of Health Metrics and Evaluation reported zero death from malaria in North America in 2015 [9,10].

PARASITOLOGY

There are four species of *Plasmodium* that infect humans. These are *Plasmodium vivax, Plasmodium ovale, Plasmodium malariae*, and *Plasmodium falciparum*. *P. falciparum* is responsible for 60% of cases of malaria, and *Plasmodium vivax* is responsible for most of the remainder. *P. ovale, P. malariae*, and *P. knowlesi* (monkey malaria) account for <1% of malarial infections. Severe life-threatening malaria is caused mostly by *P. falciparum* and *P. ovale*. The life cycles of the four parasites are similar, with sexual development (sporogony) occurring in *Anopheles* mosquito hosts and asexual maturation (schizogony) occurring in human (Figure 7.2) [11].

CLINICAL MANIFESTATIONS

Infection can occur after mosquito bite but also can be transmitted by contaminated needle, blood products, and organ transplant. The incubation period of *P. falciparum* is usually

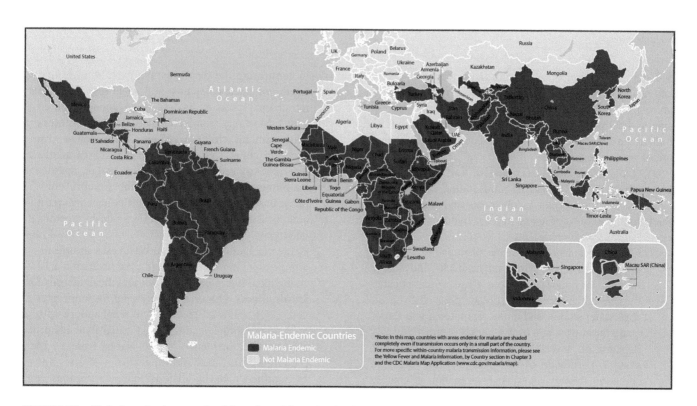

FIGURE 7.1 Malaria endemic countries. Map adapted from the CDC.

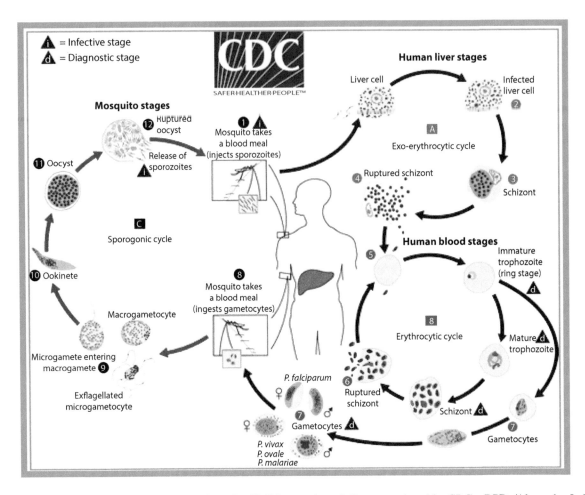

FIGURE 7.2 Life cycle of *Plasmodium*. Image from the CDC (www.cdc.gov). Image produced by CDC—DPDx/Alexander J. da Silva, Melanie Moser.

5–7 days. The onset of uncomplicated infection is insidious and results in delay in confirming the diagnosis. Patients can present with flu-like illness, fever, headache, dizziness, malaise, and body ache, but shaking chills are often absent. Fever follows tertian pattern. Jaundice is common. Splenomegaly might be inconsistent.

P. falciparum if unrecognized and left untreated, especially with high grade of parasitemia, can be complicated by multiple organ involvement and high mortality. Such manifestations of severe malaria include the following:

1. Cerebral malaria (malaria encephalopathy): Cerebral malaria is manifested by fever, headache, and change in behavior pattern. The course can be complicated by generalized seizure disorder, followed by post-ictal state, stupor, and coma. Symptoms may be of acute onset or subtle over a period of time. Severity depends on several factors such as host immune system, purulence of the parasites, and delay in initiating therapy. Physical examination is characteristic by symmetric upper motor neuron involvement with extensor posturing and dysconjugate gaze. Papilledema and retinal hemorrhage are evident in ocular exam. Lumbar puncture is essential

in confirming the diagnosis and exclusion of other causes of encephalopathy and meningitis. Raised intracranial pressure is less often encountered in adults. Mortality from cerebral edema is 80%, especially among children. Neurological deficit can occur in about 15% of children and 3% of adults. Neurological sequela includes hemiplegia, spasticity, blindness, and impaired learning. Cerebral complications are more common with other concurrent complications such as metabolic acidosis, anemia, and hypoglycemia [12,13].

2. Acute renal injury (AKI): The WHO uses serum creatinine of ≥3 mg/dL as a criterion for severe malaria. Acute renal injury can occur without the evidence of febrile illness. Oliguria and prerenal azotemia precede AKI, followed by complete renal failure with anuria, metabolic acidosis, and electrolyte abnormalities. The incidence of AKI varies from 1% to 5% in endemic areas and ranges from 25% to 50% in imported malaria. Histopathological findings of AKI in severe malaria include acute tubular necrosis, interstitial nephritis, and glomerulonephritis; however, tubular changes are the most common findings [14].

3. Hypoglycemia: It is common in children and pregnant women as the presenting symptom. Incidence ranges between 1% and 20% on admission. Hypoglycemia could be related to parasite glucose consumption and to impaired host gluconeogenesis [15]. Malnutrition is a contributing factor. Hypoglycemia is a side effect of intravenous (IV) quinine therapy.

4. Metabolic acidosis: Metabolic acidosis is usually related to lactic acidosis, dehydration, and tissue hypoperfusion. If associated with anemia (hemoglobin <5 g/mL), it is rapidly reversed by rapid blood transfusion.

5. Severe anemia: Severe anemia is usually related to hemolysis and is particularly often fatal in children and pregnant women.

6. Algid malaria: Algid malaria is an acute shock state with vascular collapse. This syndrome can be the presenting feature, occur as a result of treatment, or can be related to superimposed bacterial infection.

7. Disseminated intravascular coagulopathy (DIC): DIC is a common cause of thrombocytopenia and bleeding.

8. Idiopathic pulmonary edema: Pulmonary edema is related to severe metabolic acidosis, renal failure, and fluid resuscitation. Cardiac dysfunction can occur in severe malaria. There is evidence of increased circulating levels of cardiac enzymes, including brain natriuretic peptide (BNP) in individuals with severe malaria. Intravascular hemolysis has been shown to decrease the levels of nitric oxide and increase pulmonary pressures and myocardial wall stress [16].

9. Acute respiratory distress syndrome (ARDS): Acute respiratory distress syndrome is an important complication in severe malaria, most commonly with *P. falciparum* malaria and has also been described in *P. vivax* and *P. ovale* malaria. Incidence of ARDS in patients with severe and complicated malaria requiring CCU admission is 20%–30%. Malarial ARDS is more common in adults than in children. Pregnant women and non-immune individuals are more prone to develop this condition. Increased alveolar capillary permeability resulting in intravascular fluid loss into the lungs appears to be the key pathophysiologic mechanism. Acute respiratory distress syndrome can occur at the time of initial presentation of malaria or after initiation of therapeutic interventions. Mortality is high in severe malaria with ARDS.

10. Hemoglobinuria: Blackwater fever should be considered in presence of acute renal failure and hemoglobinuria. The condition is often a complication of quinine therapy and occurs in patients with glucose 6-phosphate dehydrogenase deficiencies.

11. Fluid and electrolytes abnormalities: Hyponatremia is the most common electrolyte abnormality. It is attributed to inappropriate secretion of antidiuretic hormone; excessive losses of sodium in sweat, vomitus, and diarrhea (sodium depletion); and administration of plain water orally or hypotonic solutions intravenously.

12. Hyperbilirubinemia: Hyperbilirubinemia may occur due to hemolysis, cholestasis, and hepatocyte dysfunction. Transaminases might not be elevated. Hypoglycemia is commonly associated with elevated transaminases in 60% of patients [13].

DIAGNOSIS

High index of suspicion is essential in the diagnosis of malaria, especially when there is a history of travel to endemic areas. The diagnosis is confirmed by the presence of *Plasmodium* parasites in the blood smears. Thick films confirm the presence of the parasites, while thin films allow the identification of the different species. Tests are available to detect malaria antigens via radioimmunoassay and enzyme-linked immunosorbent assay (ELISA) techniques such as histidine-rich protein II antigen.

P. falciparum-specific parasite lactate dehydrogenase and aldolase serum levels are elevated in infection. These methods have a limitation for assessing the degree of parasitemia. Microscopy may be negative in the initial assessment of malaria, and it is recommended to repeat testing within 48 hours if there is high clinical suspicion of malaria. Other laboratory findings include anemia, thrombocytopenia, leukocytosis, electrolyte abnormality, metabolic acidosis, transaminitis, abnormal renal function, and elevated creatine phosphokinase (CK) and aldolase.

TREATMENT

The management of severe malaria follows the same principles of organ support and the sepsis campaign guidelines. The patient should be admitted to CCU. Follow the basic principles of securing airway, adequate oxygenation, maintaining adequate circulation, and hemodynamics for sufficient organ perfusion. Implement CCU protocols regarding peptic ulcer prophylaxis, deep venous thrombosis prophylaxis, awakening and breathing coordination, delirium monitoring/management, and early mobility bundle. In addition, general measures for the prevention of nosocomial infections and malnutrition are indicated in case of all CCU patients. Antimalarial drug treatment should be instituted immediately according to national/WHO guidelines and local resistance patterns [17].

FLUID RESUSCITATION AND TREATMENT OF SHOCK

Initial recommendation is at least 30 mL/kg of IV crystalloid fluid, to be given within the first 3 hours. Additional fluids should be guided by frequent reassessment of hemodynamic status. Fluid management can be guided by invasive cardiac monitoring via pulmonary artery catheter, transpulmonary thermodilution, or transesophageal echocardiogram. Those resources might be unavailable in underdeveloped countries. Reassessment should include a thorough clinical examination and evaluation of multiple physiologic variables (heart rate, blood pressure, arterial oxygen saturation, respiratory rate, temperature, urine output, central venous oxygen saturation, and others, as available) as well as other non-invasive or invasive monitoring. Monitor lactate levels with a goal to normalize the serum lactate level. Liberal fluid management should be avoided in the management of severe malaria at best, owing to the propensity of capillary leakage in those patient populations.

Fluid resuscitation in children is controversial. The WHO malaria guidelines from 2015 advise against rapid fluid boluses of colloids or crystalloids in children. In the FEAST study, fluid boluses resulted in significant increased 48-hour mortality in critically ill children with impaired perfusion (7.3% versus 10.5% in the albumin bolus group and 10.6% in the saline bolus group). The 48-hour mortality was 10.6%, 10.5%, and 7.3% in the albumin-bolus, saline-bolus, and control groups, respectively. The 4-week mortality was 12.2%, 12.0%, and 8.7% in the respective three groups (p = 0.004 for the comparison of bolus with control). Neurologic sequelae occurred in 2.2%, 1.9%, and 2.0% of children in the respective three groups (p = 0.92), and pulmonary edema or increased intracranial pressure occurred in 2.6%, 2.2%, and 1.7% (p = 0.17), respectively [18].

Shock could be related to volume depletion and/or superimposed bacterial infection. Cultures should be obtained from blood as well as any other bodily fluid. Patient should be started on broad-spectrum antibiotic within 1 hour for both sepsis and septic shock if bacterial infection is suspected. Fluid resuscitation should begin immediately. De-escalation of antibiotic should be considered once pathogens are identified and sensitivities are available. Vasopressors are indicated for hemodynamic support if shock is unresponsive to fluid resuscitation or there is an evidence of fluid overload and pulmonary edema. Norepinephrine is the preferred vasopressor in septic shock. Intravenous hydrocortisone is recommended if adequate fluid resuscitation and vasopressor therapy are unable to restore hemodynamic stability at a maximum dose of 200 mg daily [19].

ELECTROLYTE ABNORMALITIES

Electrolyte abnormalities are common in severe malaria, as a result of gastrointestinal losses, poor oral intake, or side effect of therapeutic drugs. Quinine is a strong stimulant of insulin. Patients should be monitored closely for hypoglycemia. Hypocalcemia can be treated with 50% dextrose injection, followed by dextrose infusion, with serial monitoring of blood sugar levels. Somatostatin can be used in refractory hypoglycemia. Pregnant women and children are more susceptible to hypoglycemia.

Severe hyponatremia can cause neuromuscular disorder and seizures in those affected. Hyponatremia can be corrected with 0.9% saline or hypertonic saline solution, especially in the presence of seizure or neurological abnormalities. Sodium should be corrected at a level of 0.5 mEq/L/h and should not exceed

10 mEq/L in 24 hours or 18 mEq/L in 48 hours. Exceeding those limits can cause osmotic demyelination syndrome.

CEREBRAL EDEMA

Reducing the increased intracranial pressure is the main goal of therapeutic interventions in cerebral edema that complicate severe malaria. Osmotic diuresis lowers intracranial pressure and reduces cerebral edema. Though mannitol has historically been used to treat cerebral edema, a recent Cochrane study concluded that there are insufficient data to support the role of mannitol in decreasing mortality from cerebral malaria [20]. In addition, Mohanty et al. demonstrated that mannitol therapy in adult cerebral malaria prolongs coma duration and may be harmful [21]. In response, the WHO does not recommend mannitol in the treatment of cerebral malaria. Dexamethasone can also be delirious, with increased risk of gastrointestinal bleeding and pneumonia, and can prolong the duration of coma. General measures to reduce fever, elevation of the head of the bed, effective treatment of seizures, and hyperventilation may be helpful. Routine EEG monitoring is not indicated unless seizure activities are expected. Anti-epileptics are indicated to suppress seizure activity.

ACUTE RENAL INJURY

Initial management of acute kidney injury includes fluid replacement and correction of concomitant metabolic acidosis. Renal replacement therapy (RRT) is required in 35% of patients with malaria complicated by renal impairment. Indications for hemodialysis are acute pulmonary edema, severe acidosis, hyperkalemia, uremic encephalopathy, progressive oliguria or anuria, and pericarditis.

PULMONARY EDEMA AND RESPIRATORY FAILURE

Pulmonary edema and ARDS are late manifestations of severe malaria and could result from therapeutics interventions. Early recognition of ARDS is crucial in the management of these cases. Treatment of ARDS in severe malaria should follow the same guidelines of treating ARDS due to other etiologies. Fluid management is essential in patients with ARDS to ensure adequate organ perfusion and avoid fluid overload. Diuretics may be indicated unless there is evidence of hypovolemic shock or organ hypoperfusion. Non-invasive or invasive measurement of intravascular volume may assist in assessing the fluid status. Bedside ultrasounds can be utilized in the CCU to evaluate the intravascular volume and guide fluid resuscitation. Presence of multiple B lines on chest ultrasound and absence of respiratory variation in the diameter of the dilated inferior vena cava are indicative of fluid overload. Pulmonary artery catheters are rarely used currently.

Oxygen supplementation is required with a goal oxygen saturation of at least 88%. In some cases, oxygen can be supplied via nasal cannula, face mask, or HFNC. The advantages of non-invasive oxygenation measures include preserving airway defense mechanisms, reducing infectious complications, enhancing patient comfort, and avoiding upper airway trauma [22]. In most cases, however, oxygen supplementation will be reliant on invasive ventilation. Intubation should be considered in those with respiratory arrest, hemodynamic instability due to shock state, inability to protect an airway, altered mental status, and excessive secretions [22]. Once intubated, management of ARDS should follow guidelines outlined by the Acute Respiratory Distress Syndrome Network, which reports that tidal volume should be set in the region of 6 mL/kg predicted body weight ("lung protective ventilation") and the plateau pressures (end-inspiratory pause pressures) should be limited to 30 cm H_2O to prevent lung barotrauma [23,24]. For those patients who are unresponsive to these measures, other modalities, including prone positioning, nitrous oxide, and extracorporeal membrane oxygenation (ECMO), should be considered [25]. Daily wakening trials and evaluation for extubation are recommended for all intubated patients.

THROMBOCYTOPENIA AND HEMATOLOGICAL MANIFESTATIONS

The recommended threshold for transfusion in adults is 7 g/dL. In addition, correct coagulopathy and transfuse platelets if indicated.

HYPOGLYCEMIA

Hypoglycemia is a marker of severe malaria. Blood sugar should be routinely monitored according to CCU protocol. Glucose supplementation may be indicated. Early enteral feeding is recommended.

LEPTOSPIROSIS

EPIDEMIOLOGY

Leptospirosis is a widespread endemic and NTD that can be associated with natural disasters such as flooding and hurricanes. Leptospirosis occurs worldwide but most commonly in tropical and subtropical areas with high rainfall. The disease is often unrecognized, as its presentation can mimic other diseases such as dengue fever and viral hepatitis, resulting it to be unreported in many cases. Leptospirosis has a seasonal distribution but can be all year round leading to epidemics. Occupational and recreational exposure occur among farmers, pet shop workers, people engaging in recreational water sports such as kayaking and triathlons, and veterinarians. There has been an increase in the incidence of recreational exposure owing to rise in travel to exotic destinations and water sport activities.

The Leptospirosis Burden Epidemiology Reference Group's report in 2011 estimated the overall global annual incidence of endemic and epidemic human leptospirosis at 5 and 14 cases per 100,000 populations, respectively.

Endemic human leptospirosis rates varied by region from 0.5/100,000 population in Europe to 95/100,000 population in Africa. Annually, it is estimated that there are 1.03 million cases and 58,900 deaths due to leptospirosis worldwide. The overall mortality of hospitalized patients ranges from 4% to 52%. Mortality of patients admitted to CCU is estimated to exceed 52% [26,27].

DISEASE TRANSMISSION

Infection results from direct or indirect exposure to infected reservoir host. Poor housing with poor sanitation is a major risk factor for acquiring the disease, especially in urban areas in underdeveloped countries. The disease is mainly found wherever humans come in contact with the urine of infected animals. The natural hosts are mainly humans, domestic animals, and brown rats. Human-to-human transmission is rare and can occur through sexual contact or transplacentally. After exposure to infected animal or contaminated urine, *Leptospira* gain entry through abrasions or mucous membranes [26].

PATHOLOGY

Hematogenous spread occurs after *Leptospira* enter into the tissue through mucous membranes or abrasions. *Leptospira* persist in blood throughout the leptospiremic phase of the illness. Worse outcomes are associated with levels of >104 leptospires/mL in the blood. *Leptospira* has on its outer membrane unusual lipopolysaccharides (LPS) that activate toll-like receptor (TLR) 2. In contrast, TLR4, a central component for recognition of gram-negative LPS, is not involved in cellular responses to *Leptospira*. Mouse but not human TLR4 can recognize leptospiral LPS, suggesting that the murine innate immune response is adapted to leptospiral infection.

The systemic inflammatory responses to leptospiremia may lead to multiple-organ failure. A "cytokine storm," with higher levels of interleukin (IL)-6, tumor necrosis factor (TNF)-α, and a number of other cytokines, is seen in severe disease forms in contrast to milder forms of illness. Levels of IL-6 and IL-10 are independent predictors of mortality.

The liver is a major target organ in leptospirosis, with leptospiral infiltration of space of Disse, invasion of the perijunctional region between hepatocytes, and hepatocyte apoptosis. Leakage of bile due to damage to the hepatocellular junction results in bilirubinemia, seen in icteric forms of leptospirosis. Hemolysis is a contributory factor to rise in bilirubin.

Lung involvement is common in leptospirosis. Pulmonary hemorrhage occurs in 60% of cases, owing to hemorrhage in both the alveolar septa and intra-alveolar spaces. Petechiae are seen on the pleural surface. Severe pulmonary hemorrhage syndrome (SPHS) is a marker of severe systemic disease rather than a pulmonary manifestation of the disease.

Hypokalemia, elevated serum creatinine, shock, and the low Glasgow Coma Scale score are the risk factors for SPHS.

Bleeding in different body organs can also be a direct cause of coagulopathy associated with severe leptospirosis.

Renal involvement varies in severity from mild non-oliguric renal dysfunction to complete renal failure, a hallmark of Weil's syndrome. Renal function will recover in most patients who survive leptospirosis. Persistent renal dysfunction associated with tubular atrophy and interstitial fibrosis is a complication in some patients [26].

CLINICAL FEATURES

Leptospirosis can manifest itself as a mild form of disease such as a self-limiting acute febrile illness to a fulminant potentially lethal illness with multi-organ dysfunction in 5%–10% of patients. The incubation period is 2–30 days, and illness usually occurs 5–14 days after exposure.

Leptospirosis is characterized by two phases: The leptospiremic phase and the immunologic phase. The acute leptospiremic stage presents as a sudden onset of acute fevers with chills, non-productive cough, throbbing headache accompanied by retro-orbital pain and photophobia, conjunctival suffusion, myalgias, GI symptoms (including nausea, vomiting, diarrhea, and abdominal pain), and rarely skin rash. Laboratory abnormalities in this stage include transaminitis, anemia, thrombocytopenia, leukopenia, elevated pancreatic enzymes, elevated creatinine, and electrolyte abnormalities. Mortality of this stage is low with resolution of the symptoms.

The immunologic phase results in maximal organ injury and occurs between days 4 and 30 after the initial phase and is known as Weil's disease. In this phase, patients usually present with renal failure, hemorrhage, aseptic meningitis, meningoencephalitis, cardiac arrhythmias, pulmonary insufficiency (ARDS and massive hemoptysis), ocular pain, muscle rigidity, adenopathy, hepatosplenomegaly, vasculitis with necrosis of the extremities, and hemodynamic collapse.

Neuroleptospirosis includes meningoencephalitis and/or aseptic meningitis and is manifested by meningismus and delirium. The CT scan is normal in 67% of cases, while CT scan findings consistent with diffuse cerebral edema are present in 26% of cases. Cerebrospinal fluid analysis is consistent with pleocytosis, with lymphocytic predominance and elevated protein levels. Leptospira antibody can be detected in cerebrospinal fluid (CSF) samples. Other neurologic manifestations such as transverse myelitis, hemiplegia, and Guillain-Barré syndrome are infrequent [27].

Most patients with leptospirosis will recover without residual deficit. However, poor prognostic indicators include older age (>36 years), toxic metabolic encephalopathy, repolarization abnormalities on electrocardiogram, white blood count >12,900/mm^3, respiratory insufficiency, and oliguria. Chronic postleptospirosis is a recent well-recognized syndrome. Persistent complaints after acute leptospirosis occur in 30% of patients and include fatigue, myalgia, malaise, headache, and weakness, which can last for more than 24 months in 21% of cases [26].

DIAGNOSIS

Diagnosis of leptospirosis can be confirmed by direct detection of the organism or its components in body fluid or tissues, by isolation of leptospires in cultures, or by detection of specific antibodies. Leptospiral DNA can be detected by real-time PCR from serum, urine, aqueous humor, CSF, and a number of organs. Culture of leptospires requires specialized media and can be recovered from humans during the acute phase of the illness and during the so-called immune phase. Cultures are insensitive, and the timing of culture of different specimens depends on an accurate date of onset of symptoms. Leptospirosis is diagnosed by serology, because capacity for culture and PCR is limited. IgM antibodies, using ELISA, are detectable in the blood 5–7 days after the onset of symptoms. IgM antibodies' detection is more sensitive than microscopic agglutination test [26].

TREATMENT

Patients with severe leptospirosis need close monitoring and CCU admission for organ support. Antimicrobial agents should be started early in the course of disease. Therapy, otherwise, is essentially supportive and consists of restoration of the intravascular volume, with aggressive fluid and electrolyte replacement. Multi-organ support should be initiated early for better prognosis. Arrhythmias should be managed appropriately with correcting electrolyte abnormalities and antiarrhythmic drugs. No specific therapy is required for hepatic dysfunction. Renal dysfunction can be reversed with adequate fluid replacement and hemodynamic support, but RRT may be indicated. Mechanical ventilation, invasive or non-invasive, should be employed as required, but ECMO can be utilized in severe refractory ARDS due to pulmonary hemorrhage.

There is no need for isolation in patients with severe leptospirosis. However, level 2 biosafety measures still need to be maintained, especially with regard to exposure to body fluids, especially urine, as it is a source of transmission of disease.

DENGUE

Epidemiology

The WHO estimates that 2.5–3 billion individuals live in dengue endemic areas, with approximately 50–100 million individuals infected yearly. A recent study in 2013 suggests that is an underestimation of the global dengue infection rates, and the rate is closer to 390 million individuals infected per year [28]. Asia represented 70% of the cases, the Americas 14%, and Africa 16%. Within Asia, the largest percentage of cases was seen in India (34%) [30]. Brazil and Mexico make up over 50% of the cases within the Americas. High levels of precipitation, suitable temperature for mosquito vectors, and proximity to low-income urban/peri-urban centers were all associated with an increased risk of contracting dengue. *Aedes aegypti* mosquitoes represent the most common vector for endemic and epidemic dengue; their population is primarily confined between the latitudes of 45°N and 35°S (Figure 7.3).

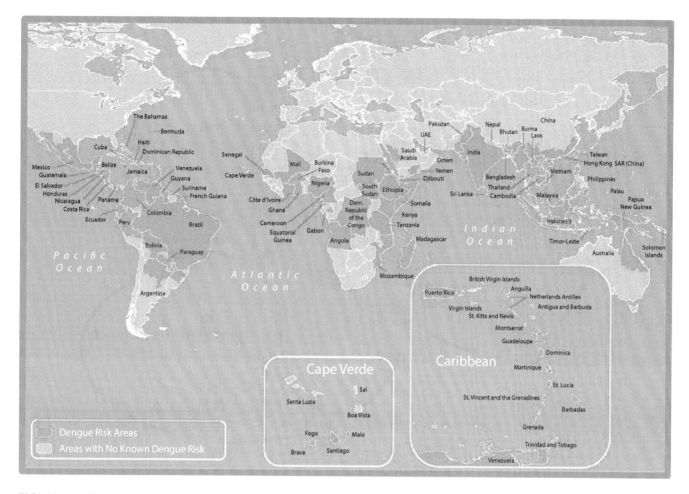

FIGURE 7.3   Epidemiology of dengue. Image from the CDC (www.cdc.gov).

PATHOGENESIS

Dengue virus is from the family Flaviviridae and genus Flavivirus [30]. Historically, four distinct serotypes have been described, with a new DENV5 serotype recently isolated [31]. DENV2 has historically been associated with progression to dengue hemorrhagic fever (DHF), but specific genotyping is not frequently performed in mild cases of dengue fever (DF) [32,33]. DENV2 serotype from Asia has been demonstrated to be increasingly virulent compared with DENV2 from other regions and has been associated with an increased risk of developing severe hemorrhagic fever [34–37].

The primary cellular targets of infection for dengue virus are unclear. Animal studies and *in vitro* studies have shown that dengue preferentially infects human dendritic cells, Langerhans cells, and macrophages [38–40]. Human autopsies show antigen-positive cells tend to cluster in lung, liver, spleen, central nervous system, kidney, and peripheral blood [41–46]. Infection with a serotype has been shown to infer lifelong immunity to that serotype; however, individuals remain susceptible to infection with another serotype in 3–6 months [47,48]. Secondary infection with a heterologous serotype has been shown to increase the risk of developing severe DHF—primary infection with dengue may also progress to dengue shock syndrome (DSS) at lower rates [49]. Secondary infection is thought to cause cross-reactivity among the various serotypes, leading to excessive cytokine production, complement system activation, and release of inflammatory markers, ultimately culminating in DHF and DSS (Figure 7.4) [39].

CLINICAL MANIFESTATIONS

Infection with dengue results in a wide spectrum of disease. Scoring systems to categorize severity are in the process of being validated but are not routinely used in clinical practice [50,51]. Infections with dengue proceed through three distinct phases—the initial febrile phase, the critical phase, and the recovery phase. Patients with simple dengue without increased permeability bypass the critical phase and pass to the recovery phase. The initial febrile phase is often non-specific, with patients experiencing fever for 2–7 days, accompanied by typical dengue symptoms [52]. These signs and symptoms include nausea, vomiting, rubelliform exanthema, headache, retro-orbital eye pain, myalgia, arthralgia, leukopenia, a positive tourniquet test, and hemorrhagic manifestations. Defervescence typically occurs during days 3–8 and marks the transition from the febrile phase to the critical phase for patients who progress to severe dengue infections. The recovery phase is characterized by resorption of

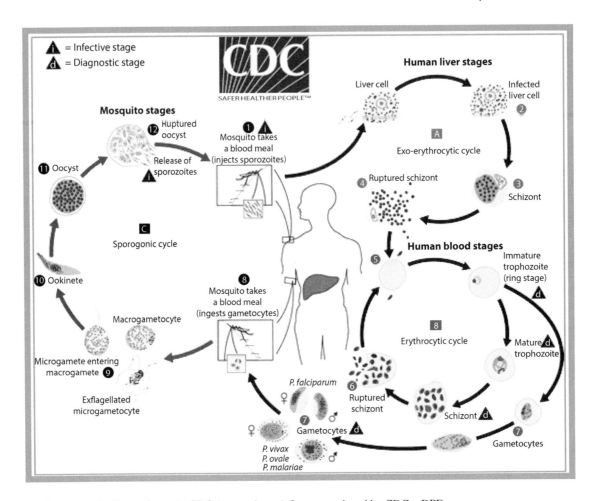

FIGURE 7.4 Dengue cycle. Image from the CDC (www.cdc.gov). Image produced by CDC—DPDx.

fluid into the intravascular space and decreased intravascular permeability. Warning signs associated with increased risk of progression to DSS include intractable vomiting, abdominal pain or tenderness, lethargy, restlessness, and hepatomegaly. Patients typically have a rapid increase in the hematocrit, reflecting increased vascular permeability, which is accompanied by worsening thrombocytopenia [52].

The WHO guidelines stratify patients with DHF into grades I–IV. The DHF grade I patients meet diagnostic criteria for DF and have evidence of hemorrhagic manifestation with positive tourniquet sign and evidence of plasma leakage. Corresponding lab values for DHF I patients include hematocrit rise of 20% from baseline or age-appropriate average and platelets less than 100,000 cells/mm^3. The DHF grade II includes criteria for DHF I but demonstrate spontaneous bleeding. The DHF grade III patients demonstrate evidence of circulatory failure, with compensated shock. The DHF grade IV patients progress to frank shock, with complete circulatory collapse [53]. Patients with prolonged shock then develop respiratory distress, pulmonary effusions, severe hemorrhage, disseminated intravascular coagulation, severe metabolic acidosis, and evidence of severe organ failure, culminating in death without intervention [54].

DIAGNOSIS

The diagnosis of dengue is clinical, with a high index of suspicion in patients presenting in dengue endemic areas or with recent travel to dengue endemic areas, as outlined in the previous section. Studies have demonstrated high positive predictive value in a clinical diagnosis in areas of high dengue prevalence [55]. A presumptive diagnosis of dengue may be made if a patient has traveled to a dengue endemic area and has two typical dengue symptoms. If there is clinical uncertainty, serum serologies, reverse transcriptase-polymerase chain reaction (RT-PCR) assays, and serum antigen studies may be performed. Patients with acute primary infections may be diagnosed with RT-PCR and NS1 antigen detection. NS1 antigen detection in serum during the acute illness phase has a sensitivity of 80%–95% for the diagnosis of dengue [56,57]. IgM serology can become positive as early as 5 days in primary infections and persist for over 90 days—the combined use of NS1 antigen testing with IgM serology has been demonstrated to successfully identify over 90% of cases of dengue [58]. In secondary infections, both IgM and IgG may be detected sooner.

TREATMENT

Physicians evaluating patients with presumptive acute dengue infection must be able to triage patients appropriately to improve their health outcomes while simultaneously utilizing limited healthcare resources appropriately. Patients with DF without warning signs or significant comorbidities can be managed with close outpatient follow-up. Thrombocytopenia and rising hematocrit are strong early indicators of plasma leakage in patients with DF. Patients with DHF without DSS can be managed initially with oral rehydration, with progression to crystalloid resuscitation if patients continue to have worsening thrombocytopenia or hematocrit despite oral resuscitation [59]. Calculated rates of IV fluid resuscitation in obese patients should be tailored to ideal body weight to avoid circulatory overload. Signs of clinical improvement with resuscitation include normalization of blood pressure, widening of the pulse pressure, decreased heart rate, improved perfusion examination, and improved respiratory rates. Decisions to adjust the infusion rates should include complete assessment of patient's clinical status, including intake, output, and laboratory findings. Patients with DHF grade III and IV (DSS) should be triaged to high-acuity-care areas and CCUs for close monitoring. Following management of the critical phase, patients will enter the convalescent phase, which is marked by improvement in clinical status with decrease in hematocrit, improved peripheral perfusion, and vital signs.

DENGUE HEMORRHAGIC FEVER I AND II

Intravenous fluid resuscitation with isotonic crystalloids should be initiated to target a urine output of 0.5–1 mL/kg/h. Initial intravenous fluids (IVF) dosing should be 5–7 mL/kg/h for 1–2 hours with titration to 3–5 mL/kg/h for 2–4 hours and finally 2–3 mL/kg/h. Hematocrit should be monitored every 4–6 hours during the critical period to ensure that it is not increasing more than 10% from baseline. Fluids should be titrated to achieve the target urine output while attempting to minimize the amount of IV fluids required to avoid circulatory overload. Patients in the critical period of illness typically require 24–48 hours of resuscitation. Strict inputs and outputs should be monitored for all patients [54].

DENGUE HEMORRHAGIC FEVER III

Patients with DHF III demonstrate the evidence of compensated hypovolemic shock, with mean arterial blood pressure being maintained primarily by diastolic blood pressure. They require an initial IV bolus of 500–1000 mL over 1 hour. Following the IV bolus, patients should be resuscitated per the WHO guidelines: 5–10 mL/kg/h for 7 hours, 3–5 mL/kg/h for the following 6 hours, 1.5–3 mL/kg/h for 7 hours, and finally 1.5 mL/kg/h for the remainder of 24 hours total [53]. If patients do not demonstrate clinical improvement, then patients should be evaluated for persistent acidosis, electrolyte abnormalities, hematocrit changes, and hypoglycemia. Patients frequently require calcium supplementation for hypocalcemia during the critical phase. Drops or plateauing of the hematocrit are potentially the indicators of occult bleeding, and patients should be transfused packed red cells at 5 mL/kg. Patients without clinical improvement who have an increase in their hematocrit should be trialed on IV colloids (Dextran 40) at similar rates to crystalloid infusion [60,61].

DENGUE HEMORRHAGIC FEVER IV

Patients with grade IV DHF present with profound shock, requiring immediate intervention to prevent death. Central or peripheral venous access should be obtained within 5 minutes, with intraosseous access if necessary. Crystalloid fluids should be given at 10 mL/kg over 10–15 minutes [59]. If blood pressure is not responsive to initial bolus, an additional 10 mL/kg should be administered, with consideration for immediate blood transfusion. Vasopressors should be administered to maintain adequate blood pressure if they are not responsive to fluid resuscitation. Once patients are stabilized, they will require IV resuscitation similar to grade III DHF. Invasive arterial blood pressure monitoring should be obtained as well as an indwelling catheter placement for hourly monitoring of urine output. Every effort should be made to localize bleeding and treat it, as these patients frequently have severe thrombocytopenia. Patients with severe end organ damage should be managed according to standard CCU protocols, i.e., RRT and mechanical ventilation.

TRANSFUSION SUPPORT

The efficacy of prophylactic platelet transfusion has been evaluated in patients with thrombocytopenia due to dengue fever and has been shown to be ineffective in preventing bleeding or correcting coagulopathies—contributing instead to circulatory overload, with longer length of stays [62,63]. Patients with severe thrombocytopenia who were transfused platelets had transient elevations in platelet counts, which reverted to pretransfusion levels at 5 hours [64]. Patients with bleeding and severe thrombocytopenia and platelet count less than 10,000 cells/mm³ may be transfused [53]. The duration of shock was the strongest predictor of acute bleeding events, highlighting the need for urgent recognition and appropriate management. Transfusion of packed red blood cells (PRBCs) should be performed for refractory shock or hemorrhage, with loss of 10% of patients' blood volume. The prophylactic use of fresh frozen plasma to correct coagulopathies has not been shown to be efficacious in DSS [65]. Patients with hemorrhage and abnormal coagulation studies due to DSS should have judicious replacement of products to improve hemostasis, with careful consideration for potential circulatory overload from transfused blood products. Vitamin K may be trialed for patients with evidence of hepatic dysfunction and prolonged prothrombin time [53].

COMPLICATIONS OF THERAPY

Owing to high volumes of fluids and blood products typically infused with DSS, patients can develop ascites, pleural effusion, pulmonary edema, and diffuse anasarca. Patients who are developing signs of peripheral volume overload but are still in the critical phase can be switched from crystalloid to colloid fluids. Diuretics should be avoided during the critical illness phase, as patients have persistent capillary leak and risk developing intravascular hypovolemia. Hypotonic fluids should be avoided in patients with DHF. If patients are in the convalescent phase and have stable blood pressure, a trial of furosemide can be attempted to diuresis patients. Patients without response to furosemide should be evaluated for intrinsic renal insult secondary to DHF and ultimately may require RRT. Patients with respiratory distress due to circulatory overload should be evaluated for non-invasive positive pressure ventilation and mechanical ventilation, if indicated. Patients with circulatory collapse from hypervolemia should be evaluated for cardiomyopathy, with potential need of inotropic support.

Dengue shock syndrome can lead to alterations in glucose metabolism, electrolyte abnormalities, and acid-base disturbances, which must be monitored during treatment. Of note, patients with DSS may develop acute liver failure, with subsequent hepatic encephalopathy. Ammonia-clearing therapies are vital acutely, as well as correction of underlying electrolyte abnormalities.

TUBERCULOSIS

EPIDEMIOLOGY

Tuberculosis is considered one of the oldest known human diseases. Genetic studies suggest its emergence about 15,000 years ago, with evidence of tuberculous spondylitis described in art as well as found in Egyptian mummies as early as 1000 BC [66]. Initially described by the spectrum of diseases it caused—including consumption, scrofula, and physitis—it wasn't until 1882 that Robert Koch discovered the pathogen responsible for TB during a time when it was reported that roughly two in three people afflicted died within 5 years of diagnosis [67]. In the following century, efforts were directed at the institution

of a curative antimicrobial regimen, and by the 1950s, the modern-day four-drug regimen for TB was established. Despite it being curative, the shear global burden of disease, its ability to remain latent with potential for reactivation in later years, and unavailability of resources in endemic countries posed obstacles that could not be overcome, and in the twenty-first century, TB remains one of the top 10 causes of death worldwide [68]. Moreover, in recent decades, this malady has seen an evolution with the emergency of drug resistance, which has exponentially increased the rates of mortality among those affected and subsequently has prompted a surge of global efforts to implement new strategies for critical management of people with TB as well universal infection control.

According to the WHO, about 25% of the world population (roughly 1.7 billion people) are estimated to be infected with *Mycobacterium tuberculosis*. In 2017, there were 10 million new cases of TB, which is equivalent to 133 cases per 100,000 people. Of those afflicted, there were 1.6 million deaths in HIV-negative people, with an additional 300,000 deaths among HIV-positive people [68].

The epidemiology of TB varies throughout the world. The most substantial number of cases—about two-thirds of those affected—was observed in eight countries: India (27%), China (9%), Indonesia (8%), the Philippines (6%), Pakistan (5%), Nigeria (4%), Bangladesh (4%), and South Africa (3%). Europe and the Americas each saw 3% of the reported cases (Figure 7.5) [68]. In these areas, the majority of infection occurred in foreign-born residents and recent immigrants from countries in which TB is endemic [71]. According to the WHO, the best estimates for 2017 were that 90% of cases were adults (aged greater than or equal to 15 years), 64% were male, and 9% has an HIV infection [68].

Globally, in 2017, there were about 558,000 new cases of rifampicin-resistant tuberculosis (RR-TB), of which almost half were predominantly India (24%), China (13%), and the Russian Federation (10%). Among RR-TB, an estimated 82% had multi-drug-resistant TB [68].

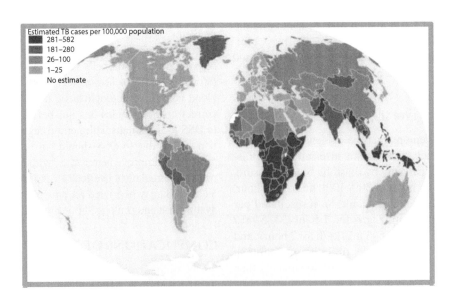

FIGURE 7.5   Incidence of tuberculosis according to the CDC.

PATHOGENESIS

Tuberculosis is caused by bacteria of the *M. tuberculosis* complex, with *M. tuberculosis* being the most common culprit, but others include *M. bovis* and *M. microti*. *M. tuberculosis* is a gram-positive, non-motile, non-spore forming, rod-shaped bacteria of 2–4 μm in length and a member of the Actinomyces family [66,74]. Mycobacteria possess a unique lipid-rich cell wall, which allows them to retain the color of arylmethane dyes when treated with diluted acid, thus giving them the "acid-fast" property by which they are known and by which they are able to resist against disinfectants and antibiotics [66,75]. Mycobacteria additionally act as a facultative intracellular parasite as well as an obligate aerobe, which supports why TB typically affects the lungs [74].

M. tuberculosis is carried in airborne particles, or droplet nuclei, and spreads when the host sneezes, coughs, or speaks. The concentration of infectious droplet nuclei in the air and the duration of exposure play a large role in whether infection develops. Within the environment, exposure in a relatively small, enclosed space with inadequate ventilation results in greater likelihood of contraction of disease [73]. Tuberculosis therefore occurs more frequently in the poorest sections of a community, among low-income people, who typically live in overcrowded areas; have poor nutrition, causing deficient immune function; and have deprived living conditions [69,70].

Transmission begins when a susceptible person inhales tuberculous-rich droplet nuclei, which then make their way through the mouth or nasal passages, upper respiratory tract, and bronchi, reaching the alveoli, where they are engulfed by phagocytic antigen-presenting cells, including alveolar macrophages, lung macrophages, and dendritic cells [73,76].

On entry into a host macrophage, and with the start of the innate immune response, *M. tuberculosis* initially resides in a phagosome. After fusion of the phagosome with a lysosome, the bacterium become exposed to acidic pH, reactive oxygen intermediates, lysosomal enzymes, and toxic peptides [67]. This innate response results in cell necrosis, apoptosis, or survival of the infected macrophages. Under cell necrosis, mycobacteria are released and may infect new macrophages. Apoptosis, on the other hand, causes destruction of the bacteria without cell membrane compromise, thereby halting any potential for dissemination. Finally, survival of the infected macrophages enables the mycobacteria to persist and even proliferate before the adaptive immune response is activated, which typically occurs 2–3 weeks after primary infection [66,79].

The adaptive immune response involves the activation of T cells, which is done largely by dendritic cells. These cells migrate to regional lymph nodes, where they present mycobacteria to naïve T cells. Activated CD4+ T cells return to the lungs and impede mycobacterial progressive growth. In HIV-positive people, the diminished CD4 cell count leads to a significant increase in susceptibility to TB [66]. The accumulation of macrophages, T cells, dendritic cells, and other host cells leads to the formation of a granuloma at the site of infection, which usually occurs within 10 weeks after initial infection [73,76].

In more than 90% of persons infected with *M. tuberculosis*, the pathogen remains latent and the host is asymptomatic [71]. In conditions such as stress, migration, poor nutrition, comorbidities (diabetes, cancer, and chronic obstructive pulmonary disease (COPD)), use of steroids, biologics, and immunotherapies, a transition occurs, where latent TB develops into active, clinical disease [72]. The risk of active disease is estimated to be approximately 5% in the first 18 months after initial infection and then approximately 5% for the remaining lifetime [71]. Persons with latent TB infection who become co-infected with HIV have approximately 8%–10% risk per year for developing active TB [73].

CLINICAL MANIFESTATIONS

Infection with TB leads to a wide range of clinical manifestations and disease severity. The most common findings associated with active pulmonary TB include chronic cough with sputum production, loss of appetite, weight loss, fever, night sweats, and hemoptysis. Extrapulmonary TB, which occurs in 10%–42% of infected persons, can affect any organ and is typically dependent on host factors such as race or ethnic background, age, presence of absence of underlying disease, and immune status, as well as genotype of the *M. tuberculosis* strain [71].

The most common reasons for CCU admission due to active TB include acute respiratory failure, septic shock, and multiorgan dysfunction. Critical illness can also result from bacterial co-infections, anti-TB drug toxicity leading to hepatic or renal failure, decreased consciousness associated with central nervous system disease, thromboembolic complications, postsurgical status, and pulmonary hemorrhage [72,77].

DIAGNOSIS

The diagnosis of TB begins with high clinical suspicion during history, taking in at-risk patients who present with concerning symptomatology. On determining that a patient is high-risk, the confirmation of TB rests upon the identification of *M. tuberculosis* from testing of an appropriate sample, based on the site of infection [66]. According to the WHO, the diagnostic tests for pulmonary TB include sputum smear microscopy, culture-based methods, and rapid molecular tests [68]. Data from these tests rely heavily on the proper collection of the specimen; if needed, sputum induction and flexible bronchoscopy can be used to obtain a sample. Sputum smear microscopy, developed over 100 years ago by Franz Ziehl and Frederick Neelson, remains the most inexpensive, simple, and rapid test for the detection of mycobacteria and works by exploiting their acid-fast property. False-positive results are common, and therefore, the Center for Disease Control and Prevention as well as the National Tuberculosis Controllers Association strongly recommend testing three specimens [80]. Though smear microscopy is highly specific for detection of mycobacteria, it is not specific for *M. tuberculosis* alone, and therefore, a confirmatory sputum culture is needed, which, owing to the slow growth of *M. tuberculosis*, takes about 4–6 weeks before resulting [66]. More recently, in the twenty-first century, the WHO has endorsed the use of rapid molecular tests, specifically Xpert® MTB/RIF assay (Cepheid, USA), for detection of the DNA of the *M. tuberculosis* complex and genetic mutations associated with resistance to rifampin in sputum samples [68,81].

THERAPY

Management of active TB begins with hospitalization of at-risk patients, followed by prompt initiation of isolation precautions and appropriate antitubercle regimen, which are associated with improved survival. The TB isolation room should consist of a single-patient room with special ventilation and negative pressure, all of which is designed to reduce the concentration of infectious droplet nuclei in the air and the escape of particles from the room. Staff should be diligent with washing their hands on entry and exit of the isolation room and wear N95 masks whenever near the patient to avoid transmission [72].

The Centers for Disease Control and Prevention and Infectious Diseases (CDC) Society of America have established guidelines for the management of pulmonary and extrapulmonary TB as well as treatment in special populations, including those with resistant strains and HIV. First-line antimicrobial therapy of pulmonary TB consists of an intensive 2-month course of isoniazid, rifampin, ethambutol, and pyrazinamide, followed by a continuation phase of daily isoniazid and rifampicin for 18 additional weeks [82]. Clinically, a clinician must consider infection with a resistant *M. tuberculosis* strain if the patient originates from a high-risk region, has undergone a treatment course of first-line anti-TB drugs, or fails to respond to standard anti-TB regimens [71,72]. If resistance is suspected, additional testing with rapid molecular tests assessing for genetic mutations should be conducted, and a new regimen should be considered, which includes at least four second-line drugs, such as fluoroquinolones, amikacin, capreomycin, kanamycin, ethionamide/prothionamide, cycloserine, linezolid, clofazimine, delamanid, bedaquiline, p-aminosalicylic acid, imipenem-cilastatin/meropenem, amoxicillin-clavulanate, thioacetazone, given over at least 18 months [72,84].

One of the most common reasons for admission to the CCU is respiratory failure, a phenomenon that occurs in about 1.5% of hospitalized patients with active TB. Respiratory failure can result from various developments of superimposed bacterial pneumonia, ARDS, or massive hemoptysis, among others. Management of these secondary processes involves directed therapy. For pneumonia, treatment consists of initiation of broad-spectrum antibiotics, which are promptly narrowed based on the data collected from sputum samples. In a patient with concomitant ARDS, standard mechanical ventilation strategies to reduce ARDS are appropriate, including lower tidal volumes and a conservative fluid strategy. In the case of massive hemoptysis, initial efforts should be directed at airway control, with the goal of maintaining adequate gas exchange, a process that typically requires endotracheal intubation and mechanical ventilation. Once the patient is stabilized, bronchoscopy should be performed to isolate the bleeding vessel, followed by treatment with topical epinephrine, among other things [72]. Mortality is high for patients with active TB and respiratory failure, with one study showing in-hospital mortality of 69% for patients requiring mechanical ventilation for treatment of TB. Risk factors for mortality in these patients include older age, duration of symptoms of more than 4 weeks, and multi-organ failure [77].

Extrapulmonary TB can affect any organ and typically occurs via hematogenous spread of the bacilli. In the central nervous system, this results in meningitis, tuberculoma of the brain or spine cord, and possible stroke. Within the pericardium, this can cause pericarditis or pericardial effusion. As with pulmonary TB, diagnosis requires high clinical suspicion, followed by identification of TB with lumbar puncture, echocardiogram, and pericardial puncture, with the latter two modalities being used for cardiac-related TB. Cerebrospinal and pericardial fluid analysis will show an increased cell count, with lymphocytic predominance, increased protein, and decreased glucose counts [72]. Treatment of extrapulmonary TB involving the pericardium and central nervous system consists of a similar course as that of pulmonary TB, with the exception of meningeal involvement, which requires a 12-month regimen. For those with meningeal and pericardial TB, steroids are also recommended with dexamethasone or equivalent doses of prednisolone for a duration of 2 months [72,78,83].

COMPLICATIONS OF THERAPY

Pathology related to TB does not necessarily only arise from direct infection with *M. tuberculosis* but can also come as a result of the adverse effects of the anti-TB drug regimen leading to drug-induced liver injury. This typically manifests as laboratory studies showing elevated liver enzymes greater than three times normal values, as well as clinical signs of liver dysfunction, which include right upper quadrant pain, jaundice, coagulopathy, hypoglycemia, and encephalopathy in its severe form. Management involves replacement of first-line drugs with second-line agents [72].

REFERENCES

1. Koplan JP, Bond TC, Merson MH, et al. Consortium of universities for global health executive board. Towards a common definition of global health. *Lancet* 2009;373:1993–1995.
2. Scutchfield FD, Michener JL, Thacker SB. Are we there yet? Seizing the moment to integrate medicine and public health. *Am J Public Health* 2012;102(suppl 3):S312–S316.
3. WHO|World malaria report—World Health Organization. Available at: https://www.who.int/malaria/publications/world_malaria_report/en/.
4. Neglected tropical diseases—World Health Organization. Report of a WHO consultation Geneva, 2018. Available at: https://www.who.int/neglected_diseases/en/.
5. Hotez PJ, Alvarado M, Basáñez M-G, et al. The global burden of disease study 2010: Interpretation and implications for the neglected tropical diseases. *PLOS Negl Trop Dis* 2014;8(7):e2865.

6. Tim Baker, Khalid K, Acicbe O, et al. On behalf of the council of the World Federation of Societies of Intensive & Critical Care Medicine. Critical care of tropical disease in low income countries: Report from the task force on tropical diseases by the World Federation of Societies of Intensive and Critical Care Medicine. *J Crit Care* 2017;42:351–354.

7. Marshall JC, Bosco L, Adhikari NK, et al. What is an intensive care unit? A report of the task force of the World Federation of Societies of Intensive and Critical Care Medicine. *J Crit Care* 2017;37:270–276.

8. WHO. World Health Statistics 2016: Monitoring health for the SDGs. https://www.who.int/gho/publications/world_health_statistics/2016/en.

9. European Centre for Disease Prevention and Control. Introduction to the Annual epidemiological report for 2015. In: ECDC. Annual epidemiological report for 2015. Stockholm: ECDC; 2017. Available at: https://ecdc.europa.eu/en/annual-epidemiological-reports-2016/methods.

10. Mace KE, Arguin PM, Tan KR. *Morbidity and Mortality Weekly Report (MMWR) Surveill Summ* 2018;67(7):1–28.

11. Chaill K, Gilles H. *Tropical Medicine: A Clinical Text.* New York, Fordham University Press.

12. Silamut K, Phu NH, Whitty C, et al. A quantitative analysis of the microvascular sequestration of malaria parasites in the human brain. *Am J Pathol* 1999;155:395–410.

13. Karnad DR, Nor MBMat, GA Richards, Baker T, Amin P. On behalf of the Council of the World Federation of Societies of Intensive and Critical Care Medicine. Intensive care in severe malaria: Report from the task force on tropical diseases by the World Federation of Societies of Intensive and Critical Care Medicine. *J Crit Care* 2018;43:356–360.

14. Barsoum RS. Malarial acute renal failure. *J Am Soc Nephrol* 2000;11:2147–2154.

15. Taylor TE, Molyneux ME, Wirima JJ, Fletcher KA, Morris K. Blood glucose levels in Malawian children before and during the administration of intravenous quinine for severe falciparum malaria. *New Engl J Med* 1988;319:1040–1047.

16. Janka JJ, Koita OA, Traore B, et al. Increased pulmonary pressures and myocardial wall stress in children with severe malaria. *J Infect Dis* 2010;202:791–800.

17. Marks M, Gupta-Wright A, Doherty JF, Singer M, Walker D. Managing malaria in the intensive care unit. *Br J Anaesth* 2014;113(6):910–921.

18. Maitland K, Kiguli S, Opoka R, et al., for the FEAST Trial Group. Mortality after fluid bolus in African children with severe infection. *N Engl J Med* 2011;364:2483–2495.

19. Rhodes A, Evans LE, Alhazzani et al. Surviving sepsis campaign: International guidelines for management of sepsis and septic shock: 2016. *Intensive Care Med* 2017;43(3):304–377.

20. Okoromah CA, Afolabi BB, Wall EC. Mannitol and other osmotic diuretics as adjuncts for treating cerebral malaria. *Cochrane Database Syst Rev* 2011;4:CD004615.

21. Mohanty S, Mishra SK, Patnaik R, et al. Brain swelling and mannitol therapy in adult cerebral malaria: A randomized trial. *Clin Infect Dis* 2011;53(4):349–355.

22. Mohana A, Sharmab SK, Bollinenic S. Review articles acute lung injury and acute respiratory distress syndrome in malaria. *J Vector Borne Dis* 2008;45:179–193.

23. Mehta S, Hill NS. Noninvasive ventilation. *Am J Respir Crit Care Med* 2001;163:540–577.

24. Acute Respiratory Distress Syndrome Network, Brower RG, Matthay MA, Morris A, Schoenfeld D, Thompson BT, Wheeler A. Ventilation with lower tidal volumes as compared with traditional tidal volumes for acute lung injury and the acute respiratory distress syndrome. *N Engl J Med* 2000;342(18):1301–1308.

25. Vandroux D, Leaute B, Hoarau N, et al. High frequency oscillation ventilation and extracorporeal membrane oxygenation during pernicious malaria. *Med Mal Infect* 2011;41:209–212.

26. Haake DA, Levett PN. Leptospirosis in humans. *Curr Top Microbiol Immunol* 2015;387:65–97.

27. Jiménez JI, Marroquin JL, Richards GA, Amin P. Leptospirosis: Report from the task force on tropical diseases by the World Federation of Societies of Intensive and Critical Care Medicine. *J Crit Care* 2018;43:361–365.

28. Bhatt S, Gething PW, Brady OJ, et al. The global distribution and burden of dengue. *Nature* 2013;496(7446):504–507.

29. Chakravarti A, Arora R, Luxemburger C, Fifty years of dengue in India. *Trans R Soc Trop Med Hyg* 2012;106(5):273–282.

30. Gubler DJ. The global emergence/resurgence of arboviral diseases as public health problems. *Arch Med Res* 2002;33(4):330–342.

31. Mustafa MS, Rasotgi V, Jain S, Gupta. Discovery of fifth serotype of dengue virus (DENV-5): A new public health dilemma in dengue control. *Med J Armed Forces India* 2015;71(1):67–70.

32. Carey DE. Chikungunya and dengue: A case of mistaken identity? *J Hist Med Allied Sci* 1971;26(3):243–262.

33. Fried JR, Gibbons RV, Kalayanarooj S, et al. Serotype-specific differences in the risk of dengue hemorrhagic fever: An analysis of data collected in Bangkok, Thailand from 1994 to 2006. *PLOS Negl Trop Dis* 2010;4(3):e617.

34. Rico-Hesse R, Harrison LM, Salas RA, et al. Origins of dengue type 2 viruses associated with increased pathogenicity in the Americas. *Virology* 1997;230(2):244–251.

35. Cologna R, Armstrong PM, Rico-Hesse R. Selection for virulent dengue viruses occurs in humans and mosquitoes. *J Virol* 2005;79(2):853–859.

36. Bennett SN, Holmes EC, Chirivella M, et al. Molecular evolution of dengue 2 virus in Puerto Rico: Positive selection in the viral envelope accompanies clade reintroduction. *J Gen Virol* 2006;87(Pt 4):885–893.

37. Vu TT, Holmes EC, Duong V, et al. Emergence of the Asian 1 genotype of dengue virus serotype 2 in Viet Nam: in vivo fitness advantage and lineage replacement in South-East Asia. *PLOS Negl Trop Dis* 2010;4(7):e757.

38. Wu SJ, Grouard-Vogel G, Sun W, et al. Human skin Langerhans cells are targets of dengue virus infection. *Nat Med* 2000;6(7):816–820.

39. Libraty DH, Pichyangkul S, Ajariyakhajorn C, et al. Human dendritic cells are activated by dengue virus infection: Enhancement by gamma interferon and implications for disease pathogenesis. *J Virol* 2001;75(8):3501–3508.

40. Kyle JL, Beatty PR, Harris E. Dengue virus infects macrophages and dendritic cells in a mouse model of infection. *J Infect Dis* 2007;195(12):1808–1817.

41. Hall WC, Crowell TP, Watts DM, et al. Demonstration of yellow fever and dengue antigens in formalin-fixed paraffin-embedded human liver by immunohistochemical analysis. *Am J Trop Med Hyg* 1991;45(4):408–417.

42. Bhoopat L, Bhamarapravati N, Attasiri C et al. Immunohistochemical characterization of a new monoclonal antibody reactive with dengue virus-infected cells in frozen tissue using immunoperoxidase technique. *Asian Pac J Allergy Immunol* 1996;14(2):107–113.

43. Couvelard A, Marianneau P, Bedel C, et al. Report of a fatal case of dengue infection with hepatitis: Demonstration of dengue antigens in hepatocytes and liver apoptosis. *Hum Pathol* 1999;30(9):1106–1110.

44. Huerre MR, Lan NT, Marianneau P, et al. Liver histopathology and biological correlates in five cases of fatal dengue fever in Vietnamese children. *Virchows Arch* 2001;438(2):107–115.

45. Miagostovich MP, Ramos RG, Nicol AF, et al. Retrospective study on dengue fatal cases. *Clin Neuropathol* 1997;16(4):204–208.

46. Ramos C, Sánchez G, Pando RH, et al. Dengue virus in the brain of a fatal case of hemorrhagic dengue fever. *J Neurovirol* 1998;4(4):465–468.

47. Halstead SB. Etiologies of the experimental dengues of Siler and Simmons. *Am J Trop Med Hyg* 1974;23(5):974–982.

48. Wilder-Smith A, Ooi EE, Vasudevan SG, et al. Update on dengue: Epidemiology, virus evolution, antiviral drugs, and vaccine development. *Curr Infect Dis Rep* 2010;12(3):157–164.

49. Halstead SB. Pathogenesis of dengue: Challenges to molecular biology. *Science* 1988;239(4839):476–481.

50. Pongpan S, Wisitwong A, Tawichasri C, Patumanond J, Namwongprom S. Development of dengue infection severity score. *ISRN Pediatr* 2013;2013:845876.

51. Pongpan S, Patumanond J, Wisitwong A, Tawichasri C, Namwongprom S. Validation of dengue infection severity score. *Risk Manag Healthc Policy* 2014;7:45–49.

52. Rigau-Pérez JG, Clark GG, Gubler DJ, Reiter P, Sanders EJ, Vorndam AV. Dengue and dengue haemorrhagic fever. *Lancet* 1998;352(9132):971–977.

53. World Health Organization, R.O.f. S.-E.A., *Comprehensive Guideline for Prevention and Control of Dengue and Dengue Haemorrhagic Fever.* WHO Regional Office for South-East Asia, 2011.

54. World Health Organization. *Dengue Guidelines for Diagnosis Treatment Prevention and Control.* 2009.

55. Kalayanarooj S, Chansiriwongs V, Nimmannitya S. *Dengue Patients at the Children's Hospital, Bangkok: 1995–1999 Review.* WHO Regional Office for South-East Asia, Dengue Bulletin, 2002. 26:33–42.

56. Guzman MG, Jaenisch T, Gaczkowski R, et al. Multi-country evaluation of the sensitivity and specificity of two commercially-available NS1 ELISA assays for dengue diagnosis. *PLOS Negl Trop Dis* 2010;4(8):e811.

57. Huits R, Soentjens P, Maniewski-Kelner U, et al. Clinical utility of the nonstructural 1 antigen rapid diagnostic test in the management of dengue in returning travelers with fever. *Open Forum Infect Dis* 2017;4(1):273.

58. Hunsperger EA, Muñoz-Jordán J, Beltran M, et al. Performance of dengue diagnostic tests in a single-specimen diagnostic algorithm. *J Infect Dis* 2016;214(6):836–844.

59. Ngo NT, Phuong CX, Kneen R, et al. Acute management of dengue shock syndrome: A randomized double-blind comparison of 4 intravenous fluid regimens in the first hour. *Clin Infect Dis* 2001;32(2):204–213.

60. Dung NM, Day NP, Tam DT, et al. Fluid replacement in dengue shock syndrome: A randomized, double-blind comparison of four intravenous-fluid regimens. *Clin Infect Dis* 1999;(4):787–794.

61. Wills BA, Dung NM, Loan HT, et al. Comparison of three fluid solutions for resuscitation in dengue shock syndrome. *N Engl J Med* 2005;353(9):877–889.

62. Lum LC, Abdel-Latif ME, Goh AY, Chan PW, Lam SK. Preventive transfusion in dengue shock syndrome—is it necessary? *J Pediatr* 2003;143(5):682–684.

63. Lye DC, Lee VJ, Sun Y, Leo YS. Lack of efficacy of prophylactic platelet transfusion for severe thrombocytopenia in adults with acute uncomplicated dengue infection. *Clin Infect Dis* 2009;48(9):1262–1265.

64. Stanworth SJ, Dyer C, Choo L, et al. Do all patients with hematologic malignancies and severe thrombocytopenia need prophylactic platelet transfusions? Background, rationale, and design of a clinical trial (trial of platelet prophylaxis) to assess the effectiveness of prophylactic platelet transfusions. *Transfus Med Rev* 2010;24(3):163–171.

65. Krishnamurti C, Kalayanarooj SI, Cutting MA, et al. Mechanisms of hemorrhage in dengue without circulatory collapse. *Am J Trop Med Hyg* 2001;65(6):840–847.

66. Heemskerk D, Caws M, Marais B, Farrar J. *Tuberculosis in Adults and Children.* London, UK: Springer, 2015.

67. Smith I. Mycobacterium tuberculosis pathogenesis and molecular determinants of virulence. *Clin Microbiol Rev* 2003;16(3):463–496.

68. World Health Organization. Global Tuberculosis Report 2018.

69. Davies PD. Tuberculosis: The global epidemic. *J Ind Med Assoc* 2000;98:100–102.

70. Zaman K. Tuberculosis: A global health problem. *J Health Popul Nutr* 2010;28(2):111–113.

71. Zumla A, Raviglione M, Hafner R. Fordham von Reyn C. Tuberculosis. *N Engl J Med* 2013;368(8):745–755.

72. Otu A, Hashmi M, Mukhtar A, et al. The critically ill patient with tuberculosis in intensive care: Clinical presentations, management and infection control. *J Crit Care* 2018;45:184–196.

73. Centers for Disease Control and Prevention. Guidelines for Preventing the Transmission of Mycobacterium tuberculosis in Health-Care Facilities, 1994.

74. Talbot E, Raffa B. Mycobacterium tuberculosis. *Mol Med Microbiol* (2nd ed.). 2015;3:1637–1653.

75. Crevel R, Hill P. Tuberculosis. *Infect Dis* (4th ed.). 2017;1:271–284.e1.

76. Ahmad S. Pathogenesis, immunology, and diagnosis of latent *Mycobacterium tuberculosis* infection. *Clin Dev Immunol* 2010;2011:814943.

77. Hagan G, Nathani N. Clinical review: Tuberculosis on the intensive care unit. *Crit Care* 2013;17:240.

78. Centers for Disease Control and Prevention. Treatment for TB Disease.

79. Saenz B, Hernandez-Pando R, et al. The dual face of central nervous system tuberculosis: A new Janus Bifrons? *Tuberculosis* (Edinb) 2013;93(2):130–135.

80. Lewinsohn D, Leonard M, LoBue PA, et al. Official American Thoracic Society/Infectious Diseases Society of America/Centers for Disease Control and Prevention clinical practice guidelines: Diagnosis of tuberculosis in adults and children. *Clin Infect Dis* 2017;64:111–115.

81. Center for Disease Control and Prevention. Availability of an assay for detecting *Mycobacterium tuberculosis*, including rifampin-resistant strains, and considerations for its use. *Morb Mortal Wkly Rep* 2013;62(41):821–824.

82. Nahid P, Dorman S, Alipanah N, et al. Official American thoracic society/centers for disease control and prevention/infectious diseases society of America clinical practice guidelines: Treatment of drug-susceptible tuberculosis. *Clin Infect Dis* 2016;63(7):e147–e195.

83. Center for Disease Control and Prevention. Treatment of tuberculosis. *Morb Mortal Wkly Rep* 2003;52(11):1–77.

84. Seaworth B, Griffith D. Therapy of multidrug-resistant and extensively drug-resistant tuberculosis. *Microbiol Spectrum* 2017;52(11):1–28.

8 Diagnostic Approach to Rash and Fever in the Critical Care Unit

Lee S. Engel, Charles V. Sanders, and Fred A. Lopez

CONTENTS

CLINICAL PERSPECTIVE

There are numerous potential etiologic agents that can cause the syndrome of fever and rash. Skin manifestations may be an early sign of a life-threatening infection. The ability to rapidly identify the cause of fever and rash in critically ill patients is essential for the proper management of the patient and protection of the healthcare worker(s) providing care for that patient.

A rapid method to narrow the potential life-threatening causes of fever and rash has been described by Cunha [1]. Patients from the community who are ill enough to be admitted to the critical care unit and have the syndrome of fever and rash from outside the hospital will most likely also have meningococcemia, Rocky Mountain spotted fever (RMSF), community-acquired toxic shock syndrome (TSS), severe drug

reactions, severe bacteremia, *Vibrio vulnificus* septicemia, gas gangrene, arboviral hemorrhagic fevers, dengue infection, or measles (Table 8.1). Patients who develop fever and rash after admission to the hospital will most commonly have drug reactions, staphylococcal bacteremia from central lines, systemic lupus erythematosus, or postoperative TSS. Multidrug-resistant gram-negative bacterial infections, including *Acinetobacter baumannii* and *Klebsiella pneumoniae*, should be considered as possible etiologies of fever and rash in patients who are hospitalized or associated with long-term care facilities [2].

The traditional approach to the patient with fever and rash is based on the characteristic appearance of the rash [3–5]. The most common types of rash include

TABLE 8.1
Etiology of Rash and Fever Based on Admission Status

Rash and Fever on Admission to the Critical Care Unit	Rash and Fever After Admission to the Critical Care Unit
Meningococcemia	Drug reaction
Rocky Mountain spotted fever	Nosocomial acquired toxic shock syndromes
Overwhelming pneumococcal or staphylococcal sepsis	Nosocomial staphylococcal sepsis
Toxic shock syndrome	"Surgical" scarlet fever
Epidemic typhus	*Vibrio vulnificus*
Typhoid fever	Cholesterol emboli syndrome
Measles	
Arboviral hemorrhagic fever	
Gas gangrene (Clostridial myonecrosis)	
Dengue	
Systemic lupus erythematosus	

Source: Data in table from text of a review by Cunha, B.A., *Crit. Care Clin.*, 14, 35–53, 1998.

petechial, maculopapular, vesicular, erythematous, and nodular. Although there can be overlap in presentation, most causes of fever and rash can be grouped into one specific form of cutaneous eruption [5].

A systematic approach requires a thorough history that includes patient age, seasonality, travel, geography, immunizations, childhood illnesses, sick contacts, medications, immune status, time of onset of symptoms, and the characteristics of the rash [4]. A detailed history, physical exam, and characterization of the rash will help the clinician reduce the number of possible etiologies. Appropriate laboratory testing will also assist in delineating the cause of fever and rash in the critically ill patient.

HISTORY

A comprehensive history of the events leading up to the development of fever and rash is essential in the determination of the etiology of the illness. Several initial questions should be answered before taking a complete history [6,7]:

1. Can the patient or someone who is with the patient provide a history?
2. Does the patient require cardiopulmonary resuscitation?
3. Are special isolation precautions needed?
   For example, patients with meningitis due to *Neisseria meningitidis* will need droplet precautions, while patients with varicella infections will need airborne and contact precautions (Table 8.2). Health care workers should always exercise universal precautions. Gloves should be worn during the examination of the skin whenever an infectious etiology is considered.

TABLE 8.2
Transmission-Based Precautions for Hospitalized Patients

Standard Precautions

Use standard precautions for the care of all patients.

Airborne Precautions

In addition to standard precautions, use airborne precautions for patients known or suspected to have serious illnesses transmitted by airborne droplet nuclei.

Examples of such illnesses include the following:

Measles

Varicella (including disseminated zoster)[a]

Tuberculosis[b]

Droplet Precautions

In addition to standard precautions, use droplet precautions for patients known or suspected to have serious illnesses transmitted by large-particle droplets. Examples of such illnesses include:

- Invasive *Haemophilus influenzae* type b disease, including meningitis, pneumonia, epiglottitis, and sepsis
- Invasive *Neisseria meningitidis* disease, including meningitis, pneumonia, and sepsis

Other serious bacterial respiratory infections spread by droplet transmission, including:

- Diphtheria (pharyngeal)
- *Mycoplasma* pneumonia
- Pertussis
- Pneumonic plague

Streptococcal pharyngitis, pneumonia, or scarlet fever in infants and young children

Serious viral infections spread by droplet transmission, including those caused by:

- Adenovirus
- Influenza
- Mumps
- Parvovirus B19
- Rubella

Contact Precautions

In addition to standard precautions, use contact precautions for patients known or suspected to have serious illnesses easily transmitted by direct patient contact or by contact with items in the patient's environment. Examples of such illnesses include:

- Gastrointestinal, respiratory, skin, or wound infections or colonization with multidrug-resistant bacteria judged by the infection control program, based on current state, regional, or national recommendations, to be of special clinical and epidemiologic significance
- Enteric infections with a low infectious dose or prolonged environmental survival, including those caused by:
  - *Clostridium difficile*
  - For diapered or incontinent patients: enterohemorrhagic *Escherichia coli* 0157:H7, *Shigella*, hepatitis A, or rotavirus
  - Respiratory syncytial virus, parainfluenza virus, or enteroviral infections in infants and young children

Skin infections that are highly contagious or that may occur on dry skin, including:

- Diphtheria (cutaneous)
- Herpes simplex virus (neonatal or mucocutaneous)
- Impetigo

(Continued)

TABLE 8.2 (Continued)
Transmission-Based Precautions for Hospitalized Patients

- Major (non-contained) abscesses, cellulitis, or decubitiPediculosis
- Scabies
- Staphylococcal furunculosis in infants and young children
- Zoster (disseminated or in the immunocompromised host)

Viral/hemorrhagic conjunctivitis

Viral hemorrhagic infections (Ebola, Lassa, or Marburg)

Source: Garner, J.S., *Infec. Control Hosp. Epidemiol.*, 17, 53–80, 1996; Centers for Disease Control and Prevention, Guidelines for preventing the transmission of *Mycobacterium tuberculosis* in health-care facilities, *Morb. Mortal. Wkly. Rep.*, 43, 1–132, 1994.

Note: CDC infection control guidelines reprinted from Garner JS and the Hospital Infection Control Practices Advisory Committee (Garner JS and hospital Infection Control Practices Advisory Committee, 1996).

a Certain infections require more than one type of precaution.

b See Centers for Disease Control and Prevention.

4. Are the skin lesions suggestive of a disease process that requires immediate antibiotic therapy?

Patients with infections suggestive of *Neisseria meningitidis*, RMSF, bacterial septic shock, TSS, or *Vibrio vulnificus* will need urgent medical and possibly surgical treatment to improve their chance of survival.

5. Does the patient have an unusual disease due to travel or bioterrorism?

Agents such as smallpox and viral hemorrhagic fevers (i.e., Ebola and Marburg) produce a generalized rash, while plague and anthrax may produce localized lesions. Isolation precautions will also need to be addressed (Table 8.2).

After the preliminary evaluation of the patient, the physician can obtain more information, including history of present illness and previous medical, social, and family histories.

Specific questions about the history of the rash itself are often helpful in determining its etiology (Table 8.3). Such questions should include time of onset, site of onset, change in appearance of the lesions, symptoms associated with the rash (i.e., itching, burning, numbness, and tingling), provoking factors, previous rashes, and prior treatments.

The physical exam should focus on the patient's vital signs; general appearance; and the assessment of lymphadenopathy, nuchal rigidity, neurological dysfunction, hepatomegaly, splenomegaly, arthritis, and mucosal membrane lesions (Table 8.4) [5,6]. Skin examination to determine the type of the rash (Table 8.5) includes evaluation of distribution pattern, arrangement, and configuration of lesions.

The remainder of this chapter will provide a diagnostic approach to patients with fever and rash based on the characteristics of the rash. Several clinically relevant causes of each type of rash associated with fever are described in brief detail.

TABLE 8.3
Fever and Rash: History

Age of patient

Season of the year

Type of prodrome associated with current illness

History of drug or antibiotic allergies

Medications taken within the past 30 days (prescription or nonprescription)

Drug ingestion

Exposure to febrile or ill persons within the recent past

Prior illness

Occupational exposures

Sun exposures

Recent travel

Exposure to wild or rural habitats

Exposure to insects, arthropods, or wild animals

Exposure to pets

Immunizations

Exposure to sexually transmitted diseases

HIV risk factors (IV drug use, unprotected sex, sexual orientation)

Site of rash onset

Factors effecting immunological status (chemotherapy, steroid use, hematological malignancy, solid organ or bone marrow transplant, asplenia)

Valvular heart disease

Rate of rash development (slow versus fast)

Direction of rash spread (centrifugal versus centripetal)

Evolution of rash (has the rash changed?)

Relationship between rash and fever

Presence or absence of pruritus

Previous treatment of the rash (topical or oral therapies)

Source: Weber, D.J. et al., The acutely ill patient with fever and rash, in: Mandell GL, Bennett JE, Dolin R eds., *Principles and Practice of Infectious Disease*, Elsevier Churchill Livingstone, Philadelphia, PA, 729–746, 2005; McKinnon, H.D., Jr. and Howard, T. Evaluating the febrile patient with a rash, *Am. Fam. Physician*, 62(4), 804–816, 2000.

PETECHIAL AND PURPURIC RASHES

Petechiae are produced by extravasation of red blood cells and are less than 3 mm in diameter. Petechiae appear as small red or brown spots on the skin. Purpura or ecchymosis are lesions that are larger than 3 mm and often form when petechiae coalesce. Neither petechial nor purpuric lesions blanch when pressure is applied.

Infections associated with diffuse petechiae are generally among the most life-threatening ones and require urgent evaluation and management. There are many infectious causes of these lesions (Table 8.6); several of the most dangerous include meningococcemia, rickettsial infections, and bacteremia [1,5,10].

ACUTE MENINGOCOCCEMIA

Neisseria meningitidis is one of the leading causes of bacterial meningitis in teens and young adults [12–14]. Bacterial meningitis associated with a petechial or purpuric rash should always suggest meningococcemia [1]. The diagnosis of meningococcemia is more difficult to make when meningitis is not present.

TABLE 8.4
Fever and Rash: Physical Examination

1. Vital signs
   a. Temperature
   b. Pulse
   c. Respiration
   d. Blood pressure
2. General appearance
   a. Alert
   b. Acutely ill
   c. Chronically ill
3. Signs of toxicity
4. Adenopathy/location of adenopathy
5. Presence of mucosal, conjunctival, or genital lesions
6. Hepatosplenomegaly
7. Arthritis
8. Nuchal rigidity/neurological dysfunction
9. Features of rash
   a. Type of primary rash lesion (Table 8.5)
   b. Presence of secondary lesions
   c. Presence of desquamation
   d. Presence of excoriations
   e. Configuration of individual lesions
   f. Arrangement of lesions
   g. Distribution pattern: Exposed areas; centripetal versus centrifugal

Source: Weber, D.J. et al., The acutely ill patient with fever and rash, in *Principles and Practice of Infectious Disease*, Mandell, G.L., Bennett, J.E. and Dolin, R. eds., Elsevier Churchill Livingstone, Philadelphia, PA, 729–746, 2005; McKinnon, H.D., Jr. and Howard, T., *Am. Fam. Physician.*, 62, 804–816, 2000.

TABLE 8.5
Type of Rash Lesions

Macule	A circumscribed flat lesion that differs from surrounding skin by color. Patches are very large macular lesions.
Papule	A circumscribed, solid, elevated skin lesion that is palpable and smaller than 0.5 cm in diameter.
Plaque	A large, solid, elevated skin lesion that is palpable and greater the 0.5 cm in diameter, often formed by confluence of papules.
Nodule	A circumscribed, solid, palpable skin lesion with depth as well as elevation.
Pustule	A circumscribed raised lesion containing pus.
Vesicle	A circumscribed elevated, fluid filled lesion less than 0.5 cm in diameter.
Bulla	A circumscribed elevated, fluid filled lesion greater than 0.5 cm in diameter.

Source: Weber, D.J. et al., The acutely ill patient with fever and rash, in *Principles and Practice of Infectious Disease*, Mandell, G.L., Bennett, J.E. and Dolin, R. eds., Elsevier Churchill Livingstone, Philadelphia, PA, 729–746, 2005; Nesbitt, L.T.J., Evaluating the patient with a skin infection-general considerations, in *The Skin and Infection: A Color Atlas and Text*, Sanders, C.V. and Nesbitt, L.T.J. eds., Williams and Wilkins, Baltimore, Maryland, 1–6, 1995.

TABLE 8.6
Etiology of Rash and Fever Based on Type of Rash

Purpura or Petechiae
- *Bacterial diseases*
  - Meningococcemia
  - Rocky Mountain spotted fever
  - Gonococcemia
  - Staphylococcal sepsis
  - Pneumococcal sepsis
  - Pseudomonal sepsis
  - Multidrug-resistant sepsis
  - Bacterial endocarditis
  - Typhus
- *Non-bacterial diseases*
  - Cytomegalovirus
  - Epstein–Barr virus
  - Echovirus 9
  - Enteroviral infections
  - Hepatitis B
  - Influenza
  - Measles
  - Rubella
- *Non-infectious diseases*
  - Allergic vasculitis
  - Acute thrombocytopenia
  - Hematologic malignancy
  - Acute rheumatic fever
  - SLE
  - Hyperglobulinemia
  - Amyloidosis

Centrally Distributed Maculopapular Rash
- *Bacterial diseases*
  - Lyme disease
  - Scarlet fever
- *Non-bacterial diseases*
  - Enteroviral infections
  - Rubeola
  - Rubella
  - Erythema infectiosum
  - Roseola
- *Non-infectious diseases*
  - Drug reactions

Peripherally Distributed Maculopapular Rash
- *Bacterial Diseases*
  - Secondary syphilis
  - Erythema multiforme (Table 8.7)
- *Non-bacterial diseases*
  - Erythema multiforme (Table 8.7)

Diffuse Erythema with Desquamation
- *Bacterial Diseases*
  - Scarlet fever
  - Scalded skin syndrome
  - Ehrlichiosis
  - Streptococcus viridans bacteremias
  - Leptospiral infections
- *Non-bacterial diseases*
  - Enteroviral disease

(Continued)

TABLE 8.6 (Continued)
Etiology of Rash and Fever Based on Type of Rash

- *Non-infectious diseases*
  - Kawasaki disease
  - TEN

Vesicular, Bullous, or Pustular Rash

- *Bacterial diseases*
  - *Staphylococcus aureus* bacteremia
  - *Vibrio vulnificus*
  - *Rickettsia akari*
- *Non-bacterial diseases*
  - Varicella
  - Herpes zoster
  - Herpes simplex
- *Non-infectious diseases*
  - Allergy
  - Plant dermatitis
  - Eczema vaccinatum

Nodular Rash

- *Bacterial diseases*
  - *Nocardia*
  - Mycobacteria
  - Erythema nodosum (Table 8.8)
- *Non-bacterial diseases*
  - Disseminated fungal infections (*Candida, Cryptococcus, Blastomycosis, Histoplasma, Coccidioides,* and *Sporothrix*)
  - Erythema nodosum (Table 8.8)
- *Non-infectious diseases*
  - Erythema nodosum (Table 8.8)

Source: Cunha, B.A., *Crit. Care Clin.*, 14, 35–53, 1998; Kang, J.H., *Infect. Chemother.*, 47, 155–166, 2015; Schlossberg, D., *Infec. Dis. Clin. N. Am.*, 10, 101–110, 1996; Weber, D.J. et al., The acutely ill patient with fever and rash, in *Principles and Practice of Infectious Disease*, Mandell, G.L., Bennett, J.E. and Dolin, R. eds., Elsevier Churchill Livingstone, Philadelphia, PA, 729–746. 2005. McKinnon, H.D., Jr. and Howard, T., *Am. Fam. Physician.*, 62, 804–816, 2000.

Abbreviations: TEN, toxic epidermal necrolysis; RMSF, Rocky Mountain spotted fever; TSS, toxic shock syndrome

Meningococcemia can occur sporadically or in epidemics and is more commonly diagnosed during the winter months. *Neisseria meningitidis* is primarily spread by respiratory droplets that require close, prolonged contact for transmission [15]. The risk of infection is highest in infants, asplenic patients, alcoholics, patients with complement deficiency, and persons who live in dormitories (coeds, military personnel, or prisoners). Initial symptoms include cough, headache, sore throat, nausea, and vomiting. Acute meningococcemia progresses rapidly, and patients typically appear ill, with high spiking fevers, tachypnea, tachycardia, mild hypotension, and a characteristic petechial rash [16,17]. Signs and symptoms of meningeal irritation such as headache, vomiting, and change in consciousness occur in up to 88% of patients with meningococcemia [16,18].

The rash associated with meningococcemia begins within 24 hours of clinical illness. The petechiae enlarge rapidly, becoming papular and then purpuric. Lesions most commonly occur on the extremities and trunk but may also be found on the head and mucous membranes [7]. The development of lesions on the palms and soles is usually a late finding [1]. Purpuric skin lesions have been described in 60%–100% of meningococcemia cases and are most commonly seen at presentation [19,20]. Histological studies demonstrate diffuse vascular damage, fibrin thrombi, vascular necrosis, and perivascular hemorrhage in the involved skin and organs. The skin lesions associated with meningococcal septic shock are thought to result from an acquired or transient deficiency of protein C and/or protein S [21]. Meningococci are present in endothelial cells and neutrophils, and smears of skin lesions are positive for gram-negative diplococci in many cases [22,23].

The diagnosis of meningococcemia is also aided by culturing the petechial lesions. Blood cultures should be drawn. Admission laboratory data usually demonstrate a leukocytosis and thrombocytopenia. Patients with meningococcemia but without meningitis will have a normal cerebrospinal fluid (CSF) profile. If meningococcal meningitis is present, the CSF culture is usually positive, although the Gram stain may be negative. Typically, the CSF-associated glucose is low, and the protein is elevated. Latex agglutination tests are available, but diagnostic sensitivity for CSF is limited [24,25]. Molecular techniques using polymerase chain reaction (PCR) assays provide rapid, sensitive and specific diagnostic testing [24,25]. Bacteriologic isolation remains the gold standard for the diagnosis of meningococcal infection [26].

CHRONIC MENINGOCOCCEMIA

Chronic meningococcemia is rare, and the associated lesions differ from those seen in acute meningococcemia. Diagnosis of chronic meningococcemia is challenging. Patients present with intermittent fever, rash, arthritis, and arthralgia, occurring over a period of several weeks to months [27,28]. The lesions of chronic meningococcemia are usually pale- to pink-colored macules and/or papules typically located around a painful joint or pressure point. Nodules may develop in the lower extremities. The lesions of chronic meningococcemia develop during periods of fever and fade when the fevers dissipate. These lesions (in contrast to those of acute meningococcemia) rarely demonstrate the bacteria on Gram stain or histology [7,10]. *Neisseria meningitidis* are internalized by endothelial cells, and the bacteria disrupt the intracellular junctions, without breaking the endothelial barrier [29]. The PCR testing of skin biopsy specimens may prove to be a valuable method of diagnosis for this rare entity [30].

ROCKY MOUNTAIN SPOTTED FEVER

Rocky Mountain spotted fever, the most lethal rickettsial disease in the United States, is caused by *Rickettsia rickettsii* [31–36]. Infection occurs approximately 7 days after a bite by a tick vector (*Dermacentor* or *Rhipicephalus*). As of 2010, cases of RMSF are reported as spotted fever rickettsiosis (SFR) to capture cases of RMSF, *R. parkeri* rickettsiosis,

Pacific Coast tick fever, and rickettsialpox [37]. The incidence of SFR has increased since 2000 from 495 reported cases to 4269 reported cases in 2016 [38]. Patients who have frequent exposure to dogs and live near wooded areas or areas with high grass may be at an increased risk of infection. The RMSF is more common in men and is most prevalent in the southern Atlantic and southern central states. North Carolina and Oklahoma are the states with the highest incidence, accounting for over 35% of the cases. Greater than 90% of patients are infected between April and September. During this season, there are increased numbers of ticks. Furthermore, research has demonstrated a link between warmer temperatures and increased tick aggressiveness [39].

Ticks spread infection most commonly through the saliva while feeding and requires tick attachment for at least 4 hours for transmission [36]. Only about 50% of patients provide a history of a tick bite. The incubation period ranges from 3 to 14 days [38]. The onset of RMSF can be abrupt with fever, headache, myalgias, shaking chills, photophobia, and nausea. Patients may have periorbital edema, conjunctival suffusion, and localized edema, involving the dorsum of the hands and feet [40]. A notable clinical finding is a pulse-temperature disparity (i.e., relative bradycardia during fever). Localized abdominal pain secondary to liver involvement, renal failure manifested by acute tubular necrosis, pancreatitis, left ventricular failure, adult respiratory distress syndrome (ARDS), and mental confusion or deafness may also be noted [40].

The rash usually begins about 2–4 days after the onset of fever and is usually not apparent until the fifth or sixth day [35]. The lesions are initially maculopapular and evolve into petechiae within 2–4 days. Characteristically, the rash starts on the wrists, forearms, ankles, palms, and soles and then spreads centripetally to involve the arms, thighs, trunk, and face. Centripetal evolution of the rash occurs 6–18 hours after the rash develops. Digital gangrene can also occur.

Prompt treatment with tetracycline decreases mortality [41,42]. Most patients' defervesce within 2–3 days, and these patients should receive treatment for at least 3 days after showing improvement [38,43]. Chloramphenicol, the only other antimicrobial agent recommended for the treatment of RMSF, causes gray baby syndrome and should not be used for pregnant women who are near term [43]. Gray baby syndrome occurs due to a lack of the necessary liver enzymes to metabolize chloramphenicol, resulting in drug accumulation, which leads to vomiting, ashen gray skin color, limp body tone, hypotension, cyanosis, hypothermia, cardiovascular collapse, and often death. Pregnant women who are near term may receive tetracycline because the risk of fetal damage or death is minimal. Previously, tetracycline is not recommended for pregnant women, in the first or second trimester, because of the effects on fetal bone and dental development [43]. However, doxycycline use during pregnancy probably does not pose substantial teratogenic risk [38]. Pregnant woman should be counseled about risks and benefits for treatment decision. Chloramphenicol can be administered in early pregnancy because gray baby syndrome is not a risk during the early period of fetal development [43].

Mortality form RMSF may be decreasing over the last decade. Initial mortality in the United States was reported to be about 20%; however, the actual case mortality rate has decreased to 0.5% [38,44]. This decrease in mortality may be related to infection with less severe rickettsioses or variations in virulence of some *R. rickettsii* strains.

Clinical diagnosis is the basis for treatment. Serological testing is sensitive but does not distinguish between infection with *R. rickettsii* and other rickettsia of the spotted fever group [38,45]. Indirect fluorescent antibody testing is the best serological method available; however, the test has poor sensitivity during the first 710 days of disease onset. Sensitivity increases to greater than 90% when a convalescent serum is available 14–21 days later [43]. Direct immunofluorescence on tissue specimens has a sensitivity of about 70%. Polymerase chain reaction is limited because of poor sensitivity for detecting *R. rickettsii* DNA in blood [45]. It may be used to amplify DNA from a biopsy of a rash lesion [38]. The Weil-Felix test is no longer recommended because of poor sensitivity and specificity. When SFR is suspected, healthcare providers can send specimens via their state health departments to the Centers for Disease Control and Prevention (CDC) for testing by indirect immunofluorescence antibody, immunohistochemical assay, PCR, and cell culture [45].

Routine admission tests may demonstrate a normal or decreased peripheral white blood cell count, hyponatremia, and thrombocytopenia. The total bilirubin and serum transaminases may be elevated. If pancreatitis is present, the serum amylase will be elevated. Patients who develop renal failure may demonstrate a rise in blood urea nitrogen (BUN) and creatinine, suggestive of pre-renal azotemia secondary to intravascular volume deficit. When the central nervous system is involved, the CSF profile will demonstrate a mild pleocytosis, normal glucose and protein concentrations, and negative Gram stain and culture. Routine blood cultures will be negative in RMSF.

SEPTIC SHOCK

The definition of sepsis was recently updated and is now described as life-threatening organ dysfunction caused by a dysregulated host response to infection [46,47]. Organ dysfunction can be identified as an acute change in the Sequential Organ Failure Assessment (SOFA) score. Parameters of the SOFA score include PaO_2/FiO_2 ration, platelet count, bilirubin, mean arterial pressure, Glasgow Coma Scale score, creatinine, and urine output. The SOFA score is not intended to be used as a tool for patient management but rather to clinically characterize a septic patient. A more rapid tool, qSOFA, allows clinicians to promptly evaluate for organ dysfunction. The parameters of qSOFA include respiratory rate greater than 22 per minute, altered mentation, and systolic blood pressure less than 100 mmHg [47].

Septic shock is defined as a subset of sepsis in which underlying circulatory and cellular metabolism abnormalities are profound enough to substantially increase mortality. Per the 2016 guidelines, patients with septic shock can be identified with a clinical construct of sepsis with persisting hypotension requiring vasopressors to maintain mean arterial pressure greater than 65 mmHg and having a serum lactate concentration greater than 2 mmol/L despite adequate volume resuscitation.

Mortality associated with sepsis remains high [48]. Based on the definitions set forth in the latest guidelines, the critical care unit (CCU) mortality rate for septic shock is 39%, about 5% higher than the mortality rate for septic shock based on the previous guideline-derived definition of septic shock [48].

Studies using older sepsis guidelines suggest that the peak incidence of septic shock occurs in patients who are in their seventh decade of life [49]. Risk factors for sepsis include cancer, immunodeficiency, chronic organ failure, and iatrogenic factors. Sepsis develops from infections of the chest, abdomen, genitourinary system, and primary bloodstream in more than 80% of cases [49–51].

Symmetric peripheral gangrene or purpura fulminans is a cutaneous syndrome most commonly associated with septic shock secondary to *Neisseria meningitidis* or *Streptococcus pneumoniae*. This syndrome is usually preceded by petechiae, ecchymosis, purpura, and acrocyanosis. Acrocyanosis denotes a grayish color to the skin that occurs on the lips, legs, nose, ear lobes, and genitalia and does not blanch on pressure. Bacteria are usually absent in smears obtained from these skin lesions.

The diagnosis of septic shock requires a causal link between infection and organ failure [45]. Some patients may have clinically obvious infection such as purpura fulminans, cellulitis, TSS, pneumonia, or a purulent wound. Blood cultures remain the gold standard for detection of bacteremia. Disadvantages of blood culture in the context of sepsis include the latency period between sample collection and culture results and the time it takes to determine antibiotic sensitivities (up to 72 hours) [52]. There are also diverse biomarkers such as lactate, procalcitonin, interleukin 6, C-reactive protein, proadrenomedullin, and soluble subtype of CD14 cell surface receptor that have been used to substantiate the diagnosis of sepsis and monitor treatment response [52].

Sepsis is the third most common cause of death in non-surgical CCUs and is the primary cause of death in surgical CCUs [52]. Overall mortality varies from 12% to 80% depending on patients' age, sex, ethnic origin, comorbidities, presence of acute lung injury or ARDS, whether the infection is nosocomial or polymicrobial, or whether the causative agent is a fungus [49,50]. Gram-negative infections are responsible for 25%–30% of cases of septic shock, while gram-positive infections now account for 30%–50% of the cases of septic shock. Multi-drug resistant bacteria and fungi are increasingly reported as causes of sepsis [49,50,53].

Updated surviving sepsis campaign guidelines were published in 2016 and provide a thorough review of treatment options for severe sepsis and septic shock [46]. Important steps to the treatment of sepsis and septic shock include the following: (1) Initial resuscitation with crystalloids with frequent hemodynamic reassessment; (2) appropriate routine microbiologic cultures, including blood, to be obtained prior to antibiotic administration; (3) administration of empiric broad spectrum IV antimicrobials as soon as possible after recognition and within 1 hour for both sepsis and septic shock; and (4) emergent source control to be identified or excluded as rapidly as possible in patients with sepsis or septic shock and any required source control intervention to be implemented as soon as medically and logistically practical after the diagnosis is made [46,54].

BACTERIAL ENDOCARDITIS

Infective endocarditis is described as acute or subacute based on the tempo and severity of the clinical presentation [55]. Categories of infective endocarditis include native valve infective endocarditis, prosthetic valve endocarditis, infective endocarditis associated with intravenous (IV) drug abuse, and nosocomial infective endocarditis [56]. The characteristic lesion is a vegetation composed of platelets, fibrin, microorganisms, and inflammatory cells on the heart valve. Patients with cardiac vegetation greater than 10 mm have increased risk of embolism and death [57]. Conditions associated with endocarditis include injection drug use, poor dental hygiene, long-term hemodialysis, diabetes mellitus, HIV infection, long-term indwelling venous catheters, mitral valve prolapse with regurgitation, rheumatic heart disease, other underlying valvular diseases, and prosthetic valves [58–61]. Organisms associated with endocarditis include *Staphylococcus aureus*, viridans streptococci, enterococci, gram-negative bacilli (including the *Haemophilus spp., Aggregatibacter actinomycetemcomitans, Cardiobacterium hominis, Eikenella corodens, Kingella spp.* [HACEK] organisms), and fungi. Staphylococci are the most common pathogen associated with endocarditis among patients in the CCU, and infection with methicillin-resistant *Staphylococcus aureus* is associated with heightened mortality [62,63].

Non-specific symptoms and signs of endocarditis include fever, arthralgia, wasting, unexplained heart failure, new heart murmurs, pericarditis, septic pulmonary emboli, strokes, and renal failure [64]. Skin lesions occur less frequently today than they once did but aid in the diagnosis if present [64]. Cutaneous manifestations of endocarditis include splinter hemorrhages, petechiae, Osler's nodes, and Janeway lesions.

Petechiae are the most common skin lesions seen during endocarditis. The petechiae are small, flat, and reddish brown and do not blanch with pressure. They frequently occur in small crops and are usually transient. They are often found on the heels, shoulders, legs, oral mucous membranes, and conjunctiva.

Osler's nodes may be seen in patients with subacute bacterial endocarditis. These nodules are tender, indurated, and erythematous. They occur most commonly on the pads of the fingers and toes, are transient, and resolve without the development of necrosis. The histology of these lesions demonstrates microabscesses and microemboli.

Janeway lesions are small, painless, erythematous macules found on the palms and soles. These lesions can be seen with both acute and subacute endocarditis. Histological analysis reveals microabscesses with neutrophil infiltration.

DISSEMINATED GONOCOCCAL INFECTION

Disseminated gonococcal infections (DGI) result from gonococcal bacteremia and occur in 1%–3% of patients with untreated *Neisseria gonorrhea*—associated mucosal infection [65–67]. It is most often seen in young women during menses or pregnancy [68]. Most patients present with fever, rash, polyarthritis, and tenosynovitis [66].

Skin lesions, which occur in 50%–70% of patients with DGI, are the most common manifestation [68]. The rash usually begins on the first day of symptoms and becomes more prominent with the onset of each new febrile episode [69]. The lesions begin as tiny red papules or petechiae (1–5 mm in diameter) that evolve to a vesicular and then pustular form. The pustular lesions develop a gray, necrotic center with a hemorrhagic base [66,69]. The rash of DGI tends to be sparse and widely distributed, and the distal extremities are most commonly involved. Gram stain of the skin lesions rarely demonstrates organisms.

Clinical clues of DGI include the symptoms of fever, rash, and arthritis/tenosynovitis. Early in the infection, blood cultures may be positive; later, synovial joint fluid aspirated from associated effusions may yield positive cultures. Smears of the cervix and urethral exudates may also yield positive results.

Strains of ceftriaxone-resistant *Neisseria gonorrhea* are emerging [70]. These strains have been found in Japan, Canada, and Australia. Therapy with ceftriaxone and azithromycin is still recommended [71].

CAPNOCYTOPHAGA INFECTION

Capnocytophaga canimorsus is a fastidious gram-negative bacillus that is part of the normal gingival flora of dogs and cats [72,73]. Human infections are associated with dog or cat bites, cat scratches, and contact with wild animals [72,73]. Predisposing factors include trauma, alcohol abuse, steroid therapy, chronic lung disease, and asplenia [72,73]. The clinical syndrome consists of fever, disseminated intravascular coagulation (DIC), necrosis of the kidneys and adrenal glands, thrombocytopenia, hypotension, and renal failure. The mortality rate approaches 25%.

Skin lesions occur in 50% of infected patients, often progressing from petechiae to purpura to cutaneous gangrene [74]. Other dermatologic lesions include macules, papules, painful erythema, and eschars. Hematogenous spread can result in endocarditis, septic arthritis, peritonitis, pneumonia, intra-abdominal abscess, meningitis, and septic shock [75].

Clinical clues include a compatible clinical syndrome and a history of a dog- or cat-inflicted wound. The diagnosis of *Capnocytophaga canimorsus* by blood culture can be difficult, and proper identification by this method may occur only 30% of the time [76,77]. More prompt diagnosis may be made by Gram staining the buffy coat. *Capnocytophaga canimorsus* is found in the neutrophil and has a characteristic, filamentous, rod-shaped morphology [76]. The CDC can assist with diagnosis using organism-specific PCR, 16S rRNA gene amplification, and matrix-assisted laser desorption/ionization time-of-flight mass spectrometry [77].

DENGUE VIRUS

Dengue is a flavivirus comprised of four serotypes, i.e., DEN-1, DEN-2, DEN-3, and DEN-4. Dengue viruses are transmitted from person to person through infected female *Aedes* mosquitoes. *Aedes albopictus* is a secondary vector that can survive cooler environments, which makes it capable of spreading dengue to North America and Europe [78]. The mosquito acquires the virus by taking a blood meal from an infected human or monkey. The virus incubates in the mosquito for 7–10 days before it can transmit the infection.

Dengue has made an enormous resurgence over the last decade and is one of the most common vector-borne diseases worldwide [79,80]. More than 2.5 billion people are at risk for dengue infections worldwide [81]. Recent estimates indicate 390 million dengue infections occur per year, of which 96 million have clinical manifestations. The number of reported cases increased from 2.2 million in 2010 to 3.2 million in 2015 [78]. The resurgence of dengue has been attributed to multiple factors, including global population growth, urbanization, deforestation, poor housing and waste management systems, deteriorating mosquito control, virus evolution, and climate change [80].

Dengue fever (also known as "breakbone fever" or "dandy fever") is a short-duration, non-fatal disease characterized by the sudden onset of headache, retro-orbital pain, high fever, joint pain, and rash [78,81,82]. The initial rash of dengue occurs within the first 24–48 hours of symptom onset and involves flushing of the face, neck, and chest [83]. A subsequent rash, 3–5 days later, manifests as a generalized morbilliform eruption, palpable pinpoint petechiae, and islands of sparing that begin centrally and spread peripherally [1]. Dengue fever lasts about 7 days. Recovery from infection provides lifelong immunity to that serotype but does not preclude patients from being infected with the other serotypes of dengue virus, i.e., secondary infections.

Dengue hemorrhagic fever and dengue TSS are two deadly complications of dengue viral infection that occur during secondary infection. Dengue hemorrhagic fever is characterized by hemorrhage, thrombocytopenia, and plasma leakage. Dengue shock syndrome includes the additional complications of circulatory failure and hypotension [79,81,82].

The incubation period for dengue virus infections is 3–14 days. If a patient presents greater than 2 weeks after visiting an endemic area, dengue is much less likely [84]. Laboratory abnormalities include neutropenia, followed by lymphocytosis, hemoconcentration, thrombocytopenia, and an elevated aspartate aminotransferase in the serum [85]. The diagnosis of dengue virus-associated infection can be accomplished by PCR, detection of anti-dengue virus immunoglobulin M (IgM), centrifugation amplification to enhance virus isolation, or flow cytometry for early detection of cultured virus [86].

A dengue vaccine was licensed in 2015 and is approved in 20 countries [78]. It is a live attenuated vaccine and appears to be safe in persons who have had previous dengue infections. However, there is an increased risk of severe dengue in patients who have been vaccinated prior to having their first natural dengue infection.

MACULOPAPULAR RASH

LYME DISEASE

Lyme disease is the most common tick vector-associated disease in the United States [87,88]. Lyme disease is caused by the spirochete *Borrelia burgdorferi*, a microbe that is transmitted by four species of the tick *Ixodes*. Lyme disease is endemic in the northeastern, mid-Atlantic, northcentral, and far western regions of the United States. The yearly incidence of Lyme disease is between 10 and 100 cases per 100,000 persons in endemic areas [89]. The disease has a bimodal age distribution, with peaks in patients younger than 15 years and older than 29 years of age [90]. Most infections occur between May and September.

Lyme disease has three stages: Early localized, early disseminated, and late disease. Early localized disease is characterized by erythema migrans (EM), which forms 1–30 days following the tick bite [91]. Erythema migrans occurs in 60%–80% of the cases and begins as a small red papule at the site of the bite. Approximately 70% of patients do not recall having a tick bite [89]. The lesion expands centrifugally and can get as large as 50 cm in diameter. The lesion develops central clearing in 30% of cases. If untreated, the lesions resolve over several weeks. Other symptoms associated with early localized disease include fatigue, myalgias, arthralgia, headache, fever, and chills.

Early disseminated disease occurs weeks to months after the tick bite. Patients may not recall having had the typical EM rash. Patients at this stage can present with lymphocytic meningitis, cranial nerve palsies, mild pericarditis, atrial-ventricular block, arthritis, generalized or regional adenopathy, conjunctivitis, iritis, hepatitis, and painful radiculoneuritis, followed by decreased sensation, weakness, and absent reflexes [87,88,92]. Disseminated skin lesions, when present, are similar to EM but smaller and usually multiple in number.

Late disease, usually developing greater than 6 months after infection, is characterized by chronic asymmetric oligoarticular arthritis that involves the large joints (most often the knee). The central nervous system may also be affected,

manifesting as subacute encephalopathy, axonal polyneuropathy, or leukoencephalopathy. Diagnosis of early localized disease is based on the history and physical exam. The standard recommended strategy for serological testing in patients with early and late disseminated disease is a two-step process [93]. The initial step is an enzyme-linked immunosorbent assay (ELISA). Positive or equivocal specimens undergo a western blot to detect the presence of IgG or IgM. ELISA may be negative during the first 4 weeks of infection. Cerebrospinal fluid should be obtained if neurological signs are present. Synovial fluid can be evaluated if arthritis is present.

Over 90% of patients diagnosed correctly with Lyme disease have successful outcomes with treatment. The *Ixodes* tick is capable of transmitting other infectious agents, *Anaplasma phagocytophilum* and *Babesia*; thus, co-infections are possible. A small number of patients may develop post-treatment Lyme disease syndrome (PTLDS) [94]. No further serologic testing is recommended for PTLDS, as IgG and IgM antibodies can persist and remain detectible for years.

DRUG REACTIONS

Drugs cause adverse skin reactions in 2%–3% of hospitalized patients [95]. Classic drug reactions include urticaria, angioedema, exanthems, vasculitis, exfoliative dermatitis/erythroderma, erythema multiforme (EM), Stevens-Johnson syndrome (SJS), and toxic epidermal necrolysis (TEN) [95,96]. There is no predilection for age, gender, or race [10]. There are, however, HLA allele associations with severe cutaneous adverse reactions such as HLA-B 5701 with abacavir and HLA-B 5801 association with allopurinol [97]. Diagnosis of a drug reaction is based on a patient's previous reaction to the drug, ruling out alternate etiological causes of the rash, timing of events, drug levels, evidence of overdose, patient reaction to drug discontinuation, or patient reaction to re-challenge.

DRUG EXANTHEMS

Exanthems are the most common skin reaction to drugs. The rash usually appears within the first 2 weeks after the offending drug is started and resolves within days after the drug is stopped. The rash is often described as a morbilliform, macular, and/or papular eruption. Pruritus is the most common associated symptom of drug-induced rash. Low-grade fever and peripheral blood eosinophilia may also occur in association with drug exanthems. Severe cutaneous adverse reactions encompass a spectrum of delayed-type hypersensitivity responses that include acute generalized exanthematous pustulosis, drug reaction with eosinophilia with systemic symptoms, and the most concerning forms, Steven-Johnson syndrome (SJS) and

TEN [97]. Differentiation of severe cutaneous adverse drug reactions from EM may be difficult during the early phase of the clinical presentation.

Erythema Multiforme

Erythema multiforme (EM) is an acute, self-limited, peripheral eruptive maculopapular rash that is characterized by a target lesion. It most often affects persons 20 years and 30 years of age and has a predilection for men. Erythema multiforme is separated from other bullous diseases, SJS and TEN, based on the pattern of individual skin lesions, including target lesions and atypical raised palpable lesions [98,99]. The rash begins as a dull-red macular eruption that evolves into papules and the characteristic target lesion. Target lesions are often found on the palms, soles, knees, and elbows (acral target lesions). Vesicles and bullae occasionally develop in the center of the papules [10]. There are many causes of this disorder (Table 8.7). Viral infections (herpes simplex virus or HSV) are the most common cause of EM [100].

Erythema multiforme may present with varying degrees of severity (previously classified as EM minor and major) [10]. Bullae and systemic symptoms are absent in less severe EM. The rash rarely affects the mucous membranes and is usually limited to the extensor surfaces of the extremities. This mild form of EM is often associated with HSV infection. Conversely, drug reactions are usually associated with more severe manifestations of EM. Erythema multiforme can be further classified into EM with mucosal involvement and EM without mucosal involvement and is further subdivided into EM minus (<1 mucosal site) and EM majus (>2 mucosal sites) [100]. Fever, cheilosis, stomatitis, balanitis, vulvitis, and conjunctivitis can also occur [95]. Diagnosis of EM is based on clinical findings. Histopathological analysis can help to differentiate EM from other mucocutaneous diseases, including pemphigus vulgaris, paraneoplastic pemphigus, mucosal bullous pemphigoid, linear IgA dermatosis, hand-foot-mouth disease, erosive lichen planus, fixed drug eruption, lupus erythematosus, and cutaneous vasculitis [100].

Stevens-Johnson Syndrome and Toxic Epidermal Necrolysis

The spectrum of SJS and TEN represents the most common and most lethal of the severe cutaneous adverse reactions [101]. The mortality rate for these entities reaches 40%. The causes of SJS and TEN are similar to the etiologies of EM (Table 8.7). Unlike EM, SJS and TEN are more frequently associated with drug reactions than with viral infections. The drug classes most frequently associated with SJS and TEN are antibiotics, antivirals, anticonvulsants, and agents that affect uric acid metabolism [101]. There is often a 4- to 28-day interval between the beginning of the causative

TABLE 8.7
Causes of Erythema Multiforme

Viral Infections	**Anticonvulsants**
Herpes simplex 1 and 2	Barbiturates
Epstein–Barr virus	Carbamazepine
Hepatitis A, B, C	Phenytoin
Varicella zoster	**Antituberculoids**
Parvovirus B19	Rifampin
Bacterial Infections	Isoniazid
Hemolytic streptococci	Pyrazinamide
Pneumococcus	**Other Drugs**
Staphylococcus species	Allopurinol
Proteus species	Fluconazole
Salmonella species	Hydralazine
Mycobacterium tuberculosis	Non-steroidal anti-inflammatory
Mycobacterium avium complex	drugs
Francisella tularensis	Estrogen
Vibrio parahaemolyticus	**Physical Factors/Contact**
Yersinia species	Sunlight
Mycoplasma pneumonia	Cold
Fungal Infections	X-ray therapy
Histoplasma capsulatum	Tattooing
Coccidioidomycosis	Poison ivy
Parasitic Infections	**Other Factors**
Trichomonas species	Pregnancy
Toxoplasma gondii	Multiple myeloma
Antibiotics	Leukemia
Penicillin	Collagen diseases
Tetracyclines	Idiopathic (50%)
Erythromycin	
Sulfa drugs	
Vancomycin	

Source: Plaza, J.A. and Prieto, V.G., Erythema Multiforme. emedicine.medscape, 2018, https://emedicine.medscape.com/article/1122915-overview#a4.

drug and the onset of signs and symptoms. The mechanism is thought to be a delayed hypersensitivity reaction mediated by Th1 cells [102]. Predisposing factors include polypharmacy, concomitant use of radiotherapy and anticonvulsants, genetic susceptibility, HIV infection, and other immunocompromised states [97,102].

Patients with SJS and TEN often present with pharyngitis, malaise, and fever [102]. These syndromes evolve over a few days with the evolution of mucous membrane erosions. Mucosal erosions and widespread purpuric macules and blisters develop, which are often confluent and eventually result in skin detachment (Nikosky's sign) [102]. Ocular involvement may be present in up to 60% of cases and may present as corneal ulcer, anterior uveitis, and pan-ophthalmitis [102]. Stevens-Johnson syndrome affects less than 10% of the total body surface, differentiating it from TEN, the most serious cutaneous drug reaction, which affects over 30% of the total body surface area. [95,98]. Older age, intestinal involvement, and pulmonary involvement predict a poor outcome [95,96].

The clinical diagnosis of SJS and TEN depends on a good history; emphasis on medication use and previous infections, combined with a thorough physical exam, is essential. Skin biopsy will demonstrate full-thickness epidermal necrosis. Because extensive skin detachment results in massive transepidermal fluid losses, patients with these adverse cutaneous drug eruptions are managed similarly to patients who have had extensive burn injuries. Sepsis can result secondary to microbial colonization of denuded skin.

SECONDARY SYPHILIS

Syphilis is a systemic disease caused by *Treponema pallidum*. Syphilis is classified into primary, secondary, early latent, late latent, and tertiary stages. The lesion of primary syphilis, the chancre, usually develops about 21 days after infection and resolves in 1–2 months. Patients with secondary syphilis can present with rash, mucosal lesions, lymphadenopathy, and fever. The rash of secondary syphilis may be maculopapular, papulosquamous, or pustular, and is characteristically found on the palms and the soles. Lues maligna is a rare form of secondary syphilis that is associated with a prodrome of fever, headache, myalgia, and ulcerating lesions [103]. Secondary syphilis can also involve any part of the body, including the lungs, kidneys, cardiovascular system, and central nervous system [104].

Diagnostic algorithms have changed over the last few years with the advancement of less expensive and rapid specific treponemal tests. A presumptive diagnosis of syphilis requires the use of two tests: A non-treponemal test (i.e., Venereal Disease Research Laboratory test and rapid plasma reagin) and a treponemal test (i.e., fluorescent treponemal antibody absorbed tests, the *T. pallidum* passive particle agglutination assay, and enzyme immunoassays) [105]. The specific treponemal tests were previously used to rule in the diagnosis of syphilis because false-positive non-treponemal tests can occur. However, with improved assays, the specific tests are now used for screening as well. Non-treponemal test antibody titers correlate with disease activity and are used to follow treatment response. Dark-field microscopic examination of skin or mucous membrane lesions can be done to diagnose syphilis definitively during the early stages as well.

MOSQUITO-VECTOR–BORNE VIRAL INFECTIONS

The flaviviruses (Zika, dengue, and West Nile) as well as the alpha virus (Chikungunya) have been reported with increasing frequency over the last decade. While most infections with these viruses are mild, there are significant cases that require CCU admission. All are transmitted by mosquito vectors, are associated with a clinical presentation of fever and rash, and present significant public health threats [37]. The rashes associated with Zika, West Nile, and Chikungunya are more frequently macular or papular, while dengue can result in a petechial rash, as discussed previously.

ZIKA VIRUS

Zika virus is transmitted by *Aedes albopictus* or *Aedes aegypti* mosquitoes and is endemic in Caribbean, Central and South America, Papua New Guinea, and the Cape Verde Islands [37]. An unusual aspect of Zika is the occurrence of sexual transmission. A pruritic macular or papular rash is common with Zika virus infection [106,107]. Zika is associated with microcephaly in newborns and Guillain-Barre syndrome in adults [106]. Diagnosis is made by real-time reverse transcriptase PCR.

WEST NILE VIRUS

West Nile virus (WNV) is transmitted to humans primarily from the bite of an infected *Culex* mosquito [108]. The virus normally circulates between mosquitoes and birds. The first reported outbreak in the United States was in New York in 1999, and since then, WNV has spread southward and westward [109–112]. It has become seasonally endemic, with peak activity for transmission from July to October in temperate zones and from April to December in warmer climates [111,112].

Though most commonly spread by infected mosquitoes, WNV may also be transmitted by organ transplantation, blood transfusion, and breast milk [113–115]. Transplacental infection from mother to fetus has also been reported [113].

West Nile virus replicates at the site of inoculation and then spreads to the lymph nodes and bloodstream [116]. The majority of human infections, i.e., 80%, are asymptomatic [117].

West Nile viral symptomatic infections range from West Nile fever to neuroinvasive disease. Most patients with symptoms have self-limited West Nile fever. West Nile fever is characterized by acute onset of fever, headache, fatigue, malaise, muscle pain, difficulty concentrating, and neck pain [118,119]. Approximately 57% of patients with West Nile fever will have a transient macular rash on the trunk of the body [118].

Neuroinvasive disease develops in less than 1% of infected patients [117]. The clinical severity of WNV encephalitis ranges from disorientation to coma to death [120,121]. Advanced age is the most significant risk factor for severe neurologic disease. Risk increases 10-fold for persons 50–59 years of age and 43 times for persons greater than 80 years of age [110,114]. Neuroinvasive disease can present as meningitis, encephalitis, or acute flaccid paralysis [117,119,121–124]. Patients with WNV encephalitis or focal neurologic findings will often have persistent deficits for months to years [110,121]. Advanced age is also the most important risk factor for death. The overall case fatality rate for neuroinvasive WNV disease is 9% [110]. Patients with acute paralysis syndrome fare the worst; mortality approaches 50% when the respiratory system is involved, and only 7% of survivors regain baseline muscle strength [124].

Diagnosis of WNV disease can be made by a high index of clinical suspicion and detection of WNV-specific IgM in serum or CSF. The serum IgM can persist for up to 8 months; therefore, nucleic amplification tests for WNV such as reverse transcriptase PCR and real-time PCR may be required to prove that the infection is acute [119,125]. Molecular diagnosis by PCR may be limited, owing to low-level and short-lived viremia [126]. West Nile virus may be detected in urine samples for longer periods of time than in plasma, serum, or CSF, owing to retention in the kidneys [127]. West Nile virus also adheres to red blood cells [128]. The WNV RNA can be detected in the whole blood (86%), serum (26%), CSF (17%), plasma (20%) and urine (58%) of WNV-infected patients [126,129]. Serological testing to detect the presence of IgM-specific antibody in the CSF remains the most widely used method to diagnose neuroinvasive WNV. Patients who have been recently vaccinated for yellow fever or Japanese encephalitis or persons recently infected with the St. Louis encephalitis virus, Zika virus, or dengue virus may have false-positive results on IgM antibody tests for WNV [129,130]. Novel methods of detection that are under investigation, including next-generation sequencing and clustered regularly interspaced short palindromic repeats (CRISPR) technology [129].

DIFFUSE ERYTHEMATOUS RASHES WITH DESQUAMATION

TOXIC SHOCK SYNDROME

Toxic shock syndrome (TSS) is characterized by sudden onset of fever, chills, vomiting, diarrhea, muscle aches, and rash. It can rapidly progress to severe hypotension and multi-organ dysfunction. The overall case fatality rate is 5%.

The microbial etiology of TSS is usually *Staphylococcus aureus*; however, coagulase-negative staphylococci, Group A streptococci, Group B streptococci, Group C streptococci, and Group G streptococci can also produce this syndrome [131–134].

Toxic shock syndrome is most commonly seen in menstruating women, women using barrier contraceptive devices, persons who have undergone nasal surgery, and patients with postoperative staphylococcal wound infections [135]. Initially, cases associated with menstruation accounted for as many as 91% of the total cases [135]. The rate of menses-associated TSS has declined significantly since 1980 [136].

Management of TSS can be summarized by the seven "Rs" [134]. These include recognition, resuscitation, removal of the source of infection, rational choice of antibiotics, role of adjunctive treatment, review progress, and reduce risk of secondary cases in close contacts. Early recognition is important, owing to the high rate of morbidity and mortality associated with TSS. Resuscitation with aggressive fluid, respiratory, and inotropic support is important to curb the rapid progression to multi-organ failure. Source control is essential to stop the persistence of infection. Broad-spectrum antibiotics should be started as soon as possible.

Benefits of adjunctive clindamycin therapy include inhibition of super-antigen production, improved tissue penetration, and an ability to overcome the "Eagle effect" associated with streptococcal infections. The "Eagle effect" occurs when stationary-growth-phase streptococci produce less penicillin-binding proteins and, in turn, render penicillin less effective [137]. Intravenous immunoglobulin has also been postulated to provide benefit; however, definitive data are lacking [138]. Household contacts of patients who suffer TSS may benefit from antibiotic prophylaxis, as there is an increased risk of invasive Group A streptococcal disease in these contacts [139].

STAPHYLOCOCCAL TOXIC SHOCK SYNDROME

Staphylococcal TSS is caused by infection or colonization with toxin-producing bacteria. One hypothesis suggests that nearly all pathogens that cause disease across mucosal and skin barriers produce inflammation by inducing epithelial cells to produce proinflammatory cytokines [140]. The most common toxins associated with TSS, toxin 1 and enterotoxin B, are super-antigens that may produce such inflammation [141–144]. Other toxins that may be involved include cytolysins (sphingomyelinase, β-toxin, α-toxin, and Panton-Valentine leukocidin) and enterotoxins (A, C, D, E, and H) [140,145].

The clinical presentation of TSS was defined by the CDC in 1981 and last updated in 2011 [146]. All patients with TSS have high fever (>39°C), hypotension, and skin manifestations. Patients may also present with headache, vomiting, diarrhea, myalgias, pharyngitis, conjunctivitis, vaginitis, arthralgias, abdominal pain, or encephalopathy [147–150]. The syndrome can progress to shock, DIC, ARDS, and renal failure.

The rash of TSS may start as erythroderma that involves both the skin and mucous membranes. The rash is diffuse, red, and macular and may resemble a sunburn. The rash can involve the palms and soles. The erythema may be more intense around a surgical wound site. Mucosal involvement can involve the conjunctiva, oropharynx, or vagina [151]. One to 3 weeks after the onset of TSS, the palms and soles may desquamate [152].

Toxic shock syndrome can be divided into menstrual versus non-menstrual. The majority of menstrual cases of TSS are associated with tampon use [153]. Non-menstrual cases are caused by abscesses, cellulitis, bursitis, postpartum infections, vaginal infections, sinusitis, burn wounds, insect bites, and surgical procedures [151,154].

The diagnosis of TSS is based on the CDC diagnostic criteria [146]. Although *S. aureus* is isolated from mucosal or wound sites in 80%–90% of patients with TSS, this criterion is not required for diagnosis. *Staphylococcus aureus* is only recovered from blood cultures 5% of the time [153]. Other laboratory abnormalities may include hypocalcemia, elevated liver enzymes, elevated creatinine, thrombocytopenia, pyuria, and proteinuria [151].

STREPTOCOCCAL TOXIC SHOCK SYNDROME

The CDC defined streptococcal TSS in 2010 as an illness with hypotension, multiple organ dysfunction, a generalized erythematous macular rash that may desquamate, soft tissue necrosis, and isolation of group A streptococcus [155]. Several elements of the clinical history are suggestive of streptococcal TSS. These include recent trauma, surgical intervention, skin lesion or NSAID use, prodromal influenza-like symptoms, digestive symptoms (vomiting, diarrhea, and abdominal pain), severe pain out of proportion to exam, signs of soft tissue infection, generalized erythematous macular rash, palmer and plantar desquamation, and multiple organ failure [131,133,156,157].

Three phases are described for streptococcal TSS [156]. Phase 1 occurs 24–48 hours before the onset of hypotension and is characterized by high fever, myalgia, headache, nausea, vomiting, diarrhea, and skin changes. These skin changes may include an early transient macular rash or violaceous bullae associated with necrotizing fasciitis. Palmar and plantar desquamation is usually a later finding associated with TSS. The second phase is characterized by tachycardia, tachypnea, and high fever and may be associated with pain in a limb, abdomen, or thorax that is out of proportion to clinical exam. Stage 3 is characterized by circulatory shock accompanied by multiple-organ failure.

The pathogenies of streptococcal TSS are similar to that cause by *Staphylococcus aureus*. Group A, C, and G streptococci produce 11 different pyrogenic enterotoxins with superantigen activity [156]. One particular difference from staphylococcal-associated TSS is that streptococci can frequently (60% of the time) be isolated from blood culture [158]. The mortality rates for streptococcal TSS are five times higher than those for staphylococcal TSS [159]. Treatment remains high-dose parenteral penicillin G combined with clindamycin [156].

STAPHYLOCOCCAL SCALDED SKIN SYNDROME

Staphylococcal scalded skin syndrome (SSSS) describes a spectrum of superficial blistering skin disorders caused by *S. aureus* strains that produce exfoliative toxins [160]. This syndrome is more commonly seen in infants and young children, with rare appearance in adults. The clinical spectrum of SSSS includes a localized form, bullous impetigo, and a generalized form, pemphigus neonatorum.

The exfoliative toxins are also known as epidermolytic toxins, epidermolysins, and exfoliatins. Production of exfoliative toxin occurs in 5% of all *S. aureus* strains [160–162]. The two main exfoliative toxins are exfoliative toxin A (ETA) and exfoliative toxin B (ETB) [160,163,164]. Bullous impetigo (also known as bullous varicella or measles pemphigoid) presents with a few localized, fragile, superficial blisters that are filled with colorless, purulent fluid [165]. The lesions re-epithelialize in 5–7 days. This form of SSSS is usually seen only in children. Typically, there are no associated systemic symptoms. The lesions are located in the area of the umbilicus and perineum in infants and over the extremities in older children [166].

The generalized form of SSSS is termed pemphigus neonatorum or Ritter's disease. Risk factors for development in adults include renal dysfunction, lymphoma, and immunosuppression [166,167]. Patients with pemphigus neonatorum present with fever, erythema, malaise, and irritability. Patients then develop large superficial blisters that rupture easily due to friction [160]. A positive Nikolsky sign refers to dislodgement of the superficial epidermis when gently rubbing the skin [168]. If untreated, the epidermis will slough off, leaving extensive areas of denuded skin that are painful and susceptible to infection. Mucous membranes are not affected in SSSS.

Complications associated with SSSS include cellulitis, guttate psoriasis, septicemia, scarring, and post-streptococcal glomerulonephritis [169]. The mortality rate in children remains below 1% in the United States [170]. Potentially fatal complications in infants and young children occur because of the loss of protective epidermis. Hypothermia, dehydration, and secondary infections are the leading causes of morbidity and mortality for these age groups affected by generalized SSSS [171]. The mortality for adults with generalized SSSS is much higher, probably due to the associated comorbidities such as renal dysfunction, immunosuppression, or malignancy found in this population [170,172,173].

Diagnosis of both generalized and localized SSSS is based on clinical characteristics. A thorough exam looking for foci of infection (pneumonia, abscess, arthritis, endocarditis, sinusitis, etc.) should be undertaken. Unfortunately, in most cases, no focus is ever found [160]. Blood cultures are usually negative because toxins are produced at a distant site [166,174].

A number of different tests, including PCR, ELISA, radioimmune assays, and reverse latex agglutination assays, can be used to demonstrate toxin production by *S. aureus* [175]. The diagnostic challenge is that bacteria must first be isolated. When the diagnosis is uncertain, a skin biopsy may be the optimal test. The biopsy typically reveals mid-epidermal splitting at the level of the zona granulosa without cytolysis, necrosis, or inflammation [176]. Staphylococci may be seen in bullous lesions of localized disease but are rarely seen in the bullous lesions of generalized disease [167].

SCARLET FEVER

Scarlet fever is the result of infection with a *Streptococcus pyogenes* strain (i.e., Group A streptococcus) that produces a pyrogenic exotoxin (erythrogenic toxin). There are three different toxins, types A, B, and C, which are produced by 90% of these strains. Scarlet fever follows an acute infection of the pharynx/tonsils or skin [10]. It is most common in children between the ages of 1 and 10 years [159,177]. There has been an increase in worldwide cases, owing to major outbreaks in Vietnam and China as well as smaller outbreaks in the United States and Canada [177].

The rash of scarlet fever starts on the neck, chest, armpits, and groin and spreads to the arms and legs [10,178]. The rash is erythematous and diffuse and blanches with pressure. There are numerous papular areas in the rash that produce a sandpaper-type quality. On the antecubital fossa and axillary folds, the rash has a linear petechial character referred to as Pastia's lines [178]. The rash varies in intensity but usually fades in 4–5 days. Diffuse desquamation occurs after the rash fades [178]. Diagnosis of scarlet fever can usually be made on a clinical basis. The Centor criteria can aid the diagnosis of Group A streptococcal pharyngitis [179]. Confirmation of the diagnosis is supported by isolation of Group A streptococci from the pharynx and serology [159]. Complications of scarlet fever include peritonsillar and retropharyngeal abscesses, glomerulonephritis, pneumonia, endocarditis, and meningitis [177].

KAWASAKI DISEASE

Kawasaki disease (KD) is an acute, self-limited, systemic vasculitis of childhood [180–182]. It was first described by Tomisaku Kawasaki in Japan in 1961 [180] and is the predominant cause of pediatric-acquired heart disease in developed countries [182]. The signs and symptoms evolve over the first 10 days of illness and then gradually resolve spontaneously in most children.

The diagnostic criteria for classical KD include the following [180]:

1. Fever for 5 days or more that does not remit with antibiotics and is often resistant to antipyretics.
2. Presence of at least four of the following conditions:
   a. Bilateral (non-purulent) conjunctivitis
   b. Polymorphous rash
   c. Changes in the lips and mouth: reddened, dry, or cracked lips; strawberry tongue; and diffuse erythema of oral or pharyngeal mucosa
   d. Changes in the extremities: Erythema of the palms or soles; indurative edema of the hands or feet; and desquamation of the skin of the hands, feet, and perineum during convalescence
   e. Cervical lymphadenopathy: Lymph nodes more than 15 mm in diameter
3. Exclusion of disease with a similar presentation, such as scalded skin syndrome, TSS, and viral exanthems

Other clinical features include intense irritability (possibly due to cerebral vasculitis), sterile pyuria, and upper respiratory symptoms [182]. The major morbidity of KD is the development of coronary artery aneurysm(s), which occur in 25% of the cases.

More recently, Kawasaki Disease Shock Syndrome (KDSS) has been described [183,184]. The incidence rate of KDSS appears to be 2%–7% [184]. Furthermore, patients requiring CCU admission were more likely to have a longer duration of fever, lower hemoglobin, lower albumin concentration, and higher C-reactive protein and be less responsive to IV immunoglobulin [184]. Differentiation of KDSS from TSS can be difficult. Patients with KDSS tend to be younger and have lower hemoglobin concentrations but higher platelet counts than patients with TSS [185]. Patients with KDSS also have more echocardiographic abnormalities [185].

There are no specific or sensitive tests that can be used to diagnose KD. The diagnosis is made by clinical assessment of the criteria discussed earlier. The cause of KD is unknown; however, an infectious etiology is still being sought. Kawasaki disease has seasonal peaks in the winter and spring months, and focal epidemics occurred in the 1970s and 1980s [187].

Treatment with IV immunoglobulin (IVIG) remains standard practice. Low IgG levels after IVIG administration appears to be a marker for patients with poor response [188]. There also appears to be a correlation between IgG levels and albumin levels after infusion of IgG in patients who fail to respond to therapy [188]. There is some evidence that resistance to IVIG may be higher during warm-weather months as compared with cold-weather months, but regional differences may need to be further studied [189]. The American Heart Association recommends low-dose aspirin until coronary artery dilation is reduced [186].

OTHER CAUSES

Streptococcus viridans bacteremia can cause generalized erythema. Ehrlichiosis can produce a toxic shock-like syndrome with diffuse erythema. Enteroviral infections, graft versus host disease, and erythroderma may all present with diffuse erythema [10].

VESICULAR, BULLOUS, OR PUSTULAR RASHES

Vesicles and bullae refer to small and large blisters, respectively. Pustules refer to a vesicle filled with cloudy fluid. The causes of vesiculobullous rashes associated with fever include primary varicella infection, herpes zoster, herpes simplex, smallpox, *Staphylococcus aureus* bacteremia, gonococcemia, *Vibro vulnificus*, *Rickettsia akari*, enteroviral infections, parvovirus B19, and HIV infection. Other causes that will not be discussed include folliculitis due to staphylococci, *Pseudomonas aeruginosa*, and *Candida*, but these manifestations would not result in admission to a critical care unit.

VARICELLA-ZOSTER

Primary infection with varicella zoster virus (VZV) (i.e., chickenpox) is usually more severe in adults and immunocompromised patients. Although it can be seen year-round, the highest incidence of infection occurs in the winter and spring. The disease presents with a prodrome of fever and malaise 1–2 days prior to the outbreak of the rash. The rash begins as erythematous macules that quickly develop into vesicles. The characteristic rash is described as "a dewdrop on a rose petal." The vesicles evolve into pustules that umbilicate and crust. A characteristic of primary varicella is that lesions in all stages may be present at one time [10].

Herpes zoster (i.e., shingles) is caused by the reactivation of VZV, which lies dormant in the basal root ganglia [190]. The incidence of zoster is greatest in older age groups because of a decline in VZV-specific cell-mediated immunity. Herpes zoster also occurs more often in immunosuppressed patients such as transplant recipients [191–193] and HIV-infected patients [194–196].

Patients often have a prodrome of fever, malaise, headaches, and dysesthesias that precede the vesicular eruption by several days [197]. The characteristic rash usually affects a single dermatome and begins as an erythematous maculopapular eruption that quickly evolves into a vesicular rash. The lesions then dry and crust over in 7–10 days, with resolution in 14–21 days [190]. Disseminated herpes zoster is seen in patients with solid-organ transplants, hematological malignancies, and HIV infection [194,195,198–202]. Thirty-five percent of patients who have received bone-marrow transplants have reactivation of VZV, and 50% of these patients develop disseminated herpes zoster [200,203,204].

Both immunocompetent and immunocompromised patients can have complications from herpes zoster; however, the risk is greater for immunocompromised patients [205]. Complications of herpes zoster include herpes zoster ophthalmicus [198,206], acute retinal necrosis [207,208], Ramsay Hunt syndrome [209], aseptic meningitis [210], peripheral motor neuropathy [210], myelitis [210,211], encephalitis [210], pneumonitis [205], hepatitis [203], and pancreatitis [200]. Severe VZV pneumonia is one of the more common and serious complications associated with primary infection with a mortality up to 43% [212].

The diagnosis of primary varicella infection and herpes zoster is often made clinically. Diagnosis of the neurological complications can be made with CSF PCR assays [213,214]. Patients with ocular involvement should be seen promptly by an ophthalmologist.

SMALLPOX

Smallpox is caused by the variola virus. The last known case of naturally acquired smallpox occurred in Somalia (1977). The World Health Organization declared that smallpox had been eradicated from the world in 1980 as a result of global vaccination [215,216]. The only known repositories for this virus are in Russia and the United States. With the threat of bioterrorism, there is still a remote possibility that this entity would be part of the differential diagnosis of a vesicular rash.

Smallpox usually spreads by respiratory droplets, but infected clothing or bedding can also spread disease [217]. The incidence of smallpox is highest during the winter and early spring. The pox virus can survive longer at lower temperatures and low levels of humidity [218,219].

After a 12-day incubation period, smallpox infection presents with a prodromal phase of acute onset of fever (often greater than 40°C), headaches, and backaches [217].

A macular rash develops and progresses to vesicles and then pustules over 1–2 weeks [220]. The rash appears on the face, oral mucosa, and arms first but then gradually involves the whole body. The pustules are 4–6 mm in diameter and remain for 5–8 days, after which time they umbilicate and crust. The lesions of smallpox are generally all in the same stage of development. "Pock" marks are seen in 65%–80% of survivors. Historically, the case-associated mortality rate was 20%–50% [217]. In the United States, almost nobody under the age of 30 years has been vaccinated; therefore, this group is largely susceptible to infection.

The diagnosis of smallpox is based on the presence of a characteristic rash that is centrifugal in progression. Laboratory confirmation of a smallpox outbreak requires vesicular or pustular fluid collection by someone who is immunized. Confirmation can quickly be made by electron microscopic examination of the fluid specimen in a high-containment (BL-4) facility. Definitive identification in the laboratory is accomplished with viral cell culture, PCR, and restriction fragment-length polymorphism analysis [221].

MONKEYPOX

Monkeypox, an emerging zoonotic disease with increased incidence since the eradication of smallpox, is an orthopox-virus that was first discovered in an outbreak of monkeys imported from Central Africa to Denmark in 1958 [222]. Possible reasons for the increased monkeypox include cessation of smallpox vaccination in 1980, more frequent exposures to the animal reservoir, increased human-to-human transmission, and advances in diagnostic testing [223]. Smallpox vaccination provides about 85% protection against monkeypox [224]. The first human case was identified in a 9-year-old child in Zaire (1970) [225]. Monkeypox is endemic in Central and West Africa, and imported cases have occurred in many countries, including the United States [223]. Transmission is thought to occur from primary animal to humans by direct contact with infected animal body fluids, bites, and scratches. Secondary human-to-human transmission is thought to occur through large respiratory droplets or contact with body fluid, lesion material, and contaminated surfaces [223].

The skin lesions of monkeypox are indistinguishable from the skin lesions of ordinary smallpox [223,226,227]. A rash appears 1–3 days after the onset of fever, with lesions developing simultaneously and evolving at a similar rate. Lesions are mainly peripheral but can cover the entire body in severe cases. The lesions progress from maculopapular to fluid-filled vesicles to pustules, followed by crusting over a 10-day period. Crusts disappear within 4 weeks. Patient with previous smallpox vaccination will have milder and more pleomorphic skin rashes than unvaccinated patients [227]. One distinguishing finding is the presence of severe peripheral lymphadenopathy that is seen during early infection with monkeypox and not with smallpox [226]. Polymerase chase reaction, antigen detection tests, ELISA, and viral cell culture are useful for diagnosis [228]. The mortality associated with monkeypox infection approaches 10% [229].

HERPES SIMPLEX

Herpes simplex virus type 1 (herpes labialis) commonly causes vesicular lesions of the oral mucosa [230]. The illness is characterized by the sudden appearance of multiple, often painful vesicular lesions on an erythematous base. The lesions last for 10–14 days. Recurrent infections in the immunocompetent host are usually shorter than the primary infection. In the immunocompromised host, infections can be much more serious. Aside from vesicular eruptions on mucous membranes, the infection can cause keratitis, acute retinal necrosis, hepatitis, esophagitis, pneumonitis, and neurological syndromes [230–239].

Herpes simplex virus type 1 can cause sporadic cases of encephalitis characterized by rapid onset of fever, headache, seizures, focal neurological signs, and impaired mental function. Herpes simplex virus type 1 encephalitis has a high rate of mortality in the absence of treatment [240]. Electroencephalography (EEG) has some prognostic use; a normal EEG has been shown to independently predict survival [241]. Diagnosis can infrequently be made by culture; PCR analysis of the CSF has become the gold-standard technique for making the diagnosis [242]. Patients with suspected encephalitis should have magnetic resonance imaging of the brain, and CSF should be obtained for nucleic acid detection by PCR and possibly serologic tests for antibodies. The PCR should be repeated in 3–7 days, and serologic tests should be repeated after 2–4 weeks in patients with severe disease that remains without a diagnosis [243].

More recently, systemic reactivation of herpes virus has been demonstrated to occur in CCU patients [244,245]. In one study, 26% of patients with septic shock were noted to have viremia with HSV-1 [245]. Although HSV viremia appears to be common among critically ill patients, no single viremic event appeared to significantly impact mortality [245].

STAPHYLOCOCCUS AUREUS BACTEREMIA

Staphylococcus aureus can cause metastatic skin infections that often manifest as pustules [5]. The pustular skin eruption due to this organism is often widespread. Risk factors for bacteremia include older age, residency at a long-term care facility, diabetes, recent surgery, mechanical ventilation, HIV, hemodialysis, neoplasm, neutropenia, and IV drug use [246–251]. Bacteremia can lead to metastatic complications, such as endocarditis and septic arthritis. Risk factors for these metastatic complications include treatment delay, presence of foreign body material such as prosthetic implants, and valvular heart disease. Patients with metastatic infections have higher mortality. The use of ^{18}F-fluorodeoxyglucose-positron emission tomography in combination with low-dose computed tomography scanning was demonstrated in one study to localize metastatic infections [252]. Metastatic foci included endocarditis, endovascular infections, pulmonary abscess, and discitis. Patients with identified metastatic foci received proper therapy and had a lower relapse rate [252].

VIBRIO VULNIFICUS

Vibrio vulnificus is a slightly curved, gram-negative bacillus that is endemic in warm coastal waters around the world. *Vibrio vulnificus* is responsible for over 95% of seafood related deaths in the United States [253,254]. There are reports that virtually all oysters and 10% of crabs harvested in the warmer summer months from the Gulf of Mexico are culture-positive for *V. vulnificus* [255]. Consequently, the illness presents mostly between March and November [256]. In the United States, most cases occur in states bordering the Gulf of Mexico or those that import oysters from the Gulf states [257]. Risk factors for infection include liver disease (most commonly alcoholic), hemochromatosis, HIV infection, steroid use, malignancy, and achlorhydria [253].

Vibrio vulnificus has been associated with two distinct syndromes: septicemia and wound infection [258,259]. A third syndrome of gastrointestinal illness has also been suggested [260]. Primary septicemia is a fulminant illness that occurs after the consumption of contaminated raw shellfish. Consumption of raw oysters within 14 days preceding the illness has been reported in 96% of the cases [261]. Wound infection occurs after a pre-existing or newly acquired wound is exposed to contaminated seawater.

The onset of symptoms is abrupt. The most common presenting signs and symptoms are fever, chills, shock, and secondary bullae [259]. Skin lesions are seen in 65% of patients and are an early sign of septicemia. The most characteristic skin manifestation is erythema, followed by a rapid development of indurated plaques. These plaques then become violaceous in color, vesiculate, and then form bullae. The necrotic skin eventually sloughs off, leaving large ulcers [262]. Gangrene of a limb can develop due to blood vessel occlusion [263].

Diagnosis is aided by clinical presentation and history. The bacteria can be readily cultured from blood and cutaneous lesions [264]. A real-time PCR assay has also been reported [265].

The mortality rate for septicemia is about 53% and is higher in patients who present with hypotension and leucopenia [266]. Median duration from hospitalization to death is about 1.6 days [259]. Failure to initiate antibiotics promptly is associated with higher mortality [257]. Doxycycline with ceftriaxone or cefotaxime is recommended as first line by the Infectious Disease Society of America [267]. Debridement of involved tissue is usually necessary.

RICKETTSIA AKARI

Rickettsialpox, which was first described in 1946 in New York City, is caused by *Rickettsia akari* [268]. *Rickettsia akari* infects house mice (*Mus musculus*) and is transmitted to humans by the house mouse–associated mite, *Liponyssoides sanguineus* [269]. Most cases have occurred in large metropolitan areas of the northeastern United States [269,270].

Rickettsialpox has an incubation period of 9–14 days [271]. The initial lesion develops into an eschar at the site of inoculation. Local lymph nodes around the eschar may become enlarged and tender. Approximately 1 week following the development of the eschar, patients will develop high fever, headaches, malaise, and myalgias. Some patients will have shaking chills and drenching sweats. Thrombocytopenia may also be noted [270]. Within 3–7 days of the fever, skin eruptions of red macules, papules, and papulovesicles will develop over the body. These lesions number between 20 and 40 and will resolve within a week. The presence of an eschar, the lack of successive crops of vesicles over time, and the presence of thrombocytopenia will help differentiate this entity from VZV infection [270].

Diagnosis can be made by comparing acute and convalescent serum antibody titers. Indirect and direct fluorescent antibody tests using anti-*Rickettsia rikettsii* antibodies have also been reported [269]. Real-time multiplex PCR has been used to identify *Rickettsia akari* in formalin-fixed, paraffin-embedded skin biopsy specimens [272]. The duration of the disease can be reduced with doxycycline, but even untreated patients typically recover without complication [269].

NODULAR RASHES

A nodule is a palpable, solid, round, or ellipsoidal lesion that may contain inflammatory cells, organisms (fungi and mycobacterium), or cancer cells [7]. Nodules usually result from disease in the dermis.

ERYTHEMA NODOSUM

Erythema nodosum is an acute inflammatory process involving the fatty tissue layer and skin. This condition is more common in women. There are several causes (Table 8.8), including sarcoid and infections with streptococci, *Chlamydia* species, and hepatitis C [273–277].

The presentation includes fever, malaise, and arthralgia. The characteristic nodules are painful rounded lumps, usually 1–6 cm in diameter. The nodules commonly develop over the anterior surface of the lower legs, knees, and arms [273,278]. The lesions do not usually undergo necrosis, and spontaneous resolution occurs within 2–8 weeks. Diagnosis is often clinical, but biopsy may be needed in atypical cases.

SYSTEMIC FUNGAL INFECTIONS

The sudden onset of dermal nodules may indicate disseminated candidiasis. Infections caused by *Candida* spp. have increased over the last several years [279,280]. Risk factors for disseminated candidiasis include malignancy, neutropenia, antimicrobial therapy, severe burn injuries, IV catheters, postoperative drain placement, hemodialysis, total parenteral antibiotics, and systemic steroid administration [281–283]. The lesions start as macules and progress to erythematous papules or nodules that are discrete, firm, and non-tender and may show a characteristic pale center. The lesions are most typically found on the trunk and extremities [283–286]. Skin

TABLE 8.8
Causes of Erythema Nodosum

Infectious	Non-infectious
Bacterial Infections	**Drug Reactions**
Streptococcus pyogenes	Oral contraceptives
Mycobacterium tuberculosis	Antibiotics
Mycobacterium leprae	Hepatitis B vaccine
Cat scratch disease	Sulfonamides
Chlamydia	**Systemic Disease**
Enteric pathogens (*Yersinia,*	Systemic lupus erythematosus
Campylobacter, and *Salmonella*)	Ulcerative colitis
Rickettsiae	Crohn's disease
Spirochetes (syphilis)	Leukemia
Systemic Fungal Infections	Lymphoma
Coccidioides immitis	Sarcoidosis
Histoplasma capsulatum	Idiopathic (55%)
Blastomycosis	
Parasites	
Amebiasis	
Giardiasis	
Ascaris	
Viral Infections	
Hepatitis B	
CMV	
EBV	

Source: Straus, S.E. et al., *Ann. Intern. Med.,* 108, 221–237, 1988; Galil, K. et al., *Arch. Intern. Med.,* 157, 1209–1213, 1997; Chowaniac, M. et al., *Reumatologia,* 54, 79–82, 2016.

Abbreviations: CMV, cytomegalovirus; EBV, Epstein–Barr virus.

biopsy and histological examination will often reveal aggregates of hyphae and spores within the dermis [286].

Candida auris, first reported in 2009, is one of the most serious emerging pathogens associated with infections of critically ill patients [280,287]. *Candida auris* is frequently resistant to fluconazole and has demonstrated an ability to develop resistance to multiple other commonly used antifungals, including echinocandins and polyenes [288,289]. Risk factors for *Candid auris* do not differ from other systemic *Candida* infections, but the incidence appears to be significantly higher in patients with primary or acquired altered immune response [290]. Furthermore, the mortality rates associated with outbreaks in the intensive care setting approach 20% [291]. The CDC has identified *Candida auris* as a nationally notifiable condition, and cases should be reported to state or local health departments [292].

Other fungi, such as blastomycosis, histoplasmosis, coccidioidomycosis, and sporotrichosis, can also produce skin nodules [7,293]. Coccidioidomycosis is associated with travel to the desert southwest or San Joaquin Valley of central California. Likewise, travel group outbreaks of histoplasmosis have been associated with exploring bat-infested caves and visiting bird dropping-contaminated renovation sites [294].

Patients with AIDS may present with umbilicated nodules that resemble *Molluscum contagiosum* but are caused by *Cryptococcus neoformans*.

RHEUMATIC FEVER

Rheumatic fever is a late inflammatory complication of acute group A streptococcal pharyngitis [295,298]. Rheumatic fever occurs 2–4 weeks following pharyngitis. This disease occurs most frequently in children between the ages of four to nine years. The disease is self-limited, but resulting damage to the heart valves may be chronic and progressive, leading to cardiac decompensation and death.

Rheumatic fever is an acute, systemic, febrile illness that can produce migratory arthritis, carditis, central nervous system deficits, and rash. The diagnosis is based on fulfilling the 2015 Jones Revised criteria, which require evidence of a recent Group A streptococcal infection and the presence of either two major criteria or one major criterion and two minor criteria, which are based on population risk [297].

Evidence of preceding Group A streptococcal infection is established by either elevated or rising antistreptolysin O antibodies, positive throat culture for Group A beta-hemolytic streptococci, or positive rapid-direct Group A streptococcus carbohydrate antigen test. The five major criteria are carditis, arthritis, chorea, erythema marginatum, and subcutaneous nodules [297,298]. For low-risk populations, the arthritis must by polyarthritis, but for moderate- and high-risk populations, the arthritis may be either monoarthritis or polyarthritis [297]. Minor criteria in low-risk populations include polyarthralgia, fever >38.0°C, erythrocyte sedimentation rate >30 mm/h and/or C-reactive peptide >30 mg/L, and prolonged PR interval on electrocardiogram. Minor criteria in moderate- to high-risk populations include monoarthralgia, fever >38.5°C, erythrocyte sedimentation rate >60 mm/h and/or C-reactive peptide >30 mg/L, and prolonged PR interval on electrocardiogram [297].

Arthritis is the most frequent and least-specific manifestation [299]. Large joints are affected most commonly. The arthritis is migratory, with the joints of the lower extremities affected first, followed by those of the upper extremities.

Carditis associated with rheumatic fever manifests as pericarditis, myocarditis, and endocarditis, most commonly involving the mitral valve, followed by the aortic valve [300,301]. Rheumatic heart disease is a late sequela of acute rheumatic fever, occurring 10–20 years after the acute attack, and is the most common cause of acquired valvular disease in the world [302]. The mitral valve is most commonly affected with resultant mitral stenosis that often requires surgical correction.

Sydenham chorea (chorea minor; St. Vitus' dance) is a neurological disorder that manifests as abrupt, purposeless, involuntary movements; muscle weakness; and emotional disturbances [303]. The abnormal movements disproportionately affect one side of the body and cease during sleep.

Skin manifestations occur in less than 10% of patients and are usually not the only manifestation of acute rheumatic fever [297]. Subcutaneous nodules are firm and painless and are seen most often in patients who have carditis [204]. The overlying skin is not inflamed. The nodules can be as large as 2 cm and are most commonly located over bony surfaces or near tendons. The nodules may be present for 1–4 weeks.

Erythema marginatum [205] is a bright-pink or faint-red, blanching non-pruritic rash that affects the trunk and proximal limbs and spares the face. Erythema marginatum occurs early in the disease and may persist or recur. The rash is usually only seen in patients with concomitant carditis.

The diagnosis of or recent scarlet fever, along with the presence of one major and two minor or two major criteria, is considered adequate to make the diagnosis.

REFERENCES

1. Cunha BA. Rash and fever in the critical care unit. *Crit Care Clin* 1998;14(1):35–53.
2. Russo A, Giuliano S, Ceccarelli G, et al. Comparison of septic shock due to multidrug-resistant *Acinetobacter baumannii* or *Klebsiella pneumoniae* carbapenemase-producing *K. pneumoniae* in intensive care unit patients. *Antimicrob Agents Chemother* 2018;62(6). doi:10.1128/AAC.02562-17.
3. Kingston ME, Mackey D. Skin clues in the diagnosis of life-threatening infections. *Rev of Infect Dis* 1986;8(1):1–11.
4. Kang JH. Febrile illness with skin rashes. *Infect Chemother* 2015;47(3):155–166.
5. Schlossberg D. Fever and rash. *Infec Dis Clin North Am* 1996;10(1):101–110.
6. Sanders CV. Approach to the diagnosis of the patient with fever and rash. In: Sanders CV, Nesbitt LTJ eds. *The Skin and Infection: A Color Atlas and Text.* Baltimore, MD: Williams and Wilkins, 1995:296–304.
7. Weber DJ, Cohen MS, Rutala WA. The acutely ill patient with fever and rash. In: Mandell GL, Bennett JE, Dolin R eds. *Principles and Practice of Infectious Disease.* Philadelphia, PA: Elsevier Churchill Livingstone, 2005:729–746.
8. Garner JS, Hospital Infection Control Practices Advisory Committee. Guideline for isolation precautions in hospitals. *Infec Control Hosp Epidemiol* 1996;17:53–80.
9. Centers for Disease Control and Prevention. Guidelines for preventing the transmission of *Mycobacterium tuberculosis* in health-care facilities. *Morb Mortal Wkly Rep* 1994;43:1–132.
10. McKinnon HD, Jr., Howard T. Evaluating the febrile patient with a rash. *Am Fam Physician* 2000;62(4):804–816.
11. Nesbitt LTJ. Evaluating the patient with a skin infection-general considerations. In: Sanders CV, Nesbitt LTJ eds. *The Skin and Infection: A Color Atlas and Text.* Baltimore, MD: Williams and Wilkins, 1995:1–6.
12. Schuchat A, Robinson K, Wenger JD, et al. Bacterial meningitis in the United States in 1995. Active surveillance team. *New Eng J Med* 1997;337(14):970–976.
13. Thigpen MC, Whitney CG, Messonnier NE, et al. Emerging infections programs network. Bacterial meningitis in the United States, 1998–2007. *N Eng J Med* 2011;364(21):2016–2025.
14. Centers for Disease Control and Prevention. Bacterial Meningitis. 2017. Available at: https://www.cdc.gov/meningitis/bacterial.html.
15. Christensen H, May M, Bowne L, et al. Meningococcal carriage by age: A systematic review and meta-analysis. *Lancet Infect Dis* 2010;10(12):853–861.
16. Yung AP, McDonald MI. Early clinical clues to meningococcemia. *MJA* 2003;178(3):134–137.

17. van Deuren M, Brandtzaeg P, van der Meer JW. Update on meningococcal disease with emphasis on pathogenesis and clinical management. *Clin Microbiol Rev* 2000;13(1):144–166.
18. Pollard AJ, Britto J, Nadel S, et al. Emergency management of meningococcal disease. *Arch Dis Child* 1999;80(3):290–296.
19. Mclean S, Caffey J. Endemic purpuric meningococcus bacteremia in early life: The diagnostic value of smears from purpuric lesions. *Am J Dis Child* 1931;42(5):1053–1074.
20. Hill WR, Kinney TD. The cutaneous lesions in acute meningococcemia: A clinical and pathological study. *JAMA* 1947;134(6):513–518.
21. Faust SN, Levin M, Harrison OB, et al. Dysfunction of endothelial protein C activation in severe meningococcal sepsis. *New Eng J Med* 2001;345(6):408–416.
22. Bernhard WG, Jordan AC. Purpuric lesions in meningococcal infections: Diagnosis from smears and cultures of the purpuric lesions. *J Lab Clin Med* 1944;29:273–281.
23. van Deuren M, van Dijke BJ, Koopman RJ, et al. Rapid diagnosis of acute meningococcal infections by needle aspiration or biopsy of skin lesions. *BMJ* 1993;306(6887):1229–1232.
24. Van Ettekoven CN, van de Beek D, Brouwer MC. Update on community-acquired bacterial meningitis: Guidance and challenges. *Clin Microbiol Infect* 2017;23(9):601–606.
25. Seth R, Murthy PSR, Sistla S, et al. Rapid and accurate diagnosis of acute pyogenic meningitis due to *Streptococcus Pneumoniae, Haemophilus influenzae* Type b and *Neisseria meningitidis* using A multiplex PCR assay. *J Clin Diagn Res* 2017;11(9):1–4.
26. Takada S, Fujiwara S, Inoue T, et al. Meningococcemia in adults: A review of the literature. *Intern Med* 2016;55(6):567–572.
27. Ploysangam T, Sheth AP. Chronic meningococcemia in childhood: Case report and review of the literature. *Ped Derm* 1996;13(6):483–487.
28. Gregory B, Tron V, Ho VC. Cyclic fever and rash in a 66-year-old woman. Chronic meningococcemia. *Arch Derm* 1992;128(12):1645–1648.
29. Dupin N, Lecuyer H, Carlotti A, et al. Chronic meningococcemia cutaneous lesions involve perivascular invasion through remodeling of endothelial barriers. *CID* 2012;54(8):1162–1165.
30. Permetier L, Garzoni C, Antille C et al. Value of a novel *Neisseria meningitidis*-specific polymerase chain reaction assay in skin biopsy specimens as a diagnostic tool in chronic meningococcemia. *Arch Dermatol* 2008;144(6):770–773.
31. Masters EJ, Olson GS, Weiner SJ, et al. Rocky mountain spotted fever: A clinician's dilemma. *Arch of Intern Med* 2003;163(7):769–774.
32. Sexton DJ, Kaye KS. Rocky mountain spotted fever. *Med Clin North Am* 2002;86(2):351–360.
33. Thorner AR, Walker DH, Petri WA, Jr. Rocky mountain spotted fever. *Clin Infec Dis* 1998; 27(6):1353–1359.
34. Jacobs RF. Human monocytic ehrlichiosis: Similar to rocky mountain spotted fever but different. *Ped Annals* 2002;31(3):180–184.
35. McFee RB, Bush L, Vasquez-Pertejo MT. Tick borne illness—Rocky mountain spotted fever. *Dis Mon* 2018;64(5):185–194.
36. Gottlieb M, Long B, Koyfman A. The evaluation and management of rocky mountain spotted fever in the emergency department: A review of the literature. *J Emerg Med* 2018;55(1):42–50.
37. Huntington MK, Allison J. Emerging vector-borne diseases. *Am Fam Phys* 2016;94(7):551–557.
38. Centers for Disease Control and Prevention. Rocky Mountain Spotted Fever, 2017. Available at: https://www.cdc.gov/rmsf/stats/index.html.

39. Parola P, Socoloschi C, Jeanjena L et al. Warmer weather linked to tick attack an emergence of severe rickettsioses. *PLoS Negl Trop Dis* 2008;2(11):1–8.
40. Cunha BA. Clinical features of rocky mountain spotted fever. *Lancet Infect Dis* 2008;8(3):143–144.
41. Holman RC, Paddock CD, Curns AT et al. Analysis of risk factors for fatal rocky mountain spotted fever: Evidence for superiority of tetracyclines for therapy. *J Infec Dis* 2001;18(11):1437–1444.
42. Kirkland KB, Marcom PK, Sexton DJ, et al. Rocky mountain spotted fever complicated by gangrene: Report of six cases and review. *Clin Infec Dis* 1993;16(5):629–634.
43. Chen LF, Sexton DJ. What's new in rocky mountain spotted fever? *Infect Dis Clin North Am* 2008;22(3):415–432.
44. Raoult D, Parola P. Rocky Mountain spotted fever in the USA: A benign disease or a common diagnostic error. *Lancet Infect Dis* 2008;8(10):587–589.
45. Dantas-Torres F. Rocky mountain spotted fever. *Lancet Infect Dis* 2007;7(11):724–732.
46. Rhodes A, Evans LE, Alhazzani M, et al. Surviving sepsis campaign: International guidelines for management of sepsis and septic shock, 2016. *Crit Care Med* 2017;45(3):486–552.
47. Singer M, Deutschman CS, Seymore CW, et al. The third international consensus definitions for sepsis and septic shock (Sepsis-3). *JAMA* 2016;315(8):801–810.
48. Driessen RGH, van de Poll MCG, Mol MF, et al. The influence of a change in septic shock definition on intensive care epidemiology and outcome: Comparison of sepsis-2 and sepsis-3 definitions. *Infect Dis* 2018;50(3):207–213.
49. Annane D, Bellissant E, Cavaillon JM. Septic shock. *Lancet* 2005;365(9453):63–78.
50. Alberti C, Brun-Buisson C, Goodman SV, et al. Influence of systemic inflammatory response syndrome and sepsis on outcome of critically Ill infected patients. *Am J Respir Crit Care Med* 2003;168(1):77–84.
51. Cunha, BA. Sepsis and septic shock: Selection of empiric antimicrobial therapy. *Crit Care Clin* 2008;24(2):313–334.
52. Richter DC, Heininger A, Brenner T, et al. Bacterial sepsis: Diagnostic and calculated antibiotic therapy. Der Anaesthesist 2018. doi:10.1007/s00101-017-0396-z.
53. Liang SY, Kumar A. Empiric antimicrobial therapy in severe sepsis and septic shock: Optimizing pathogen clearance. *Curr Infect Dis Rep* 2015;17(7):493–516.
54. Polat G, Ugan RA, Cadirci E, et al. Sepsis and septic shock: Current treatment strategies and new approaches. *Eurasian J Med* 2017;49(1):53–58.
55. Mylonakis E, Calderwood SB. Infective endocarditis in adults. *New Eng J Med* 2001;345(18):1318–1330.
56. Akpunonu BE, Bittar S, Phinney RC, Taleb M. Prevention of infective endocarditis: The new AHA guideline and the elderly. *Geriatrics* 2008;63(8):12–19.
57. Mohananey D, Mohadjer A, Pettersson G, et al. Association of vegetation size with embolic risk in patients with infective endocarditis: A systematic review and meta-analysis. *JAMA* 2018;178(4):502–510.
58. Strom BL, Abrutyn E, Berlin JA, et al. Risk factors for infective endocarditis: Oral hygiene and nondental exposures. *Circulation* 2000;102(23):2842–2848.
59. Manoff SB, Vlahov D, Herskowitz A, et al. Human immunodeficiency virus infection and infective endocarditis among injecting drug users. *Epidemiology* 1996;7(6):566–570.
60. Brown PD, Levine DP. Infective endocarditis in the injection drug user. *Infec Dis Clin N Amer* 2002;16 (3):645–665.
61. Cahil TJ. Pendergast BD. Infective endocarditis. *Lancet* 2016;387(10021):882–893.

62. Leroy O, Georges H, Devos P, et al. Infective endocarditis requiring ICU admission: Epidemiology and prognosis. *Ann Intensive Care* 2015;5(1):45–53.

63. Smid J, Scherner M, Wolfram, et al. Cardiogenic causes of fever. *Dtsch Arziebl Int* 2018;115(12):193–199.

64. Crawford MH, Durack DT. Clinical presentation of infective endocarditis. *Cardio Clinics* 2003;21(2):159–166.

65. Barr J, Danielsson D. Septic gonococcal dermatitis. *Br Med J* 1971;1(747):482–485.

66. Holmes KK, Counts GW, Beaty HN. Disseminated gonococcal infection. *Annals of Intern Med* 1971;74(6):979–993.

67. Kerle KK, Mascola JR, Miller TA. Disseminated gonococcal infection. *Am Fam Physician* 1992;45(1):209–214.

68. Handsfield HH. Disseminated gonococcal infection. *Clin Obstet & Gynecol* 1975;18(1):131–142.

69. Abu-Nassar H, Hill N, Fred HL, et al. Cutaneous manifestations of gonococcemia: A review of 14 cases. *Arch Intern Med* 1963;112(5):731–737.

70. Lahra MM, Martin I, Demczuk W, et al. Cooperative recognition of internationally disseminated ceftriaxone-resistant *Neisseria Gonorrhea* strain. *Emerg Infect Dis* 2018;24(4):735–740.

71. Centers for Disease Control and Prevention. Sexually transmitted diseases treatment guidelines, 2015. *MMWR Recomm Rep* 2015;64(No. RR-3):1–137.

72. Krol-van Straaten MJ, Landheer JE, de Maat CE. Capnocytophaga canimorsus (formerly DF-2) infections: Review of the literature. Netherlands. *J Med* 1990;6(5–6):304–309.

73. Lion C, Escande F, Burdin JC. Capnocytophaga canimorsus infections in human: Review of the literature and case report. *Eur J Epidemiol* 1996;12(5):521–533.

74. Kullberg BJ, Westendorp RG, van't Wout JW, et al. Purpura fulminans and symmetrical peripheral gangrene caused by *Capnocytophaga canimorsus* (formerly DF-2) septicemia— A complication of dog bite. *Medicine* 1991;70(5):287–292.

75. Bertin N, Brosolo G, Pistola F, et al. *Capnocytophaga canimorsus*: An emerging pathogen in immunocompetent patients-experience from an emergency department. *J Emerg Med* 2018;54(6):871–875.

76. Macrea MM, McNamee M, Martin TJ. Acute onset of fever, chills, and lethargy in a 36 year old women. *Chest* 2008;133(6):1505–1507.

77. Centers for Disease Control and Prevention. Capnocytophaga, 2016. Available at: https://www.cdc.gov/capnocytophaga/health-care-professionals/index.html.

78. World Health Organization (WHO). Dengue and severe dengue. Key facts, 2018. Available at: https://www.who.int/en/news-room/fact-sheets/detail/dengue-and-severe-dengue.

79. Centers for Disease Control and Prevention (CDC). Dengue fever clinical guidance, 2016. Available at: https://www.cdc.gov/dengue/clinicallab/clinical.html.

80. Wilder-Smith A, Gubler DJ. Geographic expansion of dengue: The impact of international travel. *Med Clin North Am* 2008;92(6): 1377–1390.

81. Guha-Sapir D, Schimmer B. Dengue fever: New paradigms for a changing epidemiology. *Emerg Themes Epidemiol* 2005;2(1):1–10.

82. Calisher CH. Persistent emergence of dengue. *Emerg Infect Dis* 2005;11(5):738–739.

83. Pincus LB, Grossman ME, Fox LP. The exanthema of dengue fever: Clinical features of two US tourists traveling abroad. *J Am Acad Dermatol* 2008;58(2):308–316.

84. Shirtcliffe P, Cameron E, Nicholson KG, et al. Don't forget dengue! Clinical features of dengue fever in returning travelers. *J Royal College of Physicians London* 1998;32(3):235–237.

85. Kalayanarooj S, Vaughn DW, Nimmannitya S, et al. Early clinical and laboratory indicators of acute dengue illness. *J Infec Dis* 1997;176(2):313–321.

86. Kao CL, King CC, Chao DY, et al. Laboratory diagnosis of dengue virus infection: current and future perspectives in clinical diagnosis and public health. *J Microbiol Immunol Infection* 2005; 38(1): 5–16.

87. Walker DH. Tick-transmitted infectious diseases in the United States. *Annu Rev Public Health* 1998; 19: 237–269.

88. Taege AJ. Tick trouble: Overview of tick-borne diseases. *Cleveland Clinic J Med* 2000; 67(4): 241, 245–249.

89. Bush LM, Vazquez-Pertejo MT. Tick borne illness—Lyme disease. *Disease a Month* 2018; 64(5): 195–212.

90. Gayle A, Ringdahl E. Tick-borne diseases. *Amer Fam Physician* 2001; 64(3): 461–466.

91. Steere AC, Coburn J, Glickstein L. The emergence of lyme disease. *J Clin Invest* 2004; 113(8): 1093–1101.

92. Edlow JA. Lyme disease and related tick-borne illnesses. *Annals Emerg Med* 1999; 33(6): 680–693.

93. Lohr B, Fingerle V, Norris DE et al. Laboratory diagnosis of lyme borreliosis: Current state of the art and future perspectives. *Crit Rev Clin Lab Sci* 2018; 55(4): 219–245.

94. Wormser GP, Dattwyler RJ, Shapiro ED. The clinical assessment, treatment, and prevention of Lyme disease, human granulocytic anaplasmosis, and babesiosis: Clinical practice guidelines by the infectious disease society of America. *Clin Infect Dis* 2006; 43(9): 1089–1134.

95. Roujeau JC, Stern RS. Severe adverse cutaneous reactions to drugs. *New Eng J Med* 1994; 331(19): 1272–1285.

96. Roujeau JC. Clinical heterogeneity of drug hypersensitivity. *Toxicology* 2005; 209(2): 123–129.

97. Mustafa SS, Ostrov D, Yerly D. Severe cutaneous adverse drug reactions: Presentation, risk factors, and management. *Curr Allergy Asthma Rep* 2018; 18(4): 26.

98. Bastuji-Garin S, Rzany B, Stern RS et al. Clinical classification of cases of toxic epidermal necrolysis, Stevens-Johnson syndrome, and erythema multiforme. *Arch Derm* 1993; 129(1): 92–96.

99. Plaza JA, Prieto VG. Erythema Multiforme. emedicine.medscape, 2018. Available at: https://emedicine.medscape.com/article/1122915-overview#a4.

100. Lerch M, Mainetti C, Beretta-Piccoli BT, Harr T. Current perspectives on erythema multiforme. *Clin Rev Allergy Immunol* 2018; 54(1): 177–184.

101. Sousa-Pinto B, Araujo L, Freitas A et al. Stevens-Johnson syndrome/toxic epidermal necrolysis and erythema multiform drug-related hospitalizations in a national administrative database. *Clin Transl Allergy* 2018; 8(2). doi:10.1186/s13601-017-0188-1.

102. Wong A, Malvestiti AA, Hafner MFD. Stevens-Johnson syndrome and toxic epidermal necrolysis: A review. *Rev Assoc Med Bras* 2016; 62(5): 468–473.

103. Angus J, Langan M, Stanway A et al. The many faces of secondary syphilis: A re-emergence of an old disease. *Clin Exp Dermatol* 2006; 31(5): 641–745.

104. Watts PJ, Greenberg HL, Khachemoune A. Unusual primary syphilis: Presentation of a likely case with review of the stages of acquired syphilis, its differential diagnosis, management, and current recommendations. *Int J Dermatol* 2016; 55(7): 714–728.

105. Workowski KA, Bolan GA. Sexually transmitted diseases treatment guidelines 2015. *MMWR* 2015; 64(3): 1–137.

106. Bozza FA, Grinsztejn B. Key points on Zika infection for the intensivist. *Int Care Med* 2016; 42(9): 1490–1492.

107. Sebastien UU, Ricardo AVA, Alverez BC et al. Zika virus-induced neurological critical illness in Latin America: Severe Guillain-Barre syndrome and encephalitis. *J Crit Care* 2017; 42: 275–281.

108. Hayes EB, Komar N, Nasci RS et al. Epidemiology and transmission dynamics of West Nile virus disease. *Emerg Infect Dis* 2005; 11(8): 1167–1173.

109. Centers for Disease Control and Prevention (CDC). West Nile virus activity—United States, 2007. *Morb Mortal Wkly Rep* 2008; 57(26): 720–723.

110. O'Leary DR, Marfin AA, Montgomery SP et al. The epidemic of West Nile virus in the United States, 2002. *Vector Borne & Zoonotic Dis* 2004; 4(1): 61–70.

111. Petersen LR, Hayes EB. Westward ho? The spread of West Nile virus. *New Eng J Med* 2004; 351(22): 2257–2259.

112. Zeller HG, Schuffenecker I. West Nile virus: An overview of its spread in Europe and the Mediterranean basin in contrast to its spread in the Americas. *Eur J Clin Micro & Infec Dis* 2004; 23(3): 147–156.

113. Hayes EB, O'Leary DR. West Nile virus infection: A pediatric perspective. *Pediatrics* 2004; 113(5): 1375–1381.

114. Kumar D, Prasad GV, Zaltzman J et al. Community-acquired West Nile virus infection in solid-organ transplant recipients. *Transplantation* 2004; 77(3): 399–402.

115. Stramer SL, Fang CT, Foster GA et al. West Nile virus among blood donors in the United States, 2003 and 2004. *New Eng J Med* 2005; 353(5): 451–459.

116. Diamond MS, Shrestha B, Mehlhop E et al. Innate and adaptive immune responses determine protection against disseminated infection by West Nile encephalitis virus. *Viral Immunol* 2003; 16(3): 259–278.

117. Mostashari F, Bunning ML, Kitsutani PT et al. Epidemic West Nile encephalitis, New York, 1999: Results of a household-based seroepidemiological survey. *Lancet* 2001; 358(9278): 261–264.

118. Watson JT, Pertel PE, Jones RC et al. Clinical characteristics and functional outcomes of West Nile fever. *Ann Intern Med* 2004; 141(5): 360–365.

119. Hayes EB, Sejvar JJ, Zaki SR et al. Virology, pathology, and clinical manifestations of West Nile virus. *Emerg Infect Dis* 2005; 11(8): 1174–1179.

120. Pepperell C, Rau N, Krajden S et al. West Nile virus infection in 2002: Morbidity and mortality among patients admitted to hospital in south-central Ontario. *CMAJ* 2003; 168(11): 1399–1405.

121. Sejvar JJ, Haddad MB, Tierney BC et al. Neurologic manifestations and outcome of West Nile virus infection. *JAMA* 2003; 290(4): 511–515.

122. Sejvar JJ, Bode AV, Marfin AA et al. West Nile virus-associated flaccid paralysis. *Emerg Infec Dis* 2005; 11(7): 1021–1027.

123. Centers for Disease Control (CDC). West Nile Virus, 2018. Available at: https://www.cdc.gov/westnile/index.html.

124. Yeung MW, Shing E, Nelder M et al. Epidemiologic and clinical parameters of West Nile virus infections in humans: a scoping review. *BMC Infect Dis* 2017; 17(1): 609–622.

125. Tilley PA, Zachary GA, Walle R et al. West Nile virus detection and commercial assays. *Emerg Infec Dis* 2005; 11(7): 1154–1155.

126. Lustig, Y, Mannasse B, Koren et al. Superiority of West Nile virus RNA detection in whole blood for diagnosis of acute infection. *J Clin Microbiol* 2016; 54(8): 2294–2297.

127. Barzon L, Pacenti M, Franchin E et al. Excretion of West Nile virus in urine during acute infection. *J Infect Dis* 2013; 208(7): 1086–1092.

128. Rios M, Daniel S, Chancey C et al. West Nile virus adheres to human red blood cells in whole blood. *Clin Infect Dis* 2007; 45(2): 181–186.

129. Lustig Y, Sofer D, Bucris ED et al. Surveillance and diagnosis of West Nile virus in the face of flavivirus cross-reactivity. *Frontiers Microbiol* 2018; 9. doi:10.3389/fmicb.2018.02421.

130. Martin DA, Biggerstaff BJ, Allen B et al. Use of immunoglobulin M cross-reactions in differential diagnosis of human flaviviral encephalitis infections in the United States. *Clin Diagn Lab Immunol* 2002; 9 (3): 544–549.

131. Reich HL, Crawford GH, Pelle MT et al. Group B streptococcal toxic shock-like syndrome. *Arch of Derm* 2004; 140(2): 163–166.

132. Todd J, Fishaut M, Kapral F et al. Toxic-shock syndrome associated with phage-group-I staphylococci. *Lancet* 1978; 2(8100): 1116–1118.

133. Stevens DL, Tanner MH, Winship J et al. Severe group A streptococcal infections associated with a toxic shock-like syndrome and scarlet fever toxin A. *New Eng J Med* 1989; 321(1): 1–7.

134. Wilkins AL, Steer AC, Smeesters PR et al. Toxic shock syndrome—The seven Rs of management and treatment. *J Infect* 2017; 74(Suppl 1): S147–S152.

135. Hajjeh RA, Reingold A, Weil A et al. Toxic shock syndrome in the United States: Surveillance update, 1979–1996. *Emerg Infect Dis* 1999; 5(6): 807–810.

136. Reduced incidence of menstrual toxic-shock syndrome—United States, 1980–1990. *Morb Mortal Wkly Rep* 1990; 39(25): 421–423.

137. Eagle H. Experimental approach to the problem of treatment failure with penicillin. *Am J Med* 1952; 13(4): 389–399.

138. Burnham JP, Kollef MH. Treatment of severe skin and soft tissue infections: A review. *Curr Opin Infect Dis* 2018; 31(1): 113–119.

139. Car J, Curtis N, Smeesters P, Steer A. Are household contacts of patients with invasive group A streptococcal disease at higher risk of secondary infection? *Aech Dis Child* 2016; 101(2): 198–201.

140. Stach CS, Herrera A, Schlievert PM. Staphylococcal superantigens interact with multiple host receptors to cause serious disease. *Immunol Res* 2014; 59(0): 177–181.

141. Bergdoll MS, Crass BA, Reiser RF et al. A new staphylococcal enterotoxin, enterotoxin F, associated with toxic-shock-syndrome *Staphylococcus aureus* isolates. *Lancet* 1981; 1(8228): 1017–1021.

142. Schlievert PM. Staphylococcal enterotoxin B and toxic-shock syndrome toxin-1 are significantly associated with non-menstrual TSS. *Lancet* 1986; 1(8490): 1149–1150.

143. Schlievert PM, Shands KN, Dan BB et al. Identification and characterization of an exotoxin from *Staphylococcus aureus* associated with toxic-shock syndrome. *J Infec Dis* 1981; 143(4): 509–516.

144. Lee VT, Chang AH, Chow AW. Detection of staphylococcal enterotoxin B among toxic shock syndrome (TSS)—and non-TSS-associated *Staphylococcus aureus* isolates. *J Infec Dis* 1992; 166(4): 911–915.

145. Lehn N, Schaller E, Wagner H et al. Frequency of toxic shock syndrome toxin- and enterotoxin-producing clinical isolates of *Staphylococcus aureus*. *Eur J Clin Micro & Infec Dis* 1995; 14(1): 43–46.

146. Centers for Disease Control. Toxic shock Syndrome (Other than streptococcal) (TSS), 2011 case definition. Available at: https://wwwn.cdc.gov/nndss/conditions/toxic-shock-syndrome-other-than-streptococcal/case-definition/2011/.

147. Barrett JA, Graham DR. Toxic shock syndrome presenting as encephalopathy. *J Infec* 1986; 12(3): 276–278.

148. Chesney RW, Chesney PJ, Davis JP et al. Renal manifestations of the staphylococcal toxic-shock syndrome. *Am J Med* 1981; 71(4): 583–588.

149. Herzer CM. Toxic shock syndrome: Broadening the differential diagnosis. *J Am Board of Family Practice* 2001; 14(2): 131–136.

150. McKenna UG, Meadows JA III, Brewer NS et al. Toxic shock syndrome, a newly recognized disease entity. Report of 11 cases. *Mayo Clinic Proceedings* 1980; 55(11): 663–672.

151. Chesney PJ, Davis JP, Purdy WK et al. Clinical manifestations of toxic shock syndrome. *JAMA* 1981; 246(7): 741–748.

152. Andrews MM, Parent EM, Barry M et al. Recurrent non-menstrual toxic shock syndrome: Clinical manifestations, diagnosis, and treatment. *Clin Infec Dis* 2001; 32(10): 1470–1479.

153. Reingold AL, Dan BB, Shands KN et al. Toxic-shock syndrome not associated with menstruation. A review of 54 cases. *Lancet* 1982; 1(8262): 1–4.

154. Reingold AL, Hargrett NT, Dan BB et al. Nonmenstrual toxic shock syndrome: A review of 130 cases. *Annals Int Med* 1982; 96(6 Pt 2): 871–874.

155. Streptococcal toxic shock syndrome (STSS) (*Streptococcal pyogenes*) 2010. Available at: https://wwwn.cdc.gov/nndss/conditions/streptococcal-toxic-shock-syndrome/case-definition/2010/.

156. Schmitz M, Roux X, Huttner B et al. Streptococcal toxic shock syndrome in the intensive care unit. *Ann Intensive Care* 2018: 8(88). Available at: https://annalsofintensivecare.springeropen.com/track/pdf/10.1186/s13613-018-0438-y.

157. Stevens DL, Bryant AE. Sever group A streptococcal infections. In: *Streptococcus Pyogenes: Basic Biology to Clinical Manifestations* (Ferretti JJ, Stevens DL, Fischetti VA eds). Oklahoma, OK: University of Oklahoma Health Sciences Center, 2016:661–665.

158. Defining the Group A streptococcal toxic shock syndrome. Rationale and consensus definition. The working group on severe streptococcal infections. *JAMA* 1993;269(3):390–401.

159. Manders SM. Toxin-mediated streptococcal and staphylococcal disease. *J Am Acad Derm* 1998;39(3):383–398.

160. Ladhani S. Recent developments in staphylococcal scalded skin syndrome. *Clin Micro Infec* 2001;7(6):301–307.

161. Adesiyun AA, Lenz W, Schaal KP. Exfoliative toxin production by *Staphylococcus aureus* strains isolated from animals and human beings in Nigeria. *Microbiologica* 1991;14(4):357–362.

162. Dancer SJ, Noble WC. Nasal, axillary, and perineal carriage of *Staphylococcus aureus* among women: Identification of strains producing epidermolytic toxin. *J Clin Path* 1991;44(8):681–684.

163. Ladhani S, Poston SM, Joannou CL, et al. Staphylococcal scalded skin syndrome: Exfoliative toxin A (ETA) induces serine protease activity when combined with A431 cells. *Acta Paediatr* 1999;88(7):776–779.

164. Papageorgiou AC, Plano LR, Collins CM, et al. Structural similarities and differences in *Staphylococcus aureus* exfoliative toxins A and B as revealed by their crystal structures. *Protein Sci* 2000;9(3):610–618.

165. Lyell A. Toxic epidermal necrolysis (the scalded skin syndrome): A reappraisal. *Br J Derm* 1979;100(1):69–86.

166. Melish ME. Staphylococci, streptococci and the skin: Review of impetigo and staphylococcal scalded skin syndrome. *Semin Dermatol* 1982;1:101–109.

167. Beers B, Wilson B. Adult staphylococcal scalded skin syndrome. *Int J Derm* 1990;29(6);428–429,

168. Moss C, Gupta E. The Nikolsky sign in staphylococcal scalded skin syndrome. *Arch Dis Childhood* 1998;79(3):290.

169. Mishra AK, Yadav P, Mishra A. A systemic review on staphylococcal scalded skin syndrome (SSSS): A rare and critical disease of neonates. *Open Microbiol J* 2016;10:150–159. Available at: https://www.benthamopen.com/contents/pdf/TOMICROJ/TOMICROJ-10-150.pdf.

170. Arnold JD, Hoek SN, Kirkorian AY. Epidemiology of staphylococcal scalded skin syndrome in the United States: A cross-sectional study, 201–2014. *J Am Acad Derm* 2018;78(2):404–406.

171. Gemmell CG. Staphylococcal scalded skin syndrome. *J Med Micro* 1995;43(5):318–3327.

172. Staiman A, Hsu DY, Silverberg JI. Epidemiology of staphylococcal scalded skin syndrome in US adults. *J Am Acad Derm* 2018;79(4):747–776.

173. Cribier B, Piemont Y, Grosshans E. Staphylococcal scalded skin syndrome in adults. A clinical review illustrated with a new case. *J Am Acad Derm* 1994;30(2 Pt 2):319–324.

174. Goldberg NS, Ahmed T, Robinson B, et al. Staphylococcal scalded skin syndrome mimicking acute graft-vs.-host disease in a bone marrow transplant recipient. *Arch Derm* 1989;125(1):85–87.

175. Ladhani S, Robbie S, Garratt RC, et al. Development and evaluation of detection systems for staphylococcal exfoliative toxin A responsible for scalded-skin syndrome. *J Clin Micro* 2001;39(6):2050–2054.

176. Gentilhomme E, Faure M, Piemont Y, et al. Action of staphylococcal exfoliative toxins on epidermal cell cultures and organotypic skin. *J Derm* 1990;17(9):526–352.

177. Basetti S, Hodgson T, Rawson TM, et al. Scarlet fever: A guide for general practitioners. *London J Primary Care* 2017;9(5):77–79.

178. Leyden JJ, Gately LE III. Staphylococcal and streptococcal infections. In: Sanders CV, Nesbitt LTJ eds. *The Skin and Infection: A Color Atlas and Text*. Baltimore, MD: Williams and Wilkins, 1995:27–38.

179. Centor TM, Witherspoon JM, Dalton HP, et al. The diagnosis of strep throat in adults in the emergency room. *Med Dec Making* 1981;1(3):239–246.

180. Kawasaki T. Acute febrile mucocutaneous syndrome with lymphoid involvement with specific desquamation of the fingers and toes in children. *Arerugi—Jpn J Allergol* 1967;16(3):178–222.

181. Burns JC, Glode MP. Kawasaki syndrome. *Lancet* 2004;364(9433):533–544.

182. Royle J, Burgner D, Curtis N. The diagnosis and management of Kawasaki disease. *J Paediatrics Child Health* 2005;41(3):87–93.

183. Dominguez SR, Friedman K, Seewald R et al. Kawasaki disease in a pediatric intensive care unit: A case-control study. *Pediatrics* 2008;122:e786–e790.

184. Kuo CC, Lee YS, Lin MR, et al. Characteristics of children with Kawasaki disease requiring intensive care: 10 years' experience at a tertiary pediatric hospital. *J Microbiol Immunol Infect* 2018;51(2):184–190.

185. Lin YJ, Chang MC, Lo MH, et al. Early differentiation of Kawasaki disease shock syndrome and toxic shock syndrome in a pediatric intensive care unit. *Pediatr Infect Dis J* 2015;34(11):1163–1167.

186. McCrindle BW, Rowley AH, Newburger JW, et al. Diagnosis, treatment, and long term management of Kawasaki disease: A scientific statement for health professional from the American Heart Association. *Circulation* 2017;135(17): e927–e999.

187. Burns JC, Cayan DR, Tong G, et al. Seasonality and temporal clustering of Kawasaki syndrome. *Epidemiology* 2005;16(2):220–225.

188. Yamazaki-Nakashimada MA, Gamez-Gonzalez LB, Murata C, et al. IgG levels in Kawasaki disease and its association with clinical outcome. *Clin Rheumatol.* doi:10.1007/s10067-018-4339-0.

189. Shimizu D, Hoshina T, Kawamura M, et al. Seasonality in clinical courses of Kawasaki disease. *Arch Dis Child.* doi:10.1136/archdischild-2018-315267.

190. Morgan R, King D. Shingles: A review of diagnosis and management. *Hosp Med* 1998;59(10):770–776.

191. Feldman S, Hughes WT, Kim HY. Herpes zoster in children with cancer. *Am J Dis Child* 1973;126(2):178–184.

192. Feldhoff CM, Balfour HH, Jr., Simmons RL, et al. Varicella in children with renal transplants. *J Pediatrics* 1981;98(1): 25–31.

193. Patti ME, Selvaggi KJ, Kroboth FJ. Varicella hepatitis in the immunocompromised adult: A case report and review of the literature. *Am J Med* 1990;88(1):77–80.

194. Veenstra J, van Praag RM, Krol A, et al. Complications of varicella zoster virus reactivation in HIV-infected homosexual men. *AIDS* 1996;10(4):393–399.

195. Buchbinder SP, Katz MH, Hessol NA, et al. Herpes zoster and human immunodeficiency virus infection. *J Infec Dis* 1992;166(5):1153–1156.

196. Gershon AA, Mervish N, LaRussa P, et al. Varicella-zoster virus infection in children with underlying human immunodeficiency virus infection. *J Infec Dis* 1997;176(6):1496–1500.

197. Straus SE, Ostrove JM, Inchauspe G, et al. NIH conference. Varicella-zoster virus infections. Biology, natural history, treatment, and prevention. *Ann Intern Med* 1988;108(2): 221–237.

198. Galil K, Choo PW, Donahue JG, et al. The sequelae of herpes zoster. *Arch Intern Med* 1997;157(11):1209–1213.

199. Levitsky J, Kalil A, Meza JL, et al. Herpes zoster infection after liver transplantation: A case-control study. *Liver Transpl* 2005;11(3):320–325.

200. Rogers SY, Irving W, Harris A, et al. Visceral varicella zoster infection after bone marrow transplantation without skin involvement and the use of PCR for diagnosis. *Bone Marrow Transplant* 1995;15(5):805–807.

201. Veenstra J, Krol A, van Praag RM, et al. Herpes zoster, immunological deterioration and disease progression in HIV-1 infection. *AIDS* 1995;9(10):1153–1158.

202. Rusthoven JJ, Ahlgren P, Elhakim T, et al. Varicella-zoster infection in adult cancer patients. A population study. *Arch Intern Med* 1988;148(7):1561–1566.

203. Tojimbara T, So SK, Cox KL, et al. Fulminant hepatic failure following varicella-zoster infection in a child. A case report of successful treatment with liver transplantation and perioperative acyclovir. *Transplantation* 1995;60(9): 1052–1053.

204. Verdonck LF, Cornelissen JJ, Dekker AW, et al. Acute abdominal pain as a presenting symptom of varicella-zoster virus infection in recipients of bone marrow transplants. *Clin Infec Dis* 1993;16(1):190–191.

205. Fleisher G, Henry W, McSorley M, et al. Life-threatening complications of varicella. *Am J Dis Children* 1981;135(10):896–899.

206. Pavan-Langston D. Herpes zoster ophthalmicus. *Neurology* 1995;45(12 Suppl 8):S50–S51.

207. Hellinger WC, Bolling JP, Smith TF, et al. Varicella-zoster virus retinitis in a patient with AIDS-related complex: Case report and brief review of the acute retinal necrosis syndrome. *Clin Infec Dis* 1993;16(2):208–212.

208. Culbertson WW, Blumenkranz MS, Pepose JS, et al. Varicella zoster virus is a cause of the acute retinal necrosis syndrome. *Ophthalmology* 1986;93(5):559–569.

209. Adour KK. Otological complications of herpes zoster. *Ann Neurol* 1994;35(Suppl):S62–S64.

210. Elliott KJ. Other neurological complications of herpes zoster and their management. *Ann Neurol* 1994;35(Suppl):S57–S61.

211. Au WY, Hon C, Cheng VC, et al. Concomitant zoster myelitis and cerebral leukemia relapse after stem cell transplantation. *Ann Hematol* 2005;84(1):59–60.

212. Mirouse A, Vignon P, Prion P, et al. Severe varicella-zoster virus pneumonia: A multicenter cohort study. *Critical Care* 2017;21(1):137–147.

213. Burke DG, Kalayjian RC, Vann VR, et al. Polymerase chain reaction detection and clinical significance of varicella-zoster virus in cerebrospinal fluid from human immunodeficiency virus-infected patients. *J Infec Dis* 1997;176(4):1080–1084.

214. Cinque P, Bossolasco S, Vago L, et al. Varicella-zoster virus (VZV) DNA in cerebrospinal fluid of patients infected with human immunodeficiency virus: VZV disease of the central nervous system or subclinical reactivation of VZV infection? *Clin Infec Dis* 1997;25(3):634–639.

215. Breman JG, Arita I. The confirmation and maintenance of smallpox eradication. *New Eng J Med* 1980;303(22): 1263–1273.

216. Henderson DA. Smallpox eradication. *Public Health Rep* 1980;95(5):422–426.

217. Dixon CW. *Smallpox.* London, UK: J & A Churchill Ltd., 1962.

218. Huq F. Effect of temperature and relative humidity on variola virus in crusts. *Bull World Health Organ* 1976;54(6): 710–712.

219. Harper GJ. The influence of environment on the survival of airborne virus particles in the laboratory. *Archiv fur die Gesamte Virusforschung* 1963;13:64–71.

220. Breman JG, Henderson DA. Diagnosis and management of smallpox. *New Eng J Med* 2002;346(17):1300–1308.

221. Henderson DA, Inglesby TV, Bartlett JG, et al. Smallpox as a biological weapon: Medical and public health management. Working group on civilian biodefense. *JAMA* 1999;281(22):2127–2137.

222. Von Magnus P, Andersion EK, Petersen KB, et al. A pox-like disease in the cynomolgus monkeys. *Acta Pathol Microbiol Scand* 1959;46(2):156–176.

223. Sklenovska N, Van Ranst M. Emergence of monkeypox as the most important orthopoxvirus infection in humans. *Front Public Health* 2018;6(241). doi:10.3389/fpubh. 2018.00241.

224. Fine PE, Jezek Z, Grab B, et al. The transmission potential of monkeypox virus in human populations. *Int J Epidemiol* 1988;17(3):643–650.

225. Marennikova SS, Seluhina EM, Malceva NN, et al. Isolation and properties of the causal agent of a new variola-like disease (monkeypox) in man. *Bull World Health Organ* 1972;46(5):599–611.

226. Cann JA, Jahrling PB, Hensley LE, et al. Comparative pathology of smallpox and monkeypox in man and macaques. *J Comp Pathol* 2013;148(1):6–21.

227. Petersen E, Abubakar I, Ihekweazu C, et al. Monkeypox— Enhancing public health preparedness for an emerging lethal human zoonotic epidemic threat in the wake of smallpox post-eradication era. *In J Infect Dis* 219;78(1):78–84.

228. Centers for disease Control and Prevention. Monkeypox 2018. Available at: https://www.cdc.gov/poxvirus/monkeypox/index.html.

229. Breman JG, Kalisa R, Steniowski MV, et al. Monkeypox, 1970–1979. *Bull World Health Organ* 1980;58(2):165–182.

230. Corey L, Spear PG. Infections with herpes simplex viruses (1). *New Eng J Med* 1986;314(11):686–691.

231. Frederick DM, Bland D, Gollin Y. Fatal disseminated herpes simplex virus infection in a previously healthy pregnant woman. A case report. *J Reprod Med* 2002;47(7):591–596.

232. Hillard P, Seeds J, Cefalo R. Disseminated herpes simplex in pregnancy: Two cases and a review. *Obstet Gynecol Surv* 1982;37(7):449–453.

233. Johnson JR, Egaas S, Gleaves CA, et al. Hepatitis due to herpes simplex virus in marrow-transplant recipients. *Clin Infec Dis* 1992;14(1):38–45.

234. Kusne S, Schwartz M, Breinig MK, et al. Herpes simplex virus hepatitis after solid organ transplantation in adults. *J Infec Dis* 1991;163(5):1001–1007.

235. Liesegang TJ. Herpes simplex virus epidemiology and ocular importance. *Cornea* 2001;20(1):1–13.

236. Muller SA, Herrmann EC, Jr., Winkelmann RK. Herpes simplex infections in hematologic malignancies. *Am J Med* 1972;52(1):102–114.

237. Priya K, Mahalakshmi B, Malathi J, et al. Prevalence of herpes simplex virus, varicella zoster virus and cytomegalovirus in HIV-positive and HIV-negative patients with viral retinitis in India. *Eur J Clin Micro Infec Dis* 2004;23(11):857–858.

238. Remeijer L, Osterhaus A, Verjans G. Human herpes simplex virus keratitis: the pathogenesis revisited. *Ocular Immunol Inflamm* 2004;12(4):255–285.

239. Siegal FP, Lopez C, Hammer GS, et al. Severe acquired immunodeficiency in male homosexuals, manifested by chronic perianal ulcerative herpes simplex lesions. *New Eng J Med* 1981;305(24):1439–1444.

240. Tyler KL. Herpes simplex virus infections of the central nervous system: Encephalitis and meningitis, including Mollaret's. *Herpes* 2004;11(Suppl 2):57A–64A.

241. Sutter R, Kaplan PW, Cervenka MC, et al. Electroencephalography for diagnosis and prognosis of acute encephalitis. *Clin Neurophysiol* 2015;126(8):1524–1531.

242. DeBiasi RL, Kleinschmidt-DeMasters BK, Weinberg A, et al. Use of PCR for the diagnosis of herpes virus infections of the central nervous system. *J Clin Virol* 2002;25(Suppl 1):S5–S11.

243. Steiner I, Budka H, Chadhuri A, et al. Viral meningoencephalitis: A review of diagnostic methods and guidelines for management. *Eur J Neurol* 2010;17(8):999–1009.

244. Lepiller Q, Sueur C, Solis M, et al. Clinical relevance of herpes simplex virus viremia in intensive care unit patients. *J Infect* 2015;71(1):93–100.

245. Ong DSY, Bonten MJM, Spitoni C, et al. Epidemiology of multiple herpes viremia in previously immunocompetent patients with septic shock. *CID* 2017;64 (99):1204–1210.

246. Gopal AK, Fowler VG, Jr., Shah M, et al. Prospective analysis of *Staphylococcus aureus* bacteremia in non-neutropenic adults with malignancy. *J Clin Oncol* 2000;18(5):1110–1115.

247. Gottlieb GS, Fowler VG, Jr., Kong LK, et al. *Staphylococcus aureus* bacteremia in the surgical patient: A prospective analysis of 73 postoperative patients who developed *Staphylococcus aureus* bacteremia at a tertiary care facility. *J Am Coll Surg* 2000;190(1):50–57.

248. Marr KA, Kong L, Fowler VG, et al. Incidence and outcome of *Staphylococcus aureus* bacteremia in hemodialysis patients. *Kidney Int* 1998;54(5):1684–1689.

249. Petti CA, Fowler VG, Jr. *Staphylococcus aureus* bacteremia and endocarditis. *Cardio Clinics* 200;21(2):219–233.

250. Shah MA, Sanders L, Lanclos K, et al. *Staphylococcus aureus* bacteremia in patients with neutropenia. *Southern Med J* 2002;95(7):782–784.

251. Tumbarello M, de Gaetano DK, Tacconelli E, et al. Risk factors and predictors of mortality of methicillin-resistant *Staphylococcus aureus* (MRSA) bacteremia in HIV-infected patients. *J Antimicrob Chemo* 2002;50(3):375–382.

252. Vos FJ, Kullberg BJ, Sturm PD, et al. Metastatic infectious disease and clinical outcome in *Staphylococcus aureus* and *Streptococcus* species bacteremia. *Medicine* 2012;91(2):86–94.

253. Mitra AK. *Vibrio vulnificus* infection: Epidemiology, clinical presentations, and prevention. *Southern Med J* 2004;97(2):118–119.

254. Baker-Austin C and Oliver JD. *Vibrio vulnificus*: New insights into a deadly opportunistic pathogen. *Environ Microbiol* 2018;20(2):423–430.

255. Ruple AD, Cook DW. *Vibrio Vulnificus* and indicator bacteria in shellstock and commercially processed oysters. *J Food Prot* 1992;55:667–671.

256. Hill MK, Sanders CV. Localized and systemic infection due to vibrio species. *Infec Dis Clin North Am* 1987;1(3):687–707.

257. Klontz KC, Lieb S, Schreiber M, et al. Syndromes of *Vibrio vulnificus* infections. Clinical and epidemiologic features in Florida cases, 1981–1987. *Ann Intern Med* 1988;109(4):318–323.

258. Chiang SR, Chuang YC. *Vibrio vulnificus* infection: Clinical manifestations, pathogenesis, and antimicrobial therapy. *J Microb Immun Infec* 2003;36(2):81–88.

259. Haq SM, Dayal HH. Chronic liver disease and consumption of raw oysters: A potentially lethal combination— A review of *Vibrio vulnificus* septicemia. *Am J Gastro* 2005;100(5):1195–1199.

260. Levine WC, Griffin PM. Vibrio infections on the gulf coast: Results of first year of regional surveillance. Gulf coast vibrio working group. *J Infect Dis* 1993;167(2):479–483.

261. Howard RJ, Bennett NT. Infections caused by halophilic marine vibrio bacteria. *Ann Surg* 1993;217(5):525–530.

262. Hsueh PR, Lin CY, Tan HJ, et al. Vibrio vulnificus in Taiwan. *Emerg Infect Dis* 2004;10(8):1363–1368.

263. Wickboldt LG, Sanders CV. *Vibrio vulnificus* infection. Case report and update since 1970. *J Am Acad Derm* 1983;9(2):243–251.

264. Koenig KL, Mueller J, Rose T. *Vibrio vulnificus*. Hazard on the half shell. *Western J Med* 1991;155(4):400–403.

265. Chen CY, Wu KM, Chang YC, et al. Comparative genome analysis of *Vibrio vulnificus*, a marine pathogen. *Genome Res* 2003;13(12):2577–2587.

266. Morris JG, Jr. *Vibrio vulnificus*—A new monster of the deep? *Ann Intern Med* 1988;109(4):261–263.

267. Stevens DL, Bisno AL, Chambers HF, et al. Practice guidelines for the diagnosis and management of skin and soft tissue infections: 2014 update by the Infectious Disease Society of America. *Clin Infect Dis* 2015;59(2):147–159.

268. Greenberg M, Pellitteri OJ, Jellison WL. Rickettsialpox—A newly recognized rickettsial disease. *Am J Public Health* 1947;37:860–868.

269. Kass EM, Szaniawski WK, Levy H, et al. Rickettsialpox in a New York city hospital, 1980–1989. *New Eng J Med* 1994;331(24):1612–1617.

270. Krusell A, Comer JA, Sexton DJ. Rickettsialpox in North Carolina: A case report. *Emerg Infec Dis* 2002;8(7): 727–728.

271. Brettman LR, Lewin S, Holzman RS, et al. Rickettsialpox: Report of an outbreak and a contemporary review. *Medicine* 1981;60(5):363–372.

272. Denison AM, Amin BD, Nicholson WL, et al. Detection of *Rickettsia rickettsia*, *Rickettsia parkeri*, and *Rickettsia akari* in skin biopsy specimens using a multiplex real-time polymerase chase chain reaction assay. *Clin Infect Dis* 2014;59(5):635–642.

273. Cribier B, Caille A, Heid E, et al. Erythema nodosum and associated diseases. A study of 129 cases. *Int J Derm* 1998;37(9):667–672.

274. Blomgren SE. Conditions associated with erythema nodosum. *NY State J Med* 1972;72(18):2302–2304.

275. James DG. Erythema nodosum. *Br Med J* 1961;5229:853–857.

276. Puavilai S, Sakuntabhai A, Sriprachaya-Anunt S, et al. Etiology of erythema nodosum. *J Med Assoc Thailand* 1995;78(2):72–75.

277. Vesey CM, Wilkinson DS. Erythema nodosum: A study of seventy cases. *Br J Derm* 1959;71(4):139–155.

278. Chowaniac M, Starba A, Wiland P. Erythema nodosum—Review of the literature. *Reumatologia* 2016;54(2):79–82.

279. Kett DH, Azoulay E, Echeverria PM, et al. Candida bloodstream infections in intensive care units: Analysis of the extended prevalence of infection in intensive care unit study. *Crit Care Med* 2011;39(4):665–670.

280. Cortegiani A, Misseri G, Fasciana T, et al. Epidemiology, clinical characteristics, resistance, and treatment of infections by *Candida auris*. *J Intensive Care* 2018;6(69). doi:10.1186/s40560-018-0342-4.

281. Maksymiuk AW, Thongprasert S, Hopfer R, et al. Systemic candidiasis in cancer patients. *Am J Med* 1984;77(4D):20–27.

282. Bodey GP. Fungal infection and fever of unknown origin in neutropenic patients. *Am J Med* 1986;80(5C):112–119.

283. Bodey GP. Candidiasis in cancer patients. *Am J Med* 1984;77(4D):13–19.

284. Balandran L, Rothschild H, Pugh N, et al. A cutaneous manifestation of systemic candidiasis. *Ann Intern Med* 1973;78(3):400–403.

285. Jacobs MI, Magid MS, Jarowski CI. Disseminated candidiasis. Newer approaches to early recognition and treatment. *Arch Derm* 1980;116(11):1277–1279.

286. Pedraz J, Delgado-Jimenez Y, Perez-Gala, et al. Cutaneous expression of systemic candidiasis. *Clin Exp Derm* 2008;34(1):106–110.

287. Satoh K, Makimura K, Haumi Y, et al. *Candida auris* sp. Nov., a novel ascomycetous yeast isolated from the external ear canal of an inpatient in a Japanese hospital. *Microbiol Immunol* 2009;53(1):41–44.

288. Lockhart SR, Etienne KA, Vallabhaneni S, et al. Simultaneous emergence of multi-drug resistant *Candida auris* on 3 continents confirmed by whole-genome sequencing and epidemiological analysis. *Clin Infect Dis* 2017;64 (2):134–140.

289. Navalkele BD, Revankar S, Chandrasekar P. *Candida auris*: A worrisome, globally emerging pathogen. *Expert Rev Anti-Infect Ther* 2017;15(9):819–827.

290. Vallabhaneni S, Kallen A, Tsay S, et al. Investigation of the first seven reported cases of *Candida auris*, a globally emerging invasive, multi-drug resistant fungus—United States, May 2013–August 2016. *Am J Transplant* 2017;17(1):296–299.

291. Eyre DW, Phil D, Sheppard AE, et al. A *Candida auris* outbreak and its control in an intensive care setting. *New Eng J Med* 2018;379(14):1322–1342.

292. Centers for Disease Control and Prevention. Tracking *Candida auris* 2018. Available at: https://www.cdc.gov/fungal/diseases/candidiasis/ tracking-c-auris.html.

293. Radentz WH. Opportunistic fungal infections in immunocompromised hosts. *J Am Acad Derm* 1989;20(6):989–1003.

294. Diaz JH. Travel-related risks of regionally-endemic systemic mycoses. *J Travel Med* 2018;25(1):1–3.

295. Hahn RG, Knox LM, Forman TA. Evaluation of poststreptococcal illness. *Am Fam Physician* 2005;71(10):1949–1954.

296. Stollerman GH. Rheumatic fever in the 21st century. *Clin Infec Dis* 2001;33(6):806–814.

297. Gewitz MH, Baltimore RS, Tani LY, et al. Revision of the Jones Criteria for the diagnosis of acute rheumatic fever in the era of Doppler echocardiography: A scientific statement from the American heart Association. *Circulation* 2015;131(20): 1806–1818.

298. Guidelines for the diagnosis of rheumatic fever. Jones Criteria. 1992 update. Special writing group of the committee on rheumatic fever, endocarditis, and Kawasaki disease of the council on cardiovascular disease in the young of the American Heart Association. *JAMA* 1992;268(15):2069–2073.

299. Feinstein AR, Spagnuolo M. The clinical patterns of acute rheumatic fever: A reappraisal. *Medicine* 1962;41:279–305.

300. Stollerman GH. Rheumatic fever. *Lancet* 1997;349(9056): 935–942.

301. Hilario MO, Andrade JL, Gasparian AB, et al. The value of echocardiography in the diagnosis and follow up of rheumatic carditis in children and adolescents: A 2 year prospective study. *J Rheumatol* 2000;27(4):1082–1086.

302. McCallum AH. Natural history of rheumatic fever and rheumatic heart disease. Ten-year report of a co-operative clinical trial of A.C.T.H., Cortisone, and aspirin. *Br Med J* 1965;2(5462):607–613.

303. Swedo SE. Sydenham's chorea. A model for childhood autoimmune neuropsychiatric disorders. *JAMA* 1994;272(22):1788–1791.

304. Baldwin JS, Kerr JM, Kuttner AG, et al. Observations on rheumatic nodules over a 30-year period. *J Pediatrics* 1960;56:465–470.

305. Burke JB. Erythema marginatum. *Arch Dis in Childhood* 1955;30(152):359–365.

9 Severe Tick-Borne Infections and Their Mimics in the Critical Care Unit

Praveen Sudhindra and Gary P. Wormser

CONTENTS

CLINICAL PERSPECTIVE

Ticks can transmit bacterial, viral, and parasitic infections. Epidemiology plays a central role in the consideration of tick-transmitted illnesses. Tick vectors are geographically limited, and transmission is usually confined to the months between spring and autumn. This chapter will focus on treatable infections that are most likely to be encountered by the intensivist.

APPROACH AND DIFFERENTIAL DIAGNOSIS

Tick-transmitted infections should be considered in the differential diagnosis of any febrile illness encountered in the critical care unit (CCU), particularly between late spring and autumn. A focused history pertaining to travel, leisure activities, and a specific history of tick exposure and tick bites may be helpful. In many cases, the tick bite may have gone unnoticed, while the exposure may have occurred in the immediate vicinity of the patient's home (backyard, etc.).

Knowledge of local tick-borne diseases is essential when considering empiric therapy and diagnostic evaluation.

In the United States, Rocky Mountain spotted fever (RMSF), babesiosis, and Lyme carditis with advanced atrioventricular nodal block probably account for the majority of critical care admissions among tick-borne infections. Other infections such as human monocytic ehrlichiosis (HME), and encephalitis due to the deer tick virus (DTV)/Powassan virus (POWV) are also occasionally encountered in the CCU. Tularemia and Q fever can be transmitted by ticks but will not be discussed here since other routes of transmission predominate. Outside the United States, Crimean-Congo hemorrhagic fever and tick-borne encephalitis virus are important causes of severe illness.

Patients may present with fever and rash, fever and prominent hematological abnormalities, or fever with neurologic involvement. Overlapping features may be seen, which can serve as a clue to the presence of co-infections. Severe manifestations such as acute respiratory distress syndrome (ARDS), seen with some of these infections, can help to narrow the differential diagnosis.

A thorough physical examination may reveal single or multiple erythema migrans skin lesions, as well as other cutaneous exanthems. Meningeal signs may also be elicited.

Tables 9.1 and 9.2 list the differential diagnostic considerations in the CCU.

EPIDEMIOLOGY AND CLINICAL FEATURES

ROCKY MOUNTAIN SPOTTED FEVER

RMSF is caused by *Rickettsia rickettsii*, which is a highly virulent member of the spotted fever group of rickettsioses. Like other members of this genus, *R. rickettsii* is an obligate intracellular gram-negative bacterium.

Dermacentor variabilis (American dog tick) is the principal vector and reservoir in the eastern two-thirds of the United States, while *Dermacentor andersonii*, along with *D. variabilis*, transmit the infection in the Western United States [1]. *Rhipicephalus sanguineus* has been recently identified as a vector in Arizona and Mexico [2]. *Amblyomma* spp. are the principal vectors in South America.

TABLE 9.1

Syndrome-Based Approach to the Diagnosis of Tick-Borne Infections

Fever and Rash	Fever and Hematological Abnormalities	Sepsis	Meningitis/Encephalitis	ARDS/Multi Organ Failure
RMSF	Babesiosis	RMSF	Powassan/deer tick virus	RMSF
HME	HME	Babesiosis	HME	Babesiosis
Lyme disease	HGA	HGA	RMSF	HME (especially in HIV/ AIDS, transplant populations)
		HME	Lyme disease	

Abbreviations: RMSF, Rocky Mountain spotted fever; HME, human monocytic ehrlichiosis; HIV/AIDS, human immunodeficiency virus/acquired immunodeficiency syndrome; HGA, Human Granulocytic Anaplasmosis.

TABLE 9.2

Differential Diagnoses and Non-Infectious Mimics of Select Tick-Borne Infections

Disease	Differential Diagnoses (Infectious)	Non-Infectious Mimics
Rocky Mountain spotted fever	Other spotted fever Rickettsioses Human monocytic ehrlichiosis Human granulocytic anaplasmosis *Ehrlichia ewingii* ehrlichiosis Tick-borne relapsing fever Murine and epidemic typhus Meningococcemia Disseminated gonococcal infection *Capnocytophaga canimorsus* infection Secondary syphilis Leptospirosis Rat bite fever Typhoid and paratyphoid fever Gastroenteritis *Mycoplasma pneumoniae* Measles Rubella	Immune complex vasculitis TTP ITP Drug eruptions Stevens-Johnson syndrome Kawasaki disease
Babesiosis	Malaria Bacterial sepsis	Autoimmune Hemolytic anemias TTP
Powassan/deer tick virus encephalitis	*Listeria* Neurosyphilis Lyme disease *Borrelia miyamotoi* disease (in immunocompromised) Herpes simplex virus West Nile virus Rabies Septic CNS emboli Other causes of viral encephalitis	CNS vasculitis Drug-induced meningitis (NSAIDs, IVIG, azathioprine, etc.) Sarcoidosis Subarachnoid hemorrhage Meningeal carcinomatosis
Lyme carditis	Infective endocarditis with perivalvular abscess Chagas' disease Syphilis Rheumatic fever	Sarcoidosis SLE Coronary artery disease Chronic structural heart disease Calcium channel blocker or beta blocker toxicity Post-coronary artery bypass grafting surgery Post-transcatheter aortic valve replacement Kawasaki disease

Abbreviations: TTP, thrombotic thrombocytopenic purpura; ITP, immune thrombocytopenic purpura; IVIG, intravenous immune globulin; SLE, systemic lupus erythematosus; NSAIDs, non-steroidal anti-inflammatory drugs.

In the United States, most cases occur in South Central and South Atlantic states. Native American reservations in Arizona, as well as certain geographic areas in North Carolina are highly endemic regions [1,3].

Peak transmission occurs in late spring and summer; however, cases do occur in the winter in warmer regions. The typical incubation period is 3–12 days after the tick bite. A sudden onset of fever, chills, headache, and myalgias herald the onset of illness. Abdominal pain, nausea, and vomiting are also frequently present (~50% of cases). Photophobia and anorexia are other common initial complaints. Approximately 2–4 days later, small, blanching, pink macules are seen on the ankles, wrists, and forearms (Figure 9.1). The palms, soles, and trunk are usually involved shortly thereafter. The face is usually spared. The rash then becomes maculopapular and subsequently petechial. The "classic" appearance may not be seen until day 5 or 6 after the onset of symptoms. The rash is present in <50% of patients when they initially seek care.

Meningoencephalitis, cutaneous necrosis, gangrene of extremities, shock, ARDS, and acute kidney injury (AKI) can manifest later in the course of severe disease. Glucose-6-phosphate dehydrogenase deficiency is a risk factor for fulminant disease, with death potentially occurring in less than 5 days. The overall mortality rate since the introduction of tetracyclines is around 3%–10% [1,3].

There are no pathognomonic laboratory findings. Mild thrombocytopenia, with an increase in immature neutrophils and elevations in hepatic transaminases, may occur. Hyponatremia and elevated lactate dehydrogenase and creatine kinase are other non-specific findings. Cerebrospinal fluid (CSF) analysis may reveal a mildly elevated protein level, normal glucose levels, as well as a mild lymphocytic or neutrophilic pleocytosis (typically <100 cells/μL) [1,3].

BABESIOSIS

Babesiosis is caused by hemoprotozoans in the genus *Babesia*. In the United States, *Babesia microti*, transmitted by *Ixodes*

scapularis, is the main causative agent, and most cases are reported from the Northeastern and upper-Midwest regions. *B. duncani* or *B. duncani*-like organisms may cause babesiosis in the Pacific Northwest. Isolated cases of disease caused by *B. divergens*-like organisms have also been reported in the United States. *B. divergens*, transmitted by *Ixodes ricinus* ticks, is a well-recognized cause of babesiosis in Europe in asplenic patients [4,5].

Other routes of transmission include blood transfusion and vertical transmission. The incubation period ranges from 1 to 6 weeks from a tick bite and up to 6 months after an infected blood transfusion. Seroprevalence rates of up to 9% have been observed in some endemic areas, suggesting that asymptomatic infections are quite common [6,7].

Fever (intermittent or persistent), chills, malaise, fatigue, arthralgias, and other non-specific symptoms are common. Mild hepatosplenomegaly and jaundice may be present on examination. Hemolytic anemia, thrombocytopenia, and elevated liver enzymes are typically found. Splenic infarcts may be seen on abdominal imaging studies. Splenic rupture has been reported, often in non-immunocompromised patients with low levels of parasitemia [8].

Severe disease and hospitalization are more common in older patients and in those with certain malignancies, asplenia, or other conditions associated with immunodeficiency. ARDS, disseminated intravascular coagulation, AKI, and heart failure are recognized complications in hospitalized patients. Severe anemia (hemoglobin level <10 g/dL) and high levels of parasitemia (>10%) are risk factors for more severe disease but are not universally present in patients who develop complications. Relapsing and persistent infections can occur in patients with certain malignancies or other immunocompromising conditions. Mortality can approach 20% in immunocompromised patients and in those that acquire infection via blood transfusion [5,9,10].

LYME CARDITIS

Lyme disease is caused by *Borrelia burgdorferi* sensu lato. *B. burgdorferi* sensu stricto is the principal cause of Lyme disease in the United States, while *B. afzelli* and *B. garinii* are the leading causes in Europe. Ticks belonging to the *Ixodes ricinus* complex transmit infection. *I. scapularis* is the principal vector in the United States. States in the Northeast and the upper Midwest have the highest incidence in the United States. Endemic regions are also present on the Pacific coast, where *I. pacificus* is the vector.

The hallmark of early infection is the cutaneous lesion, erythema migrans, which develops at the site of the tick bite typically 7–14 days after the tick is removed or falls off (Figure 9.2). The incidence of cardiac involvement is about 1%–2% among patients with Lyme disease [11] and typically occurs several weeks following the tick bite (a median of 21 days following the onset of erythema migrans) [12].

Varying degrees of atrioventricular block, with or without fever, and multiple erythema migrans lesions occurring in the summer or fall months suggest a diagnosis of Lyme

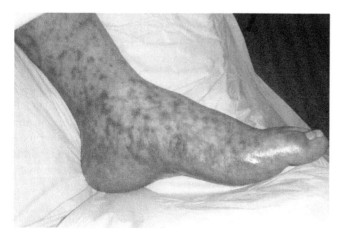

FIGURE 9.1 Late-stage petechial-purpuric rash in a patient with Rocky Mountain spotted fever. (Courtesy of CDC.)

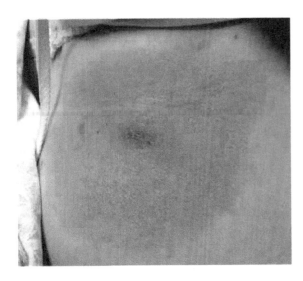

FIGURE 9.2 Erythema migrans skin lesion at the site of tick bite. (Reproduced with permission from Sanchez, E. et al., *JAMA*, 315, 1767–1777, 2016.)

carditis. A chronic cardiomyopathy has been reported in European cases of Lyme disease but not in the United States. Rare fatalities have been reported in patients with complete heart block. The usual symptoms are syncope, dizziness, and malaise. In an older case series, multiple erythema migrans lesions were present in 75% of patients with cardiac manifestations [13]. These lesions may, however, go unnoticed unless a careful head-to-toe skin examination is performed. Although meningitis and cranial nerve palsies occur in the early disseminated phase of Lyme disease, these manifestations are rarely severe enough to warrant critical care evaluation [11,12].

There are no specific abnormalities seen on routine laboratory testing; however, the presence of cytopenias may suggest the presence of other infections transmitted by *Ixodes* spp. ticks.

Human Monocytic Ehrlichiosis

Ehrlichia chaffeensis, a gram-negative intracellular bacterium, is the etiologic agent of HME. Infection occurs from the bite of an infected lone star tick (*Amblyomma americanum*). The highest incidence is in South Central and southeastern United States; however, the disease can potentially occur in any state in which this tick species is endemic [3,14].

The median incubation period is 9 days (range 5–14 days). The symptoms are similar to RMSF and include fever, headache, myalgia, abdominal pain, diarrhea, nausea, and vomiting. Rash is seen in about one-third of patients (usually around day 5 of illness) and can be maculopapular, petechial, or diffusely erythematous, involving the trunk, extremities, and occasionally the palms and soles. About 20% of infected patients develop meningitis or meningoencephalitis. HME can be particularly severe and even fatal in immunocompromised patients. ARDS, multi-organ dysfunction, and a septic shock-like state can occur [3,14]. Hemophagocytic

lymphohistiocytosis (HLH) and the macrophage activation syndrome (MAS) have been reported in association with HME [15].

Thrombocytopenia, leukopenia, and elevated liver enzymes are typical findings. A lymphocytic pleocytosis (occasionally neutrophilic) with <250 cells/μL can be seen in CSF [3].

Human Granulocytic Anaplasmosis

Human granulocytic anaplasmosis is caused by *Anaplasma phagocytophilum*, which is an obligate intracellular bacterium. As the name suggests, the organism exhibits tropism for neutrophils. The geographic distribution is generally identical to Lyme disease, since it is transmitted by the same *Ixodes* spp. tick vectors.

The clinical features are similar to RMSF and HME, with fever, headache, and myalgias being prominent. Gastrointestinal symptoms may occur, while a rash is seen in <10% of patients.

Although headache can be quite severe, meningitis is rare. About one-third of infections require hospitalization [16], with 3%–7% severe enough to warrant critical care admission [14,16]. ARDS, rhabdomyolysis, septic shock, and opportunistic infections have been reported. MAS has also been associated with HGA. Qualitative neutrophil defects may underlie the incidence of opportunistic fungal infections in some patients. Laboratory findings are virtually identical to those seen in HME.

Tick-Borne Encephalitides

Several tick-transmitted infections cause neurologic disease worldwide. HME, RMSF, and Lyme disease are known bacterial causes of meningoencephalitis. The tick-borne encephalitis group of flaviviruses is an important cause of morbidity and mortality in Europe and parts of Asia.

Powassan virus is an emerging cause of tick-borne encephalitis in North America. Two lineages of this flavivirus, which are maintained in distinct enzootic cycles, have been recognized.

Powassan virus is transmitted by *Ixodes cookei and Ixodes marxi*, with disease reported in North America and far-Eastern Russia, while DTV is transmitted by *Ixodes scapularis* and has only been described in North America thus far [17].

An incubation period of 1–5 weeks is followed by fever, sore throat, headache, and disorientation. Some individuals go on to develop neuroinvasive disease, manifesting meningitis, encephalitis, spastic or flaccid paralysis, and other focal neurologic deficits. Mortality of up to 10% has been reported in neuroinvasive disease, with about 50% of symptomatic infected patients suffering from some form of residual neurologic deficit [17,18].

The CSF analysis can be nearly normal in some cases but usually reveals a pleocytosis of up to 700 cells/μL, with neutrophilic or lymphocytic predominance. The glucose level is generally normal, while the protein level is elevated [18].

DIAGNOSIS

Laboratory investigations for tick-borne infections should include a complete blood count with a differential count, liver enzymes, bilirubin (direct and total), serum creatinine, blood urea nitrogen, electrolytes, lactate dehydrogenase, blood cultures, and, where appropriate, serum haptoglobin as well as a reticulocyte count.

The diagnosis of RMSF is clinical and epidemiological and should be strongly considered in patients with tick exposure presenting with a rapidly progressing, undifferentiated febrile illness. Obtaining the travel history and having the knowledge of the local incidence of the disease are important. The clinician should not delay treatment due to the absence of a rash, since this is present only in a minority of cases at the time of initial evaluation. *R. rickettsii* is a biosafety level 3 organism, with few laboratories undertaking isolation of the organism. Immunohistochemistry performed on skin biopsy specimens is also not widely available. Serology is the most common method of laboratory diagnosis but is usually retrospective. The indirect immunofluorescence assay (IFA) is the most sensitive and specific assay, with a titer of 1:64 and higher considered to be supportive of the diagnosis. This test cannot, however, distinguish between the various spotted fever rickettsioses. Real-time polymerase chain reaction performed on cutaneous biopsies and other specimens may prove to be a more rapid and accurate diagnostic test in the future [1,3].

A peripheral Giemsa- or Wright-stained thin and thick blood smear should be obtained when babesiosis is suspected (Figure 9.3). Real-time polymerase chain reaction performed on whole blood is highly sensitive and specific and can be useful in early disease, when parasites are difficult to visualize on a smear [5,11].

Serologic testing is usually necessary to establish a diagnosis of Lyme carditis and has >80% sensitivity in this setting. Two-step testing with an enzyme immunoassay, followed by western blot testing for IgM and IgG antibodies, is recommended. If serology is negative, and clinical suspicion

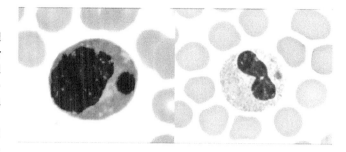

FIGURE 9.4   Wright stain of peripheral blood smear with an intra-monocytic morula seen in *Ehrlichia chaffeensis* infection (left), and an intra-granulocytic morula seen in *Anaplasma phagocytophilum* infection (right). (Reproduced from Biggs, H.M. et al., *MMWR Recomm. Rep.*, 65, 1–44.)

remains, then testing can be repeated in 2–4 weeks [11,12]. Clinicians should employ serological testing only if other clinical and epidemiologic features are suggestive of Lyme carditis. The relatively high background seroprevalence in endemic regions may lead to misattribution of conduction abnormalities to Lyme disease in some cases.

Polymerase chain reaction performed on whole blood is sensitive and specific for the diagnosis of HME. A Wright-stained peripheral smear may reveal morulae in blood monocytes. Serology (IFA) is positive in less than 50% of cases during the first week of illness [3,14].

A Giemsa-stained buffy coat smear of peripheral blood is more sensitive (20%–80%) for the diagnosis of HGA, compared with HME (<7%) (Figure 9.4). PCR of whole blood for *A. phagocytophilum* DNA is a sensitive and specific alternative to the blood smear, when available in a timely manner [3,14]. Serology is insensitive during the first week of illness.

The diagnosis of flavivirus encephalitides is usually made by demonstrating virus-specific IgM antibodies in the serum or CSF. Cross-reactivity on initial antibody screens from antibodies to multiple other flaviviruses necessitates confirmatory testing with neutralizing antibody assays [19,20].

TREATMENT

Empiric therapy is of particular importance in critically ill patients, since delay in instituting appropriate treatment can lead to worse outcomes. A high degree of clinical suspicion is necessary for the prompt initiation of therapy against treatable tick-borne infections.

Doxycycline 100 mg administered intravenously every 12 hours should be instituted without delay when RMSF is suspected (with consideration of a 200-mg loading dose). Chloramphenicol is an alternative antibiotic and can be used in pregnancy but is not as efficacious [1,3]. A study conducted among tribal communities in Arizona revealed that fatalities occurred when treatment was initiated beyond day 5 of illness, peaking at 50% on day 9 [21].

Tetracyclines are also the drugs of choice for the treatment of HME and HGA; however, rifampin has been successfully used in pregnant patients with HGA [14,22].

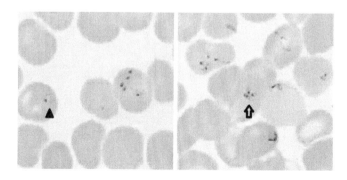

FIGURE 9.3   *Babesia microti* trophozoites in red blood cells. Arrowhead indicates a classic ring form. Asexual division yields up to four merozoites, sometimes in a tetrad, also known as the Maltese cross (arrow). (Reproduced with permission from Sanchez, E. et al., *JAMA*, 315, 1767–1777, 2016.)

TABLE 9.3

Summary of Major Causes of Severe Tick-Borne Illnesses in the United States

Disease	Causative Agent	Geographic Distribution	Vector(s)	Clinical Features	Diagnosis	Treatment	Mortality
RMSF	*Rickettsia rickettsii*	United States, Mexico, Central and South America	*Dermacentor variabilis, D. andersoni, Rhipicephalus sanguineus*	Incubation period: 3–12 days Fever, headache, myalgia, abdominal pain, nausea, vomiting, diarrhea Rash appears 2–4 days later	Clinical and epidemiological; RT PCR of skin biopsies and other specimens **Clinical clues:** Rapidly progressive febrile illness, negative blood cultures, no clear focus of infection	Doxycycline 100 mg q12h × 7–14 days, continue treating for at least 48–72 hours after defervescence Chloramphenicol can be used in pregnancy	3%–10% mortality increases greatly if treatment delayed beyond day 5 of illness
HME	*Ehrlichia chaffeensis*	United States	*Amblyomma americanum*	Incubation 5–14 days Fever, headache, myalgia, nausea, vomiting, diarrhea Rash in ~30% of adults Severe disease in immunocompromised patients, including ARDS, meningoencephalitis, HLH/MAS	PCR of whole blood, Wright stain of peripheral blood smear for intramonocytic morulae (rare), serology **Clinical clues:** Fever with leukopenia, thrombocytopenia, elevated liver enzymes	Doxycycline 100 mg q12h × 10 days	3%
HGA	*Anaplasma phagocytophilum*	United States, Europe	*Ixodes scapularis, I. ricinus complex*	Clinical features similar to HME (usually less severe, fewer GI symptoms), rash in <10%, life-threatening infection in 3%–7%; MAS, ARDS, shock, viral and fungal OIs reported CNS involvement rare	PCR of whole blood, Giemsa stain of buffy coat blood smear for intra-neutrophilic morulae (20%–80% sensitive, greater than for HME), serology (acute plus convalescent)	Doxycycline 100 mg q12h × 10 days Rifampin has been used in pregnancy	≤1%
Babesiosis	*Babesia microti, B. divergens*	United States, Europe	*Ixodes scapularis, I. ricinus* (also via blood transfusion and vertical transmission)	Asymptomatic infections common Incubation 1–6 weeks, several months in transfusion-related cases Fever, chills, myalgia, headache Persistent or relapsing infection in immunocompromised patients Severe infection in older patients, asplenia, malignancy, HIV/AIDS, and other immunocompromising conditions	Giemsa- or Wright-stained peripheral smear, PCR of whole blood **Clinical clues:** Fever, hemolytic anemia, thrombocytopenia, elevated liver enzymes	Atovaquone + azithromycin/ clindamycin + quinine × 7–10 d; >6-week course in severely immunocompromised patients Exchange transfusion for severe cases	3%–9% of hospitalized patients, up to 20% with immunocompromise

(Continued)

TABLE 9.3 (Continued)
Summary of Major Causes of Severe Tick-Borne Illnesses in the United States

Disease	Causative Agent	Geographic Distribution	Vector(s)	Clinical Features	Diagnosis	Treatment	Mortality
Lyme carditis	Borrelia burgdorferi sensu lato	United States, Eurasia	Ixodes scapularis I. ricinus complex	Varying degrees of atrioventricular block Fever and erythema migrans (often multiple) may be present	Serology—2-step testing with ELISA, followed by western blot testing for IgM and IgG antibodies	Ceftriaxone 2 g q24h initially, finish 2-week course with doxycycline 100 mg q12 h or amoxicillin 500 mg TID or cefuroxime axetil 500 mg BID	Rare
POWV/DTV encephalitis[a]	POWV/DTV	North America, far-Eastern Russia, North America	Ixodes cookei I. scapularis	Encephalitis, residual neurologic deficits Unclear if DTV and POWV have distinct manifestations	Detection of DTV/POWV specific IgM in serum with confirmatory virus specific neutralizing antibody in same or later serum specimen; virus-specific IgM in CSF; cross-reactivity with other flaviviruses occurs	Supportive; IVIG and steroids have been used in a few cases	10% fatality in patients with neuroinvasive disease

Abbreviations: OIs, opportunistic infections; ELISA, enzyme-linked immunosorbent assay; RT-PCR, real-time polymerase chain reaction; HLH = hemophagocytic lymphohistiocytosis; MAS, macrophage activation syndrome; IVIG, intravenous immunoglobulin; POVW, Powassan virus; DTV, deer tick virus.

[a] El Khoury MY, Camargo JF, White JL et al. Potential role of deer tick virus in Powassan encephalitis cases in Lyme disease-endemic areas of New York, USA. *Emerg Infect Dis* 2013; 19(12):1926–1933.

In hospitalized patients with clinical features suggestive of babesiosis (fever, hemolysis, thrombocytopenia, elevated liver enzymes, and elevated bilirubin) and a positive smear or PCR test, either intravenous azithromycin plus oral atovaquone or intravenous clindamycin plus oral quinine should be initiated. Other combinations such as clindamycin and atovaquone have also been used successfully [5,11]. There are no clinical trial data on efficacy to support one regimen over the other. Seven- to 10-day courses are usually recommended; however, more prolonged courses (of at least 6 weeks) are necessary in severely immunocompromised patients. Partial or complete RBC exchange transfusion is recommended for patients with high levels of parasitemia, particularly if there is organ dysfunction or severe anemia [5,23]. Exchange transfusion is standard therapy in Europe for splenectomized patients infected with *B. divergens* [4,5].

Patients with Lyme carditis causing high-grade second-degree or third-degree atrioventricular block should be treated with intravenous ceftriaxone initially until they are clinically stable. Therapy can then be completed with oral doxycycline, amoxicillin, or cefuroxime axetil after discharge [11]. A temporary transvenous pacemaker may be necessary in some patients.

Resolution of conduction disturbances within 1–2 weeks, either spontaneously or with treatment, is the rule [12]. Lack of response should lead the intensivist to question the diagnosis. A 14-day course is usually sufficient; however, up to 21 days of treatment is acceptable per published guidelines. Steroids are not routinely recommended in the treatment of carditis.

Treatment of flavivirus encephalitides is mainly supportive, with no evidence for specific antiviral therapy. Corticosteroids and intravenous immune globulin have been used in the treatment of POWV encephalitis with some success [18,19].

The epidemiology, clinical features, and management of the major causes of severe tick-borne illnesses in the United States are summarized in Table 9.3.

SUMMARY

Tick-transmitted illnesses are often diagnosed in endemic regions where the index of suspicion is usually high among clinicians. Considering these infections in geographic regions where transmission is sporadic or unknown can present a significant diagnostic challenge. This can result in fatal delays in instituting appropriate therapy or can result in unnecessary procedures such as permanent pacemaker implantation in patients who have Lyme carditis. Critical care practitioners need to be aware of the diagnosis and treatment of severe tick-borne infections.

REFERENCES

1. Walker DH, Blanton LS. *Rickettsia rickettsii* and other spotted fever group rickettsiae. In: Bennett JE, Dolin R, Blaser MJ eds. *Mandell, Douglas, and Bennett's Principles and Practice of Infectious Diseases* (8th ed.). Philadelphia, PA: Saunders, 2015:2198–2205.
2. Demma LJ, Traeger MS, Nicholson WL, et al. Rocky mountain spotted fever from an unexpected tick vector in Arizona. *N Engl J Med* 2005;353:587–593.
3. Biggs HM, Behravesh CB, Bradley KK, et al. Diagnosis and management of tickborne rickettsial diseases: Rocky mountain spotted fever and other spotted fever group rickettsioses, ehrlichioses, and anaplasmosis—United States. *MMWR Recomm Rep* 2016;65(2):1–44.
4. Vannier EG, Diuk-Wasser MA, Mamoun CB, Krause PJ. Babesiosis. *Infect Dis Clin North Am* 2015;29(2):357–370.
5. Gelfand JA, Vannier EG. Babesia species In: Bennett JE, Dolin R, Blaser MJ eds. *Mandell, Douglas, and Bennett's Principles and Practice of Infectious Diseases* (8th ed.). Philadelphia, PA: Saunders, 2015:3165–3172.
6. Krause PJ, McKay K, Gadbaw J, et al. Increasing health burden of human babesiosis in endemic sites. *Am J Trop Med Hyg* 2003;68:431–436.
7. Ruebush TK 2nd, Juranek DD, Chisholm ES, et al. Human babesiosis on Nantucket Island: Evidence for self-limited and subclinical infections. *N Engl J Med* 1977;297:825–827.
8. El Khoury MY, Gandhi R, Dandache P, et al. Non-surgical management of spontaneous splenic rupture due to *Babesia microti* infection. *Ticks Tick Borne Dis* 2011;2:235–238.
9. Krause PJ, Gewurz BE, Hill D, et al. Persistent and relapsing babesiosis in immunocompromised patients. *Clin Infect Dis* 2008;46:370–376.
10. Herwaldt BL, Linden JV, Bosserman E, et al. Transfusion-associated babesiosis in the United States: A description of cases. *Ann Intern Med.* 2011;155:509–519.
11. Haddad FA, Nadelman RB. Lyme disease and the heart. *Front Biosci* 2003;8:s769–s782.
12. Sanchez E, Vannier E, Wormser GP, Hu LT. Diagnosis, treatment and prevention of Lyme disease, human granulocytic anaplasmosis, and babesiosis: A review. *JAMA* 2016;315(16):1767–1777.
13. Dumler JS, Walker DH. *Ehrlichia chaffeensis, Anaplasma phagocytophilum*, and other anaplasmataceae. In: Bennett JE, Dolin R, Blaser MJ eds. *Mandell, Douglas, and Bennett's Principles and Practice of Infectious Diseases* (8th ed.). Philadelphia, PA: Saunders, 2015:2227–2233.
14. Kumar N, Goyal J, Goel A, et al. Macrophage activation syndrome secondary to human monocytic ehrlichiosis. *Indian J Hematol Blood Transfus* 2014;30(suppl 1):145–147.
15. Ebel GD. Update on Powassan virus: Emergence of a North American tick-borne flavivirus. *Annu Rev Entomol* 2010;55:95–110.
16. Piantadosi A, Rubin DB, McQuillen DP, et al. Emerging cases of Powassan virus encephalitis in New England: Clinical presentation, imaging, and review of the literature. *Clin Infect Dis* 2016;62(6):707–713.

17. Buitrago MI, Ijdo JW, Rinaudo P, et al. Human granulocytic ehrlichiosis during pregnancy treated successfully with rifampin. *Clin Infect Dis* 1998;27:213–215.

18. Spaete J, Patrozou E, Rich JD, et al. Red cell exchange transfusion for babesiosis in Rhode Island. *J Clin Apher* 2009;24:97–105.

19. Regan JJ, Traeger MS, Humpherys D, et al. Risk factors for fatal outcome from rocky mountain spotted fever in a highly endemic area—Arizona, 2002–2011. *Clin Infect Dis* 2015;60:1659–1666.

20. El Khoury MY, Camargo JF, White JL, et al. Potential role of deer tick virus in Powassan encephalitis cases in lyme disease-endemic areas of New York, USA. *Emerg Infect Dis* 2013;19(12):1926–1933.

21. Lindquis L, Vapalahti O. Tick-borne encephalitis. *Lancet* 2008;371(9627):1861–1871.

22. Steere AC, Batsford WP, Weinberg M, et al. Lyme carditis: Cardiac abnormalities of lyme disease. *Ann Intern Med* 1980;93:8–1623.

23. Dahlgren FS, Mandel EJ, Krebs JW, et al. Increasing incidence of *Ehrlichia chaffeensis* and *Anaplasma phagocytophilum* in the United States, 2000–2007. *Am J Trop Med Hyg* 2011;85:124–131.

Section II

*Clinical Syndromic Approach
in the Critical Care Unit*

10 The Clinical Approach to Sepsis and Its Mimics in the Critical Care Unit

Abdullah Chahin and Steven M. Opal

CONTENTS

CLINICAL PERSPECTIVE

Sepsis is a life-threatening organ dysfunction due to dysregulated host response to an infective process. In sepsis, the infection triggers a complex network of interactions between the host response and microbial invasion and replication. The infected host's innate and adaptive immune response features an array of pro- and anti-inflammatory cytokines and chemokines, along with complement-mediated defenses and pro- and anti-coagulation mediators [1]. If the infection is not controlled locally, sepsis continues to propagate, leading to dysfunction in multiple organ systems.

The initial immune host response manifests as systemic inflammatory response syndrome (SIRS), a term first coined by Roger Bone and associates in 1992. It consists of four readily available clinical and laboratory parameters (elevated body temperature, pulse rate, respiratory rate, and white blood cell count), thought to embody the signs and symptoms seen with the body's innate immune reaction to the inflammatory process. The SIRS criteria were intended to be used to standardize the terminology and the reproducibility of patient populations enrolled in new therapeutic trials in sepsis. However, their ease of use and face validity were rapidly adopted by clinicians as a diagnostic tool for the early recognition of sepsis in the emergency room, medical floors, and the critical care unit.

Despite the fact that the cutoff values for the SIRS criteria were set by expert opinion, they seemed reasonable and quickly became established as the criteria to diagnose sepsis expeditiously and to begin management as soon as possible [2]. Clinical experience soon began to appreciate that the SIRS plus infection definition of sepsis had some major practical limitations. A large study found that infection accounted for only 26% of SIRS patients in the emergency room setting in the United States [3]. Another recent study in the critical care unit (CCU) found a sensitivity of 88% for SIRS in patients with confirmed sepsis [4]. The SIRS criteria are therefore a reasonably sensitive but highly non-specific measure, as it can be caused by ischemia-reperfusion injury, sterile inflammation, tissue trauma, burns, necrosis, or several insults combined. In Table 10.1, the initial category of illness causing SIRS in adults, when presenting to emergency departments in the United States (2007–2010) [3]. Mimics of sepsis are a common cause of misdiagnosis in acute settings, as all of these clinical conditions present with symptoms and signs that meet the definition of SIRS. It is of critical importance to differentiate between infection-mediated sepsis and its common clinical mimics in the intensive care settings. The failure to recognize these mimics as separate entities from sepsis carries the potential for increased mortality and morbidity.

THE NEW SEPSIS DEFINITIONS

In response to the increasingly recognized, clinically evident shortcomings of the SIRS-sepsis-severe sepsis-septic shock definitions, as purposed by the Bone criteria in 1992, an international sepsis definition consensus conference was organized in 2001 [2]. At this meeting, the investigators widely agreed that the lack of precision in the current diagnostic criteria was problematic for both clinicians and clinical investigators

TABLE 10.1

Distinguishing Features Between the 1991/2001 and the 2106 Version 3 Sepsis Definitions

Definition Terms	1991/2001 Versions 1/2	2016 (Version 3)
Colonization	Not stated	Contact with a potential pathogen but no host response
Infection	Contact with a pathogen inducing a local host immune response	Contact with a pathogen inducing a local host immune response
Severe infection	Not stated	Contact with a pathogen inducing systemic host inflammatory response
Sepsis	Infection accompanied by SIRS	Severe infection accompanied by one or more damaging host-induced organ dysfunction(s)
Severe sepsis	Contact with a pathogen inducing SIRS and one or more damaging host-induced organ dysfunction(s)	Term no longer used, as all sepsis is considered severe and life-threatening
Septic shock	Subset of severe sepsis with fluid-non-responsive hypotension necessitating vasopressors	Subset of sepsis with fluid-non-responsive hypotension necessitating vasopressors to maintain MAP >65 mmHg and blood lactate >2 mmol/L

alike. The participants acknowledged that the lack of clear diagnostic criteria for sepsis terminology was a hindrance to progress, but no concrete proposals were agreed upon to move the field ahead. The conference participants added a number of organ dysfunctions and biomarkers that were highly associated with sepsis. They also proposed the idea of categorizing patients by using the PIRO method. PIRO stands for Predisposing factors; Infection; host Response, and Organ dysfunction. The logic was to categorize septic patients into a system akin to the TNM (T-tumor size, N-nodal involvement, M-metastasis) classification used so effectively in clinical oncology as a guide to staging, optimal treatment, and prognostication. This concept is still an intriguing framework to approach sepsis from a logical, graded format but has not been extensively developed to analyze its clinical relevance in sepsis research [2].

Recently, another international group of sepsis researchers organized a meeting in a further attempt to improve the clinical applicability of sepsis definitions for improved clinical utility and for greater recognition of the basic pathophysiological processes that underlie sepsis. According to the new 2016 definition, also called Sepsis-3, sepsis is defined a life-threatening organ dysfunction due to dysregulated host response to infection. Septic shock is a subset of sepsis accompanied by the following: (1) Persistent hypotension; (2) requirement for vasopressors to maintain a mean arterial pressure of 65 mmHg or higher; and (3) a serum lactate level greater than 2 mmol/L (18 mg/dL) despite adequate volume resuscitation. The combination of hyperlactatemia and hypotension a hospital mortality rates of more than 40% [5], in addition to prolonging their stay in the CCU. Table 10.2 outlines the components of what constituted the sepsis definitions in various stages of the

TABLE 10.2

Sepsis Mimics

Condition	Features Mimicking Sepsis	Distinctive Features
Macrophage activation syndrome	High fever, lymphadenopathy, altered mental status, cytokine elevation, pancytopenia, multi-organ failure	Pancytopenia on presentation, mucocutaneous findings (purpura, easy bruising, mucosal bleeding), hepatosplenomegaly, elevated ferritin
Pancreatitis	Low grade fever, leukocytosis, tachycardia, lung infiltrates	Severe, epigastric pain, elevated amylase and lipase, abdominal computerized tomography findings consistent with pancreatitis
Aspiration pneumonitis	Dyspnea, tachypnea, fever, lobar infiltrate on chest X-ray	Witnessed aspiration of gastric contents, pneumonitis comes on suddenly while pneumonia builds up gradual symptoms. Infiltrates in dependent areas of lung
Adrenal insufficiency	Fatigue, hypotension, hyperdynamic state with low SVR	Positive response to hydrocortisone stress dose
Hypovolemia	Tachypnea, tachycardia, hypotension, low-grade fever	Clinical signs of dehydration. External signs of volume loss (hemorrhage, trauma, vomiting, diarrhea)
Pulmonary embolism	Fever, tachycardia, leukocytosis	Hypoxemia with respiratory alkalosis, unilateral leg swelling, hemoptysis, obstructive shock picture
Anaphylaxis	Hypotension, tachycardia	Abrupt onset, mucocutaneous manifestations, eosinophilia, exposure to allergens, upper respiratory tract swelling. Elevated histamine and tryptase levels in serum
Non-infectious hyperlactatemia	Altered mental status, tachypnea, hypotension, oliguria	No signs of infection found, search for drugs implicated as possible cause of lactic acidosis
Diabetic ketoacidosis	Altered mental status, tachycardia, tachypnea and hypotension	Clinical signs of dehydration (dry tongue and skin), ketosis, hyperglycemia, and elevated serum osmolarity and beta-hydroxybutyrate

process. It should be noted that even today, sepsis is a syndrome with no validated criterion that confirms the diagnosis. Because of its significant impact on clinical outcome, the new sepsis definition changes the focus from the SIRS criteria to screening for organ dysfunction. In an attempt to quantify organ damage, the Sequential Organ Failure Assessment (SOFA) score is calculated for patients with sepsis in a critical care unit [6]. According to the new definition, organ dysfunction can be identified as an acute change in total SOFA score ≥2 points, consequent to the infection. This acute change in SOFA reflects an overall inpatient mortality risk of approximately 10% [7].

A new measure, developed from detailed analyses from large clinical databases, was developed into the term qSOFA (for quick SOFA). This effort was an attempt to use data-driven endpoints rather than expert opinion to establish diagnostic endpoints and cutoff values. The qSOFA was derived from readily available vital signs and measures of mentation that most effectively predicted which patients would rapidly progress to septic shock and death. The quick SOFA parameters chosen from a large database comprised hundreds of thousands of patient data. The final score was whittled down to only 3, independent, predictive criteria consisting of altered mentation, systolic blood pressure of ≤100 mmHg, and respiratory rate ≥22/min. The qSOFA provides a simple bedside criterion to identify adult patients outside the CCU with suspected infection who are likely to have poor outcomes. The sensitivity of this tool, however, has come under some question of its validity, and some follow-up studies find suboptimal performance in terms of sensitivity in predicting severe sepsis and mortality [8]. Additional studies are warranted to validate and improve these criteria. The consensus committee members fully acknowledge that the optimal diagnostic criterion for sepsis and septic shock is, and likely will be, a continuously evolving process. New diagnostic methodologies using real-time genomics for both the microbial pathogen detection and the dynamics of the host response will likely improve over time, rendering existing definitions obsolete, and will necessitate periodic updates (e.g., sepsis definitions 4, 5, 6... or 3.1, 3.2, etc.).

EPIDEMIOLOGY OF SEPSIS

A retrospective analysis of an international database reported that, between the years 1995 and 2015, the global incidence for sepsis was 437 per 100,000 person-years. It is thought that this rate was not reflective of contributions from low- and middle-income countries. One large study estimated approximately 16.6 million emergency department visits of adult with SIRS per year nationally in the United States [3].

Sepsis has been a leading cause of death in the United States, and the most common cause of death among critically ill patients in non-cardiac CCUs. The steady increase in the rate of sepsis is being attributed to advancing age, immunosuppression, and multidrug-resistant infections.

SEPSIS WORKUP: APPROACH CONSIDERATIONS

INTRAVENOUS FLUID RESUSCITATION

Hypotension is commonly seen in patients with sepsis. Low blood pressure is typically caused by a combination of increased vascular permeability, decreased systemic vascular resistance (SVR), and intravascular hypovolemia. Intravenous fluid resuscitation continues to be recommended as the first-line resuscitative therapy for all patients with sepsis and septic shock. However, there is no established evidence demonstrating benefit to fluid resuscitation as a therapy in isolation. It is presumed that fluid resuscitation in septic patients help resolve tissue hypoperfusion, usually evidenced by increased lactate, oliguria, and delivery-dependent oxygen consumption, each finding attributed to inadequate blood flow. This linear clinical reasoning is now viewed to be too simplistic. Lactate production and clearance during sepsis is complex and remains poorly understood. The current evidence suggests that elevated blood lactate level is not a reliable indicator of tissue hypoxia during sepsis [9]. Similarly, observational studies on murine models of sepsis strongly suggest that oliguria is not a function of decreased renal perfusion during sepsis. More importantly, clinical studies both in sepsis and in other conditions such as burns have shown that fluid resuscitation based on oliguria often has minimal to no effect on urine output and fails in reversing renal dysfunction [10].

In conclusion, there are no randomized controlled trials that assess fluid resuscitation as an intervention for septic shock. An increasing number of studies now link fluid overload in septic patients to worse outcomes. Positive fluid balance has been associated with increased mortality in septic patients. Furthermore, fluid de-resuscitation—where a negative mean daily fluid balance is achieved—was consistently associated with improved clinical outcomes in the RENAL trial. On the other hand, a conservative fluid management strategy can potentially improve patient outcomes, as was demonstrated in the "fluids and catheters treatment trial" (FACTT). Therefore, clinicians should determine which patient would benefit from fluid therapy and tailor their treatment accordingly. A recent study showed that changes in stroke volume, pulse pressure, and peak velocity of femoral artery flow triggered by passive leg raising are shown to be helpful indices for predicting fluid responsiveness in patients with sepsis or pancreatitis.

EMPIRIC ANTIMICROBIAL THERAPY

Appropriate empiric antimicrobial therapy must be administered as soon as possible in patients with suspected sepsis, as delayed antimicrobial therapy is strongly associated with increased mortality in severe infections [11]. Therefore, empiric antimicrobial therapy should be started immediately (preferably within 30 min) of making the presumptive clinical diagnosis. The objective is the rapid reduction of total microbial load before progression to irreversible shock. Efforts to optimize antimicrobial therapy in clinical practice can be divided into (a) early achievement of therapeutic drug concentrations and (b) optimizing cidality of the drug regimen. For the former objective, special attention should be paid to the existence of renal or hepatic insufficiency and the tissue penetration. As for the later objective, the choice of empiric antimicrobial regimen should always take into consideration the location of the infectious process, as each anatomic location has a different spectrum of flora that can become pathogenic when organ function is impaired. Inappropriate antimicrobial therapy in CCU patients has historically been reported in 15%–30% and is associated with increased hospital mortality [12]. Inappropriate antimicrobial choice carries a five-fold increase in mortality (52% vs. 10.3%). However, apart from the treatment of endocarditis and meningitis, the perceived superiority of bactericidal vs. bacteriostatic antimicrobials in treating many infections *in vivo* has not been demonstrated.

Combination therapy (a β-lactam combined with another agent) is generally thought to be most beneficial in the sickest patients. De-escalation of antimicrobial therapy based on microbiological culture, susceptibility testing, and clinical improvement is associated with improved outcomes in serious infections, as well as promoting antimicrobial stewardship [13].

Blood Pressure and Organ Support

Circulatory support in suspected sepsis is required, not only for hypotension or shock but also to prevent complications in patients at risk of organ failure. If tissue hypoperfusion persists, the function of vital organs will be impaired. Assessment of tissue perfusion can be performed clinically, by looking at skin color and temperature, capillary refill, pulse volume, and sweating. Raised lactate and decreased urine outputs are other indicators of poor perfusion but are not as accurate in the setting of sepsis as explained earlier.

Surviving Sepsis Guidelines to target an initial mean arterial pressure (MAP) target of 65 mmHg was based on limited evidence. Some evidence suggests that increasing the mean pressure up to 85 mmHg (using norepinephrine) may be more appropriate. Therefore, there is no established cutoff for MAP that is supported by evidence in individual patients. The main objective for organ support should always focus on restoring oxygen delivery to the tissues while addressing the underlying cause. Delays in initiating treatment, along with suboptimal resuscitation, contribute to the development irreversible dysfunction of vital organs. Preload volume optimization and vasopressor agents are the most efficient way of increasing cardiac output and restoring tissue perfusion.

Drainage and Source Control

Source control is the constitution of measures taken in the process of care to control the foci of infection and to restore optimal function of the site of infection. Source-control measures can be categorized into three broad modalities: Drainage of liquid component of an infection; debridement of solid

necrotic tissue; and excision or amputation of an infected foci, an organ, or an infected hardware. The utility of source control is heavily dependent on the site and nature of the underlying infection, the patient's health status at baseline, and the availability of human and technological resources. Appropriate source-control intervention can rapidly alter the course of sepsis to a more favorable direction [14].

MIMICS OF SEPSIS

A myriad of medical disease can have a clinical presentation that mimics that of sepsis. The differentiation is vital, because if these conditions are not considered, increased mortality and morbidity could be anticipated. Table 10.3 summarizes some of the main sepsis mimics and outlining both the features mimicking sepsis along with their distinctive features.

Macrophage Activation-Like Syndrome

About 5% of critical care unit patients who are diagnosed with sepsis/septic shock likely have a related hyperinflammatory state, now known as macrophage activation-like syndrome (MALS) [15,16]. MALS is a subgroup of a spectrum of syndromes referred to as primary or secondary hemophagocytic lymphohistiocytosis (HLH). Primary HLH is an early-onset, hereditary dysfunction of cytotoxic activity of natural killer (NK) cells or CD8 T cells [17]. The hallmark finding in making the diagnosis HLH is determined by bone marrow biopsy with the evidence of hemophagocytosis. Secondary acquired forms of HLH are much more akin to MALS. MALS is generally seen in older children and adults and is frequently associated with systemic autoimmune, autoinflammatory states, neoplastic disorders, or occasionally with systemic infections. Infectious causes are generally attributable to systemic herpes virus infections (e.g., Epstein–Barr virus or cytomegalovirus) or bacterial sepsis.

This is a devastating hyperinflammatory state with a high mortality rate. MALS is accompanied by fever, cytopenias, cytokine release, hepatic dysfunction, acute kidney injury, and signs of macrophage activation. Macrophage-driven hyperinflammation is manifest by inflammasome-driven increases in interleukin (IL)-1 beta and IL-18, along with striking

TABLE 10.3
Types of Shock and the Distinguishing Circulatory Derangements

Type of Shock	PCWP	Cardiac Output	Volume Status	Systemic Vascular Resistance	Tissue Perfusion (Mixed Venous O$_2$ Saturation)
Hypovolemic	↓↓	↓	↓	↑	↓
Cardiogenic	↑↑	↓	↔	↑↑	↓
Distributive	↓ or ↔	↑	↔	↓	↑
Obstructive	↑	↓	↔	↑	↓

increases in serum ferritin (>4420 ng/mL), elevations in serum triglycerides, and other plasma markers of macrophage activation such as sCD163 and sCD25 [15]. Ferritin is stored in macrophage cells and is released into the circulation during acute inflammatory states. Since bone marrow biopsies are rarely done in critically ill patients, and hemophagocytosis is not needed to make a diagnosis, the term MALS is now used to define this clinical syndrome of sepsis-induced MALS. The overlapping associations with systemic infection and the multi-organ dysfunction that typifies both MALS and sepsis make MALS difficult to recognize in a septic patient population. The distinction between the two syndromes is based on cytopenias, markedly elevated ferritin levels, and early-onset and persistent hyperinflammation. These features are indicative of MALS rather than sepsis. The distinction is important, as refractory cases of MALS will often be amenable to treatment with high-dose steroids, etoposide-containing regimens, immunomodulators, and possibly IL-1 receptor antagonist or similar inflammasome inhibitors [16,17]. Eradication of the causative microbial pathogen will often reduce the risk of death from sepsis-induced MALS and is the primary treatment priority [15].

PANCREATITIS

Pancreatitis, particularly when it is acute, severe, and associated with tissue necrosis, can easily be confused with sepsis on its initial presentation. The acute systemic inflammatory changes and hemodynamic consequences induced by "sterile" inflammation of the pancreas from the release of damage-associated molecular pattern substances look clinically very similar to sepsis induced by pathogen-associated molecular patterns [18]. Often, the pain associated with pancreatitis is poorly localized and can lead to initial diagnostic uncertainty. Radiographic evidence showing pancreatic swelling and necrosis, along with elevated amylase and lipase levels, usually confirms the diagnosis. Predisposing factors for pancreatitis, such as biliary and pancreatic duct obstruction, alcohol excess, hypercalcemic states, drugs known to induce pancreatitis, etc., should prompt a search for pancreatic inflammation.

To further complicate matters, the pancreatic bed can be the primary source of sepsis when the intestinal microbiota contaminates necrotic tissue left behind from severe pancreatitis. Pre-existing pancreatic pseudocysts can also become infected and complicate the course of necrotizing pancreatitis, leading to sepsis and septic shock [19].

A major, unsolved debate continues over the wisdom of administering an empiric regimen of broad-spectrum antibiotics such as carbapenems with an aim of preventing secondary infection of the necrotic pancreatic tissue. Detailed meta-analyses of the clinical trials attempting to answer this question have failed to verify the benefits of this strategy, and this approach is generally not recommended. However, if a needle aspiration of the pancreatic tissue, cyst, or pseudocyst or surrounding peritoneal fluid reveals inflammatory cells and microbial pathogens, then antimicrobial therapy directed at enteric aerobic and anaerobic pathogens is warranted. Optimal source control with removal of necrotic tissue, enteral nutrition, and supportive care, along with antibiotics, if indicated by objective evidence of infection, is the preferred management strategy for severe necrotizing pancreatitis [20].

ASPIRATION PNEUMONITIS

Aspiration of small quantities of nasogastric contents is a commonplace occurrence in patients with neurologic impairment and in heavily sedated persons. This process is of little consequence, unless large volumes of either gastric acid contents or particulate material occur. Low-pH gastric fluid rapidly induces essentially a chemical burn in the lower airways that impairs gas exchange and disrupts mucociliary airway clearance mechanisms. Particulate aspiration of food particles can obstruct large and small airways, inducing ventilation-perfusion mismatches and impairment of lung clearance mechanisms. Both types of aspiration can facilitate infection of the distal airways and develop into secondary infectious complications. The major diagnostic challenge to the clinician is recognizing non-infected lung injury from secondary infection. This process can occur in the community, in long-term care settings, or in critically ill patients with impaired levels of consciousness [21].

Acid aspiration induces a robust acute inflammatory response with fever and release of cytokines, drawing neutrophils into the lung in response to tissue injury. Acute, asymmetric but often bilateral infiltrates are commonplace within a few hours to 24 hours after aspiration and often resolve quickly if secondary infection does not intervene. Secondary bacterial infection after the onset of aspiration pneumonitis usually occurs several days after the initial aspiration event. Symptoms and radiographic evidence of worsening occur and should alert the clinician to re-investigate the patient. The microbiology of the secondary pneumonia is largely dependent on the location of the patient (community-acquired or hospital acquired) and the baseline health status of the patient at the time of the aspiration. Treatment with antibiotics is only indicated if secondary pneumonia occurs and should be directed at the pathogen identified as the most likely causative organism [22].

ADRENAL INSUFFICIENCY

Acute adrenal insufficiency (AI) is an infrequently encountered problem that may mimic overwhelming sepsis. This condition typically presents with abdominal pain, nausea, vomiting, and diarrhea, frequently confused for an intra-abdominal sepsis. It also causes weakness, fatigue, hypoglycemia, salt craving, and hypotension resistant to IV fluids and vasopressors. The AI is remarkable for elevated cardiac output and low SVR, consistent with a distributive shock [23]. Risk factors for developing AI include corticosteroid use for more than 2 weeks, cancer, and tuberculosis.

Diagnosis of acute adrenocortical insufficiency should be considered when a patient manifests with septic shock picture without any obvious infectious cause and is not improving despite receiving considerable intravenous fluid therapy resuscitation. Baseline cortisol testing can be performed in patients with AI but is not mandatory [23]. To establish the diagnosis of acute AI—and for treatment—stress-dose hydrocortisone or dexamethasone is initiated in the patient, with improvement of hypotension and abdominal symptoms confirming the diagnosis.

Hypovolemia

Hypovolemia is the state of decrease in blood volume or a decrease in intravascular component. This loss leads to volume contraction. Causes are loss of blood, loss of plasma (severe burns and oozing wounds), or loss of sodium with consequent loss of intravascular and extravascular water (diarrhea, vomiting, heat stroke, etc.). For hypovolemia to result in hypotension, around 30%–40% of intravascular volume would typically be lost [24].

Fluid depletion can cause tachycardia, tachypnea, systemic inflammation, increasing WBCs, and temperature elevation, meeting two or more SIRS criteria. External signs of volume loss (hemorrhage, trauma, vomiting, or diarrhea) should be looked for. Medication change, especially diuretics, can be the underlying etiology in elderly. Exam can reveal lethargy, dry mucous membranes, turgor, delayed capillary refill, weak rapid distal peripheral pulses, hypotension, and tachypnea. Volume repletion (oral or intravenous) is the mainstay of treatment [25], along with the reversal of the primary etiology behind the volume loss.

Pulmonary Embolism

Pulmonary emboli (PE) usually arise from thrombi that originate in the deep venous system of the lower extremities. Patients may present with sudden-onset, tachycardia, dyspnea, and hypoxia, but this "classic presentation" is infrequently seen in practice. Occasionally, patients may have fever, often low-grade; abdominal pain; cough; lethargy; and syncope. Clinician should inquire about recent travel history, history of thrombosis, family history of thrombosis, pregnancy, and history of cancer. Leg swelling has poor sensitivity and specificity in diagnosing deep venous thrombosis (DVT)/PE (sensitivity of 10%–54% and specificity of 39%–89%). The Pulmonary Embolism Rule Out Criteria (PERC) rules out patients who are considered low-risk for PE, based on clinical criteria alone [26]. Massive PE can result in an obstructive shock, where increased cardiac preload is seen in conjunction with low cardiac output.

Computerized tomographic angiogram of the chest must be considered in patients with moderate to high risk. Ventilation-perfusion scan can be alternatively used if the baseline chest radiograph is unremarkable. Cardiac echocardiography is helpful in assessing right ventricle size and pulmonary artery pressure, both of which are increased with PE. It can also identify the presence of right-chamber emboli. Serum troponin and brain natriuretic peptide, although seemingly marginal for purposes of diagnosis of PE, may contribute significantly to the ability to stratify patients by risk for short-term death [27].

Anaphylaxis

Anaphylaxis is an acute life-threatening condition with multisystemic manifestations due to the rapid release of inflammatory mediators. It, therefore, must be identified and treated quickly. Patient could present with anaphylactic shock, an immediate hypersensitivity reaction that is mediated by the interaction of IgE on mast cells and basophils with an encountered antigen. This type of shock resembles the hemodynamics of distributive shock but is also associated with cutaneous (hives, edema, and pruritus), respiratory (bronchospasm and tongue and laryngeal edema), and gastrointestinal (vomiting, diarrhea, and abdominal distension) manifestations [28]. Identifying allergic exposures aid in establishing the diagnosis and initiating treatment.

A simplified way to diagnose is with acute onset of illness and involvement of two organ systems (including skin, mucosa, respiratory, GI symptoms, and hemodynamic instability). No fever is typically seen. A known exposure to a suspected drug allergy agent with hypotension also meets criteria. Epinephrine—intravenous or intramuscular—is the first line of treatment. Injection in a large muscle (e.g., lateral thigh) results in better absorption of the medication and does not require insertion of intravenous access. Corticosteroids IV and histamine H1/H2 antagonist IV are frequently used, but data proving their efficacy is lacking [29,30].

Lactic Acidosis

Lactic acidosis is an acid-base disorder resulting from elevated lactate levels. The use of lactic acid as a clinical diagnostic and prognostic tool has been steadily increasing lately over the last decade. Failure to achieve lactate clearance beyond the first 6 hours despite circulatory restoration suggests the need for therapeutic interventions that differ from those used in early sepsis management [31]. In some patients, causes other than sepsis should be explored. Clinicians must be aware of the many potential causes of lactic acid elevation, as the clinical and prognostic importance of an elevated lactate varies widely by underlying etiology.

Elevated lactic acid commonly results from tissue hypoperfusion resulting from hypovolemia, sepsis, or cardiac failure (type A). In type B lactic acidosis, the underlying mechanisms include toxin-induced impairment of cellular metabolism and regional areas of ischemia. This type is seen in diabetes mellitus, malignancy, alcoholism, HIV infection, and mitochondrial dysfunction or is medication induced. A much less common form (D-lactic acidosis) is caused by its overproduction by bacteria in the colon in patients with short bowel syndrome or other forms of GI malabsorption.

Mechanisms of drug-induced metabolic acidosis include drugs acting as exogenous acid loads, leading to loss of bicarbonate in the GI tract or kidneys, increasing endogenous acid production, or decreasing renal acid excretion [32]. The causative medications include metformin, propofol, linezolid, beta-agonists, nucleoside reverse transcriptase inhibitors, biguanides, iron, isoniazid, zidovudine, salicylates, and many others [33].

Despite its substandard sensitivity and specificity, the lactic acid assay remains a clinically useful test to alert clinicians of underlying hypoperfusion, critical tissue hypoxia, and the need for immediate treatment or an etiology not readily apparent on initial evaluation. Clinicians need to be aware of the many potential etiologies of lactic acid elevation.

Diabetic Ketoacidosis

Diabetic ketoacidosis (DKA) is an acute life-threatening complication of diabetes (mainly type I but seen frequently with type II diabetes). It is characterized by hyperglycemia, ketoacidosis, and ketonuria. Patients with DKA frequently present with a clinical picture that mimics sepsis. They are often tachycardic and confused and have elevated lactic acid. Occasionally, patients with DKA are hypotensive on presentation, due to osmotic diuresis and hypovolemia. In addition, infection, ischemia, medication non-compliance, drug abuse, pancreatitis, trauma, and many other causes can precipitate DKA [34]. In fact, concomitant infection is seen in roughly 40% of patients admitted with DKA.

Diagnosing DKA requires the detection of ketosis (either in urine or in serum), acidosis or acidemia, and hyperglycemia. In the setting of DKA, it is reasonable to initiate empiric antibiotics for assumed infection until it is ruled out. Fluid resuscitation is a crucial part of management and is required, along with electrolyte management (closely monitor potassium). Insulin treatment—frequently in the form of an intravenous infusion—is initiated after proper fluid resuscitation [35]. If properly treated, the prognosis of patients with DKA is excellent.

CARDIOGENIC VS. SEPTIC SHOCK

Shock is defined as a circulatory failure that results in inadequate cellular oxygen delivery or utilization. It is prevalent in critical care setting, where approximately one-third of patients are affected. Assessment of the causes of shock can be challenging. In the SOAP II, 62% of approximately 1700 patients had septic shock; 17% had cardiogenic shock; 16% had hypovolemic shock, anaphylaxis, or other non-septic distributive shock in 4%; and only 2% had obstructive shock [36]. Septic shock is the most commonly encountered type of shock, with reported case-fatality rates ranging between 40% and 80% [37]. Cardiogenic shock is the second most common and has been mainly studied in the setting of acute myocardial infarction. However, mechanisms of shock can co-exist. In Table 10.4, different types of shock and the various circulatory parameters derangements are outlines. It is not uncommon that determining the type of shock is not an easy clinical task. Therefore, trying to determine or measure some of those parameters can help not only the institution of stabilization measures (such as IV fluid resuscitation and initiation of

TABLE 10.4
Adults with SIRS and Initial Category of Illness When Presenting to Emergency Departments in the United States (2007–2010)

Causes of SIRS in the Emergency Room

Unrecognized	56%
Infection	26%
Trauma	10%
Ischemia	3%
Hemorrhage	3%
Toxins	1%
Pancreatitis	1%
Anaphylaxis	<1%
Burn	<1%

Source: Horeczko, T. et al., *West. J. Emerg. Med.*, 15, 329–336, 2014.

vasopressors), but also better identifying and managing the underlying etiology causing shock.

Identifying the main mechanism behind shock—hypovolemic, cardiogenic, obstructive, or distributive—is of high importance. The diagnosis of acute shock is based on a combination of clinical, hemodynamic, and biochemical markers. The context of the presentation (infection, trauma, chest pain, etc.) is usually helpful but leads to complex situations where more than one etiology of shock is present. Arterial hypotension (although this is not always present), altered mental status, oliguria, and cold clammy skin are the cardinal clinical features of shock.

Distributive shock usually presents with elevated cardiac output, while the other types of shock are associated with low cardiac output. Cardiogenic shock is associated with high blood pressures and volumes, unlike hypovolemic shock. Obstructive shock is associated with elevated pulmonary artery pressure and dilated right-sided heart chambers.

Echocardiography may reveal unsuspected reasons for shock by evaluating cardiac output, cardiac function, and cardiac preload and therefore should be performed whenever possible [38]. In cases of severe shock and in complex conditions, advanced hemodynamic monitoring can be helpful but should not be resorted to in non-severe cases of shock that rapidly respond to initial therapy.

SUMMARY

Sepsis is a major challenge for clinicians and for patients in critical care units worldwide. Septic shock can rapidly progress, with potentially lethal consequences if not recognized and treated promptly. The lack of a single confirmatory diagnostic test for sepsis can lead to delayed diagnosis from an array of clinical entities that mimic sepsis. A high index of suspicion for the possibility of sepsis is needed, and a new generation of molecular diagnostic capabilities will hopefully find their way into standard critical care unit medicine in the near future to assist in diagnosis and appropriate therapy.

REFERENCES

1. Aziz M, Jacob A, Yang W-L, Matsuda A, Wang P. Current trends in inflammatory and immunomodulatory mediators in sepsis. *J Leukoc Biol* 2013;93(3):329–342.
2. Levy MA, Ramsey G, Fink M, et al. The 2001 SCCM/ESICM/ACCP/ATS/SIS international sepsis definitions conference. *Crit Care Med* 2003;31(4):1250–1256.
3. Horeczko T, Green JP, Panacek EA. Epidemiology of the systemic inflammatory response syndrome (SIRS) in the emergency department. *West J Emerg Med* 2014;15(3):329–336.
4. Kaukonen KM, Bailey M, Pilcher D, Cooper DJ, Bellomo R. Systemic inflammatory response syndrome criteria in defining severe sepsis. *N Engl J Med* 2015;372:1629–1638.
5. Singer M, Deutschman CS, Seymour CW, et al. The third international consensus definitions for sepsis and septic shock (Sepsis-3). *JAMA* 2016;315(8):801–810.
6. Vincent JL, de Mendonça A, Cantraine F, Moreno R, Takala J, Suter PM, Sprung CL, Colardyn F, Blecher S. Use of the SOFA score to assess the incidence of organ dysfunction/failure in intensive care units: Results of a multicenter, prospective study. Working group on "sepsis-related problems" of the European society of intensive care medicine. *Crit Care Med* 1998;26(11):1793–1800.
7. Seymour CW, Liu V, Iwashyna TJ, et al. Assessment of clinical criteria for sepsis. *JAMA* 2016;315(8):762–774.
8. Park HK, Kim WY, Kim MC, Jung W, Ko BS. Quick sequential organ failure assessment compared to systemic inflammatory response syndrome for predicting sepsis in emergency department. *J Crit Care* 2017;42:12–17.
9. James JH, Luchette FA, McCarter FD, Fischer JE. Lactate is an unreliable indicator of tissue hypoxia in injury or sepsis. *Lancet* 1999;354(9177):505–508.
10. Bihari S, Prakash S, Bersten AD. Post resuscitation fluid boluses in severe sepsis or septic shock: Prevalence and efficacy (price study). *Shock* 2013;40(1):28–34.
11. Lodise TP, McKinnon PS, Swiderski L, Rybak MJ. Outcomes analysis of delayed antibiotic treatment for hospital-acquired Staphylococcus aureus bacteremia. *Clin Infect Dis.* 2003;36:1418–1423.
12. Ibrahim EH, Sherman G, Ward S, Fraser VJ, Kollef MH. The influence of inadequate antimicrobial treatment of bloodstream infections on patient outcomes in the ICU setting. *Chest* 2000;118:146–155.
13. Joung MK, Lee JA, Moon SY, et al. Impact of de-escalation therapy on clinical outcomes for intensive care unit-acquired pneumonia. *Crit Care* 2011;15:R79.
14. Marshall JC, Maier RV, Jimenez M, et al. Source control in the management of severe sepsis and septic shock: An evidence-based review. *Crit Care Med* 2004;32: S513–S526.
15. Kyriazopoulou E, Leventogiannis K, Norby-Teglund A, et al. Macrophage activation-like syndrome: An immunologic entity associated with rapid progression to death in sepsis. *BMC Med* 2017;15:172.
16. Shakoory B, Carcillo JA, Chatham W, et al. Interleukin-1 blockade reduces mortality in sepsis patients with features of macrophage activation syndrome. *Crit Care Med* 2016;44(2):275–281.
17. Janka, GE, Lehmberg K. Hemophagocytic syndrome: An update. *Blood Rev* 2014;28(4):135–142.
18. Cinel I, Opal SM. Molecular biology of inflammation and sepsis: A primer. *Crit Care Med* 2009;37(1):291–304.
19. Bakker OJ, Santvooort HC, Brunschot S, et al. Endoscopic transgastric vs. surgical necrosectomy for infected necrotizing pancreatitis: A randomized trial. *JAMA* 2012;307:1053–1061.
20. Tenner S, Baillie J, DeWitt J, Vege SS. Management of acute pancreatitis. *Am J Gastroenterol* 2013;108:1400–1415.
21. Reza Shariatzadeh M, Huang JQ, Marrie TJ. Differences in the features of aspiration pneumonia according to the site of acquisition: Community of continuing care facility. *J Am Geriatr Soc* 2006;54:296–302.
22. El-Solh AA, Pietrantoni C, Bhat A, et al. Microbiology of severe aspiration pneumonia in institutionalized elderly. *Am J Resp Crit Care Med* 2003;167:1650–1654.
23. Tintinalli JE, Stapczynski J, Ma O, et al. eds. *Tintinalli's Emergency Medicine: A Comprehensive Study Guide.* New York: McGraw-Hill, 2011.
24. Greaves I, Porter K, Hodgetts T, et al. eds. *Emergency Care: A Textbook for Paramedics.* Elsevier Health Sciences, 2006:229. ISBN 9780702025860.
25. Krausz MM. Initial resuscitation of hemorrhagic shock. *World J Emerg Surg* 2006;1:14.
26. Kline JA, Courtney DM, Kabrhel C, et al. Prospective multi-center evaluation of the pulmonary embolism rule-out criteria. *J Thromb Haemost* 2008;6:772–780.
27. Konstantinides S. Clinical practice. Acute pulmonary embolism. *N Engl J Med* 2008;359(26):2804–2813.
28. Webb LM, Lieberman P. Anaphylaxis: A review of 601 cases. *Ann Allergy Asthma Immunol* 2006;97(1):39–43.
29. Sheikh A, Ten Broek V, Brown SG, et al. H1-antihistamines for the treatment of anaphylaxis: Cochrane systematic review. *Allergy* 2007;62(8):830–837.
30. Choo KJL, Simons E, Sheikh A. Glucocorticoids for the treatment of anaphylaxis: Cochrane systematic review. *Allergy* 2010;65(10):1205–1211.
31. Chertoff J, Chisum M, Garcia B, Lascano J. Lactate kinetics in sepsis and septic shock: A review of the literature and rationale for further research. *J Intens Care* 2015;3:39.
32. Pham AQT, Xu LHR, Moe OW. Drug-induced metabolic acidosis. *F1000Research* 2015;4:F1000 Faculty Rev-1460.
33. Mégarbane B, Brivet F, Guérin JM, Baud FJ. Lactic acidosis and multi-organ failure secondary to anti-retroviral therapy in HIV-infected patients. *Presse Med* 1999;28(40):2257–2264.
34. Savage MW, Datary KK, et al. Joint british diabetes societies guideline for the management of diabetic ketoacidosis. *Diabet Med* 2011;28(5):508–515.
35. Perilli G, Saraceni C, Kilvert A, et al. Diabetic ketoacidosis: A review and update. *Curr Emerg Hosp Med Rep* 2013;1:10–17.
36. De Backer D, Biston P, et al. Comparison of dopamine and norepinephrine in the treatment of shock. *N Engl J Med* 2010;362(9):779–789.
37. Jawad I, Luksic I, Rafnsson SB. Assessing available information on the burden of sepsis: Global estimates of incidence, prevalence and mortality. *J Glob Health* 2012;2:010404.
38. Labovitz AJ, Noble VE, Bierig M, et al. Focused cardiac ultrasound in the emergent setting: A consensus statement of the American society of echocardiography and American college of emergency physicians. *J Am Soc Echocardiogr* 2010;23:1225–1230.

11 Acute Bacterial Meningitis and Its Mimics in the Critical Care Unit

Burke A. Cunha

CONTENTS

CLINICAL PERSPECTIVE

There are several diagnostic difficulties in patients presenting with the possibility of acute bacterial meningitis (ABM). Meningitis may be mimicked by a variety of infectious and non-infectious disorders. The mimics of meningitis are readily ruled out on the basis of the history/physical exam, and lumbar puncture (LP) with cerebrospinal fluid (CSF) analysis will exclude the diagnosis of ABM. Early and appropriate empiric antimicrobial therapy of ABM in the critical care unit (CCU) may be lifesaving. In contrast to differential of diagnostic problem of encephalitis in the CCU, ABM in the CCU is not usually a diagnostic problem but is primarily a therapeutic problem.

Acute bacterial meningitis is primarily caused by bacterial neuropathogens. It occurs in normal and compromised hosts and may be acquired naturally or as a complication of open head trauma or neurosurgical procedures. Regardless of the pathogen or mode of acquisition, the definitive diagnosis of ABM rests on CSF analysis and Gram stain/culture of the CSF. In normal and compromised hosts, ABM clinically presents with fever and meningeal irritation, i.e., nuchal rigidity. Nuchal rigidity must be differentiated from other causes of neck stiffness, i.e., meningismus. There are relatively few non-bacterial causes of meningitis, but it is therapeutically important to differentiate aseptic or viral meningitis from bacterial meningitis. In general, patients with aseptic or viral meningitis are less critically ill than those with ABM. Aseptic viral meningitis may be inferred from CSF analysis and diagnosed by viral polymerase chain reaction (PCR). Patients with acute meningitis, either bacterial or viral,

will have various degrees of neck stiffness and intact mental status. In general, patients with mental confusion, i.e., encephalopathy, encephalitis but these patients do not have nuchal rigidity. Central nervous system (CNS) infection caused by a few organisms, i.e., herpes simplex virus (HSV), *Mycoplasma pneumoniae*, and *Listeria monocytogenes*, may present with a combination of stiff neck and mental confusion, i.e., meningoencephalitis. Any patient with fever and otherwise-unexplained neck stiffness should have an LP performed to confirm or rule out the diagnosis of ABM. If ABM is suspected, LP should be performed prior to head imaging studies [1–6].

Therefore, the challenge of ABM in the CCU is to rapidly arrive at a correct presumptive diagnosis by ruling out the non-infectious mimics of meningitis and aseptic viral meningitis. Patients with signs of meningeal irritation and mental confusion, i.e., meningoencephalitis, are diagnosed by CSF profile and extra-CNS signs, symptoms, and laboratory abnormalities. The objective of rapidly deriving at a presumptive diagnosis of ABM is to begin appropriate empiric antibiotic therapy as soon as possible. Appropriate empiric therapy for ABM is determined by predicting the likely pathogen. In ABM, the most likely pathogen is determined by patient age; acuteness of onset; epidemiological history; predisposing factors; physical signs, e.g., rash; deafness; and cranial nerve abnormalities. In compromised hosts, specific host defense defects are associated with the underlying immune defect which predicts the likely pathogen, e.g., multiple myeloma, a pure β-lymphocyte humoral immunity (HI) defect, predisposes only to encapsulated neuropathogens, e.g., *Streptococcus pneumoniae, Neisseria meningitidis, Haemophilus influenza,* and *Listeria monocytogenes,* and is confirmed by morphology/arrangement of organisms seen on the CSF Gram stain [1–9].

CLINICAL DIAGNOSTIC APPROACH IN THE CCU

Excluding open CNS trauma or neurosurgical procedures, bacteria causing ABM reach the CSF hematogenously. Acute bacterial meningitis primarily involves the leptomeninges. Leptomeningeal irritation is responsible for nuchal rigidity, Kernig's and Brudzinski's signs associated with ABM [7,8]. Because the leptomeninges cover the brain parenchyma, ABM is not associated with changes in mental status, which involves brain parenchyma, as in encephalitis. Most ABM pathogens are respiratory tract pathogens.

Acute bacterial meningitis may also result from contiguous spread from a local source in close proximity to the brain, e.g., sinusitis and mastoiditis. Cracks in the cribriform plate is another mode of entry to the CNS. Acute bacterial meningitis may also be due to CNS seeding of non-respiratory pathogens, e.g., *Listeria monocytogenes, Escherichia coli,* and *Staphylococcus aureus.* Acute bacterial endocarditis (ABE) due to *S. aureus* is not infrequently complicated by purulent ABE [1,2,8]. The CNS shunts for hydrocephalus/increased intracranial pressure may be complicated by ABM or ventriculitis due to either skin flora introduced during the insertion process, or distal shunt flora, i.e., coliforms with ventricular peritoneal (VP) shunt. Open head trauma or external ventricular drains (EVDs) may introduce CCU flora into the CSF [1–5,10–13].

L. monocytogenes ASM or meningoencephalitis is common in the elderly and in those with malignancies. *M. pneumoniae* meningoencephalitis is recognized as part of the clinical presentation of *M. pneumoniae* CAP. The clue to *M. pneumoniae* meningoencephalitis in patients with *Mycoplasma pneumoniae* community-acquired pneumonia is that it is accompanied by very high cold agglutinin levels (>1:512) [1,2,5] (Table 11.1).

Relatively few viruses, e.g., enteroviruses, cause aseptic meningitis. Some viruses, i.e., HSV, cause a spectrum of CNS infections, from aseptic meningitis to encephalitis.

Partially treated bacterial meningitis (PTBM), following treatment of meningitis, is diagnosed by history and CSF findings, i.e., moderate pleocytosis with variably decreased glucose and a moderately elevated CSF lactic acid (4–6 mmol/L). Partially treated bacterial meningitis requires re-treatment (14 days total) for ABM [1,5,6,14,15].

DIFFERENTIAL DIAGNOSTIC CONSIDERATIONS: MENINGITIS MIMICS

Because a stiff neck or nuchal rigidity is the hallmark of ABM, any condition that is associated with neck stiffness may mimic meningitis. In patients, acute torticollis, muscle spasm of the head/neck, cervical arthritis, and meningismus due to a variety of head and neck disorders can mimic bacterial meningitis but are not accompanied by fever. Fever plus otherwise-uncomplicated nuchal rigidity is the distinguishing hallmark of ABM. Elderly patients may have fever due to a variety of non-CNS causes and may have a stiff neck due

TABLE 11.1
Diagnostic Approach: Acute Infections of the Central Nervous System

	Acute Bacterial Meningitis	Meningoencephalitis	Acute Viral Encephalitis
Clinical presentation	Fever *plus* nuchal rigidity	Fever *plus* neck stiffness *plus* some mental confusion	Fever *plus* mental confusion
Usual pathogens	**Bacteria** *S. pneumoniae* *N. meningitidis* *H. influenzae*	*M. pneumoniae* *Listeria monocytogenes* HSV VZV	**Viruses** Enteroviruses VZV HSV
Diagnostic tests	LP with CSF profile Gram stain and culture	LP with CSF profile Gram stain & culture PCR for viral neuropathogens, e.g., HSV VZV, enteroviruses	LP with CSF profile EEG Head CT/MRI PCR for viral neuropathogens, e.g., HSV, VZV, enteroviruses
CSF lactic acid level	**Highly elevated (>6 nmol/L)**	**Elevated (4-6 nmol/L)**	**Unelevated (<4 nmol/L)**
Empiric therapy[b]	***S. pneumoniae,* etc.:** Ceftriaxone[a] or meropenem (PCN allergic)[b]	***Listeria:*** Ampicillin[b] or meropenam[b] ***M. pneumoniae*:** Doxycycline	**HSV/VZV:** Acyclovir

[a] If *Listeria* suspected, add ampicillin.

[b] Use "meningeal doses."

TABLE 11.2
Non-Infectious Mimics of Meningitis

- **Drug-induced aseptic meningitis**
  - NSAIDs
  - TMP–SMX
- **Systemic rheumatic disorders**
  - CNS vasculitis
  - SLE cerebritis
  - Sarcoid meningitis
- **CNS emboli**
  - Bland emboli from SBE or marantic endocarditis
  - (non-bacterial thrombocytic endocarditis) from malignancies
  - Meningeal carcinomatosis
  - AML
  - ALL
  - lymphomas
  - Melanoma
  - Breast carcinoma
  - Bronchogenic carcinomas
  - Hypernephroma (renal cell carcinomas)
  - Germ cell tumors

Abbreviations: NSAIDs, non-steroidal anti-inflammatory drugs; TMP–SMX, trimethoprim–sulfamethoxazole; SLE, systemic lupus erythematosus; SBE, subacute bacterial endocarditis; AML, acute myelogenous leukemia; ALL, acute lymphoblastic leukemia; CNS, central nervous system.

to cervical arthritis. For other ABM mimics, CSF analysis will readily distinguish the mimics of meningitis from ABM, particularly the CSF lactic acid level [1,4,5,18] (Table 11.2).

Other mimics of ABM include drug-induced meningitis (DIM), meningeal carcinomatosis, CNS, granulomatous angiitis (GA), Beçhet's disease, systemic lupus erythematosus (SLE), and neurosarcoidosis [1,7,14–17]. The diagnostic approach to meningitis mimics is related to the clinical context in which they occur. For example, lupus cerebritis rarely presents as the initial or sole manifestation of SLE. With Beçhet's disease, patients with neuro-Beçhet's disease have established Beçhet's, with characteristic, e.g., oral/genital ulcers, which should lead the clinician to suspect the diagnosis. With neurosarcoidosis, the presentation is usually subacute rather than acute, and usually occurs primarily in patients with a history of sarcoidosis [1,4,5,19–24]. In patients on drugs associated with drug-induced medications, the DDx should include DIM.

DRUG-INDUCED MENINGITIS

Drug-induced meningitis (DIM) may present with a stiff neck and fever. The time of meningeal symptoms after consumption of the medication is highly variable. The most common drugs associated with DIM include non-steroidal anti-inflammatory drugs. Among the antibiotics, trimethoprim–sulfamethoxazole (TMP–SMX) is the most common cause of DIM. The CSF leukocytosis with a polymorphonuclear predominance is typical with DIM. The clinical clue to DIM is eosinophils in the CSF. In DIM, the CSF has increased protein, but the CSF glucose is rarely decreased. Treatment of DIM is discontinuation of the offending agent [1,5,16,17].

RHEUMATIC DISEASES

Systemic lupus erythematosus often presents with CNS manifestations, ranging from meningitis to cerebritis. The most frequent CNS manifestation of SLE is aseptic meningitis. The CNS manifestations of SLE usually occur in patients who have established multisystem manifestations of SLE. The CNS SLE is usually present as part of a flare of SLE. The SLE flare may be manifested by fever, an increase in the signs/symptoms of SLE present in previous flares. Laboratory tests suggesting flare include new or more severe leukopenia, thrombocytopenia, increased erythrocyte sedimentation rate (ESR) and decreased serum complement (C_3). The CSF in patients with SLE includes a lymphocytic predominance (usually <100 WBCs/mm³). Polymorphonuclear neutrophils (PMNs) may predominate early in SLE aseptic meningitis. The CSF RBCs are not present with SLE aseptic meningitis. The CSF lactic acid level is also normal. The definitive test for diagnosing CNS SLE cerebritis is to demonstrate a decreased C4 level. Importantly, patients with an SLE flare of CNS lupus are predisposed to bacterial meningitis. The CCU clinicians must be careful to be sure that the patient with an SLE flare with CNS manifestations does not have an associated ABM [1,8,19–24].

Granulomatous angiitis of the CNS is a rare cause of aseptic meningitis. The fever and encephalopathy are the most common manifestations of granulomatous angiitis of the CNS, but the focal abnormalities, including seizures and cranial nerve palsies, may mimic bacterial meningitis. Systemic laboratory tests are unhelpful. The ESR is usually elevated. The CSF profile of GA includes a lymphocytic predominance (usually <200 cells/mm³); a low CSF glucose may occur; and RBCs are rarely present. Such findings are also compatible with the diagnosis of HSV meningoencephalitis or aseptic meningitis. The diagnosis of GA of the CNS is made by head CT/MRI, demonstrating vasculitic lesions in the CSF [19,20].

Behçet's disease is a multisystem disorder characterized by oral ulcers, genital ulcers, and eye findings. Neurologic manifestations are present in up to one quarter of patients. The CNS presentation of Behçet's may rarely be the presenting finding. Neuro-Behçet's disease is characterized by fever, headache, and meningeal signs that closely mimic ABM. Features of meningoencephalitis or encephalitis may also be present. The CSF profile is indistinguishable from aseptic/viral meningitis/encephalitis. There are no distinguishing features on the electroencephalography (EEG) or head CT/MRI. The diagnosis of neuro-Behçet's disease is based on recognizing that the patient has Behçet's disease and has neurologic manifestations not attributable to another process [20,21].

Neurosarcoidosis is a common manifestation of sarcoidosis. Signs of CNS sarcoid include headaches, mental confusion, and cranial nerve palsies. Any of the cranial nerves may be affected. Patients with sarcoidosis may often present with polyclonal gammopathy on serum protein electrophoresis, an elevated ESR, leukopenia, mild anemia, and increased levels of serum angiotensin-converting enzyme (ACE). Chest X-ray shows one of the four stages of sarcoidosis, ranging from bilateral hilar adenopathy to parenchymal reticular nodular fibrotic changes. In neurosarcoidosis, the CSF is usually abnormal. A lymphocytic pleocytosis (≤300 cells/mm) is usual. Protein levels in the CSF are usually elevated. About 20% have a decreased CSF glucose level. The RBCs are not a feature of neurosarcoidosis. Aseptic meningitis with sarcoidosis may mimic viral aseptic meningitis. Patients usually have a history of sarcoidosis, which is a clue to the diagnosis. Diagnosis of neurosarcoidosis is a diagnosis of association and exclusion. Neurosarcoidosis occurs in the setting of systemic sarcoidosis and is characterized by elevated ACE levels and negative CSF Gram stain/culture. Multiple cranial nerve palsies are usual. Treatment is with corticosteroids/immunosuppressives [1,20,23,24] (Table 11.3).

PREDICTING THE PATHOGEN IN ABM

In compromised hosts, pathogen prediction of ABM depends on correlating the underlying disorder with its host defense defect, which predicts the pathogen. Compromised hosts with impaired cellular-mediated immunity (CMI) usually present with intracellular pathogens, e.g., *Listeria*. With ABM, compromised hosts with impaired CMI are afflicted with the same pathogens as normal hosts. Compromised hosts are not exempt from the usual/common infectious diseases that affect immunocompetent hosts. Compromised

---

TABLE 11.3
Mimics of Meningitis

ABM Mimics	Differential Features and Diagnostic Clues

Enteroviral meningitis	**Seasonal distribution**: Summer (recent fresh water/sick person exposure)
	History: Sore throat, facial/maculopapular rash, loose stools/diarrhea
	Onset: Subacute; not as ill as bacterial meningitis
	Clinical features: Subacute
	CSF:
	  • Gram stain: –
	  • Lactic acid: Normal (<3 mmol/L)

HSV-1	**Season**: Non-seasonal
	History: Antecedent not concurrent herpes labialis
	Onset: Aseptic meningitis/meningoencephalitis (subacute)
	Clinical Features: Viral/aseptic meningitis, meningoencephalitis
	CSF:
	  • Gram stain: –
	  • RBCs: –
	  • WBCs:
	    ↑ PMNs (early); lymphocytic response (later)
	  • Glucose: Normal or ↓
	  • Lactic acid: 2–4 nmol/L (~RBCs in CSF)

Meningeal carcinomatosis	**History**: Leukemias, lymphomas, carcinomas, or without known primary neoplasm; mental status changes: ±
	Onset: Subacute
	Clinical features: Most have multiple cranial nerve palsies, (CNs III, IV, VI, VII, or VIII most common)
	CSF:
	  • Gram stain: –
	  • RBCs: ±
	  • Protein: Highly ↑
	  • Lactic acid: Variably ↑
	  • Cytology: Diagnostic in 90%

Brain abscess
(with ventricular leak)
	History: Suppurative lung disease (bronchiectasis), cyanotic heart disease (R → L shunts)
	Onset: Acute, mastoiditis, dental abscess, etc.
	Head MRI/CT: Brain abscess
	CSF: Brain abscess *with ventricular leak* mimics ABM
	  • Protein: Highly ↑
	  • WBCs:
	    Without leak: Usually <200 WBCs/hpf
	    With leak: ≤100,000 WBCs/hpf

(Continued)

TABLE 11.3 (*Continued*)
Mimics of Meningitis

ABM Mimics	Differential Features and Diagnostic Clues
Tuberculous meningitis	**Onset:** Subacute **Clinical Features**: Basilar meningitis; unilateral CN VI abducens palsy (chest X-ray negative in 50%) **Fundi:** Choroidal tubercles **Head MRI/CT scans:** Hydrocephalus/arachnoiditis **CSF**: • WBCs: <500/hpf • PMNs (early); lymphocytic predominance (later) • Glucose: ↓ (may be normal) • RBCs: + • TB smear/culture + ~80% • TB PCR: + • ADA: + **Serial LPs:** • Over time: ↓ glucose/↑ protein • Lactic acid: ↑ (variably elevated)
Neurosarcoidosis	**History**: Systemic sarcoidosis (bilateral hilar adenopathy/interstitial infiltrates, skin lesions, uveitis, erythema nodosum, arthritis, hypercalciuria, ↑ ACE levels **Onset**: Subacute **Clinical presentation**: Cranial nerves: Unilateral/bilateral CN VII (facial nerve palsy characteristic also CN palsies II, VII, VIII, IX, X **Fundi**: "Candle wax drippings" **CSF**: • Lymph: ↑ • Glucose: ↓ • WBCs: <100/hpf • RBCs: None (vs. TB or malignancy)
SLE cerebritis	**History:** SLE, pneumonitis, nephritis, or skin lesions **Onset:** Subacute **Clinical Features**: Aseptic meningitis **Fundi**: Cytoid bodies/cotton wool spots **CSF**: • CSF: ANA: + • CSF: C_4: ↓

Abbreviations: CSF, cerebrospinal fluid; CNS, central nervous system; SLE, systemic lupus erythematosus; PMNs, polymorphonuclear leukocytes; LCM, lymphocytic choriomeningitis; RMSF, Rocky Mountain spotted fever; HSV, herpes simplex virus; ACE, angiotensin-converting enzyme; SGOT, serum glutamate oxaloacetate transaminase; SGPT, serum glutamate pyruvate transaminase; EEG, electroencephalogram; MRI, magnetic resonance imaging; CT, computed tomography.

hosts with defects in HI or those with combined CMI and HI defects, e.g., multiple myeloma, are predisposed to meningitis due to encapsulated organisms, *Streptococcus pneumoniae, Haemophilus influenzae*, or *Klebsiella pneumoniae* [1–6,8,18] (Tables 11.4–11.7).

The critical laboratory test in ABM is the analysis of the CSF. In ABM, there is usually a pleocytosis of the CSF. In ABM, nearly all cells in the CSF are PMNs. As the meningeal infection is treated, the number of PMNs decreases and there is a parallel rise in the number of CSF lymphocytes. Bacterial meningitis begins with a PMN predominance and ends with a lymphocytic predominance. Other CNS infections, e.g., tuberculosis (TB), viral infections, fungal infections, and syphilis, may all present initially with a PMN-predominant pleocytosis. These disorders are characterized by a lymphocytic CSF pleocytosis, but initially, they may present with a PMN predominance. Importantly, with the exception of HSV-1, ≥90% PMNs in the CSF initially always indicate ABM. A PMN predominance of <90% is compatible with a wide variety of CNS pathogens and does not, of itself, indicate a bacterial etiology. In patients with fever and nuchal rigidity, an LP should always be performed before a head CT/MRI scan is obtained. Patients with bacterial meningitis are acutely ill and have a potentially rapidly fatal disorder. Wasting valuable time in obtaining a head CT/MRI can result in a fatal outcome. Fear of supratentorial herniation is the main reason why head imaging studies are done before LP, which is appropriate if a mass lesion is suspected but not if the diagnosis includes ABM. Far more people will die from a delay in therapy than have died from supratentorial herniation [1–5,18,25,26] (Table 11.8).

TABLE 11.4
Host-Pathogen Association in Meningitis

Host	Pathogen
• Sinopulmonary dysfunction	*Streptococcus pneumoniae*
	Haemophilus influenzae
	Neisseria meningitidis
• Elderly	*H. influenzae*
	Listeria monocytogenes
	Brain abscess (2° dental focus)
• Sickle cell disease	*S. pneumoniae*
	Salmonella
	N. meningitidis
	H. influenzae
• Hyposplenism	*S. pneumoniae*
	H. influenzae
	N. meningitidis
	Klebsiella pneumoniae
• HIV	HIV
	CMV
	Toxoplasma gondii
	Listeria monocytogenes
	Cryptococcus neoformans
• Complement deficiencies	*S. pneumoniae*
	N. meningitidis
• CSF leak	*S. pneumoniae*
• IVDAs	*Staphylococcus aureus (MSSA/MRSA)*
	Aerobic GNBs
• Alcoholism/cirrhosis	*S. pneumoniae*
	Klebsiella pneumoniae
	TB
• Hypogammaglobulinemia	*S. pneumoniae*
	H. influenzae
	N. meningitidis
	Enteroviruses
• CNS shunts	
VA Shunts	*S. epidermidis* (CoNS)
	S. aureus (MSSA/MRSA)
VP Shunts	Aerobic GNBs
• Recurrent ABM (2° to *immune or anatomic* defects)	*S. pneumoniae*
	H. influenzae
	N. meningitidis
	Recurrent non-infectious CNS diseases
	SLE cerebritis
	Neurosarcoidosis
	Neuro-Beçhet's
	CNS Vasculitis
• ABE	MSSA/MRSA
• Brain abscess (with ventricular leak)	Oral anaerobes

Abbreviations: IVDAs, IV drug abusers; VA, ventriculoatrial; VP, ventriculoperitoneal; ABE, acute bacterial endocarditis; CoNS, coagulase-negative staphylococcal; CMV, cytomegalovirus; CNS, central nervous system; SLE, systemic lupus erythematosus; MAI, mycobacterium arium-intracellulare; TB, tuberculosis; GNB, gram-negative bacilli.

TABLE 11.5
Complications of Meningitis

Complications	Associated Organisms
• Acute Deafness	*Haemophilus influenzae*
	Neisseria meningitidis
• New seizures	*Streptococcus pneumoniae*
	H. influenzae
	HSV-1
	Brain abscess
• Subdural effusions	*S. pneumoniae*
• New hydrocephalus	*H. influenzae*
	TB
	Neurosarcoidosis
	Neurocysticercosis
• Cranial nerve abnormalities	*N. meningitidis* (CN VI, VII, VIII)
	CNS tuberculosis (CN VI)
	Neurosarcoidosis (CN VII)
	Meningeal carcinomatosis
• Herpes labialis	*N. meningitidis*
	S. pneumoniae
• Panophthalmitis	*N. meningitidis*
	S. pneumoniae
	H. influenzae
• Purpura/petechiae	*N. meningitidis*
	S. pneumoniae
	Listeria monocytogenes
	Staphylococcus aureus (ABE)

Abbreviations: TB, Tuberculosis; CNS, central nervous system; HSV, herpes simplex virus; ABE, acute bacterial endocarditis.

TABLE 11.6
Central Nervous System Infections in Normal Versus Immunocompromised Hosts

CNS Infections in Normal Hosts
- Usually *acute* onset of ABM
- *Single* pathogen
- *Pathogen predictable* (based on epidemiology host features)
- ***Meningitis* Most Frequent Manifestation of CNS Infections**

CNS Infections in Immunocompromised Hosts
Subacute onset of CNS infections
- *Single* or *sequential pathogens* (not simultaneous or multiple pathogens)
- *Pathogen determined by immune defect and degree of immunosuppression*
- **Encephalitis or mass lesions (brain abscess) most common manifestations of CNS infection**

Abbreviations: CNS, central nervous system; ABM, acute bacterial meningitis.

TABLE 11.7

CNS Disorders Associated with Impaired B-Lymphocyte–Mediated Humoral Immunity Deficiency

Disorders Associated with Impaired B-Lymphocyte Function/ Humoral Immunity

- Multiple myeloma
- B-cell lymphoma
- Advanced age
- Waldeström's macroglobulinemia
- Immunoglobulin deficiencies
- CLL

Hyposplenia/Decreased Splenic Function

- Congenital asplenia
- Hyposplenism of the elderly
- Chronic alcoholism
- Sickle cell trait of disease
- Amyloidosis
- Splenic infarcts
- Splenic malignancies
- Systemic mastocytosis
- IgA deficiency
- Sezary syndrome
- Splenectomy
- Rheumatoid arthritis
- Intestinal lymphangiectasia
- Myeloproliferative disorders
- Waldeström's macroglobulinemia
- Steroid therapy
- Non-Hodgkin's lymphoma
- γ-Globulin therapy
- Celiac disease
- Regional enteritis
- Ulcerative colitis

CNS Disorders Associated with Impaired T-Lymphocyte Cellular-Mediated Immunity Deficiency

- HIV
- Lymphoreticular malignances
- lymphomas
- Chronic immunosuppressive therapy
- Chronic corticosteroid therapy
- Organ transplantation
- CMV

Abbreviations: CNS, central nervous system; CMV, cytomegalovirus; VZV, varicella zoster virus; HSV, herpes simplex virus; PML, progressive multifocal leukoencephalopathy.

TABLE 11.8

Diagnostic Approach in Compromised Hosts with Symptoms/Signs of Central Nervous System Infection

Syndrome Presentation	Diagnostic Procedures	Comments
ABM	CSF: • WBC cell count/ • differential • RBC count • Glucose/protein • Lactic acid • Cytology • Gram stain and culture	• Host defense *defect predicts the most likely CNS pathogen* • Rule out meningitis mimics • Selection of empiric therapy is based on host factors and CSF fluid findings
Encephalitis/ encephalopathy or mass lesion	Head CT/MRI: To rule out cerebritis, mass lesions, hydrocephalus, CNS hemorrhage LP (if papilledema not present) CSF: • WBC cell count/ differential • Glucose/protein • RBCs • Lactic acid • Cytology • Gram stain If viral etiology suspected, viral PCR If TB suspected • AFB smear/culture • ↑ ADA levels • TB PCR	• Host defense *defect predicts most likely CNS pathogen* • Rule out non-infectious mimics by history/ physical exam, and CT/MRI appearance • Empiric therapy for the most likely pathogen

Abbreviations: CNS, central nervous system; CSF, cerebrospinal fluid; MRI, magnetic resonance imaging; CT, computed tomography; AFB, acid-fast bacilli; LP, lumbar puncture.

CSF PROFILE IN ABM

The evaluation of the CSF is the definitive diagnostic test in ABM. Microscopic examination of the CSF by Gram stain provides rapid information regarding the CSF cellular response as well as the concentration, morphology, and arrangement of neuropathogenic bacteria. The typical "purulent profile" in the CSF of bacteria causing ABM includes an early PMN predominance, a decreased CSF glucose, a variably CSF protein, no RBCs, and a highly elevated CSF lactic acid level of >6 nmol/L [1,3–6]. The CSF Gram stain positivity depends on the concentration and type of organism. The CSF Gram stain is negative half the time with *L. monocytogenes* ABM but is virtually always culturable from the CSF with 3 days. With ABM due to the meningococcus, no organisms may be seen on CSF Gram stain, even in the presence of overwhelming infection, because of autolysis. The CSF may appear turbid or cloudy due to the abundance of WBCs present, but the organisms may not be visible on CSF Gram stain. However, CSF culture is invariably positive for *Neisseria meningitidis* [1,8,27].

Viral/aseptic meningitis is uniformly associated with a normal CSF glucose, with a few important exceptions. The presence of a normal CSF glucose in a patient with suspected ABM meningitis suggests a viral or non-infectious mimic of meningitis. Viruses capable of decreasing the CSF glucose include HSV, lympho-cytic choriomeningitis (LCM), mumps, and occasionally entero-viruses. These exceptions aside, a normal CSF glucose virtually excludes a bacterial etiology of ABM [1,5,8,14,18,28,29].

Similarly, RBCs are not a feature of ABM. Excluding a traumatic tap, CNS leaking aneurism, etc., RBCs in the CSF, effectively limits the diagnostic possibilities to *L. monocy-togenes*, amebic meningoencephalitis, leptospirosis, tubercu-lous meningitis, and HSV. The RBCs alone in the CSF can decrease CSF glucose and mildly increase the CSF lactic acid. The abnormalities in CSF glucose and lactic acid are propor-tional to the number of RBCs present in the CSF [1,5,8,18,27].

The WBC response in the CSF is typically early and brisk with ABM. Characteristically, many CNS infections associated with a lymphocytic predominance may present acutely with a PMN pre-dominance, e.g., TB, fungi, syphilis, and viruses. With the excep-tion of HSV-1, only ABM presents with a CSF PMNs ≥90%. Patients with PTBM have a mixed picture, with both PMNs and lymphocytes, as well as a moderately decreased glucose (versus the profoundly decreased glucose of untreated ABM), and CSF lactic acid levels that are intermediate between aseptic/viral men-ingitis and ABM [1,5,8,30] (Tables 11.9 and 11.10).

TABLE 11.9
CSF Gram Stain Clues in Meningitis

- **Purulent CSF/no organisms seen**
  Neisseria meningitidis
  Streptococcus pneumoniae
- **Cloudy CSF/without WBCs**
  S. pneumoniae
- **Gram positive bacilli**
  Listeria monocytogenes
  Pseudomeningitis (*Bacillus*,
    Corynebacterium, etc.)
- **Gram-negative bacilli**
  Haemophilus influenzae (small
    encapsulated, pleomorphic)
  Enteric aerobic GNBs (larger,
    unencapsulated)
- **Gram-positive cocci**
  Group A, B streptococci (pairs and chains)
  S. pneumoniae (pairs)
  Staphylococcus aureus (clusters)
  Staphylococcus epidermidis (clusters)
    VA/VP shunt infections only
- **Gram-negative cocci**
  N. meningitidis
- **Mixed organisms/polymicrobial**
  Pseudomeningitis
  Brain abscess (with meningeal leak)
  VP shunt infection
  Disseminated *Strongyloides stercoralis*
  Meningitis (2° to penetrating head trauma)

- **Clear CSF/no organisms seen**
  Viral aseptic meningitis
  TB/fungal meningitis
  Neurosarcoidosis meningitis
  Early ABM
  Partially treated bacterial meningitis
  ABM (leukopenic hosts)
  Meningeal carcinomatosis
  Brain abscess
  Parameningeal infection
  Bland emboli (2° to SBE)
  SLE cerebritis
  Neuroborreliosis
  LCM
  L. monocytogenes
  HIV
  Leptospirosis

Abbreviations: SBE, subacute bacterial endocarditis; HIV, human immunodeficiency virus; VA, ventriculoatrial; VP, ventriculoperitoneal; LCM, lymphocytic choriomeningitis.

TABLE 11.10
Differential Diagnosis of CSF with a Negative Gram Stain

Predominantly PMNs/Decreased Glucose	Predominantly Lymphocytes/Normal Glucose
Partially treated bacterial meningitis	Viral (aseptic) meningitis
Listeria monocytogenes	Partially treated bacterial meningitis
HSV-1	Neurosarcoidosis
Tuberculosis (early)	Neuroborreliosis
Syphilis (early)	HIV
Neurosarcoidosis	Leptospirosis
Septic emboli (2° to ABE)	RMSF
Amebic meningoencephalitis	Bland emboli (2° to SBE)
(*N. fowleri*)	Parameningeal infection
Syphilis (early)	TB/fungal meningitis
Posterior fossa syndrome	Meningeal carcinomatosis

Predominantly Lymphocytes/ Decreased Glucose
L. monocytogenes
Partially treated bacterial meningitis
LCM
Viral (aseptic) meningitis
Mumps
Leptospirosis
TB/fungal meningitis
Neurosarcoidosis
Meningeal carcinomatosis

CSF Protein
Elevated (any CNS infection/inflammation)
Very highly elevated
Brain tumor
Brain abscess
TB (with subarachnoid block)
Demyelinating CNS disorders
Multiple sclerosis

RBCs
Traumatic tap
Posterior fossa syndrome
CNS bleed/tumor
HSV-1
L. monocytogenes
Leptospirosis
TB meningitis
Amebic meningoencephalitis
(*Naegleria fowleri*)
meningoencephalitis
Meningeal carcinomatosis

CSF Eosinophils
CNS vasculitis
DIM (NSAID, TMP-SMX)
Coccidioidomycosis
Neurocysticercosis
Angiostrongyliasis
Gnathostomiasis
Paragonimiasis
Shistosomiasis
Toxocara canis/cati (VLM)
CNS lymphomas
VA/VP shunts

CSF Lactic Acid
- **<4 mmol/L**
  Aseptic "viral" meningitis
  Parameningeal infections
- **4–6 mmol/L**
  Partially treated meningitis
  RBCs
  TB/fungal meningitis
- **6 mmol/L**
  Bacterial meningitis

Abbreviations: CSF, cerebrospinal fluid; HSV, herpes simplex virus; CNS, central nervous system; ABE, acute bacterial endocarditis; LCM, lymphocytic choriomeningitis; SBE, subacute endo-carditis; PMNs, polymorphonuclear leukocytes; RMSF, Rocky Mountain spotted fever; VA, ventriculoatrial; VP, ventriculoperitoneal; NSAIDs, nonsteroidal inflammatory drugs; TB, tuberculosis; VLM, visceral larva migrans.

DIAGNOSTIC SIGNIFICANCE OF CSF LACTIC ACID LEVELS IN ABM AND EVD-ASSOCIATED ABM

In the diagnosis of ABM, the CSF lactic acid levels are second only to the CSF Gram stain as a rapid and reliable indicator of ABM. The CSF glucose levels and CSF lactic acid levels are inversely proportional to each other. As the CSF glucose decreases, the CSF lactic acid increases. With successful antibiotic treatment, CSF lactic acid levels and CSF glucose levels are the first to normalize. It takes days for the initial PMN predominance in the CSF to become lymphocytic, and lymphocytic pleocytosis may persist in the CSF for weeks. The CSF lactic acid level decreases more rapidly and acutely than does the CSF glucose. If a patient has *S. aureus* ABE and has seeded the CSF, resulting in an early ABM, the CSF lactic acid level will be elevated before the Gram stain is positive or the CSF glucose levels have decreased, and CSF cultures are reported positive later. The CSF lactic acid test is invaluable in separating viral from ABM as well as for identifying patients with PTBM [1,30–32].

The CSF lactic acid levels are also useful in assessing the significance of RBCs in the CSF in patients with a decreased CSF glucose. If the diagnosis is between HSV-1 and *L. monocytogenes*, CSF lactic acid levels in *L. monocytogenes* meningoencephalitis will be highly elevated, i.e., ≥ 6 mmol/dL, but CSF lactic acid levels will be normal/near normal in HSV-1. A normal CSF lactic acid level in the absence of RBCs from a bleed or traumatic tap is the best way to differentiate aseptic from ABM. If the Gram stain is negative and CSF lactic acid levels are normal, then the clinician can confidently wait for CSF cultures to be reported as negative. Importantly, no empiric antimicrobial therapy is needed if the CSF lactic acid level is normal. The CSF lactic acid levels may be obtained serially to determine if antimicrobial therapy of ABM is effective and also may be used at the end of therapy as a test of cure [1,30–34] (Table 11.11).

OTHER CSF TESTS IN ABM

The CSF C-reactive protein (CRP) is elevated in bacterial meningitis but is not as highly elevated as in viral/aseptic meningitis. The CSF procalcitonin (PCT) levels are highly elevated in ABM but not in aseptic/viral meningitis [35].

Other CSF parameters have been used, i.e., lactate dehydrogenase, to differentiate the various types of meningitis, but they lack sensitivity and specificity [1,3–5,8].

Other tests are useful in selected CNS disorders. The CSF C4 level is decreased and CSF ANA is increased in SLE meningitis. Cerebritis monoclonal bands in the CSF may be present in SLE as well as multiple sclerosis. Cytology of the CSF is diagnostic of meningeal carcinomatosis, which may mimic ABM [1,19–21,28,29].

The RBCs are also present in multiple cranial nerve palsies. The PCR technique is useful in the diagnosis of enteroviral, HSV-1/2, and HHV-6 aseptic meningitis [1,5,25,27,36].

TABLE 11.11

CSF Diagnostic Criteria for EVD-Associated ABM

EVD-Associated ABM (4CSF Diagnostic Criteria for EVD-Associated ABM)

- Highly elevated CSF lactic acid level (>6 nmol/L)
  plus
- Marked CSF pleocytosis (>50 WBCs/hpf)
  plus
- Positive CSF Gram stain (with some morphology as the cultures neuropathogen)
  plus
- Positive CSF culture of the neuropathogen (same morphology on Gram stain)

EVD Associated CSF Colonization or Non-Infectious Disorder[a] (<4 CSF Diagnostic Criteria)

Source: Cunha, C.B. and Cunha, B.A., *Antibiotic Essentials*, 17th ed., JayPee Medical Publishers, New Delhi, India, 2020; Munoz-Gomez, S, et al., *Heart Lung*, 44, 158–160, 2015.

Abbreviations: LA, CSF lactic acid; ABM, acute bacterial meningitis; EVD, external-ventricular drain

[a] CNS malignancy, intracranial bleed, post-craniotomy, and brain trauma.

SERUM TESTS IN ABM

The serum CRP has also been useful to differentiate ABM from aseptic/viral meningitis. In ABM, serum CRP levels are higher than those in viral/aseptic meningitis [35,37,38].

Highly elevated serum ferritin levels appear to be a marker for West Nile encephalitis (WNE). In WNE, serum ferritin levels are highly elevated but are unelevated/minimally elevated in aseptic/viral and bacterial meningitis [39,40].

IMAGING IN ABM

Neuroimaging tests are primarily valuable for ruling out the mimics of ABM, e.g., malignancies, brain abscess, and vasculitis. In ABM, head CT/MRI scans are of limited value and are done to rule out a parameningeal suppurative focus or brain abscess or CNS mimics of meningitis. If the diagnosis of ABM is being considered, e.g., fever and stiff neck, mental confusion takes precedence over neuroimaging. The EEG is primarily useful in diagnosing encephalitis. The EEG abnormalities are diffuse with most causes of acute viral encephalitis but are localized early with HSV-1 encephalitis, which is an important diagnostic clue [1–5,26,27,41].

ANTIBIOTIC THERAPY OF ABM

Empiric therapy of ABM depends on predicting or demonstrating the CNS pathogen, so that an appropriate antibiotic may be selected. If the pathogen can be demonstrated by Gram stain or inferred from aspects of the history, epidemiological data, systemic laboratory tests, or physical findings, then an antibiotic with an appropriate spectrum can be selected to begin treatment. Early treatment with an appropriate antibiotic is crucial to the outcomes in patients [1,42–50].

Not only must the antimicrobial selected be effective against the pathogen, but it must reach bactericidal concentrations in the CSF with the usual "meningeal doses." Certain antibiotics achieve a therapeutic CSF concentration when being in the "usual dose," e.g., chloramphenicol, TMP–SMX, doxycycline, and minocycline. Others require higher-than-usual doses, i.e., "meningeal doses," to effectively penetrate the CSF, e.g., cefepime and meropenem. Most other antimicrobials do not achieve sufficient CSF concentration even with high dosing, e.g., first-/second-generation cephalosporins [1–3,42–45] (Table 11.12).

Patients are ordinarily treated for a total of 2 weeks. The main determinants of antibiotic penetration of the CSF are antibiotic size and the lipid solubility. In general, highly lipid-soluble antibiotics penetrate the CSF in the presence or absence of inflammation. β-Lactam antibiotics do not penetrate the CSF well in the absence of inflammation. Third- and fourth-generation cephalosporins given in "meningeal doses" do not penetrate the CNS well but penetrate sufficiently with sufficiently high degree of activity, so that they are effective against common neuropathogens (except *L. monocytogenes*) [1,42–48].

TABLE 11.12
Empiric Therapy of CNS Infections

Subset	Usual Pathogens	Preferred IV Therapy	Alternate IV Therapy	IV-to-PO Switch
Normal host	*N. meningitidis* *H. influenzae* *S. pneumoniae*	Ceftriaxone 2 g (IV) q12h × 2 weeks	Meropenem 2 g (IV) q8h × 2 weeks	Chloramphenicol 500 mg (PO) q6h × 2 weeks
Elderly or malignancy	*Listeria monocytogenes* *N. meningitidis* *H. influenzae* *S. pneumoniae*	**Before culture results:** Ceftriaxone 2 g (IV) q12h **plus** ampicillin 2 gm (IV) q4h **Listeria present after culture results:** Ampicillin 2 gm (IV) q4h × 3 weeks **Listeria not present:** Ceftriaxone 2 g (IV) q12h × 2 weeks	**Listeria present after culture results:** TMP-SMX 5 mg/kg (IV) q6h × 3 weeks **or** meropenem 2 g (IV) q8h × 3 weeks **or** **Listeria not present:** Ceftriaxone 2 g (IV) q12h × 2 weeks	**For Listeria meningitis only:** TMP-SMX 5 mg/kg (PO) q6h × 3 weeks **or** linezolid 600 mg (PO) q12h × 3 weeks **For usual meningeal pathogens:** Chloramphenicol 500 mg (PO) q6h × 2 weeks
CNS shunt infections (VA shunts)	*S. aureus* *S. epidermidis* (CoNS)	**MSSA/MSSE** Meropenem 2 g (IV) q8h **MRSA/MRSE** Linezolid 600 mg (IV) q12h	**MSSA/MSSE** Cefepime 2 g (IV) q8h **MRSA/MRSE** Vancomycin 2 g (IV) q12h **plus** Vancomycin 20 mg (IT) q24h (until shunt removal)	**MSSE/MRSE** Linezolid 600 mg (PO) q12h **MSSA/MRSA** 200 mg (PO) × 1, then 100 mg (PO) q12h **or** linezolid 600 mg (PO) q12h
CNS shunt infections (VP shunts)	*E. coli* *K. pneumoniae* *Enterobacter* sp. *S. marcescens*	Certriaxone 2 g (IV) q12h × 2 weeks (after shunt removal)	TMP-SMX 5 mg/kg (IV) q6h × 2 weeks (after shunt removal)	TMP-SMX 5 mg/kg (PO) q6h × 2 weeks (after shunt removal)
Ventriculitis (EVD associated)	MDR *P. aeruginosa*	Meropenem 2 g (IV) q8h ± colistin 5 mg/kg (IV) q8h **plus** colistin 10 mg (IT) q24h × 2 weeks (after shunt removal)	Meropenem 2 g (IV) q8h plus Amikacin 1 g (IV) q24h **and** amikacin 10 mg (IT) q24h × 2 weeks (after shunt removal)	
	MDR *Acinetobacter* sp.	Ampicillin/sulbactam 4.5 g (IV) q6h × 2 weeks (after shunt removal **plus either** meropenem 2 g (IV) q8h × 2 weeks (after shunt removal) **or** colistin 10 mg (IT) q12h × 2 weeks (after shunt removal)	Meropenem 2 g (IV) q8h × 2 weeks (after shunt removal) **or** ampicillin/sulbactam 4.5 g (IV) q6h × 2 weeks (after shunt removal **plus** colistin 10 mg (IT) q12h × 2 weeks (after shunt removal)	

Source: Cunha, C.B. and Cunha, B.A., *Antibiotic Essentials*, 17th ed., Jay Pee Medical Publishers, New Delhi, India, 2020.
Abbreviations: MSSA/MRSA, methicillin-sensitive/-resistant *S. aureus*; MSSE/MRSE, methicillin-sensitive/-resistant *S. epidermidis*.

Listeria monocytogenes meningitis is ordinarily treated with "meningeal doses" of ampicillin, i.e., 2 g (IV) q4h, in penicillin-tolerant patients. In patients with penicillin-intolerant *Listeria monocytogenes* ABM, TMP–SMX or meropenem may be used. For the treatment of staphylococcal meningitis due to methicillin-sensitive *S. aureus* (MSSA), "meningeal doses" of an anti-staphylococcal penicillin, e.g., nafcillin, may be given as a 2 g (IV) q4h dose. Drugs used to treat methicillin-resistant *S. aureus* (MRSA) ABM include minocycline and linezolid. Vancomycin does not penetrate the CSF well, and CSF concentrations are ~15% of simultaneous serum concentrations. Therefore, at the usually used dose of 1 g (IV) q12h (15 mg/kg/day), CSF concentrations may be inadequate. If vancomycin is selected to treat MRSA CNS infections, then either 30–60 mg/day of vancomycin is necessary or the usual dose of vancomycin [15 mg/kg/day (IV)] may be supplemented with 20 mg of intrathecal (IT) vancomycin daily. Oral linezolid and minocycline penetrate the CSF well and achieve therapeutic concentrations [42].

The treatment of shunt-related ventriculoatrial/ventriculoperitoneal (VA/VP) infections usually requires shunt removal and the administration of an antibiotic that has a high degree of activity against *Staphylococcus epidermidis* (CoNS) or *S. aureus* (depending on the pathogen isolated that penetrates the CSF in therapeutic concentrations). In patients with ABM secondary to open CNS trauma, the antibiotics selected should have a high degree of aerobic gram-negative bacillary coverage as well as sufficient anti-staphylococcal activity [1,42,51,52]. The preferred drugs for each pathogen-causing meningitis are presented in Table 11.12 [1,42].

In the CCU, neurologic patients post craniotomy or post open brain trauma are at risk for EVD associated ABM. The diagnosis of EVD associated ABM is problematic and based on combined CSF profile criteria.

The use of steroids as an adjunctive measure to treat ABM remains controversial. Steroids have long been used, together with antituberculous therapy in acute tuberculous meningitis, but there is relatively little information on the use of steroids in the treatment of ABM in adults. Steroids have been shown to be beneficial in the treatment of meningitis in children due to *H. influenzae* but have been limited to *H. influenzae*. Because steroids affect blood-brain barrier permeability, if used, steroids should be given after antimicrobial therapy has been initiated [46–50].

ROLE OF REPEAT LUMBAR PUNCTURE IN ABM

The diagnosis of ABM rests on the analysis of the CSF and demonstration of the putative organism in the CSF by Gram stain or culture. Corroborative evidence includes a PMN predominance in the CSF, a decreased CSF glucose, and a highly increased CSF lactic acid level. A repeat LP is indicated if the patient has not responded to therapy within 72 hours. If the antibiotic is ineffective, the CFS profile will remain relatively unchanged, and most importantly, the CSF lactic acid levels will have not decreased. The CSF lactic acid levels decrease rapidly with appropriate antimicrobial therapy, and CSF glucose levels also quickly return to normal. If the patient is clinically not responding to antimicrobial therapy and the repeat LP shows the same or only slightly increased CSF glucose levels with the same or only slightly decreased lactic acid levels, then the clinician should re-assess the antimicrobial regimen [1,5,30–33,45].

Re-evaluation of the antibiotic should include a re-assessment of its spectrum, degree of activity, dosage, and CSF penetration, to determine if a change in therapy is warranted. The only CNS infection that may present with ABM that would change quickly as the result of appropriate therapy would be a brain abscess that has ruptured into the ventricular system. Such a large number of organisms released from the brain abscess into the CSF would be overwhelming to the host, and in spite of appropriate antimicrobial therapy, this would not change the CSF parameters within 3 days without drainage of the brain abscess. There is no need to repeat the LP if the patient is responding to therapy, suggesting that the proper antibiotic has been chosen and given in the correct dose and that it is effectively cidal at CNS concentrations, resulting in a rapid clinical response and a rapid response to the key CSF parameters of the lactic acid/CSF glucose [1–5,45,53].

REFERENCES

1. Schlossberg D. *Infections of the Nervous System.* New York: Springer-Verlag, 1990.
2. Scheld WM, Whitley RJ, Durack DT. *Infections of the Central Nervous System.* New York: Raven Press, 1991.
3. Tunkel AR. *Bacterial Meningitis.* Philadelphia, PA: Lippincott Williams & Wilkins, 2001.
4. Roos KL. *Central Nervous System Infectious Diseases and Therapy.* New York: Marcel Dekker Inc., 1997.
5. Wood M, Anderson M. *Neurologic Infections.* London, UK: W.B. Saunders, 1988.
6. Quagliarello V, Scheld WM. Bacterial meningitis: Pathogenesis, pathophysiology, and progress. *N Engl J Med* 1992;327:864–872.
7. Thomas K, Hasbun R, Jekel J, et al. The diagnostic accuracy of Kernig's and Brudzinski's signs in a prospective cohort of adults with suspected meningitis. *Clin Infect Dis* 2002;35:46–52.
8. Attia J, Hatala R, Cook DJ, et al. Does this adult patient have acute meningitis? *JAMA* 1999;282:175–181.
9. Swartz MN. Bacterial meningitis: A view of the past 90 years. *N Engl J Med* 2004;351:1826–1828.
10. Tunkel AR, Hartman BJ, Kaplan SL. Practical guidelines for the management of bacterial meningitis. *Clin Infect Dis* 2004;39:1267–1284.
11. Spanos A, Harrell FE Jr, Durack DT. Differential diagnosis of acute meningitis. An analysis of the predictive value of initial observation. *JAMA* 1989;262:2700–2707.
12. Short WR, Tunkel AR. Changing epidemiology of bacterial meningitis in the United States. *Curr Infect Dis Rep* 2000;2:327–331.
13. Logan SA, MacMahon E. Viral meningitis. *B Med J* 2008;336:36–40.
14. Eisenstein L, Calio F, Cunha BA. Herpes simplex virus type 1 (HSV-1) aseptic meningitis. *Heart Lung* 2004;33:196–197.
15. Hasbun R. The acute aseptic meningitis syndrome. *Curr Infect Dis Rep* 2000;2:345–351.

16. Chaudry HJ, Cunha BA. Drug-induced aseptic meningitis. *Postgrad Med* 1991;90:65–70.

17. Rodriguez SC, Olguin Am, Miralles CP, et al. Characteristics of meningitis caused by Ibuprofen: Report of 2 cases with recurrent episodes and review of the literature. *Medicine* 2006;85:214–220.

18. Roos KL. Pearls and pitfalls in the diagnosis and management of the central nervous system in infectious diseases. *Semin Neurol* 1998;18:185–196.

19. Warnatz K, Peter HH, Schumacher M, et al. Infectious CNS disease as a differential diagnosis in systemic rheumatic diseases: Three case reports and a review of the literature. *Ann Rheum Dis* 2003;62:50–57.

20. Carsons SE, Belilos E. Mimics of central nervous system infections. In: Cunha BA ed. *Infectious Diseases in Critical Care Medicine*. New York: Marcel Dekker, 1998:181–189.

21. Sanna G, Bertolaccini ML, Mathieu A. Central nervous system lupus: A clinical approach to therapy. *Lupus* 2003;12:935–942.

22. Hadfield MG, Aydin F, Lippman HR, et al. Neuro-Behçet's disease. *Clin Neuropathol* 1997;16:55–60.

23. James DG, Williams WJ. *Sarcoidosis and Other Granulomatous Disorders*. Philadelphia, PA: W.B. Saunders, 1985.

24. Sharma OP. *Sarcoidosis—Clinical Management*. London, UK: Butterworths, 1984.

25. Durand ML, Calderwood SB, Weber DJ, et al. Acute bacterial meningitis in adults. A review of 493 episodes. *N Engl J Med* 1993;328:21–28.

26. Hasbun R, Abrahams J, Jekel J, et al. Computed tomography of the head before lumbar puncture in adults with suspected meningitis. *N Engl J Med* 2001;345:1727–1733.

27. Tyler KL, Martin JB. *Infectious Diseases of the Central Nervous System. Philadelphia*, PA: FA Davis Company, 1993.

28. Pruitt AA. Nervous system infections in patients with cancer. *Neurol Clin* 2003;21:193–219.

29. Dropcho EJ. Remote neurologic manifestations of cancer. *Neurol Clin* 2002;20:85–122.

30. Cunha BA. The diagnostic significance of the CSF lactic acid. *Infect Dis Pract* 1997;21:57–60.

31. Bailey EM, Domenico P, Cunha BA. Bacterial versus viral meningitis. The importance of CSF lactic acid. *Postgrad Med* 1990;88:217–223.

32. Cunha BA. The usefulness of CSF lactic acid levels in central nervous system infections with decreased cerebrospinal fluid glucose. *Clin Infect Dis* 2004;39:1260–1261.

33. Latcha S, Cunha BA. *Listeria monocytogenes* meningoencephalitis: The diagnostic importance of the CSF lactic acid. *Heart Lung* 1994;23:177–179.

34. Cunha BA, Fatehpuria R, Eisenstein LE. *Listeria monocytogenes* encephalitis mimicking herpes simplex (HSV) encephalitis: The differential diagnostic importance of CSF lactic acid levels. *Heart & Lung* 2007;36:226–231.

35. Shimentani N, Shimetani K, Mori M. Levels of three inflammation markers, C-reactive protein, serum amyloid A protein and procalcitonin, in the serum and cerebrospinal fluid of patients with meningitis. *Scand J Clin Lab Invest* 2001;61:567–574.

36. Fishman RA. *Cerebrospinal Fluid in Diseases of the Nervous System* (2nd ed.). Philadelphia, PA: W.B. Saunders, 1992.

37. Knudsen TB, Larsen K, Kristiansen TB, et al. Diagnostic value of soluble CD163 serum levels in patients suspected of meningitis: Comparison with CRP and procalcitonnin. *Scand J Infect Dis* 2007;39:543–553.

38. Dubos F, Moulin F, Gajdos V, et al. Serum procalcitonin and other biologic markers to distinguish between bacterial and aseptic meningitis. *J Pediatr* 2006;149:72–76.

39. Cunha BA, Sachdev B, Canario D. Serum ferritin levels in West Nile encephalitis. *Clin Microbiol Infect* 2004;10:184–186.

40. Cunha BA. West Nile encephalitis: Clinical diagnostic and prognostic indicators in compromised hosts. *Clin Infect Dis* 2006;42:117.

41. McCullers JA, Lakeman FD, Whitley RJ. Human herpesvirus 6 is associated with focal encephalitis. *Clin Infect Dis* 1995;21:571–576.

42. Cunha BA. *Antibiotic Essentials* (8th ed.). Sudbury, MA: Jones & Bartlett, 2009.

43. Aronin SI. Bacterial meningitis: Principles and practical aspects of therapy. *Curr Infect Dis Rep* 2000;2:337–344.

44. Quagliarello VJ, Scheld WM. Treatment of bacterial meningitis. *N Engl J Med* 1997;336:708–716.

45. van de Beek D, de Gans J, Tunkel AR, et al. Community-acquired bacterial meningitis in adults. *N Engl J Med* 2006;354:44–53.

46. Schut ES, de Gans J, van de Beek. Community-acquired bacterial meningitis in adults. *Pract Neurol* 2008;8:8–23.

47. Mace SE. Acute bacterial meningitis. *Emerg Med Clin North Am* 2008;26:281–317.

48. Weisfelt M, de Gans J, van de Beek D. Bacterial meningitis: A review of effective pharmacotherapy. *Expert Opin Pharmacother* 2007;8:1493–1504.

49. Girgis NI, Farid Z, Mikhail IA, et al. Dexamethasone treatment for bacterial meningitis in children and adults. *Pediatr Infect Dis J* 1989;8:848–851.

50. van de Beek D, de Gans J. Dexamethasone in adults with community-acquired bacterial meningitis. *Drugs* 2006;66:415–427.

51. Gardner P, Leipzig T, Phillips P. Infections of central nervous system shunts. *Med Clin North Am* 1985;69:297–314.

52. Krol V, Hamid NS, Cunha BA. Neurosurgically related nosocomial *Acinetobacter baumannii* meningitis: Report of two cases and literature review. *J Hosp Infect* 2009;71:176–180.

53. Foerster BR, Thurnher MM, Malani PN, et al. Intracranial infections: Clinical and imaging characteristics. *Acta Radiol* 2007;48:875–893.

54. Cunha CB, Cunha BA. *Antibiotic Essentials* (17th ed.). New Delhi, India: Jay Pee Medical Publishers, 2020.

55. Munoz-Gomez S, Wirkowski E, Cunha BA. Post-craniotomy extra-ventricular drain (EVD) associated nosocomial meningitis: CSF diagnostic criteria. *Heart & Lung* 2015;44:158–160.

12 Encephalitis and Its Mimics in the Critical Care Unit

John J. Halperin

CONTENTS

CLINICAL PERSPECTIVE

A critically ill patient presents to the emergency department with a low-grade fever and altered mental status. Is this a brain infection? Is it a stroke? Is it the "toxic metabolic" encephalopathy so commonly seen in patients who are septic, hypotensive, hypoxic, or otherwise severely compromised? How far must one go to exclude the possibility of a central nervous system (CNS) damaging process? How does one most rationally approach this all too frequent occurrence? This chapter will attempt to provide a framework to address these frequent and challenging questions.

The neurologist's approach to the patient with impaired nervous system function is firmly rooted in the classic clinical approach of characterizing the disease process in space and time. Although technology, including magnetic resonance imaging (MRI) and electroencephalography (EEG), can augment the neurologic examination, important initial information can be quickly ascertained by performing a limited but directed bedside assessment.

A basic premise of clinical neurology is that CNS-damaging processes cause constant or progressive impairment of specific neurologic functions related to the location of the responsible CNS damage. In contrast, many systemic illnesses will cause impairments that wax and wane in both time and space—deficits may appear focal but improve, only to be followed by transient impairment of other functions. Simple and repeated clinical assessments of brainstem function, and of specific cortical functions such as language, memory, and vision, can raise or lower the index of suspicion for a primary CNS process.

BRAIN INFECTION OR NOT?

The clinical approach to these patients begins with differentiating among three distinct entities—encephalopathy, meningitis, and encephalitis. All may initially present in strikingly similar fashion, with systemic symptoms accompanied by changes in level of alertness and cognitive function.

Encephalopathy is by far the most common of the three, and, from a neurologic perspective, the most benign. Although the word can be defined to include any abnormality of brain function, it is most commonly used to describe alterations of consciousness and cognition in response to systemic disorders, without necessarily any underlying structural brain damage. Common causes of "toxic metabolic encephalopathy" include hyper- or hypoglycemia, hyponatremia, hypoxia, hyperthermia, sepsis, and organ system failure such as significant renal or hepatic insufficiency. The unifying theme of these disorders is that, by altering the brain's physiologic milieu, they alter brain function. Although all can result in nervous system damage if sufficiently severe or prolonged, each can cause transient neurobehavioral changes that are completely reversible.

Meningitis refers to inflammation in the subarachnoid space—the fluid filled space that surrounds the brain and spinal cord. Infections that remain limited to this space, such as viral meningitis, are medically benign, though symptomatically less so. "Aseptic meningitis," a term dating to a time when only bacterial pathogens could be readily identified, typically causes severe headaches and systemic symptoms but rarely has serious sequelae. Changes in neurologic function are generally non-focal and simply reflect the fact that the patient is ill and very uncomfortable.

Bacterial meningitis, in contrast, can be devastating. This infection starts in the subarachnoid space, but bacteria then invade and damage the arteries and veins passing into the adjacent brain and invade the brain directly. It is this vascular related damage, combined with focal cerebritis and abscess formation, as well as the effects of having a purulent exudate in the subarachnoid space obstructing cerebrospinal fluid (CSF) flow, that leads to severe neurologic sequelae. This, in combination with the systemic effects of the bacteremia, can result in a lethal outcome.

Finally, encephalitis refers to inflammation within the substance of the brain itself. This can lead to severe parenchymal CNS damage, resulting in irreversible neurologic impairment or death. Most often infectious, there are also rare disorders in which this occurs on a primarily immunologic basis.

Brain infections of all types are uncommon, in large part because the nervous system is so well protected—both mechanically and at the cellular level. Bacterial infection occurs primarily in three settings—mechanical injury to the skull (traumatic or surgical), contiguous untreated infection in the sinuses or mastoids, eroding through bone, or bacteremia with an organism able to cross the blood-brain barrier.

Some organisms, particularly neurotropic viruses, have developed unique strategies to enable CNS invasion. Herpes simplex virus (HSV) can invade the CNS by at least two mechanisms—crossing through the olfactory epithelium, then migrating along the olfactory tracts to the medial temporal lobes, or binding peripheral sensory nerve terminals and entering the axons and then being transported intra-axonally to the sensory ganglia, from which it can track centrally along trigeminal branches, innervating the meninges [1]. Poliovirus specifically binds receptors on motor neuron terminals and then migrates centrally within axons [2]. Other microorganisms have developed mechanisms to cross the blood-brain barrier but lack the ability to bind to neurons or glia; these cause infections limited to the meninges, but not encephalitis. In the absence of such specialized mechanisms, very few microorganisms are capable of invading and infecting the CNS.

CLINICAL APPROACH

Given the low incidence of encephalitis (10,000–20,000 cases per year in the United States), only a small subset of febrile patients with altered mental status will actually have encephalitis. In most instances, alterations of consciousness and cognitive function will be a nonspecific response to the febrile state, probably caused by circulating cytokines or other small molecules that cross the blood-brain barrier and are then neuroactive [3].

Differentiating between such encephalopathies and primary brain processes involves two key elements. From the systemic perspective, identification of a specific underlying medical abnormality is key. Neurologically, it is essential to establish whether the observed changes are focal or not—brain disorders resulting from localized damage to the brain cause abnormalities of function related to the site of damage.

Damage to the cerebral cortex can cause seizures, an altered level of consciousness and cognitive difficulty. Damage to the deep white matter causes spasticity, ataxia, visual, and sensory problems but not seizures and has a less severe impact on alertness and cognition. Damage to the brainstem can affect level of consciousness, long tracts that pass through the brainstem, and, important diagnostically, cranial nerve function.

Within the brain, different functions have discrete localization as well. Damage to the temporal lobes can cause memory and olfactory problems, frontal lobe damage affects behavior, occipital lobe damage affects vision, etc. In brief, location dictates the specific functions that are affected. Typically, if there is a brain damaging process, functions that are affected remain affected. In contrast, in patients with encephalopathy, abnormalities fluctuate in space and time. Hence, a detailed clinical neurologic assessment can help differentiate between a structural process, i.e., potentially an encephalitis, and a systemic abnormality altering the brain's metabolic milieu, that secondarily induces a time-varying abnormality of brain function.

In assessing patients' mental status, one of the first steps must be to assess language. Without establishing meaningful communication with the patient, further assessment of brain function can be uninterpretable. Aphasic patients are commonly described as "confused" because what they say makes no sense. If a patient's language sounds fluent but its content is incomprehensible, it is understandable to interpret this as evidence of confusion. However, several simple steps—asking the patient to follow several simple verbal commands (without helpful gesticulations), asking him/her to name a few objects or repeat a few words—should readily differentiate between a language disorder and a confusional state.

Similarly, the behavior of a patient with psychosis may seem inexplicable and be interpreted as evidence of confusion. Remarkably, although psychotic patients may demonstrate extraordinarily bizarre behavior, they almost always retain orientation and memory. Testing these simple functions usually will be very helpful.

Many disorders other than infections can produce focal brain damage—strokes and tumors being the most common. Differentiating between these disorders and infections should usually be straightforward based on the clinical context. Stroke usually has a virtually instantaneous onset and causes abnormalities related to the specific artery involved. Tumors typically cause symptoms that develop insidiously (over weeks or longer) and are not usually accompanied by systemic symptoms of infection.

Often most challenging are epileptic disorders. If there is no history of epilepsy and if no motor seizure activity was witnessed, these can be particularly perplexing. Post-ictal confusional states usually clarify themselves by resolving over minutes to hours. However non-convulsive status epilepticus, in which part of the brain seizes continuously but with no corresponding motor activity, can result in a patient with profoundly altered cognitive function, but with a cause only identifiable by EEG monitoring. Although, as with patients with brain tumors, these patients do not typically have systemic symptoms of infection, assuming that this excludes encephalitis can be dangerous—not all patients with encephalitis have systemic signs at the onset, and encephalitis can present as non-convulsive status!

INFECTIOUS ENCEPHALITIS

All encephalitides, regardless of cause, share several key characteristics. All are inflammatory processes involving the substance of the brain, resulting in at least a transient alteration of brain function, but ultimately potentially causing irreversible CNS damage. All are potentially devastating and much feared diseases—think of rabies or "sleeping sickness" as just two examples. On the other hand, most of the viruses that can cause encephalitis cause many more asymptomatic infections than symptomatic ones; usually even among patients with symptomatic infection only a small subset develop neuroinvasive disease [2].

The initial presentation of these infections is often unimpressive—typically much less dramatic than that of meningitis, where infection of the brain lining causes severe pain, sensitivity to light and sound, and reflex protective neck stiffness. The meninges and cortical blood vessels have nociceptive receptors, so inflammation is painful; the brain itself has no nociceptors. Fever, often low grade, is common—but less so in the very young, the elderly and the immunocompromised. Neurologic changes are often initially limited to subtle alterations of consciousness or cognition—easily confused with the mild changes typically seen as a non-specific result of systemic infection. Specific etiologic agents may cause more specific symptoms. Enteroviruses and *Listeria* often cause prominent associated gastrointestinal symptoms. Some arboviruses similarly can present with GI or other non-localizing symptoms.

Most CNS bacterial infections do not need to be considered further in this discussion, as affected patients generally present acutely toxic with little doubt about the diagnosis. However, some bacteria, typically more slow-growing ones that elicit a less dramatic immunologic response, cause much more indolent CNS infections—typically spirochetes, listeria, and mycobacteria.

SPECIFIC ENCEPHALITIDES

A consideration of the specific infections (Table 12.1) that cause encephalitis should begin with those that are most treatable—spirochetoses, mycobacteria, and herpes viruses—all of which cause meningitis with varying degrees of parenchymal brain involvement. Consideration should next turn to disorders with significant prevalence—primarily arthropod-borne agents such as the flaviviruses West Nile in the United States and tick-borne encephalitis (TBE) common in Europe and Asia. Zika and Chikungunya are highly prevalent outside the United States and occasionally cause neuroinvasive disease; although neither is endemic in the United States both are worth considering in travelers returning from the Caribbean, South America, and elsewhere. Powassan and the closely related deer tick virus remain rare but are increasingly recognized. Finally, there is a broad array of other

TABLE 12.1
Common Etiologic Agents and Diagnostic Approach

Acute Bacterial Meningitis
   Brain imaging
   Blood cultures
   CSF examination
   Identify source (skin, sinuses, mastoids, dental, cardiac, other)

Indolent Bacterial

Tuberculosis
   Chest X-ray
   Brain MRI with contrast (basal cisterns)
   CSF examination

Neuroborreliosis (Lyme disease)
   Peripheral blood serologic testing
   Consider CSF examination, including Lyme ELISA

Neurosyphilis
   Serum reaginic and specific serologic testing
   CSF reaginic and specific serologic testing

Listeria
   Brain MRI with contrast (brainstem)
   CSF examination

Mycoplasma
   Chest X-ray
   Serum cold agglutinins
   IgM mycoplasma ELISA

Viral

Herpes simplex
   Brain MRI with contrast (frontal and temporal lobes)
   CSF with PCR

West Nile virus
   Brain MRI with contrast (brainstem)
   Serum IgG and IgM specific serologies (acute and convalescent)
   CSF serology and PCR

Rabies
   Immunofluorescence for virus in skin biopsy
   Serology
   Saliva PCR

Abbreviations: CSF, cerebrospinal fluid; ELISA, enzyme linked immunosorbent assay; IgG, immunoglobulin G; IgM, immunoglobulin M; MRI, magnetic resonance imaging; PCR, olymerase chain reaction.

agents that must be identified—if for no other reason than for epidemiologic recognition and prevention of additional victims (e.g., rabies).

BACTERIAL BRAIN INFECTIONS

Tuberculosis

Worldwide, tuberculosis (TB) remains a significant public health problem, particularly in the less developed world. In the United States, it occurs primarily in patients who have immigrated from Southeast Asia, Africa, and eastern Europe and in the immunocompromised, particularly among patients with HIV infection. Tuberculosis, caused by *Mycobacterium tuberculosis*, is spread primarily by airborne droplets, initially causing pulmonary infection. Although this infection is typically controlled by hosts' cell-mediated immunity, some degree of hematogenous dissemination occurs frequently. Bacilli can seed the CNS, where tuberculomas most commonly occur along the meninges but can occur at typical intraparenchymal sites of hematogenously disseminated infection such as the subcortical gray-white junction. At some point long after initial infection, a tuberculoma may rupture into the subarachnoid space causing meningitis. This meningitis tends to involve the meninges at the base of the brain, regardless of where the tuberculoma was, where involvement of the cranial nerves and blood vessels that pass through the subarachnoid space is commonplace. This results in cranial neuropathies, obstructive hydrocephalus, and strokes [4].

In the absence of obvious chest X-ray findings, diagnosis can be challenging. In a small percentage of patients, brain imaging will demonstrate thick enhancement of the basilar meninges. Skin tests are usually but not invariably positive. T spot® tests, which measure peripheral blood mononuclear cells' response to synthetic peptides, can avoid some of the pitfalls of skin test interpretation. Cerebrospinal fluid analysis typically demonstrates a significant lymphocytic pleocytosis (cell count in the 100s–1000s) with increased protein, low glucose (sometimes unmeasurably so) and elevated adenosine deaminase concentration [5]. The latter, indicative of a vigorous T-cell response, is said to have approximately 90% sensitivity and specificity. Culture, acid-fast stain, and polymerase chain reaction (PCR)-based testing for mycobacteria are available but of incomplete sensitivity, and initial empiric treatment is necessary in up to half of the affected patients.

Outcome is heavily dependent on the patient's level of function at the time treatment is initiated. If treatment begins while the patient is neurologically normal, outcomes are excellent. If initiated in comatose individuals, outcomes are predictably quite poor. Although treatment for TB in general has been well studied, fewer studies have specifically addressed TB meningitis [6]. If multi-drug resistant (MDR) TB is unlikely, three drug regimens with isoniazid, rifampin, and pyrazinamide are usually given for 2 months; at the end of that time, pyrazinamide is usually stopped, and the other drugs are continued for up to 10 additional months. If MDR TB is likely, ethambutol or streptomycin is typically added for the first 2 months. Corticosteroids are often added initially (except in HIV-infected individuals) and seem to improve outcomes [4]. Neurologic sequelae are common.

Spirochetal Infections

Two spirochetal infections commonly involve the nervous system – neurosyphilis (*Treponema pallidum*) and neuroborreliosis. Neuroborreliosis, or nervous system Lyme disease, is typically caused by *Borreliella* (formerly *Borrelia*) *burgdorferi* in North America, by the closely related organisms *B. afzelii*, *B. garinii*, and others in Eurasia. Both commonly cause meningitis quite early in infection. In both, the basilar

meningitis can be accompanied by cranial neuropathies. Both may develop parenchymal nervous system involvement later in infection, although this appears to be far more common in neurosyphilis.

Lyme Disease

Borreliella burgdorferi infection, transmitted virtually exclusively by bites of hard shelled *Ixodes* ticks, often begins with a typically asymptomatic skin lesion at the site of inoculation, known as erythema migrans (EM). Prevalent in areas of the northeast and upper Midwest United States [7], as well as much of temperate Europe, this is a multisystem infectious disease that involves the nervous system in 10%–15% of untreated patients [8]. Meningitis occurs in up to 10% of patients, who also can develop cranial neuritis and peripheral nerve involvement. Only rarely is the brain or spinal cord parenchyma directly involved, although many patients with systemic infection may develop a "toxic metabolic" encephalopathy as a result of the systemic inflammatory response [9–11].

This encephalopathy well exemplifies the difficulty many non-neurologists have differentiating between brain infection and the physiologic effects systemic infection (and the immune response to it) can have on the nervous system. Affected patients often describe cognitive slowing, memory difficulty and other non-specific symptoms reflecting the ongoing presence of a chronic indolent infection—symptoms which typically resolve with successful treatment. Unfortunately, many patients and physicians conclude that these symptoms mean that the spirochetes have infected the brain and fear that this will lead to inevitable and progressive neurologic decline. It is now quite clear that most of these patients do not have CNS infections [12,13] and that simple oral antimicrobial regimens will cure virtually all.

Very rare patients with neuroborreliosis will develop infection within the parenchyma of the brain or spinal cord—encephalomyelitis. Such individuals, who generally have abnormal neurologic examinations, abnormal MRI scans, and abnormal spinal fluid, are similarly responsive to conventional courses of antimicrobials [14].

Diagnosis in general is confirmed with two-tiered antibody testing. An initial screen is performed using an enzyme-linked immunosorbent assay (ELISA); sera judged to be borderline or positive (antibody concentration 2 and 3 standard deviations above the mean, respectively) are then assessed for specificity with a western blot [15]. The serologic response may take 4 to 8 weeks to be measurable so in patients suspected of having very early disease, if the initial test is negative a follow-up ELISA in 1–2 months is reasonable. However, EM is virtually pathognomonic; in endemic areas patients with this rash should be treated regardless of serologic results (which can be negative in up to 50% of these individuals) [16].

In patients without parenchymal involvement (a group which includes those with meningitis), oral doxycycline 200 mg daily for 2–4 weeks is generally effective. In children (in whom the dose of any medication must be adjusted for weight) under 8 years of age, in pregnant women and in patients allergic to doxycycline, amoxicillin 500 mg three times daily or cefuroxime axetil 500 mg twice daily is probably as effective, though less well studied. In those with parenchymal CNS involvement or those who fail these oral regimens, intravenous ceftriaxone (2 g daily), cefotaxime (2 g three times daily), or penicillin 24 million units daily is highly effective, all for 2–4 weeks [14].

Neurosyphilis

Transmitted almost exclusively by sexual contact, syphilis typically begins with a chancre, a painless skin lesion at the site of inoculation. Spirochetes disseminate quite early in infection, with seeding of the neuraxis in about 40% of individuals [17]. Almost all of these patients develop meningitis, which can be variably symptomatic. However, virtually all develop CSF changes including a lymphocytic pleocytosis, modest elevation of protein, and minimal changes in glucose. In most, non-treponemal "reaginic" (anticardiolipin) antibodies are detectable in the CSF; treatment success can be monitored by measuring the decline in these antibodies as well as in the cell count.

Parenchymal CNS involvement is grouped into three syndromes. Meningovascular syphilis occurs on average 7 years after initial infection and results from inflammatory damage to the blood vessels in the subarachnoid space. This causes a series of primarily small-artery strokes, often somewhat slowly evolving, typically accompanied by chronic headaches from the meningitis. One to two decades after disease onset, other patients will develop "general paresis of the insane," a more diffuse picture thought to result from a combination of chronic hydrocephalus and parenchymal gummas. Finally, some patients will develop tabes dorsalis two to three decades after initial infection—primarily a disorder of the dorsal roots (which cross through the chronically inflamed subarachnoid space). These same patients often develop parenchymal inflammation in the midbrain, causing Argyll Robertson pupils.

Diagnosis is primarily serologic, using both reaginic antibody tests such as the rapid plasma reagin (RPR) and Venereal Disease Research Laboratory assays and more specific tests such as the fluorescent treponemal antibody and more recently ELISA technology. Historically, reaginic antibodies—present in high concentration and easily measurable with inexpensive, technically simple methods—have been used as screening tests, with confirmation by the more specific but technically demanding treponeme-specific assays. Recent work has questioned this approach with evidence that reversing the sequence—performing treponeme specific assays first with confirmation with assays for reaginic antibodies—may actually be more sensitive and specific [18]. Although there continues to be considerable debate as to the best testing paradigm, including use of PCR [19], most of this relates to positive and negative predictive values for screening for early syphilis. In secondary and tertiary neurosyphilis, both reaginic and treponemal tests are virtually always positive [20].

Treatment when the CNS parenchyma is involved is typically with parenteral penicillin, usually 18–24 million units daily for 10–14 days. Oral doxycycline (200 mg daily for 4 weeks) is recommended and used as an alternative in penicillin allergic patients, despite a paucity of supportive studies.

Listeria

Listeria is a widely prevalent organism that only rarely causes human disease. Infection most often occurs by exposure to contaminated food, most often dairy products. The organism is ingested by, and survives within, a number of types of cells. It seems particularly able to invade the placenta and the CNS, probably hiding intracellularly within trafficking monocytes [21].

Initial symptoms are primarily gastrointestinal. Infections are particularly problematic in pregnant women (causing miscarriages) and newborns (causing disseminated infection). Neurologic involvement takes several forms, most typically meningitis, being the commonest cause of bacterial meningitis in the immunocompromised and the second most common in otherwise healthy adults over age 50. The clinical picture of this meningitis is often more indolent than in other meningitides; patients appear less ill, and the time course is more protracted. A subset of patients— often younger and otherwise healthy—develop a brainstem encephalitis, or rhombencephalitis, with cranial nerve and long tract signs (ataxia, paresis) referable to this anatomic segment of the CNS [22]. Mortality in neurolisteriosis is greater in individuals with demonstrated bacteremia and in those taking corticosteroids or other immunosuppressives prior to infection [23].

Magnetic resonance imaging (MRI) can demonstrate microabscesses, particularly in the brainstem. Diagnosis is typically by culture of blood or CSF. The organism is very sensitive to ampicillin and penicillin, but perhaps because of its intracellular location, may be slow to respond. Consequently, gentamicin is often added for synergy, and treatment is typically prolonged. Meningitis is typically treated for 3 weeks; rhombencephalitis for 6 weeks.

Mycoplasma Pneumonia

Most patients with mycoplasma pneumonia have prominent headaches [24]; however actual CNS involvement, or even alterations of cognitive function or alertness, is quite rare. When encephalitis does occur, there are few specific features. Diagnosis is generally by measuring either cold agglutinins or specific antibody titers. Prognosis is generally excellent.

Viral Encephalitis

Viral encephalitides are typically divided into those transmitted by vectors and those that primarily infect humans. Most of the former fall under the rubric of arboviruses, a grouping that persists because of its clinical utility despite its being meaningless from a virologic perspective. Arthropods— subsuming both insects (e.g., mosquitoes) and arachnids (ticks and others)—can transmit zoonoses, infections that require specific non-human hosts and supportive environmental conditions. As a result, the likelihood of these infections in any given patient depends on both geography and timing. Although West Nile virus, now responsible for 95% of all arboviral disease in the United States, is the most common arboviral encephalitis, other agents include La Crosse, St. Louis encephalitis, Jamestown Canyon, Powassan, and Eastern equine encephalitis viruses, which cause sporadic cases and outbreaks [25]. Of agents uniquely infecting humans, herpes and enteroviruses are the most common.

Herpes Simplex Encephalitis

Human herpes viruses, similar to polioviruses, differ from many other encephalitis-causing viruses in that they have just one host—humans. Because of this, it is at least theoretically possible to eliminate these pathogens entirely—primarily through effective vaccines. While sufficiently potent vaccines are not yet available for herpes simplex, this strategy has eliminated smallpox and hopefully will eliminate polio in the not-too-distant future. Unfortunately, this approach cannot eliminate the innumerable other viruses, such as West Nile and rabies, which exist as zoonoses in multiple species. Even with successful vaccination, the best that can be hoped for with zoonotic infections is temporary protection of the immunized individuals, not permanent elimination of the virus and therefore the disease.

Herpes virus is the most commonly identified agent of sporadic encephalitis [26]. Herpes simplex virus (HSV) 1 and 2 are ubiquitous. Following initial infection, primarily via the mucous membranes, the virus generally establishes permanent residence in the innervating dorsal root ganglion neurons. Periodically, virus will migrate back down the axon, causing a recurrent cutaneous eruption. A similar mechanism is thought to underlie HSV1 encephalitis, the cause of the vast majority of herpes simplex encephalitis. The sensory neurons of the trigeminal nerve, which innervate the lips, also innervate the meninges of the middle and anterior cranial fossa. Experimentally, reactivating virus can be shown to migrate centrally, affecting the medial temporal and frontal lobes, the primary site of involvement in herpes simplex encephalitis.

HSV1 encephalitis is potentially a devastating illness, with mortality approaching 90% in the pretreatment era. Initial presentation can be as a non-specific febrile prodrome with headaches. Often, mild personality changes are noted for a few days. Two important (and probably inter-related) functions of the medial temporal lobes are olfaction and memory. Early manifestations of this necrotizing, localized infection often include focal seizures that manifest as olfactory hallucinations and perceptions of déjà vu or jamais vu. Often, a diagnosis is not made until the patient has a generalized or at least focal motor seizure.

The diagnosis should be considered in a previously healthy individual with abrupt onset of altered mental status and fever; headache is present in most. Clinically evident seizures are a presenting symptom in up to half of people. Since other brain infections can be clinically similar, confirmatory testing is necessary. Imaging, particularly MRI scans, classically will demonstrate changes in the medial temporal lobes, though this may take a few days to be evident. The EEG can show paroxysmal periodic discharges—but again usually only after several days. The CSF examination is the most helpful. Although cases have been reported in which CSF is initially normal, typically it shows a modest lymphocytic pleocytosis, with a significant number of erythrocytes, and mild hypoglycorrhachia. Most importantly, CSF PCR for herpes viruses is highly sensitive and specific.

Speed is of the essence in treating herpes simplex encephalitis—there is a much higher probability of successful outcome if treatment is initiated when the patient is awake and unimpaired than if it is started when the patient is comatose [27]. Therefore, it is common practice to perform an MRI and lumbar puncture rapidly, initiate treatment immediately, and then stop treatment if PCR and other testing do not support the diagnosis. Treatment consists of acyclovir 10 mg/kg every 8 hours for 21 days. Its major complication is renal toxicity; this risk can be decreased with aggressive hydration. However, the requisite fluid load can be problematic, since patients with herpes simplex encephalitis frequently develop significant hyponatremia and cerebral edema, both requiring fluid restriction. Most patients require anticonvulsants. Although animal studies and a small retrospective study suggest that corticosteroid use might be beneficial [28], the role of steroids remains unclear.

Other Herpes Viruses

Neurologic complications used to accompany about 1 of every 10,000 cases of chickenpox [26]. With widespread vaccination, this is now rarely seen. Cytomegalovirus can cause ventriculoencephalitis and dementia in the immunocompromised. HSV 6 can cause an encephalitis similar to HSV 1 and has been associated with febrile seizures in infants. Epstein–Barr virus has been associated with a similar clinical picture but has not been shown to respond to acyclovir or other antivirals.

West Nile Virus

With over 1300 cases of neuroinvasive disease in 2017 [29], West Nile virus is now probably the commonest cause of diagnosed encephalitis in the United States (with virtually the same number of cases as HSV1). This arthropod-borne zoonosis appears to have been brought to the United States in infected birds and was originally recognized for being highly lethal in some but not all bird species.

Key to the transmissibility of any zoonosis is its production of prolonged viremia in some host species, and the presence of mosquitoes or other vectors that feed on both this infected reservoir species and on humans [30]. This interspecies promiscuity is essential to the transmission of this large group of pathogens, which can persist in the environment in reservoir hosts, and periodically infect humans when a large group of non-immune individuals is exposed. Since there are hundreds of asymptomatic or minimally symptomatic infections for every neuroinvasive case, "herd immunity" normally takes over after the infection is present in the environment for a period of time—presumably the reason the incidence of cases has moved like a wave across the United States from east to west since its initial introduction (see Figure 12.1).

West Nile is a flavivirus (the family that includes and is named for Yellow Fever virus), a broad group that includes dengue, TBE, Japanese encephalitis, St Louis encephalitis, and Powassan viruses. It was first detected in North America in 1999. In the Middle East, serologic studies indicate up to 40% of the population has had asymptomatic infection. Studies in the United States suggest 80% of infections are asymptomatic with most of the remainder developing non-specific symptoms with fever, head and back pain, and GI symptoms, all occurring with some frequency. Neuroinvasive disease develops in fewer than 1% of infected individuals. Mortality among these is about 10%. Disease severity increases with age, with most mortality occurring in individuals over 50. Over half the survivors of neuroinvasive disease have sequelae [30].

Neuroinvasive disease causes meningitis; a syndrome of flaccid lower motor neuron type weakness resembling polio occurs in about half. Involvement of the brainstem and basal ganglia appears to be common, with extrapyramidal syndromes, tremors, and ataxia occurring with some frequency. Patients often have a peripheral leucopenia and CSF lymphocytosis. Diagnosis is by serologic testing (IgG and IgM antibodies in serum and CSF) and PCR. Magnetic resonance imaging has shown abnormalities in the spinal cord, brainstem, and basal ganglia. No specific treatment is available.

Powassan and Deer Tick Virus

Powassan virus, another flavivirus, is transmitted by bites of *Ixodes* ticks, as are the related Eurasian TBE viruses and the agents of Lyme borreliosis. While still numbering only about 100 reported patients since it was first identified in 1958 (in Powassan, Ontario [31]), cases are now being increasingly recognized in Lyme-endemic areas of the northeast United States, where the virus is referred to as Powassan lineage II or deer tick virus [32,33]. Clinical presentation resembles other viral encephalitides, starting with fever, headaches, and altered consciousness. Seizures and focal neurologic deficits are not uncommon. Brain MRIs have demonstrated areas of abnormal T2, fluid-attenuated inversion recovery (FLAIR), and diffusion weighted signal, primarily in deep gray matter structures, with similar changes in cortical gray matter in some patients as well. The CSF findings are typical of viral encephalitis, with a lymphocyte predominant pleocytosis ranging up to the mid-100s/mm^3, protein ranging up to the low-200-mg/dL range, and normal glucose. Diagnosis has generally been serologic, with identification of IgM antibodies in CSF and/or serum, an evolving IgG serology, or, occasionally, virus isolation. The virus is highly neurotropic; autopsies have demonstrated virus in neurons and glia. Involvement of brainstem and spinal cord motor neurons has been prominent [31] (much like TBE). Seroprevalence studies suggest that many infections are either asymptomatic or non-specific; 80% of diagnosed cases have had neuroinvasive disease [31]. Mortality

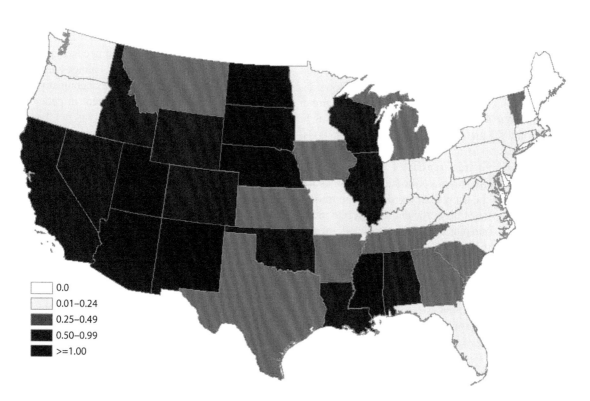

0.0
0.01–0.24
0.25–0.49
0.50–0.99
>=1.00

FIGURE 12.1 This map shows the incidence of human West Nile virus neuroinvasive disease (e.g., meningitis, encephalitis, and acute flaccid paralysis) by state for 2017, with shading ranging from 0.01 to 0.24, 0.25 to 0.49, 0.50 to 0.99, and greater than 1.00 per 100,000 population. (Courtesy of the Centers for Disease Control and Prevention.)

rates have generally been reported to be about 10%–15%, with neurologic sequelae in many survivors [33].

Zika and Chikungunya

While Zika (another flavivirus) remains extremely rare in the United States, it has become widely prevalent elsewhere in the Americas. Most feared because of the sequelae of *in utero* infection, it is not uncommonly associated with peripheral nerve involvement (Guillain Barre syndrome [GBS]) and occasionally meningoencephalitis and transverse myelitis [34]. In the largest series reported to date [34], of 40 patients diagnosed with nervous system-affecting Zika, 29 had GBS, 1 had chronic inflammatory demyelinating polyneuropathy, 7 had encephalitis, and 3 had transverse myelitis. Most had a viral prodrome. Two of the 40 (including 1 of the encephalitis patients) died. Magnetic resonance imaging has generally shown nerve root and meningeal enhancement with limited parenchymal CNS abnormalities.

Chikungunya similarly remains very rare in the United States but is widely prevalent elsewhere in the Americas. Unlike most of the other viruses discussed, most patients infected with this alphavirus are symptomatic [35]. Most are febrile with severe, widespread arthralgias symmetrically affecting multiple joints. While neurologic involvement occurs in only about 10%–15% of cases, primarily affecting individuals above the age of 60, encephalitis is a relatively common nervous system manifestation. Specific details remain unclear, particularly since encephalopathy is very common in these patients and encephalitis and encephalopathy have not always been clearly distinguished in reported series.

Rabies

Fortunately, human rabies is extremely rare in the United States, with typically one case per year nationwide. However, there is a significant incidence among animals; when human cases occur, there often is some delay in diagnosis, resulting in additional individuals being exposed, requiring prophylaxis. This too is a zoonosis, existing in innumerable mammalian species. Transmission requires transfer of virus-containing secretions or tissue through mucosa or broken skin. Since the virus has an affinity for the acetylcholine receptor on muscle endplates, infection is particularly efficient when a bite introduces the virus directly into muscle. Once introduced, virions are transported back within axons, where they multiply, and then on to the spinal cord and brainstem. This asymptomatic incubation period last weeks to years [36]. Once the virus is in the nervous system patients develop fever, anxiety, muscle aches, and non-specific symptoms. Neuropathic symptoms ranging from itching to pain may develop at the inoculation site. Ultimately patients develop either paralytic rabies or the encephalitic form. In the former, patients develop a Guillain-Barre–like picture, with fever, sensory and motor symptoms, facial involvement, and sphincter dysfunction. More common is the encephalitic form in which patients develop inspiratory spasms, precipitated by any contact with the face, including trying to drink (hydrophobia). Hallucinations and fluctuating consciousness proceed to coma, paralysis, and death within a week.

Diagnosis can be challenging. Presence of antibodies in serum (if unvaccinated) or CSF is diagnostic but not terribly sensitive. Immunofluorescence can often detect virus in nerve twigs surrounding hair follicles in skin biopsied from the nape of the neck. PCR has been used to detect virus in saliva. Despite numerous attempts at treatment, only one or two individuals have survived [37].

ENCEPHALITIS MIMICS

Mental status changes are common in many patients with systemic infections, particularly in older individuals—typically in the absence of nervous system infection. Confusional states in septic patients—even with sources as localized as urinary tract infections or pneumonia—are so commonplace that clinicians rarely question the underlying pathophysiology. However, in some infections CNS changes can be disproportionately prominent; in these a number of mechanisms may underlie these changes.

Patients with rickettsia (particularly Rocky Mountain spotted fever [RMSF]) and ehrlichia/anaplasma (particularly human monocytic and granulocytic ehrlichiosis) infected patients can have severe headaches and prominent mental status changes. In both, the disorder caused by these intracellular organisms probably is less an encephalitis than an infectious vasculitis. Rocky Mountain spotted fever in particular can be associated with significant cerebral edema and stupor. Cerebrospinal fluid typically demonstrates a modest lymphocytic pleocytosis and increased protein; CSF glucose is most often normal. Autopsy studies demonstrate perivascular inflammatory infiltrates and occasionally intravascular thrombi in the brain, pathologic changes that could easily explain the seizures that sometime accompany RMSF. Focal CNS findings are relatively infrequent in patients with these infections, and survivors typically do not have prominent neurologic sequelae. Whether ehrlichia infections have significant neurologic involvement remains unclear—although headaches and alterations of consciousness are described frequently, only a few case reports have described focal brain abnormalities.

Diagnosis can be quite challenging. Organisms can sometimes be identified in buffy coat isolates, using special stains. Serologic studies using immunofluorescence or ELISA can be useful, but titers may be negative very early in infection and often comparison of acute and convalescent sera is necessary for diagnosis. Treatment with doxycycline is quite effective.

Legionnaire's, disease similarly does not infect the brain but causes altered cognitive function with remarkable frequency—out of proportion to any associated hypoxia or other metabolic abnormalities. This infection can often be suspected clinically by its multisystem involvement—often with prominent early gastrointestinal symptoms (diarrhea and abdominal pain), bradycardia, and hepatic and renal involvement. Diagnosis typically rests on the combination of rapidly worsening changes on chest radiograms, and either serologic or urinary antigen testing.

Patients with bacterial endocarditis similarly can have CNS manifestations related more to involvement of the cerebral vasculature than of the brain itself. Signs and symptoms are typically non-specific—except when a septic embolism causes either a stroke or a mycotic aneurysm which ruptures. CSF examination can demonstrate minor abnormalities. Diagnosis can be quite challenging.

Similarly, non-infectious inflammatory disorders can affect the CNS—most prominently CNS systemic lupus erythematosus. Again, findings are typically non-focal, either on exam or imaging, but cerebral edema can be prominent. Since many of these patients are on chronic immunosuppression, one of the greatest diagnostic challenges can be differentiating between insufficiently controlled lupus and a superimposed opportunistic infection in an immunocompromised patient.

DIAGNOSTIC APPROACH

Given the broad array of disorders considered, what is the most straightforward approach to the ill patient with altered mental status? As illustrated in Figure 12.2, the first step is a clinical assessment, focusing on the history. Where has the patient been? What were the earliest symptoms and how did the disorder evolve? If neurologic involvement is evident

from the outset (seizures and persisting focal deficits), the possibility of neurologic disease must be assessed simultaneously with the assessment of the patient's overall medical status.

A general examination should initially focus on vital signs—remembering that fever may not be evident at either end of the age spectrum or in those with compromised immunity. The examination must seek evidence of pulmonary, hepatic or renal compromise. Finally, a limited neurologic assessment, focusing on language, orientation, and cranial nerve function, is essential. Key biochemical markers, including glucose, sodium, liver, and renal function, and, if relevant, blood gases, should similarly be assessed immediately. If none of this reveals significant extra-neurologic disease, focus should shift to the nervous system.

If either the history or examination suggests a primary CNS process, brain imaging (usually, in the interest of timeliness, with computerized tomography) is usually rapidly completed. If this does not demonstrate significant focal mass effect and the picture does not clearly suggest a non-infectious cause, a lumbar puncture should be performed. Spinal fluid studies should include cell count, differential, protein, glucose (with simultaneous blood glucose), bacterial culture, and Gram stain. Depending on the context, additional studies may include mycobacterial cultures and PCR, fungal cultures, CSF RPR, paired serum and CSF Lyme serologies, PCR for herpes viruses, serologic and PCR testing for

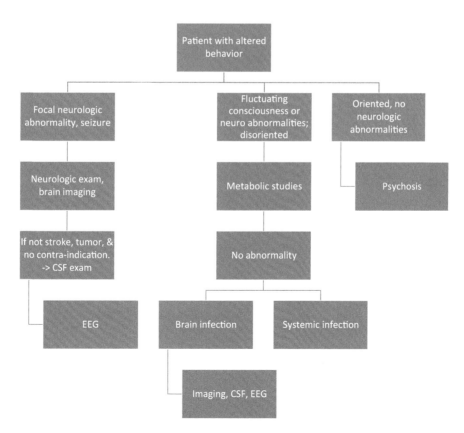

FIGURE 12.2 Clinical approach to the patient with altered brain function.

West Nile virus, etc. The recent introduction of multiplexed PCR testing for a large battery of CNS pathogens [38] can be extremely helpful, rapidly providing information about the most common bacterial, fungal, and viral agents. As with any laboratory test, though, it is crucial to keep in mind both that the test sensitivity is high but not 100%, varying somewhat from pathogen to pathogen, and that there are uncommon pathogens for which it does not test. Blood cultures should normally be obtained as well if there is serious consideration of a nervous system bacterial infection. Initial treatment is often started empirically, depending on the context to cover likely pathogens.

CONCLUSIONS

Although alterations of nervous system function can arise from a broad range of disorders, a logical clinical approach can lead to rapid diagnosis in most. Fortunately, CNS infection is statistically rare. However, when encephalitis does occur, its results can be devastating; generally, the earlier the treatment can be initiated, the better the likelihood of a favorable outcome.

REFERENCES

1. Whitley R, Kimberlin D, Roizman B. Herpes simplex viruses. *Clin Infect Dis* 1998;26:541–553.
2. Halperin J. Viral encephalitis. In: Halperin J, ed. *Encephalitis: Diagnosis and Treatment*. New York: Informa, 2007:115–132.
3. Heyes MP, Lackner A. Increased cerebrospinal fluid quinolinic acid, kynurenic acid and L-kynurenine in acute septicemia. *J Neurochem* 1990;55:338–341.
4. Garcia-Monco J. Tuberculosis of the central nervous system. In: Halperin J, ed. *Encephalitis: Diagnosis and Treatment*. New York: Informa, 2007:283–304.
5. Lopez-Cortes L, Cruz-Ruiz M, Gomez-Mateos J, et al. Adenosine deaminase activity in the CSF of patients with aseptic meningitis: Utility in the diagnosis of tuberculous meningitis or neurobrucellosis. *Clin Infect Dis* 1995;20:525–530.
6. Horsburgh C, Jr, Feldman S, Ridzon R. Practice guidelines for the treatment of tuberculosis. *Clin Infect Dis* 2000;31:633–639.
7. Bacon RM, Kugeler KJ, Mead PS. Surveillance for Lyme disease—United States, 1992–2006. *Morb Mortal Wkly Rep* 2008;57:1–9.
8. Pachner AR, Steere AC. The triad of neurologic manifestations of Lyme disease. *Neurology* 1985;35:47–53.
9. Halperin JJ, Krupp LB, Golightly MG, Volkman DJ. Lyme borreliosis-associated encephalopathy. *Neurology* 1990;40:1340–1343.
10. Krupp LB, Fernquist S, Masur D, Halperin JJ. Cognitive impairment in Lyme disease. *Neurology* 1990;40:304.
11. Halperin JJ, Heyes MP. Neuroactive kynurenines in Lyme borreliosis. *Neurology* 1992;42:43–50.
12. Dersch R, Sommer H, Rauer S, Meerpohl JJ. Prevalence and spectrum of residual symptoms in Lyme neuroborreliosis after pharmacological treatment: A systematic review. *J Neurol* 2016;263:17–24.
13. Wills AB, Spaulding AB, Adjemian J, et al. Long-term follow-up of patients with Lyme disease: Longitudinal analysis of clinical and quality-of-life measures. *Clin Infect Dis* 2016;62:1546–1551.
14. Halperin JJ, Shapiro ED, Logigian EL, et al. Practice parameter: Treatment of nervous system Lyme disease. *Neurology* 2007;69:91–102.
15. Anonymous. Recommendations for test performance and interpretation from the Second National Conference on Serologic Diagnosis of Lyme Disease. *Morb Mortal Wkly Rep* 1995;44:590–591.
16. Wormser GP, Dattwyler RJ, Shapiro ED, et al. The clinical assessment, treatment, and prevention of Lyme disease, human granulocytic anaplasmosis, and babesiosis: Clinical practice guidelines by the Infectious Diseases Society of America. *Clin Infect Dis* 2006;43:1089–1134.
17. Halperin J. Spirochetal infections of the nervous system. In: Aminoff M, ed. *Neurology and General Medicine*, 4th ed. Philadelphia, PA: Harcourt Health Sciences, 2008:789–802.
18. Park IU, Chow JM, Bolan G, Stanley M, Shieh J, Schapiro JM. Screening for syphilis with the treponemal immunoassay: Analysis of discordant serology results and implications for clinical management. *J Infect Dis* 2011;204:1297–1304.
19. Vanhaecke C, Grange P, Benhaddou N, et al. Clinical and biological characteristics of 40 patients with neurosyphilis and evaluation of *Treponema pallidum* nested polymerase chain reaction in cerebrospinal fluid samples. *Clin Infect Dis* 2016;63:1180–1186.
20. Knaute DF, Graf N, Lautenschlager S, Weber R, Bosshard PP. Serological response to treatment of syphilis according to disease stage and HIV status. *Clin Infect Dis* 2012;55:1615–1622.
21. Winston A, Marriott D, Brew B. Early syphilis presenting as a painful polyradiculopathy in an HIV positive individual. *Sex Transm Infect* 2005;81:133–134.
22. Hirsch B. Listeria infections and the central nervous system. In: Halperin JJ, ed. *Encephalitis: Diagnosis and Treatment*. New York: Informa, 2007:273–282.
23. Charlier C, Perrodeau E, Leclercq A, et al. Clinical features and prognostic factors of listeriosis: The MONALISA national prospective cohort study. *Lancet Infect Dis* 2017;17:510–519.
24. Cunha B, Halperin JJ. Clinical approach in encephalitis. In: Halperin JJ, ed. *Encephalitis: Diagnosis and Treatment*. New York: Informa, 2007:1–18.
25. Krow-Lucal E, Lindsey NP, Lehman J, Fischer M, Staples JE. West Nile virus and other nationally notifiable arboviral diseases—United States, 2015. *Morb Mortal Wkly Rep* 2017;66:51–55.
26. King N, Roos K. Herpesvirus encephalitis. In: Halperin JJ, ed. *Encephalitis: Diagnosis and Treatment*. New York: Informa, 2007:167–194.
27. Whitley R, Alford C, Hirsch M, al. e. Vidarabine versus acyclovir therapy in herpes simplex encephalitis. *N Engl J Med* 1986;314:144–149.
28. Kamei S, Sekizawa T, Shiota H, et al. Evaluation of combination therapy using aciclovir and corticosteroid in adult patients with herpes simplex virus encephalitis. *J Neurol Neurosurg Psychiatry* 2005;76:1544–1549.
29. Wilson MR, Naccache SN, Samayoa E, et al. Actionable diagnosis of neuroleptospirosis by next-generation sequencing. *N Engl J Med* 2014;370:2408–2417.
30. Asnis D, Crupi R. West Nile virus. In: Halperin JJ, ed. *Encephalitis: Diagnosis and Treatment*. New York: Informa, 2007:133–156.
31. Doughty CT, Yawetz S, Lyons J. Emerging causes of arbovirus encephalitis in North America: Powassan, chikungunya, and Zika viruses. *Curr Neurol Neurosci Rep* 2017;17:12.
32. El Khoury MY, Camargo JF, White JL, et al. Potential role of deer tick virus in Powassan encephalitis cases in Lyme disease-endemic areas of New York, U.S.A. *Emerg Infect Dis* 2013;19:1926–1933.

33. Piantadosi A, Rubin DB, McQuillen DP, et al. Emerging cases of Powassan virus encephalitis in New England: Clinical presentation, imaging, and review of the literature. *Clin Infect Dis* 2016;62:707–713.

34. da Silva IRF, Frontera JA, Bispo de Filippis AM, Nascimento O, Group R-G-ZR. Neurologic complications associated with the Zika virus in Brazilian adults. *JAMA Neurol* 2017;74:1190–1198.

35. Brizzi K. Neurologic manifestation of chikungunya virus. *Curr Infect Dis Rep* 2017;19:6.

36. Halperin JJ. Rabies. *Encephalitis: Diagnosis and Treatment.* New York: Informa, 2007:195–206.

37. Willoughby RJ, Tieves K, Hoffman G, et al. Survival after treatment of rabies with induction of coma. *N Engl J Med* 2005;352:2508–2514.

38. Hanson KE, Couturier MR. Multiplexed molecular diagnostics for respiratory, gastrointestinal, and central nervous system infections. *Clin Infect Dis* 2016;63:1361–1367.

13 Severe Community-Acquired Pneumonia in the Critical Care Unit

Burke A. Cunha

CONTENTS

CLINICAL PERSPECTIVE

Community-acquired pneumonia (CAP) may present as mild, moderate, or severe pneumonia. Patients with severe CAP require hospital admission and usually are admitted to the critical care unit (CCU). Patients with severe CAP in the CCU are those requiring ventilatory support. Clinically in immunocompetent patients, CAP is severe, primarily because of the underlying cardiopulmonary status. While some pathogens are inherently more virulent than others, e.g., *Legionella* is more virulent than *Moraxella catarrhalis*, clinical severity is primarily determined by host rather than by microbial factors. A patient with Legionnaire's disease and good cardiopulmonary function may present with severe CAP, as may a patient with severe chronic obstructive pulmonary disease with *M. catarrhalis* CAP. Patients with bacterial CAP and various degrees of hyposplenism often present with severe CAP [1–7].

Community-acquired pneumonia occurs in normal or compromised hosts. The clinical approach is to determine the cause of severe CAP, which depends on assessing cardiopulmonary status and degree of splenic dysfunction and identifying the disorders associated with specific immune defects, e.g., β-lymphocyte (humoral immunity [HI]). Analysis of host defense defects by history is combined with the chest X-ray findings and degree of hypoxemia [1,8]. After non-infectious causes of severe CAP are ruled out, i.e., mimics of CAP, the physician should then consider the DDx of non-infectious disorders resembling CAP [8–10].

Optimal empiric therapy is based on covering the usual pathogens associated with CAP, based on correlating chest X-ray (CXR) and clinical findings. Selection of empiric

antimicrobial therapy of severe CAP is done in the same way as for non-severe CAP. However, severe CAP patients may have a longer length of stay (LOS), stormy clinical course, and longer courses of antibiotic therapy. Therapy is continued as the diagnostic workup is in progress. If the causative pathogen is identified, there is no rationale for changing the antibiotics to one with a narrower spectrum. It is a popular antibiotic myth that de-escalation to a narrower spectrum has some advantages. Antibiotic resistance potential is related to specific antibiotics and not antibiotic class. Changing to a narrow-spectrum antibiotic is of no benefit, and, if chosen wisely, e.g., using a "low resistance potential," antibiotic has no effect on antibiotic resistance. With *Streptococcus pneumoniae*, there is no rationale to change from ceftriaxone to penicillin because of a narrower spectrum. Therapy of severe CAP is usually for 2–3 weeks in total [10–12]. Ceftriaxone is as effective as penicillin and may be given less frequently. Importantly, there is no increased resistance with *S. pneumoniae*, even with prolonged use.

DETERMINANTS OF SEVERE CAP

MICROBIAL VIRULENCE

The clinical spectrum of *S. pneumoniae* CAP ranges from mild in ambulatory adults to fulminating/overwhelming sepsis in asplenics. Because of severe lung disease, even low-virulence organisms, e.g., *M. catarrhalis*, may decrease borderline respiratory function. Microbial virulence and host factors are the important determinants of severe CAP clinical presentation (Table 13.1).

TABLE 13.1
Determinants of Severe CAP

Microbial/Host Factors	Host Defense Factors
Microbial factors	***Impaired B lymphocyte function/HI***
• **Bacterial virulence**	• **Disorders associated with ↓ HI**
Legionella sp.	SLE
S. pneumoniae	Multiple myeloma
• **Encapsulated**	Cirrhosis
respiratory pathogens	Hyposplenia
S. pneumoniae	Asplenia
H. influenzae	***Impaired T lymphocyte function***
K. pneumoniae	***cell-mediated immunity (CMI)***
• **Viral virulence**	• **Disorders associated with ↓ CMI**
Influenza A	T cell lymphomas
Avian influenza (H5N1)	High/dose chronic steroid therapy
Swine influenza (H1N1)	Immunosuppressive therapy
SARS	TNF-α antagonists
MERS	HIV
COVID-19	***Impaired combined B and T lymphocyte***
HPS	***function*** (*HI/CMI immunity*)
Pulmonary factors	• **Disorders associated with ↓ HI and**
• *Severe lung disease*	**↓ CMI**
Emphysema	CLL
Chronic bronchitis	SLE with flare
Interstitial fibrosis	SLE with flare/immunosuppressive
Cardiac factors	therapy
• CHF	Advanced age
• Severe valvular disease	
• Severe cardiomyopathy	
• CAD	
Systemic factors	
• Advanced age (CNS/	
esophageal dysfunction)	
• Hepatic insufficiency	
• Renal insufficiency	

Abbreviations: SLE, systemic lupus erythematosus; CLL, chronic lympho-cytic leukemia; CAP, community-acquired pneumonia; CHF, congestive heart failure; HI, humoral immunity, CAD, coronary artery disease; CNS, central nervous system; CMI, cell-mediated immunity.

Bacteremias associated with CAPs are reflective of the bacteremic potential of the organism and are not per se a marker of clinical severity. Bacteremia frequently accompanies *S. pneumoniae* or *Hemophilus influenzae* CAP and is part of the clinical presentation. It is not related to CAP severity [1,13–20].

CARDIOPULMONARY FUNCTION

Elderly adults with decreased lung function have diminished pulmonary reserve, and pulmonary function is further impaired with superimposed CAP. In patients with advanced lung disease/borderline pulmonary function, even with low-virulence organisms causing CAP the CAP presents as severe CAP, since lung function is a key determinant of CAP severity [1,2,10–21].

In patients with CAP with borderline cardiac function, cardiac decompensation is common. The fever from CAP increases the heart rate and alone may be sufficient to precipitate acute myocardial infarction (MI) or congestive heart failure (CHF). The heart rate (pulse) increases 10 beats/min for each degree Fahrenheit of temperature elevation above normal. Fever often precipitates CHF, mimicking the clinical presentation of severe CAP [2,10,22–25].

The heart and lung are physiologically interrelated, and decompensation of one will adversely affect the other. Elderly patients often have advanced lung and heart disease. Elderly patients with CAP, with limited cardiopulmonary reserve, often present clinically as severe CAP [1,2,5,9,10,26].

CLINICAL APPROACH TO SEVERE CAP

The history and physical examination coupled with the CXR appearance/distribution of infiltrates determines the DDx, e.g., bilateral perihilar/interstitial infiltrates points to a viral or non-infectious etiology, while a focal segmental lobar suggests a bacterial pneumonia [1,2,8,10] (Tables 13.2 through 13.7).

DISORDERS WITH ASSOCIATED IMMUNE DEFECTS DETERMINE PROBABLE CAP PATHOGEN

SCAP in compromised .hosts, as in normal patients, are most often due to the usual CAP pathogens. However, clinical severity may be increased due to impaired host defenses. Compromised hosts have specific immune defects that predispose to limited-potential pathogen causing CAP. It is a common clinical misconception that because a patient is immunocompromised, the pathogen range is more extensive. Excluding the usual CAP pathogens in normal hosts, the range of CAP pathogens in compromised hosts is limited by the immune defect, i.e., CAP patients with multiple myeloma are prone to CAP due to the same typical encapsulated bacterial pathogens, not viruses, as normal hosts. If the patient has multiple myeloma, then the pulmonary pathogens are predictable and are not extensive or unusual. The clinical approach, therefore, rests on the relationship between the disorder, which is the determinant of the immune defect, which, in turn, limits the potential pathogen range. The potential pathogens determine what constitutes appropriate empiric antimicrobial coverage in normal/immunocompromised patients with severe CAP [1,2,8–10]. The immune defect while having no effect on CAP pathogen DDx, does effect severity, duration of therapy and prognosis.

TABLE 13.2

Diagnostic Approach to Severe CAP with Hypotension/Shock

Infectious Causes	Non-infectious with Infectious Causes
• CAP (with hyposplenia)[a]	• Acute MI (with CAP)
• CAP (with asplenia)[b]	• Acute gastrointestinal bleed (with CAP)
• Zoonotic CAP (tularemia, plague, Q fever)	• Acute pancreatitis (with CAP)
• Human influenza A	• Decompensated lung function (with CAP)
• Avian influenza (H5N1)	
• Swine influenza (H1N1)	• Severe CAD, severe cardiomyopathy, or severe valvular disease (with CAP)
• Severe influenza A (with simultaneous *S. aureus* CAP)	
• SARS	
• MERS	
• COVID-19	
• HPS	
• Adenovirus	
• CMV[c]	
• PCP (HIV)	

Infectious Mimics of CAP	Non-infectious Mimics of CAP
• TV ABE (with septic pulmonary emboli)	• ARDS
• Anthrax (hemorrhagic mediastinitis)	• Due to pegylated interferon-α
	• Due to TNF-α antagonists
	• Due to acute pancreatitis
	• Interstitial fibrosis
	• Radiation pneumonitis
	• BOOP

Abbreviations: CAD, coronary artery disease; MI, myocardial infarction; SARS, severe acute respiratory syndrome; CMV, cytomegalovirus; ARDS, acute respiratory distress syndrome; TV, tricuspid valve; ABE, acute bacterial endocarditis; TNF, tumor necrosis factor; HPS, hantavirus pulmonary virus; BOOP, bronchiolitis obliterans organizing pneumonia; MERS, Middle East respiratory syndrome.

[a] Howell-Jolly bodies on peripheral blood smear. Look for disorders associated with hyposplenism (see Table 13.3).

[b] Surgically removed or congenitally absent.

[c] In normal hosts.

TABLE 13.3

Disorders Associated with Functional/Anatomic Hyposplenia

Splenic Disorders	Extra-Splenic Disorders
• Splenectomy	• Sickle cell anemia
• Congenital asplenia	• Sickle/Thalassemia
• Splenic atrophy	• Hemoglobin SC disease
• Impaired splenic blood flow	• Rheumatoid arthritis
• Amyloidosis	• SLE
• Infiltrative disorders of the spleen	• Cirrhosis

Abbreviation: SLE, systemic lupus erythematosus.

TABLE 13.4

Clinical Approach to Severe CAP

I. Presumptive Diagnosis of Severe CAP
- Infiltrate pattern on CXR
- Clinical severity (ABGs on RA)
- Sputum/blood cultures
- Ventilatory and vital organ support

II. Consider Disorders That Mimic Severe CAP
- Chest CT scan to r/o CAP and limit differential diagnostic mimics of severe CAP
- Treat medical disorders mimicking severe CAP

III. Empiric Therapy of Severe Bacterial CAP
- Initiate empiric antibiotic therapy ASAP
- Order additional diagnostic laboratory tests to identify specific CAP pathogens
- Select an agent active against both typical/atypical CAP pathogens
  Moxifloxacin or levofloxacin
  Tigecycline
  Ceftriaxone *plus* doxycycline or azithromycin
- If influenza A pneumonia presents with early focal/segmental infiltrates and rapid cavitation <72 hours, DX = MSSA/CA-MRSA CAP
  Linezolid
  Tigecycline
- If influenza A pneumonia improves/resolves after 5–7 days, followed by subsequent focal/segmental infiltrates after 10–14 days, then *H. influenzae* or *S. pneumoniae* is the likely CAP pathogen
  Moxifloxacin or levofloxacin
  Ceftriaxone

Abbreviations: CAP, community-acquired pneumonia; CXR, chest X-ray; CT, computed tomography.

DISORDERS ASSOCIATED WITH IMPAIRED B LYMPHOCYTE/HUMORAL IMMUNITY

The disorders associated with impaired B lymphocyte function are those that decrease HI. The pathogens predisposed to by impaired B lymphocyte function are the same, regardless of the underlying disorder. The CAP pathogens associated with impaired HI are the encapsulated pulmonary pathogens, i.e., *S. pneumoniae* and *H. influenzae*. The conditions associated with decreased HI commonly encountered in clinical practice include hyposplenia/asplenia, multiple myeloma, cirrhosis, systemic lupus erythematosus (SLE), and chronic lymphocytic leukemia (CLL) (combined B/T lymphocyte disorder: HI > cell-mediated immunity [CMI]). The degree of hyposplenism may be inferred from the CBC by noting the concentration of Howell-Jolly bodies (percentage) in the peripheral smear. The number of Howell-Jolly bodies is inversely proportional to the degree of splenic dysfunction. The most common clinical presentation of CAP associated with hyposplenism is an "apparently normal" host with good cardiopulmonary function that presents as otherwise-unexplained severe CAP. SCAP often

TABLE 13.5

Epidemiologic Clues to the Etiology of Severe CAP

Epidemiologic Clues[a]	CAP Pathogen Associations
• Air travel	Legionnaire's disease
	Influenza A COVID-19
	Avian influenza (H5N1)
	Swine influenza (H1N1)
• Rodent exposure	SARS
	HPS
	Plague
• Recent contact with influenza/ILI	Influenza A ILIs
• Deer/rabbit/ticks	Tularemia
• Birds/poultry	Avian influenza (H5N1)
• Closed populations/crowded exposures	Adenovirus
• Cats	Q fever
	Tularemia
	Plague
• Camels	MERS
• Pigs	Swine influenza (H1N1)
• Construction/water/air conditioning	Legionnaire's disease
• HIV/organ transplants/	PCP
immunosuppressive drugs/steroids	Legionnaire's disease

Abbreviations: SARS, severe acute respiratory syndrome; CAP, community-acquired pneumonia; HPS, hantavirus pulmonary syndrome; PCP, *Pneumocystis (carinii) jirovecii* pneumonia; MERS, Middle East respiratory syndrome.

[a] Recent close contact history.

TABLE 13.6

Clinical Clues to the Causes of Severe CAP

Clinical Clues	CAP Pathogen Associations
• Hyperacute onset	Influenza A COVID-19
	Avian influenza (H5N1)
	Swine influenza (H1N1)
	MERS
	SARS
	Tularemia
	Plague
• Relative bradycardia	Legionnaire's disease
	Q fever
• Severe myalgias	Influenza A COVID-19
	Avian influenza (H5N1)
	Swine influenza (H1N1)
• Mental confusion	Legionnaire's disease
• Prominent headache	Tularemia
	Q fever
• Conjunctival suffusion	Adenovirus
	Influenza A COVID-19
	Legionnaire's disease
• Sore throat	Avian influenza (H5N1)
	Swine influenza (H1N1)
• *H. labialis*	*S. pneumoniae*
• Chest pain	
Substernal	HPS
Pleuritic	Influenza A COVID-19
• Watery diarrhea/abdominal pain	Legionnaire's disease
	Swine influenza (H1N1)
• Splenomegaly	Q fever
	CMV

Abbreviations: SARS, severe acute respiratory syndrome; CAP, community-acquired pneumonia; CMV, cytolomegalovirus; HPS, hantavirus pulmonary syndrome.

due to host factors e.g.,impaired cardiopulmonary function or decreased immune rather than pathogen virulence, per se Patients presenting with CAP and hypotension/shock have impaired splenic function, influenza alone or with superimposed *Staphylococcus aureus* pneumonia, or unrelated systemic disorder causing hypotension/shock, i.e., acute MI and pulmonary embolus. Virulent viral/zoonotic pathogens aside, normal hosts do not present with severe CAP with hypotension/shock [1,8–10,26–30].

DISORDERS ASSOCIATED WITH IMPAIRED T LYMPHOCYTE FUNCTION CELL-MEDIATED IMMUNITY

Patients with impaired T lymphocyte/macrophage function have decreased CMI. Disorders associated with impaired CMI predispose to CAP due to intracellular pathogens, i.e., viruses, *Rickettsiae*, systemic mycoses, and intracellular bacteria. Impaired CMI does not, per se, predispose to bacterial CAP pathogens. However, all compromised hosts may be infected with the same usual CAP pathogens of normal hosts. Therefore, the intracellular pathogens associated with severe CAP with decreased CMI are predominantly intracellular pathogens, i.e., *Pneumocystis (carinii) jirovecii* (PCP), cytomegalovirus (CMV), and *Legionella* sp. The most common disorders associated with decreased CMI include chronic/

high-dose corticosteroid therapy, immunosuppressive therapy, tumor necrosis factor (TNF)-α antagonists, organ transplants, and HIV [1,8,10,31–35].

DISORDERS ASSOCIATED WITH COMBINED IMPAIRED B AND T LYMPHOCYTE FUNCTION (HI AND CMI)

Excluding CLL, most disorders with combined immune defects are those with underlying B lymphocyte disorders, combined with an immunosuppressant drug, which, in addition, decreases CMI, i.e., inflammatory bowel disease treated with monoclonal antibody therapy, steroids, or immunosuppressives. The clinician should appreciate the additive effects of combined immune defects. For example, SLE is a pure B lymphocyte defect with decreased HI, but SLE patients with flare resemble CLL with predominantly impaired HI and decreased CMI. However, SLE patients with flare on

TABLE 13.7

Non-Specific Laboratory Clues to the Etiology of Severe CAP

Non-specific Laboratory Test Clues	CAP Pathogen Associations
• Leukopenia	Influenza A, COVID-19, SARS, MERS, adenovirus, CMV
• Relative lymphopenia	Legionnaire's disease, adenovirus, CMV, SARS, MERS, influenza A, COVID-19, HPS, PCP
• Acute thrombocytopenia	Adenovirus, CMV, SARS, HPS, influenza A, COVID-19, MERS
• Acute thrombocytosis	Q fever, *M. pneumoniae*
• ↑↑↑ LDH	PCP
	Avian influenza (H5N1)
• ↑↑↑ Ferritin levels	COVID-19
	Legionnaire's disease
• ↓ Serum sodium	Legionnaire's disease
• ↓ Serum phosphorus	Legionnaire's disease
• ↑ Cold agglutinins	*M. pneumoniae*
	Adenovirus
	Q fever
• ↑ AST/ALT	Legionnaire's disease, Q Fever, CMV, adenovirus, HPS, SARS, MERS, influenza A, COVID-19
• ↑ 1,3 β-glucan	PCP

Abbreviations: CAP, community-acquired pneumonia; SARS, severe acute respiratory syndrome; PCP, *Pneumocystis (carinii) jirovecii* pneumonia; CMV, cytomegalovirus; HPS, hantavirus pulmonary syndrome.

corticosteroids/immunosuppressive therapy add to the "net immunosuppression," further impairing CMI, a markedly impaired T lymphocyte function not unlike that of transplant patients [1,4,17,36,37].

CLINICAL APPROACH TO SEVERE CAP BY PATTERN OF INFILTRATES ON CXR AND DEGREE OF HYPOXEMIA

Normal hosts with CAP and without significant pre-existing cardiopulmonary disease usually are due to typical pulmonary pathogens and present with focal or segmental/lobar defects with/without small pleural effusion. Pleural effusion is pathogen dependent and with CAP. The CAP with pleural effusion DDx includes group A streptococci, commonly with *H. influenzae,* and uncommonly with *S. pneumoniae.* The CAP with ill-defined non-segmental/lobar infiltrates usually due to atypical CAP organisms, i.e., *Mycoplasma pneumoniae,* which may present as severe CAP in compromised hosts. Radiographically, *Legionella* characteristically presents with rapidly progressive bilateral asymmetric infiltrates. Importantly, it is the behavior

of the CXR infiltrates rather than the location/description of the infiltrates, per se, which suggests the possibility of Legionnaire's disease [1,8,10].

If the CAP patients' infiltrates are perihilar/interstitial, the diagnosis is not due to usual typical/atypical CAP pulmonary pathogens. Bilateral symmetrical/interstitial infiltrates suggest an intracellular pathogen, e.g., PCP, CMV, influenza A, avian influenza (H5N1, H3N2), and swine influenza (H1N1). Excluding CAP mimics, bilateral interstitial infiltrates CAP presenting as severe CAP are due to intracellular pathogens, associated with various degrees of hypoxemia. A combination of bilateral perihilar/interstitial infiltrates, and hypoxemia, with a ↓ DLCO (carbon monoxide diffusing capacity)/↑ A-a gradient indicates a diffusion defect due to interstitial process, e.g., PCP and viral CAP. There are many non-infectious mimics of CAP that may present with bilateral infiltrates that are not infectious. In the CCU, the common mimics of CAP include acute pulmonary edema (due to fluid overload/acute MI), pulmonary emboli/infarcts, SLE pneumonitis, pulmonary vasculitis, pulmonary drug reactions, bronchiolitis obliterans organizing pneumonia (BOOP), pulmonary leukostasis, pulmonary hemorrhage, and acute respiratory distress syndrome (ARDS). Excluding viral pneumonias or PCP, most mimics of severe CAP may have impressive pulmonary infiltrates but are *not* accompanied by severe hypoxemia, i.e., ↓ DL_{CO}/↑ A-a gradient (>30) [1,8,10] (Table 13.8).

TABLE 13.8

Diagnostic Approach to Diffuse Pulmonary Infiltrates and Hypoxemia with Severe CAP in the CCU

	Bilateral/Diffuse Pulmonary Infiltrates	
Acute	Hypoxemia (A-a Gradient <35)	Severe Hypoxemia (A-a Gradient >35)
Non-infectious causes	• Congestive heart failure • Pulmonary embolus/infarction • Pulmonary hemorrhage	• ARDS
Infectious causes	• Legionnaire's disease • Bacterial CAP • TB	• Influenza • ILI viral pneumonias • CMV • HSV • Adenovirus • MERS
Subacute		
Non-infectious causes	• Drug induced pneumonitis	• BOOP • Sarcoidosis • Idiopathic pulmonary fibrosis • Lymphangitic spread

Source: Cunha, B.A., *Inf. Dis. Clin. N. Am.,* 15, 591–612, 2001.

SEVERE CAP WITH CAVITATION

Cavitation on the CXR/chest CT scan is an important diagnostic finding in determining the etiology of severe CAP. Acute CAPs with cavitation indicates a necrotic/hemorrhagic pneumonia, e.g., *P. aeruginosa* and *S. aureus*. The DDx of severe CAP with cavitation may be approached clinically by the rapidity of the cavitary process. Cavitation is not a feature of *S. pneumoniae* or *H. influenzae* CAP. Rarely, severe *S. pneumoniae* with cavitation may occur only with HIV or TNF-α antagonists. Clinically, cavitation <72 hours occurring in a patient with CAP the DDx is limited to *S. aureus* (with concomitant influenza) pneumonia (Table 13.8).

In adults, human seasonal influenza A may usually present as influenza pneumonia alone and less commonly with superimposed *S. aureus* pneumonia with focal segmental/lobar infiltrates. The *S. aureus* (methicillin-susceptible *S. aureus* [MSSA]/CA-MRSA) CAP occurs only with influenza pneumonia and not alone. The third clinical presentation of influenza A pneumonia is that of initial influenza pneumonia, followed by a period of improvement (~1 week), which is then followed by *S. pneumoniae* or *H. influenzae* pneumonia with new fevers and focal/segmental infiltrates on CXR. Patients presenting with influenza pneumonia A may have an unremarkable CXR early, even with hypoxemia present. Bilateral segmental interstitial infiltrates may appear in 48 hours and are accompanied by severe hypoxemia. The *S. pneumoniae* and *H. influenzae* CAPs following influenza A pneumonia sequentially after improvement are not, unlike *S. aureus*, accompanied by cavitation. However, if influenza pneumonia A presents simultaneously with focal/segmental infiltrates and rapid cavitation in <72 hours, the likely pathogen is *S. aureus* (MSSA or MRSA). Avian influenza (H5N1 and H3N2) pneumonia and swine influenza (H1N1) pneumonia have not been complicated by simultaneous subsequent bacterial pneumonia.

With CAP, cavitation occurring after 3–5 days points to *Klebsiella pneumoniae* as the pathogen, which occurs almost exclusively in patients with alcoholism. Therefore, the clinical history plus the speed of cavitation points to the diagnosis, easily confirmed by Gram stain/culture of the sputum/blood. The *K. pneumoniae* CAP often presents as severe CAP. Acute CAP with cavitation after 5–7 days is most often due to aspiration pneumonia. Unless the aspiration is bilateral/massive, such patients do not present as severe CAP [29,30,38]. These patients usually present with CAP that becomes more severe as cavitation becomes apparent after more than 1 week with bilateral massive aspiration [8,10] (Table 13.9).

OTHER RADIOLOGIC CLUES: MEDIASTINAL ADENOPATHY AND ROUND PNEUMONIAS

Some radiologic findings on CXR or chest CT scans are helpful when present. "Round pneumonias" have round or oval infiltrates and limit DDx possibilities. Although the DDx includes non-infectious etiologies, if the patient has SCAP,

TABLE 13.9
Severe CAP with Cavitation

Rapid cavitation (<3 days)[a]
- *S. aureus*[a] (MSSA/CA-MRSA,[b] CO-MRSA)

Moderately rapid cavitation (3–5 days)
- *K. pneumoniae*

Slow cavitation (>5 days)
- Aspiration pneumonia (oral anaerobes)

Abbreviations: CAP, community-acquired pneumonia; MSSA, methicillin-susceptible *S. aureus*; CA-MRSA, community-acquired methicillin-resistant *S. aureus*.
[a]   Only in patients with influenza A pneumonia, or an influenza-like illness (ILI) pneumonia or adenovirus.
[b]   Only *S. aureus* and *P. aeruginosa* cause rapid cavitation in <3 days. *P. aeruginosa* is not a CAP pathogen except with cystic fibrosis/chronic bronchiectasis.

TABLE 13.10
Differential Diagnosis of "Round Pneumonia" in Hospitalized Adults

Infectious Causes
Legionella species
Streptococcus pneumoniae
Haemophilus influenzae
Q fever
RSV
Septic pulmonary emboli

Non-Infectious Causes[a]
Bronchogenic carcinoma
Round atelectasis
Bronchiolitis obliterans organizing pneumonia
Wegener's granulomatosis
Rheumatoid nodules

Source: Cunha, B.A. et al., *Respir. Care*, 58, 80–82, 2013.
[a]   Chronic infiltrates present on CCU admission.

then diagnoses are limited to Legionnaire's disease, Q fever, or *S. pneumoniae* (Table 13.10).

Mediastinal adenopathy in hospitalized adults with SCAP has a DDx that includes PCP, Legionnaire's disease, *S. pneumoniae*, or *M. pneumoniae*. Primary tuberculosis (TB) does not present as SCAP but rather is in the DDx of CAP (Table 13.11).

EMPIRIC THERAPY FOR SEVERE CAP

Appropriate empiric therapy depends on identifying the most likely pathogen. The pathogen range is predictable by host factors [8,10,39]. Severe CAP may present with focal segmental lobar infiltrates or bilateral interstitial infiltrates, with or without accompanying hypoxemia. The patient's history is important in identifying previously diagnosed disorders associated with specific immune defects. Combined with the

TABLE 13.11

Differential Diagnosis of Legionnaire's Disease with Mediastinal Adenopathy in the CCU

Infectious Causes of Mediastinal Adenopathy	Non-Infectious Causes of Mediastinal Adenopathy
• Legionnaire's disease[a]	**Malignant Causes**
• *S. pneumoniae*[a]	• Hodgkin's lymphoma
• *M. pneumoniae*[a]	• Acute lymphoblastic leukemia
• Primary tuberculosis[a]	• Chronic lymphatic leukemia
• HIV (PCP)	• Lymphosarcoma
	• Giant follicular lymphoma
	• Bronchogenic carcinoma
	• Metastases
	Benign Causes
	• Sarcoidosis

Source: Cunha, B.A. et al., *Eur. J. Clin. Micro. Inf. Dis.*, 2018.
[a] Unilateral hilar adenopathy.

CXR appearance, the appearance/distribution of infiltrates and the presence or absence of hypoxemia limit the DDx possibilities [8,10,40,41].

An apparently normal host presenting with severe CAP with focal/segmental infiltrates should be treated for the usual typical and atypical CAP pathogens. Appropriate empiric therapy should be started as soon as the diagnosis of CAP is suspected [2,10,12,42–45].

Apparently, normal hosts presenting with near-normal CXR and profound hypoxemia should be considered as having viral pneumonia or PCP. If severe pneumonia occurs during influenza season, then influenza is a likely diagnostic possibility. A clue to otherwise-unsuspected HIV is often one or more isolated cytopenias, and PCP is likely if accompanied by an otherwise-unexplained, highly elevated serum lactic dehydrogenase (LDH) and β 1, 3, glucan levels. The PCP is an HIV-defining illness and is not an uncommon cause of CAP in HIV patients. Patients on steroids/immunosuppressive therapy, and organ transplants, when present with acute CAP with focal, segmental lobar infiltration unaccompanied by severe hypoxemia should be treated for the usual pathogens affecting normal hosts with CAP. Organ transplants presenting with bilateral symmetrical/interstitial infiltrates may be approached as those with mild/moderate hypoxemia versus those with severe hypoxemia. In such CAP patients, the absence of a significant diffusion defect (A-a gradient <35) suggests pulmonary hemorrhage, pulmonary embolus, or another non-infectious process. Those with bilateral infiltrates, accompanied by a profound oxygen diffusion defect (A–a gradient >35), viral pneumonias, or PCP, are the most likely diagnostic infectious possibilities. The common non-infectious causes of bilateral pulmonary infiltrates with severe hypoxemia and no fever include BOOP and ARDS [1,8,10,47,48].

The clinicians should not use the "shot gun" approach to treating severe CAP cases based on the mistaken notion that there are many potential pathogens. The diagnostic process is based on a syndromic approach utilizing history, physical, and laboratory abnormalities; CXR/chest CT appearance; and findings of severity of hypoxemia with limited diagnostic possibilities. Rapid cavitation (<72 hours) with severe CAP points to MSSA or MRSA CAP superimposed on underlying influenza A pneumonia. Treat all such patients for MRSA [10,19,35,49–58]. Excluding patients with impaired CMI, severe cases of CAP with focal, segmental/lobar defects should be treated the same way as normal hosts with antibiotics directed against the usual typical/atypical CAP pathogens (Table 13.12).

Subacute/chronic CAP with focal/segmental infiltrates (days/weeks) in patients with decreased CMI does not present as severe CAP. Clinicians should be aware of the non-infectious mimics of CAP both in the normal and compromised hosts. The mimics of CAP are common and can usually be easily diagnosed by physical findings, CXR or chest CT appearance, and routine laboratory tests. In CAP patients unresponsive "to therapy" either remain febrile or" no regression in infiltrates to apparently appropriate antibiotic therapy, transbronchial or open lung biopsy may be necessary for a definitive diagnosis. Compromised hosts respond more slowly than normal hosts to effective antibiotic therapy. Normal hosts with severe CAP usually show some improvement in 3–5 days, but in compromised hosts, ~7–10 days may be needed before clinical improvement is noted. The duration of antibiotic therapy, IV/PO, for CAP in normal hosts is 1–2 weeks, whereas in compromised hosts, 2–3 weeks are often necessary because of impaired host defenses [1,8,10].

The prognosis in severe CAP is also a function of host factors, i.e., cardiopulmonary reserve/impaired immunity. Inappropriate/delayed empiric therapy lengthens LOS and is associated with a worse prognosis [1,10,59].

CLINICAL SUMMARY

Patients presenting with severe CAP often require ventilatory, volume, or pressor support. The clinician's first task is to support vital functions and rapidly consider the treatable/reversible causes of severe CAP mimics. The cause of CAP mimics is usually fairly straightforward based on history, physical findings, and routine laboratory tests. The CXR/chest CT scan is helpful in eliminating diagnostic possibilities, in limiting diagnostic possibilities, and sometimes in making a specific diagnosis.

If the mimics of severe CAP can be reasonably ruled out, the clinician's next task is to determine the likely pathogen based on history, physical findings, routine laboratory tests, and aspects of the clinical presentation, including assessment of cardiopulmonary function, HI/CMI status, and the degree of hypoxemia.

The most common cause of severe CAP in normal hosts is viral pneumonias. In adults, the classic severe viral pneumonia is influenza A pneumonia. As mentioned previously, influenza A pneumonia most commonly occurs alone. Alternately, it may be complicated by bacterial CAP, either simultaneously

TABLE 13.12

Differential Diagnostic Findings in Severe CAP in the CCU

	LD	Mycoplasma pneumoniae	Streptococcus pneumoniae	Plague	Anthrax	Tularemia	Influenza	COVID-19	Mers	RSV	HPS	Adenovirus	PCP
Symptoms													
Headache	+	+	−	−	−	+++	+++	++	+	−	−	++	−
Fever/Chills	+++	+	+++	+++	+	+	+++	+++	+++		+	++	−
Prominent Fatigue	−	−	−				+++	+++					−
Myalgias	+	−	−	+		+++	+++	++	+++	+	+	+	−
Dry cough	+	+++	−				+++	+++	++	+++	+	+++	+
Shortness of breath	+	+	−	+++	+++	+	+++	+++	+++	+++	+++	+++	+++
Sore throat	−	+	−	−	−	+	+++	++	+++	+++	−	++	−
Nausea/Vomiting	−	−	−	+	+	−	+	+	+	−	−	+	−
Diarrhea	+	+	−	−	−	−	+	+	−	−	−	+	−
Abdominal pain	+	−	−	−	−	−	−	−	−	−	−	−	−
Hemoptysis	+	−	−	+	+	+	+	+	−	−	−	−	−
Signs													
Relative bradycardia	+	−	−	−	−	−	−	−	−	−	−	−ᵃ	−
Tachycardia	−	−	−	+	+	−	+	+	+	−	+	+	+
Conjunctival suffusion	−	−	−	−	−	+	+	−	+	−	−	−	−
Diminished breath sounds	−	−	+	+	−	−	+++	+++	+++	+++	−	++	+++
Acute renal failure (ARF)	+	−	−	−	−	−	−	−	−	−	+	+	−
Laboratory tests													
Normal WBC count	−	−	−	−	−	−	+	+	+	+	−	−	+
Leukopenia	−	−	−	−	−	−	+++	+	+++	+++	+	+++	+++ᵇ
Relative lymphopenia	+++	−	−	−	−	−	+++	+++	+++	+	−	+++	+++ᵇ
Thrombocytopenia	−	−	−	−	−	−	+	+	+++	+	+	+++	+++ᵇ
Highly elevated ESR	+	−	+	−	−	−	−	−	−	−	−	−	−
Highly elevated CRP	+	−	−	−	−	−	−	+	−	−	−	+	−
Elevated serum transaminases	+	−	−	−	−	−	+	+	+	−	−	+	+ᵇ
Elevated LDH	+	−	−	−	−	−	+	+	+	−	−	+	+++
Elevated CPK	+++	−	−	−	−	−	+++	+++	−	−	−	−	−
↑ β 1,3 glucan	−	−	−	−	−	−	−	−	−	−	−	−	+
↑ A-a gradient (>35)	−	−	−	−	−	−	+	+	+	+	+	+	+
Chest film													
Normal/minimal basilar infiltrates (early)	−	−	−	−	−	−	+	+	+	+	+	−	+
Unilateral infiltrate (early)	+	+	+	−	−	+	−	−	+	+	−	−	−
Bilateral infiltrates (late)	+	−	−	+	+	−	+	+	+	+	+	+	+
Pleural effusion	−	+	−	−	+	+	−	−	−	−	−	+	−
Cavitation	−												
ARDS (severe cases)	−	−	−	−	−	−	+	+	+	+	+	+	+

Source: Cunha, B.A., *Pneumonia Essentials*, 3rd ed., Jones & Bartlett, Sudbury, MA, 2010; Cunha, C.A., and Opal, S.M., *Virulence*, 5, 650–654, 2014.

Abbreviations: LD, Legionnaire's disease; RSV, respiratory syncytial virus; HPS, hantavirus pulmonary syndrome; MERS, Middle Eastern respiratory syndrome; CPK, creatine phosphokinase; ARDS, acute respiratory distress syndrome; CRP, C-reactive protein; PCP, *Pneumocystis (carinii) jirovecii* pneumonia.

ᵃ   No bradycardia/relative bradycardia unless on high dose ribavirin.

ᵇ   Due to underlying HIV, not PCP.

initially (with MSSA/CA-MRSA) or sequentially after a 5- to 7-day interval of improvement with subsequent CAP due to *S. pneumoniae* or *H. influenzae*. In cases without bacterial superinfection, prognosis is related to degree and duration of hypoxemia. In pandemic influenza A, as in 1918–1919, the majority of the deaths occurred in young, healthy adults without comorbidities and were due to severe hypoxemia uncomplicated by bacterial pneumonia. Unlike influenza A, avian influenza (H5N1) is not efficiently transmitted from person to person and for this reason does not, as yet, have pandemic potential. However, in contrast to human influenza A, avian influenza (H5N1) is fatal in the majority of cases and affects primarily young healthy adults. Similarly, with Middle East respiratory syndrome, deaths from avian influenza (H5N1, H3N2) occurs from severe hypoxemia uncomplicated by bacterial pneumonia.

In the spring of 2009, the swine influenza (H1N1) pandemic began in Mexico and quickly spread throughout the world. Although large numbers of the population were affected by swine influenza (H1N1), there were relatively few mortalities. In the fatal cases of swine influenza (H1N1) pneumonia, patients died from severe hypoxemia uncomplicated by bacterial pneumonia. The majority of fatalities with swine influenza (H1N1) pneumonia were young healthy adults without comorbidities [60–65].

SUMMARY

The diagnosis of CAP is clinical and based on imaging and clinical findings. Presumptive clinical diagnosis is the basis for initial appropriate antimicrobial therapy (Table 13.12). Accurate diagnosis, not adequate therapy, is paramount in medicine and infectious disease. Diagnosticians are readily able to work through differential diagnostic possibilities. Recognizing and associating (linking) the key characteristic clinical findings of the most likely pneumonias in the differential diagnosis are the most important tasks of the diagnostician. Recognizing key diagnostic eliminators to rule out diagnoses is nearly as important, i.e., narrowing the differential diagnosis, thereby eliminating unnecessary excessive diagnostic testing as airway microbiologic diagnosis. In all adults presenting with CAP, the CXR is important as a diagnostic eliminator, i.e., the CXR does not diagnose the causative organism, i.e., does not indicate a specific diagnosis, but it is most helpful as a diagnostic eliminator of diagnoses. With adult hospitalized CAP patients, the lack of a segmental/lobar infiltrate at the pleura effectively eliminates typical bacterial CAP pathogens and suggests a possible viral pneumonia. The only viral CAP that mimics a typical bacterial CAP is adenoviral pneumonia. A febrile, hypoxemic hospitalized adult with a clear CXR with mild peripheral/diffuse fuzzy infiltrates limits the diagnostic possibilities to influenza, an influenza-loke illness (ILI) pneumonia, or PCP.

The task of the diagnostician is a clinical correlation of CXR findings with clinical findings looking for associative findings. A hospitalized adult with CAP and a fuzzy non-segmented/

lobar infiltrate(s) limits diagnosis to *M. pneumoniae* and Legionnaire's disease, which cannot be easily differentiated on CXR. Associated clinical findings readily separate these entities, i.e., fever of Legionnaire's disease is accompanied by relative bradycardia, while mycoplasma CAP is not. If transaminases are elevated, Legionnaire's disease is favored, since hepatic involvement is not a feature of mycoplasma CAP. Furthermore, an otherwise-unexplained highly elevated ESR and/or ferritin again points to a diagnosis of Legionnaire's disease and not features of mycoplasma CAP. Conversely, with the CXR findings described, the presence of highly elevated cold agglutinins (>1:64) eliminates Legionnaire's disease and points to mycoplasma as the correct diagnosis period deferred testing.

PNEUMONIA BIOMARKERS (ESR, CRP, AND FERRITIN)

Aside from CXR's appearances and clinical correlations, e.g., CAP with height of fever, relative bradycardia, headache, mental confusion, sore throat, severe myalgias, microscopic hematuria, hypophosphatemia, hyponatremia, elevated CPK, elevated ferritin, elevated transaminases, and splenomegaly.

The diagnostic significance of non-specific findings is increased if several are present. Also, diagnostic significance is increased by the company they keep, e.g., adult hospitalized with influenza CAP may have an elevated CPK and transaminitis but not a highly elevated ESR or ferritin level. Degree of abnormality, of itself, increases the diagnostic specificity; e.g., many disorders are associated with elevated ESR, but if the ESR >100 mm/h in an adult CAP, the diagnosis is narrowed to *S. pneumoniae* and Legionnaire's disease (easily differentiated by the presence of absence of relative bradycardia).

Similarly, no/minimal ferritin elevations may occur in a variety of disorders, but if it is highly elevated (>2 xn) in an adult with CAP, diagnostic possibilities are narrowed to Legionnaire's disease. Since clinicians may not be familiar with the diagnostic significance of characteristic clinical findings in adults hospitalized with CAP, there has been an attempt to use biomarkers as a substitute for clinical diagnostic reasoning. With few notable exceptions, e.g., highly elevated ESR, CRP, and ferritin levels, other biomarkers have not been very useful in the diagnosis or prognosis of CAP, e.g., procalcitonin (PCT) levels. Relying on biomarkers also readily leads to excessive/unnecessary empiric treatment at the expense of a carefully considered diagnostic approach. As mentioned previously, the most useful biomarkers for CAP have been the ESR and CRP. In hospitalized adults with CAP, mild to moderate elevations of ESR and CRP are unhelpful, but an otherwise-unexplained high elevation, i.e., ESR >100 mm/h and/or CRP >35, points to Legionnaire's disease. Highly elevated ESR with a CRP <35 suggests *S. pneumoniae*.

Serum PCT levels have been used to bypass the diagnostic process in CAP. There are several interpretational difficulties with PCT. First, PCT is not commonly elevated (>0.15 ng/mL) with infection, e.g., CAP some have contended that PCT levels of >0.25 ng/mL should warrant "antimicrobial therapy". Unfortunately, PCT levels (>10 ng/mL) may be elevated due to a variety of non-infectious disorders commonly encountered in the CCU in severe CAP patients, e.g., renal insufficiency (AKI/ATN), recent surgery, hypotension, shock, pancreatitis, immunosuppressive medications, steroids, and febrile neutropenia, and are a normal variant in the elderly.

In summary, PCT initial or serial elevations are all too frequently false positive or more disturbingly false negative. Needless to say, PCT is not useful as a marker for disease severity resolution of infection. The PCT levels or serial PCT levels certainly are not a marker for discontinuation of antibiotics therapy, which remains a clinical determination.

CONCLUSIONS

Optimal empiric therapy is based on correlating epidemiologic and clinical findings to rapidly arrive at a presumptive clinical diagnosis directed at the most likely pulmonary pathogen. Empiric therapy is continued, as less likely diagnostic possibilities are eliminated. If clinically effective, empiric therapy should be continued and a full course of therapy (1–2 weeks).

REFERENCES

1. Cunha BA. Severe community-acquired pneumonia. *Crit Care Clin* 1998;14:105–118.
2. Cunha BA. Severe community-acquired pneumonia: Determinants of severity and approach to therapy. *Infect Med* 2005;22:53–58.
3. Wilson PA, Ferguson J. Severe community-acquired pneumonia: An Australian perspective. *Intern Med J* 2005;35:699–705.
4. Moine P, Vercken J-P, Chevret S, et al. Severe community-acquired pneumonia. *Chest* 1994;105:1487–1495.
5. Lim WS, van der Eerden M, Laing R, et al. Defining community-acquired pneumonia severity on presentation to hospital: An international derivation and validation study. *Thorax* 2003;58:377–382.
6. Marrie TJ, Shariatzadeh MR. Community-acquired pneumonia requiring admission to an intensive care unit: A descriptive study. *Medicine* 2007;86:103–111.
7. Restrepo MI, Mortensen EM, Velez JA, et al. A comparative study of community-acquired pneumonia patients admitted to the ward and the ICU. *Chest* 2008;133:610–617.
8. Cunha BA. Pulmonary infections in the compromised host. *Infect Dis Clin* 2001;16:591–612.
9. Cunha BA. Infections in acutely ill non-leukopenic compromised hosts with diabetes mellitus, SLE, asplenia, or on steroids. *Crit Care Clin* 1998;8:263–282.
10. Cunha BA, ed. *Pneumonia Essentials* (3rd ed.). Sudbury, MA: Jones & Barlett, 2009.
11. Cunha BA. Community-acquired pneumonia: Reality revisited. *Am J Med* 2000;108:436–437.
12. Dean NC, Silver MP, Bateman KA, et al. Decreased mortality after implementation of a treatment guideline for community-acquired pneumonia. *Am J Med* 2001;110:451–457.
13. Jennings LC, Anderson TP, Beynon KA, et al. Incidence and characteristics of viral community-acquired pneumonia in adults. *Thorax* 2008; 63:42–48.
14. Lee N, Rainer TH, IP M, et al. Role of laboratory variables in differentiating SARS-coronavirus from other causes of community-acquired pneumonia within the first 72 h of hospitalization. *Eur J Clin Microbiol Infect Dis* 2006;25:765–772.
15. Rainer TH, Lee N, Ip M, et al. Features discriminating SARS from other severe viral respiratory tract infections. *Eur J Clin Microbiol Infect Dis* 2007;26:21–29.
16. Cunha BA, Pherez F, Walls N. Severe cytomegalovirus (CMV) community-acquired pneumonia (CAP) in an immunocompetent host. *Heart Lung* 2009;38:243–248.
17. Cunha BA. Severe adenovirus mimicking Legionella community-acquired pneumonia (CAP). *Eur J Clin Microbiol Infect Dis* 2009;28:313–315.
18. Cunha BA, Nausheen S, Busch L. Severe Q fever mimicking legionella community acquired pneumonia (CAP): The diagnostic importance of cold agglutinins, anti-smooth muscle antibodies, and thrombocytosis. *Heart Lung* 2009;38:354–362.
19. Cunha BA. Viral & mycoplasma pneumonias. In: Rackel ER, Bope ED, eds. *Conn's Current Therapy* (60th ed.). Philadelphia, PA: W.B. Saunders, 2008.
20. Cunha BA. Influenza: Historical aspects of epidemics and pandemics. *Infect Dis Clin* 2004;38:141–156.
21. Janssens JP, Gauthey L, Hermmann F, et al. Community-acquired pneumonia in older patients. *J Am Geriatr Soc* 1996;44:539–544.
22. MacFarlane JT, Finch RG, Ward MJ, et al. Hospital study of adult community-acquired pneumonia. *Lancet* 1982;2:255–258.
23. Klimek JJ, Ajemian E, Fontecchio S, et al. Community-acquired bacterial pneumonia requiring admission to hospital. *Am J Infect Control* 1983;11:79–82.
24. Leroy O, Santre C, Beuscart C, et al. A five-year study of severe community acquired pneumonia with emphasis on prognosis in patients admitted to an intensive care unit. *Intensive Care Med* 1995;21:24–31.
25. Angus DC, Marrie TJ, Obrosky DS, et al. Severe community-acquired pneumonia. *Am J Respir Crit Care Med* 2002;166:717–723.
26. Wara DW. Host defense against *Streptococcus pneumoniae*: The role of the spleen. *Rev Infect Dis* 1981;3:299.
27. Gopal V, Bisno AL. Fulminant pneumococcal infection in "normal" asplenic hosts. *Arch Intern Med* 1977;137:1526.
28. Cunha BA. Community-acquired pneumonias in SLE. *J Crit Illn* 1997;13:779–783.
29. de Roux A, Cavalcanti M, Marcos MA, et al. Impact of alcohol abuse in the etiology and severity of community-acquired pneumonia. *Chest* 2006;129:1219–1225.
30. Johnson DH, Cunha BA. Infections in alcoholic cirrhosis. *Infect Dis Clin* 2001;16:363–372.
31. van Risemsdijk, van Overbeeke IC, van den Berg B. Severe Legionnaire's disease requiring intensive care treatment. *Neth J Med* 1996;49:185–188.
32. Pedro-Botet ML, Sopena N, Garcia-Cruz A, et al. *Streptococcus pneumoniae* and *Legionella pneumophila* pneumonia in HIV-infected patients. *Scand J Infect Dis* 2007;39:122–128.
33. Cunha BA. Community-acquired pneumonia in HIV patients. *Clin Infect Dis* 2001;16:363–372.
34. Cunha BA. Clinical manifestations and antimicrobial therapy of methicillin resistant *Staphylococcus aureus* (MRSA). *Clin Microbiol Infect* 2005;11:33–42.
35. Cunha BA. Simplified clinical approach to community acquired MRSA (CA-MRSA) infections. *J Hosp Infect* 2008;68:271–273.

36. Zimmer C, Beiderlinden M, Peters J. Lethal acute respiratory distress syndrome during anti-TNF alpha therapy for rheumatoid arthritis. *Clin Rheumatol* 2006;25:430–432.

37. Gotoh S, Nishimura T, Takahashi O, et al. Adrenal function in patients with community-acquired pneumonia. *Eur Respir J* 2008;31:1268–1273.

38. Jong GM, Hsiue TR, Chen CR, et al. Rapidly fatal outcome of bacteremic *Klebsiella* pneumonia in alcoholics. *Chest* 1995;107:214–217.

39. Hohenthal U, Vainionpaa R, Meurman O, et al. Etiological diagnosis of community acquired pneumonia: Utility of rapid microbiological methods with respect to disease severity. *Scand J Infect Dis* 2008;40:131–138.

40. Bruns AH, Oosterheert JJ, Prokop M, et al. Patterns of resolution of chest radiograph abnormalities in adults hospitalized with severe community-acquired pneumonia. *Clin Infect Dis* 2007;45:983–991.

41. Shorr AF, Khashab MM, Xiang JX, et al. Levofloxacin 750-mg for 5 days for the treatment of hospitalized fine risk class III/IV community-acquired pneumonia patients. *Respir Med* 2006;100:2129–2136.

42. Cunha BA. Empiric therapy of community-acquired pneumonia. *Chest* 2004;125:1913–1919.

43. Cunha BA. Clinical relevance of penicillin resistant Streptococcus pneumoniae. *Semin Respir Infect Dis* 2002; 17:204–214.

44. Cunha BA. Empiric antibiotic therapy for community-acquired pneumonia: Guidelines for the perplexed? *Chest* 2004;125:1913–1921.

45. Martinez FJ. Monotherapy versus dual therapy for community-acquired pneumonia in hospitalized patients. *Clin Infect Dis* 2004;38:328–340.

46. Oosterheert JJ, Bonten MJ, Schneider MM, et al. Effectiveness of early switch from intravenous to oral antibiotics in severe community acquired pneumonia: Multicentre randomised trial. *BMJ* 2006;333:1193.

47. Cunha BA. Oral and IV-to-PO switch antibiotic therapy of hospitalized patients with serious infections. *Scand J Infect* 2008;40:1004–1006.

48. Cunha BA. Oral antibiotic therapy of serious systemic infections. *Med Clin North Am* 2006;90:1197–2222.

49. Hageman JC, Uyeki TM, Francis JS, et al. Severe community-acquired pneumonia due to *Staphylococcus aureus*, 2003–04 influenza season. *Emerg Infect Dis* 2006;12:894–899.

50. Centers for Disease Control and Prevention (CDC). Severe methicillin-resistant *Staphylococcus aureus* community-acquired pneumonia associated with influenza—Louisiana and Georgia, December 2006-January 2007. *Morb Mortal Wkly Rep* 2007;56:325–329.

51. Magira EE, Zervakis D, Routsi C, et al. Community-acquired methicillin-resistant *Staphylococcus aureus* carrying Panton-Valentine leukocidin genes: A lethal cause of pneumonia in an adult immunocompetent patient. *Scand J Infect Dis* 2007;39:466–469.

52. Vayalumkal JV, Whittingham H, Vanderkooi O, et al. Necrotizing pneumonia and septic shock: Suspecting CA-MRSA in patients presenting to Canadian emergency departments. *CJEM* 2007;9:300–303.

53. Martino JL, McMillian WD, Polish LB, et al. Community-acquired methicillin-resistant *Staphylococcus aureus* pneumonia. *Respir Med* 2008;102:932–934.

54. Mohan SS, McDermott BP, Cunha BA. Diagnostic and prognostic significance of relative lymphopenia in adult patients with influenza A. *Am J Med* 2005;118:1307–1309.

55. Cunha BA. Amantadine may be lifesaving in severe influenza A. *Clin Infect Dis* 2006;43:1574–1575.

56. Cunha BA. The clinical diagnosis of severe viral influenza A. *Infection* 2008;36:92–93.

57. Saner FH, Heuer M, Rath PM, et al. Successful salvage therapy with tigecycline after linezolid failure in a liver transplant recipient with MRSA pneumonia. *Liver Transpl* 2006;12:1689–1692.

58. Shakil S, Akram M, Khan AU. Tigecycline: A critical update. *J Chemother* 2008;20:411–419.

59. Heath CH, Grove DI, Looke DF. Delay in appropriate therapy of *Legionella* pneumonia associated with increased mortality. *Eur J Clin Microbiol Infect Dis* 1996;5:286–290.

60. Harper SA, Bradley JS, Englund JA, et al. Seasonal influenza in adults and children–diagnosis, treatment, chemoprophylaxis, and institutional outbreak management: Clinical practice guidelines of the Infectious Diseases Society of America. *Clin Infect Dis* 2009;48:1003–1032.

61. Hayden FG, Palese P. Influenza virus. In: Richman DD, Whitley RJ, Hayden FG eds. *Clinical Virology* (3rd ed.). Washington, DC: ASM Press, 2009:943–976.

62. Thomas JK, Noppenberger J. Avian influenza: A review. *Am J Health System Pharm* 2007;64:149–165.

63. Uyeki TM. Human infection with highly pathogenic avian influenza A (H5N1) virus: Review of clinical issues. *Clin Infect Dis* 2009;49;279–290.

64. Hien ND, Ha NH, Van NT, et al. Human infection with highly pathogenic avian influenza virus (H5N1) in Northern Vietnam, 2004–2005. *Emerg Infect Dis* 2009;15:19–23.

65. Centers for Disease Control and Prevention (CDC). Outbreak of swine-origin influenza A (H1N1) virus infection—Mexico, March-April 2009. *Morb Mortal Wkly Rep* 2009;58:467–470.

66. Stolz D. Procalcitonin in severe community acquired pneumonia. Some precision medicine ready for prime time. *Chest* 2016;150:769–771.

67. Cunha BA, Gran A, Simon J. Round pneumonias. *Respir Care* 2013;58:80–82.

68. Cunha BA, Dieguez B, Varantsova A. Lessons learned from splenic infarcts with fever of unknown origin (FUO): Culture-negative endocarditis (CNE) or malignancy? *Eur J Clin Micro Inf Dis* 2018.

69. Cunha CB, Opal SM. Middle East respiratory syndrome (MERS): A new zoonotic viral pneumonia. *Virulence* 2014;5:650–654.

14 Legionnaire's Disease and Severe Pneumonia Mimics in the Critical Care Unit

Burke A. Cunha

CONTENTS

CLINICAL PERSPECTIVE

In the differential diagnosis (DDx) of severe community-acquired pneumonia (CAP) in the critical care unit (CCU), there are some other causes of severe CAP that may have, besides severity, some features in common with severe Legionnaire's disease, i.e., may clinically mimic Legionnaire's disease. With severe CAP (SCAP), various etiologies may have radiographic and/or have overlapping clinical features or non-specific laboratory test abnormalities present with Leionnaires disease. In the DDx of severe CAP in the CCU, the pneumonias most likely to resemble Legionnaire's disease include influenza, influenza-like illnesses (ILIs) due to RSV, hMPV, HPIV-3, adenovirus, *M. pneumoniae*, and *S. pneumoniae*. Infectious determinants of severe CAP in hospitalized adults, depends on microbiologic, host factors, and cardiopulmonary function (Table 14.1). Microbiologic factors are related to inocular size and pathogen virulence. All other factors being equal, influenza has more potential inherent virulence than the ILI viral causes of CAP. Inocular size determines the incubation period and likelihood of infection transmission but has less, if any, impact on the clinical severity of CAP. Among the typical bacterial pathogens causing CAP, clearly *S. pneumoniae* remains potentially the most virulent, i.e., vs. *H. influenzae* [1–7].

Host factors are the key determinants of severity and prognosis in adult CAP. In patients with severe cardiopulmonary disorders, even a relatively low virulence pulmonary pathogen may present as severe CAP, e.g., *M. catarrhalis* ILI viral

TABLE 14.1

Legionnaire's Disease: Characteristic Clinical Findings in Adults Hospitalized with Pneumonia

Clinical Findings[a]
- New onset of pneumonia symptoms
- Fever greater than 38.9°C (102°F) (with relative bradycardia)

Chest Film Features[a]
- New rapidly progressive unilateral or bilateral interstitial/nodular infiltrates
- New rapidly progressive bilateral multifocal infiltrates

Laboratory Test Abnormalities[a]
- Leukocytosis
- Relative lymphopenia
- Highly elevated ESR (>90 mm/h) or highly elevated CRP (>180 mg/L)
- Highly elevated ferritin levels (>2 × normal)
- Hypophosphatemia (on admission/early)
- Highly elevated CPK (>2 × normal)
- Microscopic hematuria (on admission)

Source: Cunha, B.A. et al., *Am. J. Med.*, 128, e21–e22, 2015.
[a] Otherwise unexplained.

pneumonias. Adults with congestive heart failure (CHF) and/or chronic obstructive pulmonary disease with superimposed CAP will likely present as severe CAP, independent of the pathogen's inherent virulence [8–14].

All CAP pathogens have a spectrum of clinical presentation from "walking pneumonia" to severe CAP, requiring

CCU care. Excluding zoonotics CAP, e.g., Middle Eastern respiratory syndrome and tularemic pneumonia, the pathogens that most likely present as severe CAP in hospitalized adults among the viruses are influenza, adenovirus, and RSV; among typical bacterial CAP pathogens, *S. pneumoniae*; among the atypical CAP pathogens, *M. pneumoniae* and Legionnaire's disease; and among the fungi, pneumocystosis pneumonia (PCP) [2,7,15–20].

NON-INFECTIOUS MIMICS OF SEVERE CAP IN THE CCU

Patients presenting clinically as severe CAP may have pre-existing disorders that impair immune function or cardiopulmonary function. Impaired host defenses particularly impaired B-lymphocyte function, i.e., impaired humoral immunity (HI) (e.g., multiple myeloma and systemic lupus erythemosis [SLE]), not only predispose to infection by encapsulated pulmonary pathogen, e.g., *S. pneumoniae* but also predicts a severe/prolonged pneumonia. Since CHF is so common, it is not surprising that CHF not only may radiologically resemble CAP but also may make any cause of CAP clinically appear more severe. Non-infectious mimics of CAP may present as radiologic

mimics or clinical mimics with symptoms/signs or laboratory abnormalities of an infectious pneumonia. Obviously, DDx possibilities are compounded when a patient presents with an pulmonary disorder that radiologically mimics CAP and, in addition, may have a superimposed pneumonia, i.e., both factors combining to present as a severe CAP in the CCU [7,18–20].

The non-infectious mimics of CAP with or without superimposed pneumonia likely to present as CAP include SLE pneumonitis, CHF, bronchiolitis obliterans organizing pneumonia (BOOP), radiation pneumonitis, COPD (particularly chronic bronchitis or bronchiectasis), bronchogenic carcinomas, pulmonary sarcoidosis, pulmonary hemorrhage, pulmonary lymphomas, pulmonary metastasis, pulmonary drug reactions, Wegener's granulomatosis, hypersensitivity pneumonitis, fibrosis, interstitial pulmonary embolus/infarction and acute respiratory distress syndrome (ARDS) [7].

The aforementioned pulmonary disorders not only may radiographically mimic CAP but are also likely to present as severe CAP, with bacterial or viral pneumonia superimposed on pre-existing lung/heart disease. The diagnostic challenge is to sort out the underlying and superimposed components that have come together to present as severe CAP in the CCU (Table 14.2).

TABLE 14.2

Legionnaire's Disease: Clinical Mimics in Hospitalized Adults

	Fever >102°F (with Relative Bradycardia)	Dry Cough	Headache and or Mental Confusion	Loose Stools or Watery Diarrhea
Bacterial LD Clinical Mimics	• Q fever • Psittacosis • Leptospirosis • Any typical bacterial CAP (with drug fever)	• *M. pneumoniae* • *C. pneumoniae* • Pertussis	• Psittacosis • Q fever • Tularemia • Leptospirosis • *M. pneumoniae*[a]	• *M. pneumoniae* • Any pneumonia (on stool softeners or laxatives)

Viral LD Clinical Mimics	• Any viral CAP (with drug fever)
	• hMPV
	• COVID-19
		• Influenza
		• COVID-19
		• Respiratory non-influenza ILI viruses
		  RSV
		  HPIV-3
		  hMPV
		• Adenovirus
			• Influenza
			• COVID-19
			• Respiratory non-influenza ILI viruses
			  RSV
			  HPIV-3
			  hMPV
			  Adenovirus
				• Influenza
				• COVID-19
				• Respiratory non-influenza ILI viruses
				  RSV
				  HPIV-3
				  hMPV
				• Adenovirus

Non-Infectious LD Clinical Mimics	• Hypersensitivity pneumonitis[b] • SLE pneumonitis[b] • Pulmonary hemorrhage[b] • Lymphoma with pulmonary involvement • Any pulmonary disorder (with drug fever)	• Bronchogenic carcinomas • CHF	• Bronchogenic carcinomas (with CNS metastases) • SLE cerebritis • Pulmonary sarcoidosis with basilar meningitis	• Any pulmonary disorder (on stool softeners or laxatives)

Abbreviations: LD, Legionnaire's disease; ILI, influenza-like illnesses; SLE, systemic lupus erythematosus; hMPV, human metapneumovirus; CHF, congestive heart failure; CAP, community acquired pneumonia; HPIV-3, human parainfluenza virus-3.

[a] With meningoencephalitis (cold agglutinin titers >1:512).

[b] On β-blockers, verapamil, diltiazem, heart block or pacemaker rhythm.

CLINICAL DIAGNOSTIC APPROACH TO LEGIONNAIRE'S DISEASE MIMICS

IMPORTANCE OF THE HISTORY IN THE DDx OF DIAGNOSIS

The first step for the diagnostician is to obtain an accurate past medical history (PMH) and a recent timeline of events. Combined, these points are key determinants of the DDx, i.e., underlying disorders by PMH, and tempo of infection, i.e., subacute, acute, and hyperacute. For example, if a patient's PMH is positive for SLE, the clinician should try to determine if the patient has had flares and or SLE episodes of SLE pneumonitis. Does the current presentation resemble previous episodes? Are there previous chest films of SLE pneumonitis episodes? Is the SLE patient currently on steroids/immunosuppressives? Importantly, are there current clinical features unexplained by SLE that may provide clues to the possibly etiology of a possible superimposed pneumonia [7].

IMPORTANCE OF PHYSICAL FLUIDS IN THE DDx OF LEGIONNAIRE'S DISEASE MIMICS

The physical examination (PE) has a limited value but an important significance in the setting of severe CAP. First, like the PMH, the PE may reveal previously unappreciated findings of SLE, CHF, sarcoidosis, abdominal pain (acute pancreatitis), which may be a clue to the etiology of ARDS. Generalized wheezing may be a clue to CHF as well as RSV. Unilateral pleural effusion may suggest a bacterial pneumonia, primary pulmonary tuberculosis (TB), bronchogenic carcinoma, SLE pneumonitis, etc. Bilateral pleural effusion suggests CHF. On chest auscultation, localized rales suggest a typical bacterial pneumonia vs. viral pneumonia. In contrast, in an adult with severe CAP and no rales, decreased breath sounds, an unremarkable CXR, and profound hypoxia essentially limit the DDx possibilities to influenza or PCP [7,20–31].

Severe myalgias with fever/chills point to influenza. Other CAP may be accompanied by chills but not of the severity/duration as in viral influenza. Profound fatigue is also a cardinal finding in severe influenza but not a clinical feature of other causes of CAP [7,32].

DIAGNOSTIC IMPORTANCE OF CHEST FILM FINDINGS

The chest X-ray (CXR) is most important in either limiting DDx possibilities or eliminating diagnostic possibilities, i.e., a diagnostic eliminator. The CXR findings may not suggest a specific diagnosis but is most helpful in eliminating diagnostic possibilities.

As mentioned, an essentially unremarkable initial CXR in an adult with profound hypoxemia and severe CAP limits the DDx possibilities to viral pneumonia, e.g., influenza or PCP. Later in progression of pneumonia, both influenza and PCP will develop bilateral perihilar/peripheral interstitial infiltrates with small or no pleural effusions. These CXR findings point to influenza or PCP but also importantly, diagnostically, function as a diagnostic eliminator, i.e., eliminates all typical and atypical CAPs from further diagnostic consideration.

Segmental/lobar infiltrates point to a typical bacterial pneumonia and essentially rule out influenza (without secondary bacterial pneumonia) and PCP. Unilateral pleural effusion may be present and supports the diagnosis of a typical bacterial CAP pathogen [7,32].

Some pneumonia etiologies may have CXR findings with a focal/localized but are not confirmed to a particular lung segment/lobe. Such "localized" but not lobar infiltrates are common with RSV, adenovirus, and Legionnaire's disease. While the appearance of Legionnaire's disease on the CXR is non-diagnostic, its radiologic behavior is that of a rapidly progressive unilateral/bilateral pneumonia with fluffy or nodular interstitial infiltrates. Consolidation occurs with typical bacterial CAP, e.g., *S. pneumoniae*. However, consolidation is not uncommon with viral pneumonias, e.g., RSV, adenovirus, and Legionnaire's disease. Excluding *K. pneumoniae* in alcoholics and lung abscesses (from massive aspiration), cavitation is an uncommon but important diagnostic clue in severe CAPs, if due to influenza with simultaneous *S. aureus* pneumonia (Table 14.3).

Cavitation rates are also diagnostically helpful. The speed of cavitation has important DDx significance, e.g., rapid cavitation of infiltrates in severe influenza in <72 hours limits the DDx possibility to superimposed *S. aureus* CAP [33,34].

In an alcoholic presenting with severe CAP and cavitation on CXR after 3–5 days is characteristic of *K. pneumoniae* CAP. Late cavitation (after 5 days) suggests lung abscesses due to aspiration pneumonia. Because these patients are, in general, less critically ill, than *S. aureus* or *K. pneumoniae*

TABLE 14.3
Legionnaire's Disease: CAP Radiologic Mimics

Non-infectious CAP CXR Mimics		Bacterial CAP LD CXR Mimics	Viral CAP LD CXR Mimics
With Fever	**Without Fever**		
• SLE pneumonitis	• CHF (no MI)	• *S. pneumoniae*[a]	• Adenovirus
• CHF (due to MI)	• BOOP	• Q fever[a]	• Influenza
• Pulmonary embolus/ infarction	• Bronchogenic carcinomas	• *Legionella* sp.[a]	• COVID-19
• Pulmonary hemorrhage	• Pulmonary sarcoidosis	• Pertussis	• Some respiratory viral non-influenza ILIs
• Hypersensitivity pneumonitis	• Pulmonary alveolar proteinosis		HPIV-3[b]
• Lymphoma (involving the lungs)	• Lung metastases		hMPV[b] RSV[b]

Abbreviations: SLE, systemic lupus erythematosus; ILIs, influenza like illnesses CHF, congestive heart failure; RSV, respiratory syncytial virus; BOOP, bronchiolitis obliterans organizing pneumonia; HPIV-3, human parainfluenza virus-3; CXR, chest X-ray; hMPV, human metapneumovirus; MI, myocardial infarction; LD, Legionnaire's disease.

[a] May have nodular infiltrates.

[b] May have asymmetrical infiltrates.

cavity pneumonias, the clinical presentation is not as acute/early as with *S. aureus* or *K. pneumoniae* CAP [7].

CLINICAL FEATURES OF LEGIONNAIRE'S DISEASE AND ITS SCAP MIMICS

Legionnaire's disease is usually accompanied by a variety of extrapulmonary findings, e.g., headache (HA), mental confusion, loose stools, and abdominal pain. Influenza may also present with HA and mental confusion; otherwise-unexplained loose stools in a CAP patient suggests influenza or *M. pneumoniae* as a diagnostic possibility. While Legionnaire's disease is accompanied by fever (usually >102°F) + chills, influenza is characterized by severe rigors and myalgias with profound fatigues, not features of Legionnaire's disease [31,32,35].

An important clue to the presence of Legionnaire's disease in the context of an SCAP, in those with fevers >102°F, is the presence of a pulse-temperature deficit, i.e., relative bradycardia. Of course, if present, relative bradycardia must not be due to medications, i.e., β-blockers, diltiazem, verapamil, or pacemaker rhythms. With temperature >102°F, relative bradycardia is virtually always present in Legionnaire's disease, and its absence acts as a key diagnostic eliminator, arguing strongly against the diagnosis of Legionnaire's disease.

Neither *S. pneumoniae or M. pneumoniae* nor influenza, the common SCAP mimics of Legionnaire's disease, is accompanied by relative bradycardia. In contrast to Legionnaire's disease with fevers typically >102°F, fever with *M. pneumoniae* CAP rarely exceeds 102°F. Like Legionnaire's disease, the chills and fatigue in *M. pneumoniae* are mild and not prominent, as with influenza [7,36–39].

IMPORTANCE OF NON-SPECIFIC LABORATORY ABNORMALITIES

The clinical diagnostic significance of non-specific findings is enhanced when combined in the appropriate clinical setting. Some CAP pathogens, e.g., atypical pneumonias, have particular characteristic, non-specific findings. The more characteristic findings related to a particular pathogen are present, the more likely a clinical syndromic diagnosis [20,31,40]. The diagnostician's first task is to know and then recognize the characteristic findings of each cause of atypical CAP and viral CAP [41,42].

Otherwise-unexplained leukopenia in a CAP patient suggests a viral etiology, particularly if accompanied by thrombocytopenia. Alternately, in acute HIV, leukopenia is not an uncommon early finding in those with PCP. Typical bacterial pneumonias are not accompanied by leukopenia/thrombocytopenia. Importantly, either marked leukopenia or thrombocytopenia is essentially diagnostic eliminator for Legionnaire's disease. An otherwise-unexplained highly elevated ESR and or CRP in an adult patient with CAP points to either *S. pneumoniae* or Legionnaire's disease. Modest elevations in serum transaminases may occur with some causes of severe CAP but not *M. pneumoniae, S. pneumoniae,* or PCP. Highly elevated CPK levels in severe CAP adults, if not drug induced, e.g., statins, may occur with influenza, RSV, and Legionnaire's disease [7,42–49] (Table 14.4).

TABLE 14.4
Legionnaire's Disease: Pneumonia with Non-Specific Laboratory Abnormalities

	Non-infectious LD Laboratory Mimics	Bacterial LD Laboratory test	Viral LD Laboratory Test Mimics
Leukocytosis	• Any pulmonary disorder (with fever)	• Any bacterial pneumonia	• Influenza • Respiratory viral non-influenza ILI RSV hMPV HPIV-3 • Adenovirus
Relative lymphopenia	• Any pulmonary disorder (on steroids or immuno-suppressive drugs)	• None	• Influenza • COVID-19 • Respiratory viral non-influenza ILIs RSV hMPV HPIV-3 • Adenovirus
Highly ↑ ESR (>100 mg/L) and or highly ↑ CRP (>180 mg. L)	• Pulmonary emboli/infarction	• *S. pneumoniae*	• None
Highly ↑ serum ferritin levels (>2 × n)	• Any malignancy involving the lungs • Any cause of renal insufficiency (with pulmonary infiltrates)	• Q fever • PCP	• hMPV • Adenovirus
Hyponatremia	• Any pulmonary disorder	• Any bacterial pneumonia	• Any viral pneumonia
Hypophosphatemia	• None	• None	• hMPV (rare) • Adenovirus (rare)
Highly elevated CPK	• SLE	• Leptospirosis • Tularemia	• Influenza • HPIV-3 • Adenovirus
Mildly elevated serum transaminases	• EBV infectious mononucleosis (with pulmonary involvement)	• Q fever • Psittacosis • Tularemia • Leptospirosis	• Influenza • COVID-19 • Respiratory viral non-influenza ILIs RSV hMPV HPIV-3 • Adenovirus

Abbreviations: ESR, erythrosedimentation rate; CPK, creatinine phosphokinase; CRP, C-reactive protein; ILI, influenza-like illnesses; LD, Legionnaire's disease; CAP, community acquired pneumonia; hMPV, human metapneumovirus; HPIV-3, human parainfluenza virus-3; PCP, *Pneumocystis (carinii) jirovecii* pneumonia; SLE, systemic lupus erythematosus.

When ferritin levels are highly elevated (not minimal/transient elevated as an acute-phase reactant) in severe CAP patients, Legionnaire's disease is most likely. No other SCAP etiology is regularly associated with such highly elevated ferritin levels (>2 × n) (Table 14.5).

Otherwise-unexplained microscopic hematuria may only occur with Legionnaire's disease and not other CAPs. Acute kidney injury (AKI) is a frequent accompaniment of Legionnaire's disease, excluding unrelated hypotension. AKI is not a feature of other severe CAP pathogens [42–51].

TABLE 14.5

Pneumonias with Increased Ferritin Levels and Other Infectious and Non-Infectious Disorders

Infectious Causes[a,b]

Pneumonias	Non-Pneumonias
• Legionnaire's disease	• WNE
• Adenovirus	• EBV
• PCP	• CMV
	• Toxoplasmosis
	• S. aureus ABE
	• Malaria
	• Babesiosis
	• Ehrlichiosis/anaplasmosis

Non-Infectious Causes

May Have Lung Involvement	No Lung Involvement
• Chronic renal failure (fluid overload)	• Non-pulmonary malignancies
• Rheumatoid arthritis (rheumatoid lung)	• Myeloproliferative disorders
• Bronchogenic carcinomas (any pulmonary malignancy)	• Adult Still's disease
	• SLE
	• TA
	• AOCD
	• Hemochromatosis
	• Chronic hepatitis (HCV)

Source: Cunha, C.B., Infectious disease differential diagnosis, In: Cunha, C.B., Cunha, B.A. (Eds.), Antibiotic Essentials (17th ed.), JayPee Medical Publishers, New Delhi, India, 2020; Kroll, V., Cunha, B.A., Infect Dis Pract., 27, 199–192.

Abbreviations: SLE, systemic lupus erythematosus; TA, temporal arteritis; AOCD, anemia of chronic disease; WNE, West Nile encephalitis; CMV, cytomegalovirus; EBV, Epstein–Barr virus; HCV, hepatitis C virus, PCP, pneumocystosis pneumonia.

[a] Otherwise unexplained and not due to other disorders associated with increased ferritin levels.

[b] Acute-phase ferritin elevations (n < 186 ng/mL) are transient minimal elevations, e.g., 187–200 ng/mL. In contrast, diagnostically important non-acute-phase ferritin elevations are much higher, e.g., >2 × n (>375 ng/mL) and persist for days.

TABLE 14.6

Diagnostic Criteria for Relative Bradycardia: Temperature-Pulse Relationships

Temperature, °F (°C)	Appropriate Pulse Response for Temperature, /min	Relative Bradycardia Present[a] If Pulse, /min
106°F (41.1°C)	150 beats/min	140 beats/min
105°F (40.6°C)	140 beats/min	130 beats/min
104°F (40.7°C)	130 beats/min	120 beats/min
103°F (39.4°C)	120 beats/min	110 beats/min
102°F (38.9°C)	110 beats/min	100 beats/min

Source: Cunha, C.B. and Cunha, B.A. (Eds.), Antibiotic Essentials (17th ed.), JayPee Medical Publishers, New Delhi, India, 2020.

[a] Relative bradycardia refers to heart rates that are inappropriately slow relative to body temperature (pulse must be taken simultaneously with temperature elevation). Applies to adult patients with temperature >102°F; does not apply to patients with second-/third-degree heart block, pacemaker-induced rhythms, or those on beta-blockers, diltiazem, or verapamil.

In summary, non-specific findings, when considered together, increase diagnostic probability, the greater the number of findings are present, i.e., five or six findings are more likely to limit diagnostic possibilities than two or three findings. Importantly, findings representing "diagnostic eliminators" have diagnostic significance by eliminating a diagnosis from further diagnostic consideration; e.g., Legionnaire's disease is effectively ruled out in an adult patient with severe CAP and a fever >102°F if no relative bradycardia is present [31,32,41] (Table 14.6).

DIAGNOSTIC SYNOPSIS OF LEGIONNAIRE'S DISEASE AND ITS SCAP MIMICS

Legionnaire's disease is likely in a severe CAP patient when several non-specific but characteristic findings are present e.g., otherwise-unexplained, highly elevated ESR, CRP, ferritin, CPK, and microscopic hematuria. The other clinical clues suggesting Legionnaire's disease are patchy nodular lobular infiltrates or the lack of response to β-lactam antibiotic therapy [49,50]. Legionnaire's disease improves over 5–7 days (decrease in daily fever spikes). However, as with other pneumonias, radiographic resolution is slower than clinical improvement. Since Legionnaire's disease requires antibiotics, with anti-Legionella sp., a presumptive clinical diagnosis is essential [7,31,32] (Tables 14.7–14.9).

Based on a clinical syndromic diagnosis, as described earlier, early empiric therapy for Legionnaire's disease should be started if diagnostic probability is high and should be initiated pending test results (Table 14.10). The diagnosis of Legionnaire's disease may be confirmed by Legionella sp. titers or Legionella urinary antigen (LUA). The limitation of

TABLE 14.7
Legionnaire's Disease: Diagnostic Clinical Clues in Adults Admitted with CAP[a, b]

Diagnostic Clues	Diagnostic Eliminators
Clinical Clues	**Clinical Eliminators**
• Mental confusion	• Fever (>102°F) *without relative*
• Fever (>102°F) *with relative bradycardia*	*bradycardia*
• ABG clues: Moderate hypoxemia (A-a gradient <35)	• Severe myalgias
Radiologic Clues	
Rapidly progressive asymmetrical patchy/nodular infiltrates	
Laboratory Clues[b]	**Laboratory Eliminators**
• Highly elevated ESR (>90 mm/h) or	• Negative chest X-ray (no infiltrates)
• highly elevated CRP (>35 mg/L)	• No relative lymphopenia
• Highly elevated serum ferritin levels (>2 × n)	• Leukopenia
	• Thrombocytopenia
• Hypophosphatemia (on admission/	• Unelevated or minimally
• early)	elevated ferritin levels
• Hyponatremia	
• Highly elevated CPK (>2 × n)	
• Microscopic hematuria (on admission)	
Legionnaire's disease **very likely if >3 clinical clues present**	Legionnaire's disease **very unlikely if <3 clinical clues or if diagnostic eliminators present**

Source: Cunha, B.A. (Ed.), *Pneumonia Essentials*, 3rd ed., Jones & Bartlett, Sudbury, MA, 2010; Cunha, B.A. et al., *Am. J. Med.*, 128, e21–e22, 2015.

[a] Pulmonary symptoms: Shortness of breath, cough, etc., with fever and a new focal/segmental infiltrate on chest film.

[b] Otherwise unexplained. If finding is due to an existing disorder, it should not be used as a clinical predictor.

TABLE 14.8
Severe CAP: Diagnostic Clues

Symptoms

• Headache	Influenza
	Legionnaire's disease
	M. pneumoniae
	Tularemia
• Mental Confusion	Tularemia
	Plague
	M. pneumoniae
	Legionnaire's disease
• Wheezing	RSV
• Chest pain (pleuritic)	*S. pneumoniae*
	Influenza
	Plague
	Anthrax (substernal)
• Watery eyes	Adenovirus
	(Continued)

TABLE 14.8 *(Continued)*
Severe CAP: Diagnostic Clues

Symptoms

• Conjunctival suffusion	Influenza
	Adenovirus
	MERS
	Leptospirosis
• Hemoptysis	Plague
	Legionnaire's disease
• Hoarseness	Influenza
	RSV

Signs

• Relative bradycardia	Legionnaire's disease
	Psittacosis
	Q fever
• Epistaxis	Influenza
	Plague
	Leptospirosis
	Psittacosis
• *H. labialis*	*S. pneumoniae*
• Parotid enlargement	Adenovirus
	Influenza
• Abdominal pain	Legionnaire's disease
• Splenomegaly	Psittacosis
	Q fever

Laboratory Tests

• Normal WBC count	RSV
	COVID-19
• Leukopenia	Influenza
	Viral
• Relative lymphopenia	Legionnaire's disease
	influenza
	MERS
• Hemoconcentration	HPS
• Normoblasts	HPS
• Thrombocytosis	*M. pneumoniae*
	Q fever
• ↑ CPK	Legionnaire's disease
	Influenza
	COVID-19
• ↑ LDH	Legionnaire's disease
	PCP
	COVID-19
• Highly elevated serum ferritin	Legionnaire's disease
• ↓ Phosphorus	Legionnaire's disease
• Microscopic hematuria	Legionnaire's disease
• AKI	Legionnaire's disease
• Highly elevated cold agglutinins	*M. pneumonia*

Imaging

• Spontaneous pneumothorax	Legionnaire's disease
	PCP
• Round "nodular" patchy infiltrates	Legionnaire's disease
	RSV
	MERS
	COVID-19
• Mediastinal adenopathy	Legionnaire's disease
• Rapidly progressive asymmetric patchy/nodular infiltrates	Legionnaire's disease

TABLE 14.9

Differential Diagnostic Findings in Severe CAP in the CCU

	LD	Mycoplasma pneumoniae	Streptococcus pneumoniae	Plague	Anthrax	Tularemia	COVID-19	Influenza	MERS	RSV	HPS	Adenovirus	PCP
Symptoms													
Headache	+	+	−	−	−	+++	++	+++	++	−	−	+	−
Fever/chills	+++	+	+++	+++	+	+	+++	+++	++	−	+	+++	−
Prominent Fatigue	−	−	−	−	−	−	+++	+++	−	−	−	−	−
Myalgias	+	+	−	+	−	+++	++	+++	+	+	+	+++	+
Dry cough	+	+++	−	−	−	−	+++	+++	+++	+++	+	++	+++
Shortness of breath	+	+	−	+++	+++	+	+++	+++	+++	+++	+++	+++	+++
Sore throat	−	+	−	−	−	+	++	+++	++	+++	−	+++	−
Nausea/vomiting	−	−	−	−	+	−	+	+	+	−	−	−	−
Diarrhea	+	+	−	−	−	−	+	+	+	−	+	+	+
Abdominal pain	+	−	−	−	−	+	−	−	−	−	−	−	−
Hemoptysis	+	−	−	−	+	−	−	+	−	−	+	+	−
Signs													
Relative bradycardia	+	−	−	−	−	−	−	−	−[a]	−	−	−	+
Tachycardia	−	−	−	+	+	+	+	−	+	+	+	+	+
Conjunctival suffusion	−	−	−	−	−	+	−	−	−	−	+	+	−
Diminished breath sounds	−	−	+	+	−	−	+++	+++	++	+++	−	+++	+++
Acute renal failure (ARF)	+	−	−	−	−	−	−	−	+	−	+	−	−
Laboratory Tests													
Normal WBC count	−	−	−	−	−	−	+	+	−	+	−	+	+
Leukopenia	−	−	−	−	+	+	+	+++	+++	+++	+	+++	+++[b]
Relative lymphopenia	+++	−	−	−	−	−	+++	+++	+++	+	−	+++	+++[b]
Thrombocytopenia	−	−	−	−	−	+	−	+	+++	+	+	+++	+++[b]
Highly elevated ESR	+	−	+	−	−	−	−	−	+	−	−	+	−
Highly elevated CRP	+	−	−	−	−	−	−	−	+	−	−	+	−
Elevated serum transaminases	+	−	−	−	−	−	−	+	+	+	−	+	+[b]
Elevated LDH	+	−	−	−	−	−	+++	+	+	−	−	+	+++
Elevated CPK	+++	−	−	−	−	−	+++	+++	−	−	−	−	−
↑ β 1,3 glucan	−	−	−	−	−	−	−	−	−	+	−	+	+
↑ A-a gradient (>35)	−	−	−	−	−	−	+	+	+	−	−	+	+
Chest Film													
Normal/ minimal basilar infiltrates (early)	−	−	−	−	−	−	+	+	−	+	+	+	+

(Continued)

TABLE 14.9 (Continued)
Differential Diagnostic Findings in Severe CAP in the CCU

	LD	Mycoplasma pneumoniae	Streptococcus pneumoniae	Plague	Anthrax	Tularemia	COVID-19	Influenza	MERS	RSV	HPS	Adenovirus	PCP
Unilateral infiltrate (early)	+	+	+	−	−	+	+	−	−	+	−	+	−
Bilateral infiltrates (late)	+	−	−	+	+	−	−	+	+	+	+	+	+
Pleural effusion	−	+	−	−	+	+	−	−	+	−	−	−	−
/Cavitation	−												
ARDS (severe cases)	−	−	−	−	−	−	+	+	+	+	+	+	+

Source: Cunha, B.A., *Pneumonia Essentials* (3rd ed.), Jones & Bartlett, Sudbury, MA, 2010; Cunha, C.A. and Opal, SM., *Virulence*, 5, 650–654, 2014.

Abbreviations: LD, Legionnaire's disease; RSV, respiratory syncytial virus; HPS, hantavirus pulmonary syndrome; MERS, Middle Eastern respiratory syndrome; CPK, creatine phosphokinase; ARDS, acute respiratory distress syndrome; CRP, C-reactive protein; PCP, *Pneumocystis (carcini) jirvecii* pneumonia.

[a] No bradycardia/relative bradycardia unless on high dose ribavirin.
[b] Due to underlying HIV not PCP.

TABLE 14.10

Diagnostic Approach to Diffuse Pulmonary Infiltrates and Hypoxemia with Severe CAP in the CCU

	Bilateral/Diffuse Pulmonary Infiltrates	
Acute	Hypoxemia (A-a Gradient <35)	Severe Hypoxemia (A-a Gradient >35)
Non-Infectious Causes	• Congestive heart failure • Pulmonary embolus/infarction • Pulmonary hemorrhage	• ARDS
Infectious Causes	• Legionnaire's disease • Bacterial CAP • TB	• Influenza • COVID-19 • ILI viral pneumonias • CMV • HSV • Adenovirus • MERS
Subacute		
Non-Infectious Causes	• Drug-induced pneumonitis	• BOOP • Sarcoidosis • Idiopathic pulmonary fibrosis • Lymphangitic spread

Source: Cunha, B.A., *Infect Dis Clin North Am.*, 2001.

LUA testing is that results may be negative early and the test only detects *L. pneumophilia* (serotype 01) and not other serotypes or species [30–32].

EMPIRIC THERAPY FOR LEGIONNAIRE'S DISEASE AND ITS SCAP MIMICS

Optimal antibiotic therapy for Legionnaire's disease is with doxycycline, tigecycline, a quinolone, or azithromycin. In immunocompromised hosts, Legionnaire's disease may be treated with two drugs, e.g., levofloxacin plus wither doxycycline or azithromycin. Depending on severity, treatment should be for 2–3 weeks [7].

Selecting optimal empiric treatment for SCAP depends on the likely pathogen. If SCAP is likely due to a non-zoonotic atypical CAP pathogen, i.e., Legionnaire's disease or *mycoplasma pneumoniae*, then monotherapy with a quinolone, e.g., levofloxacin or doxycycline, is optimal therapy. If SCAP is likely due to a zoonotic atypical pathogen, i.e., tularemia, anthrax, or plague, then doxycycline or a quinolone (+ gentamicin or streptomycin) is an excellent therapy [7,52] (Tables 14.11–14.14).

TABLE 14.11

Antimicrobial Therapy: Severe Typical Bacterial Community-Acquired Pneumonia in the CCU

Subset	Usual Pathogens	IV Therapy	PO Therapy or IV-to-PO Switch
Typical Bacterial CAP Pathogens	*S. pneumoniae* *H. influenzae* *M. catarrhalis*	Levofloxacin 750 mg (IV) q24h × 5 days or moxifloxacin 400 mg (IV) q24h × 1–2 weeks or ceftriaxone 1 g (IV) q24h × 1–2 weeks or tigecycline 200 mg (IV) × 1 dose, then 100 mg (IV) q24h × 1–2 weeks or doxycycline[b] (IV) × 1–2 weeks or ertapenem 1 gm (IV) q24h × 1–2 weeks	Levofloxacin 750 mg (PO) q24h × 5 days or quinolone[a] (PO) q24h × 1–2 weeks or doxycycline[b] (PO) × 1–2 weeks
	K. pneumoniae	Meropenem 1 gm (IV) q8h × 2 weeks or ertapenem 1 gm (IV) q24h × 2 weeks or levofloxacin 750 mg (IV) q24h × 5 days or moxifloxacin 400 mg (IV) q24h × 2 weeks or ceftriaxone 1 gm (IV) q24h × 2 weeks	Levofloxacin 750 mg (PO) q24h × 5 days or moxifloxacin 400 mg (PO) q24h × 2 weeks
MDR *K. pneumoniae*		Meropenem 1 gm (IV) q8h × 2 weeks or tigecycline 200 mg (IV) × 1 dose, then 100 mg (IV) q24h × 1–2 weeks	Levofloxacin[a] 750 mg (PO) q24h × 5 days or moxifloxacin[a] 400 mg (PO) q24h × 2 weeks

Source: Cunha, C.B. and Cunha, B.A., *Antibiotic Essentials* (14th ed.), JayPee Medical Publishers, New Delhi, India, 2017.

Note: Duration of therapy represents total time IV, PO, or IV + PO.

[a] Levofloxacin 500 mg or moxifloxacin 400 mg.

[b] Doxycycline 200 mg (IV or PO) q12h × 3 days, then 100 mg (IV or PO) q12h × 4–11 days.

TABLE 14.12

Antimicrobial Therapy: Severe Non-Zoonotic Atypical Community Acquired Pneumonia in the CCU

Subset	Usual Pathogens[a]	Preferred IV Therapy	Alternate IV Therapy	PO Therapy or IV-to-PO Switch
Non-Zoonotic Atypical CAP Pathogens	Legionella sp. Mycoplasma pneumoniae	Levofloxacin 500 mg (IV) q24h × 1–2 weeks **or** moxifloxacin 400 mg (IV) q24h × 1–2 weeks **or** doxycycline 200 mg (IV) q12h × 3 days, then 100 mg (IV) q12h × 4–11 days **or** tigecycline 200 mg (IV) × 1 dose, then 1000 mg (IV)q24h × 1–2 weeks	Azithromycin 500 mg (IV) q24h × 1–2 weeks	Levofloxacin 500 mg (PO) q24h × 1–2 weeks **or** moxifloxacin 400 mg (PO) q24h × 1–2 weeks **or** doxycycline 200 mg (PO) q12h × 3 days, then 100 mg (PO) q12h × 4–11 days **or** azithromycin 500 mg (PO) q24h × 1–2 weeks

Source: Cunha, C.B. and Cunha, B.A. *Antibiotic Essentials* (14th ed.), JayPee Medical Publishers, New Delhi, India, 2017.

Note: Duration of therapy represents total time IV, PO, or IV + PO.

[a] *Legionella* (2–3 weeks); *Mycoplasma* (2 weeks).

TABLE 14.13

Antimicrobial Therapy: Severe Zoonotic Atypical Community-Acquired Pneumonia in the CCU

Subset	Usual Pathogens[a]	Preferred IV Therapy	Alternate IV Therapy	PO Therapy or IV-to-PO Switch
Zoonotic Atypical CAP Pathogens	C. psittaci (psittacosis) Coxiella burnetti (Q fever) Francisella tularensis (tularemia)	Doxycycline 200 mg (IV) q12h × days, then 100 mg (IV) q12h × 11 days	Levofloxacin 500 mg (IV) × 2 weeks **or** moxifloxacin 400 mg (IV) × 2 weeks	Doxycycline 200 mg (PO) q12h × 3 days, then 100 mg (PO) q12h × 11 days **or** levofloxacin 500 mg (PO) × 2 weeks **or** moxifloxacin 400 mg (PO) × 2 weeks

Source: Cunha, C.B. and Cunha, B.A., *Antibiotic Essentials*, 14th Ed., JayPee Medical Publishers, New Delhi, India, 2017.

Note: Duration of therapy represents total time IV, PO, or IV + PO.

[a] Compromised hosts may require longer courses of therapy.

TABLE 14.14

Antimicrobial Therapy: Severe Viral Community-Acquired Pneumonia in the CCU

Subset	Usual Pathogens	Preferred IV Therapy	Alternate IV Therapy	PO Therapy or IV-to-PO Switch
Viral CAP Pathogens				
Influenza	Influenza A	Peramivir 600 mg (IV) × 1 dose		
Influenza (with simultaneous bacterial CAP)	S. aureus (MSSA/ MRSA)	Linezolid 600 mg (IV) q12h × 2 weeks **or** Vancomycin 1 g (IV) q12h × 2 weeks		Linezolid 600 mg (PO) q12h × 2 weeks **or** minocycline 100 mg (PO) q12h × 2 weeks
Influenza (followed by subsequent bacterial CAP) after ~1 week	S. pneumoniae H. influenzae	Quinolone (IV q24h × 2 weeks)	Ceftriaxone 1 g (IV) q24h × 2 weeks	Quinolone (PO) q24h × 2 weeks
COVID-19	SARS-CoV-2	Remdesavir 200 mg (IV) x 1, then 100 mg (IV) q24th x 10 days		Hydroxychoroquine 400 mg (PO) x 1 day, then 200mg (PO) q12h x 4 days plus Azithromycin 500 mg (PO) x 1, then 250 mg (PO) q24h x 4 days
CMV	CMV	Ganciclovir 5 mg/kg (IV) q12h × 12 weeks, then q24h **or** complete therapy with valganciclovir 900 mg (PO) q24h until cured		
RSV	RSV	Ribavirin 2 g (aerosol) q8h until cured		

REFERENCES

1. Chahin A, Opal S. Severe pneumonia caused by *Legionella pneumophila*: Differential diagnosis and therapeutic considerations. *Infect Clin North Am* 2017;31:111–122.
2. Ruuskanen O, Lahti E, Jennings LC, Murdoch DR. Viral pneumonia. *Lancet* 2011;377:1264–1275.
3. Cesairo TC. Viruses associated with pneumonia in adults. *Clin Infect Dis* 2012;55:107–113.
4. Kroll JL, Weinberg A. Human metapneumovirus. *Semin Respir Crit Care Med* 2011;32:447–453.
5. Johnstone J, Majumdar SR, Fox JD, Marrie TJ. Human metapneumovirus pneumonia in adults: Results of a prospective study. *Clin Infect Dis* 2008;46:571–574.
6. Volling C, Hassan K, Mazzulli T, et al. Respiratory syncytial virus infection associated hospitalization in adults: A retrospective cohort study. *BMC Infect Dis* 2014;14:655.
7. Cunha BA (Ed). *Pneumonia Essentials* (3rd ed.). Sudbury, MA: Jones & Bartlett, 2010.
8. Lanternier F, Ader F, Pilmis B, Catherinot E, Jarraud S, Lortholary O. Legionnaire's disease in compromised hosts. *Infect Dis Clin North Am* 2017;31:123–136.
9. Htwe TH, Khardori N. Legionnaire's disease and immunosuppressive drugs. *Infect Dis Clin North Am* 2017;31:29–42.
10. Souza JS, Watanabe A, Carraro E, Granato C, Beliei N. Severe metapneumovirus infections among immunocompetent and immunocompromised patients admitted to hospital with respiratory infection. *J Med Virol* 2013;85:530–536.
11. Falsley AR, McElhaney JE, Beran J, et al. Respiratory syncytial virus and other respiratory viral infections in older adults with moderate to severe influenza-like illness. *J Infect Dis* 2014;209:1873–1881.
12. Ong DS, Faber TE, Klein Klouwenberg PM, et al. Respiratory eyncytial virus in critically ill adult patients with community acquired respiratory failure: A prospective observational study. *Clin Microbiol Infect* 2014;20:505–507.
13. Falsey AR, Walsh EE. Viral pneumonia in older adults. *Clin Infect Dis* 2006;42:518–524.
14. Basri Mat Nor M, Richards G, McGloughlin S, Amin P. Pneumonia in the tropics; Report from the task force on tropical diseases by the world federation of Societies of Intensive and critical care medicine. *J Crit Care* 2017;42:360–365.
15. Nor MBM, Richards GA, McGloughlin S, Amin PR, Council of the World Federation of Societies of Intensive and Critical Care Medicine. Pneumonia in the tropics: Report from the Task Force on Tropical diseases by the World Federation of Societies of Intensive and Critical Care Medicine. *J Crit Care* 2017;42:360–365.
16. Cunha CB, Opal S. Middle East respiratory syndrome (MERS). *Virulence* 2014;5:650–654.
17. Hui DS, Memish ZA, Zumla A. Severe acute respiratory syndrome vs. the Middle East Respiratory Syndrome. *Curr Opin Pulm Med* 2014;20:233–241.
18. Cunha BA, Quintiliani R. The atypical pneumonias: A diagnostic and therapeutic approach. *Postgrad Med* 1979;66:95–102.
19. Cunha BA. Atypical pneumonias: Current clinical concepts focusing on Legionnaire's disease. *Curr Opin Pulm Med* 2008;14:183–194.
20. Cunha BA. Legionnaire's disease: Clinical differentiation from typical and other atypical pneumonias. *Infect Dis Clin North Am* 2010;24:73–105.
21. Lattimer GL, Rhodes LV. Legionnaire's disease. Clinical findings and one-year follow-up. *JAMA* 1978;240:169–171.
22. Woodhead MA, Macfarlane JT. The protean manifestations of Legionnaire's disease. *J R Coll Physicians* 1985;19:224–230.
23. Woodhead MA, Macfarlane JT. Legionnaire's disease: A review of 79 community acquired cases in Nottingham. *Thorax* 1986;41:635–640.
24. Strampfer MA, Cunha BA. Clinical and laboratory aspects of Legionnaire's disease. *Semin Respir Infect* 1987;2:228–234.
25. Woodhead MA, Macfarlane JT. Comparative clinical and laboratory features of legionella with pneumococcal and mycoplasma pneumonias. *Br J Dis Chest* 1987;81:133–139.
26. Cotton LM, Strampfer MJ, Cunha BA. Legionella and mycoplasma pneumonia: A community hospital experience. *Clin Chest Med* 1987;8:441–453.
27. Gacouin A, Revest M, Letheulle J, el al. Distinctive features between community acquired pneumonia due to *Chlamydophila psittaci* and CAP due to *Legionella pneumophila* admitted to the intensive care unit. *Eur J Clin Microbiol Infect Dis* 2012;31:2713–2718.
28. Cunha BA. Clinical features of Legionnaire's disease. *Semin Respir Infect* 1998;13:116–127.
29. Cunha BA, Burillo A, Bouza E. Legionnaire's' disease. *Lancet* 2016;387:376–385.
30. Dunne WM, Picot N, van Belkum A. Laboratory tests for Legionnaire's disease. *Infect Dis Clin North Am* 2017;31:167–178.
31. Cunha BA, Cunha CB. Legionnaire's disease: A clinical diagnostic approach. *Infect Dis Clin North Am* 2017;31:81–94.
32. Cunha BA, Cunha CB. Legionnaire's disease and its mimics: A clinical perspective. *Infect Dis Clin North Am* 2017;31:95–109.
33. Coletta FS, Fein AM. Radiological manifestations of Legionella/Legionella-like organisms. *Semin Respir Infect* 1998;13:109–115.
34. Mittal S, Singh A, Gold M, et al. Thoracic imaging features of Legionnaire's disease. *Infect Dis Clin North Am* 2017;31:43–54.
35. Rizzo C, Caporali MG, Rota MC. Pandemic influenza and pneumonia due to *Legionella pneumophila*: A frequently underestimated coinfection. *Clin Infect Dis* 2010;51:115.
36. Magira E, Zakynthinos S. Legionnaire's disease and influenza. *Infect Dis Clin North Am* 2017;31:1337–1154.
37. Cunha BA, Klein NC, Strollo S, Syed U, Mickail N, Laguerre M. Legionnaire's disease mimicking swine influenza (H1N1) pneumonia during the "herald wave" of the pandemic. *Heart Lung* 2010;39:242–248.
38. Cunha BA. Swine Influenza (H1N1) pneumonia: Clinical considerations. *Infect Dis Clin North Am* 2010;24:203–228.
39. Cunha BA. Severe adenovirus mimicking legionella community-acquired pneumonia (CAP). *Eur J Clin Microbiol Infect Dis* 2009;28:313–315.
40. Cunha BA, Irshad N, Connolly, JJ. Adult human metapneumonovirus (hMPV) pneumonia mimicking Legionnaire's disease. *Heart Lung* 2016;45:270–272; Cunha BA. The clinical diagnosis of Legionnaire's disease: The diagnostic value of combining non-specific laboratory tests. *J Infect* 2008:56:395–397.
41. Cunha BA. Characteristic predictors that increase the pretest probability of Legionnaire's disease: "Don't' order a test just because you can" revisited. *South Med J* 2015;108:761.
42. Cunha CB. Infectious disease differential diagnosis. In: Cunha CB, Cunha BA eds. *Antibiotic Essentials* (17th ed). New Delhi, India: Jay Pee Medical Publishers, 2020.
43. Cunha BA. The diagnostic significance of relative bradycardia in infectious disease. *Clin Micro Infect* 2000;6:633–634.

44. Cunha BA, Strollo S, Schoch P. Extremely elevated erythrocyte sedimentation rates (ESRs) in Legionnaire's disease. *Eur J Clin Microbiol Infect Dis* 2010;29:1567–1569.

45. Cunha BA. Highly elevated serum ferritin levels as a diagnostic marker for Legionella pneumonia. *Clin Infect Dis* 2008;46:1789–1791.

46. Cunha BA. Hypophosphatemia: A diagnostic significance in Legionnaire's disease. *Am J Med* 2006;119:e5–e6.

47. Cunha BA, Strollo S, Schoch P. *Legionella pneumophila* community-acquired pneumonia (CAP): Incidence and intensity of microscopic hematuria. *J Infect* 2010;61:275–276.

48. Brewster UC. Acute renal failure associated with legionellosis. *Ann Intern Med* 2004;140:406–407.

49. Cunha BA, Gran A, Simon J. Round pneumonia. *Respir Care* 2013;58:e80–e82.

50. Wan YL, Kuo HP, Tsai YH, et al. Eight cases of severe acute respiratory syndrome presenting as round pneumonia. *Am J Roentgenol* 2004;182:1567–1570.

51. Cunha BA, Wu G, Raza M. Clinical diagnosis of Legionnaire's disease: Six characteristic criteria. *Am J Med* 2015:128:e21–e22.

52. Cunha BA, Cunha CB. Antimicrobial therapy for Legionnaire's disease: Antibiotic stewardship implications. *Infect Dis Clin North Am* 2017;31:179–192.

53. Kroll V, Cunha BA: Diagnostic significance of serum ferritin levels in infectious and non-infectious diseases. *Inf Dis Prac* 27:199–192.

54. Cunha BA. Pneumonias in the Compromised Host. *Inf Dis Clinics of N Amer.* 2001.

55. Cunha CB, Cunha BA. *Antibiotic Essentials* (14th ed.) JayPee Medical Publishers, New Delhi, India, 2017.

15 Severe Influenza Pneumonia and Its Mimics in the Critical Care Unit

Eleni E. Magira

CONTENTS

CLINICAL PERSPECTIVE

The big five global conditions that primarily contribute to the respiratory disease burdens are acute infections, chronic obstructive pulmonary disease (COPD), asthma, tuberculosis, and lung cancer [1].

Respiratory infections are the leading cause of death in the developing countries [2]. In a multinational study among the 5500 patients, 12% had severe acute respiratory infections. Gram-positive and gram-negative bacteria were found in 30% and 26% of patients, respectively, but atypical bacteria were rarely found (1%). Viruses were present in 7.7% of patients [3]. Another prospective population study in 2320 hospitalized adults with community-acquired pneumonia (CAP) estimated the annual incidence rates of pathogens. Viruses were detected in 27% of the patients. Among them, influenza A or B virus was the second most common pathogen causing pneumonia, detected after the human rhinovirus [4].

The respiratory illnesses caused by influenza virus infections are difficult to distinguish from other respiratory pathogens, since the clinical signs and symptoms are often overlapping. The vast majority of patients affected by this viral infection will develop mild upper respiratory symptoms or only mild pneumonia. However, other will progress their infection to severe respiratory failure. Identifying these patients is of utmost importance, since the mortality rate is usually very high [5]. In addition, influenza infection can be complicated by subsequent bacterial pneumonia or could initially present as a coinfection of bacterial pneumonia. Besides the infectious mimics of influenza, there are non-infectious diseases that mimic influenza pneumonia. The objective of this chapter is to provide comprehensive data regarding the clinical syndromic diagnosis, the differential diagnosis, and the mimics of the severe influenza pneumonia requiring critical care unit (CCU) admission.

PATHOGENESIS, INCUBATION PERIOD, CLINICAL SYNDROMES, AND AGE PATTERNS OF INFLUENZA INFECTION

WHY INFLUENZA WILL SUSTAIN ITS VIRULENCE

Influenza viruses are members of the family *Orthomyxoviridae*, with three known types: A, B, and C. They all possess single-stranded ribonucleic acid (RNA) segments to replicate. Different genomic RNA segments facilitate reassortment and swapping between different influenza virus strains. This leads to the rapid exchange of RNA segments and to new influenza subtypes. A strain such as the novel H1N1, the pandemic influenza A (H1N1) 2009, or swine influenza H1N1 virus rapidly spread from person to person because of its absence of immunity. Every new influenza subtype resulted after a genome reassortment was capable of causing an unpredictable pandemic in term of spreading, difficulty treating infection, and mortality rates. This phenomenon is called "antigenic shift" and is observed only in influenza virus A. In contrast, the "antigenic drift" involves all influenza types, and the new virus is usually easy to treat [6,7].

Depending on the type of the hemagglutinin (HA) and the neuraminidase (NA) glycoproteins that are located on the external layer of the virus structure, the influenza A virus can be subdivided into different serotypes. The subtypes H1N1 and H3N2 are the most common ones that infect humans. Inhibiting NA with oseltamivir suppresses both viral infection and viral release from the human airway epithelial cells [7].

INFLUENZA TYPES THAT MAY CAUSE SEVERE PNEUMONIA AND THE ASSOCIATED CLINICAL SYNDROMES

All influenza viruses can infect the respiratory epithelium, from the upper airways to alveoli [8,9]. However, swine influenza A H1N1 virus can progress rapidly to acute respiratory distress syndrome (ARDS) with a greater percentage of deaths. H3N2 influenza A, the prevalent subtype during the 2014–2015 season in the United States, caused record-high numbers of influenza outbreaks, with increased hospitalizations and deaths in the 2017 winter season in Australia [10].

Type B influenza, although generally regarded as having a lower morbidity and mortality in healthy people compared with type A influenza, severe respiratory failure could occur. Influenza B mainly affects children but can cause a substantial number of seasonal flu infections in adults as well. Interestingly, the most serious or fatal cases of influenza B virus-associated pneumonia were unlinked with chronic medical conditions [11]. Influenza C is much milder than types A and B.

Avian-influenza viruses (which infect birds) rarely infect humans. Currently, H7N9 influenza became a great concern in global public health due to a new outbreak that occurred in China in April 2013 [12]. Clinical presentation of the H7N9 influenza infection includes severe pneumonia, ARDS, and multiple-organ failures as the most common causes of death [13].

The clinical syndromes of the patients with influenza-associated pneumonia include primary influenza pneumonia, secondary bacterial pneumonia, and concomitant viral and bacterial pneumonia. These syndromes have been historically categorized almost as above by Louria DS et al. in studies on influenza in the pandemic of 1958 [14].

INCUBATION, SHEDDING PERIODS, AND AGE PATTERNS

Prodromal symptoms such as fever, malaise, and nausea are due to the response of the host to the influenza genome replication phase, known as the incubation period. The incubation period for influenza is in the range of 1–4 days [15]. There is also the influenza shedding period, which refers to the transmissibility of the virus from an infected person to other people. Knowledge of this time is crucial for the implementation of prevention measures within a healthcare environment and for the prompt administration of the antiviral medications. Shedding period begins 1 day before the symptoms start and last from 5–7 days. Peak shedding day is between the second day and third day after the infection. However, immunocompromised people of any age with influenza virus infection may shed viruses for weeks to months, even without fever or respiratory symptoms [16].

There is also a certain age pattern predilection in the pandemic waves of influenza. Severe pneumonia and influenza mortality in 2009 peaked at the age group of 45–54 years for both sexes, a pattern that is reminiscent of the W-shaped curve seen only during the pandemic (H1N1)1918 (Figure 15.1) [17]. Also, severe disease and mortality are affecting relatively healthy adolescents and adults between the ages of 10 years and 60 years. In contrast, in the well-characterized pandemics of the previous century, mostly children and young adults have been infected, with increased mortality at a very young age in the pattern of a U-shaped curve [17].

EPIDEMIOLOGICAL CLUES AND CLINICAL SYNDROMIC CHARACTERISTICS OF INFLUENZA PNEUMONIA

The following description refers mainly to swine influenza H1N1 virus as the most severe and dangerous manifestation of the influenza-related respiratory infection syndromes.

Patients with suspected swine H1N1 virus pneumonia on admittance require the investigation of certain epidemiological clues. Physicians must be aware that influenza A virus is present

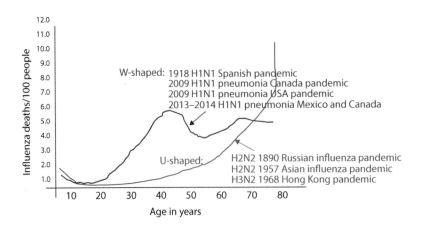

FIGURE 15.1 Predominant age groups in W- and U-shaped mortality curves showing the young adults and the very "young-elderly" people affected throughout the influenza pandemics, respectively.

in their area. The Centers for Disease Control and Prevention's (CDC) Influenza Division collects and analyses information on influenza activity year-round in the United States and produces the weekly FluView surveillance report available at https://www.cdc.gov/flu/weekly. Accordingly, for Europe and Canada, the sources are http://www.flunewseurope.org/ and https://www.canada.ca/en/public-health/services/diseases/flu-influenza/fluwatcher.html, respectively.

Key medical history questions should be of priority as well. Respiratory symptoms after an "aircraft travel" raises the possibility of Legionnaire's disease or avian influenza H5N1 or swine H1N1 influenza. Rodent exposure points to hantavirus pneumonia or plague. Deer, rabbit, and ticks raise concerns about tularemia. Close contact with people with the same symptomatology may relate to human influenza A, swine influenza H1N1 virus, or adenovirus. Flooding and constructions history may relate to *Legionella* pneumonia [18].

CLINICAL SYNDROMIC STEPWISE APPROACH OF A PATIENT WITH THE SUSPECT OF PRIMARY INFLUENZA PNEUMONIA

Although the most common over-represented risk factors (pregnant and postpartum women, immunosuppression, body mass index above 30 kg/m², asthma or COPD, diabetes mellitus, tobacco smoking, alcoholism, etc.) [19,20] are expected to be associated with severe swine 2009 H1N1 infection, establishing a clinical suspicion of a primary influenza viral respiratory tract infection, especially in the critically ill, is extremely difficult and complicated, mainly because of the poor specificity of the clinical diagnosis and the poor sensitivity of the clinical findings. Also, primary swine H1N1 influenza pneumonia can affect young adults without any underlying comorbidities.

For these reasons, the syndromic diagnostic approach that identifies a consistent group of symptoms associated with a certain likelihood of influenza infection is of major assistance in the clinical practice. The primary respiratory influenza infection may be approached in the following clinical syndromes:

1. Acute onset of high fever with cough on admittance: The clinical presentation of primary influenza A respiratory infection is abrupt and dramatic, and usually, the patient can recall the exact moment of the onset of symptoms. The majority of patients report a preceding short period of 1–2 days, with influenza-like illnesses (ILIs) characterized by intense, excruciating, and violent dry cough, high fevers more than 102°F with chills, severe forehead-over-the-brows headache, prominent myalgias in limbs and back, and prostration. Basic clinical pictures of patients diagnosed with influenza A H1N1 include cough, fever, and headache (Figure 15.2, day 1). Approximately, in one-third of patients, symptoms appear before the onset of high fever and patients usually report feeling feverish. Mainly, this happens in the older patient, who may present only with lethargy, confusion, anorexia, and cough and also in the severely immunocompromised group of patients. In this acute phase, auscultation of the lungs is clear, and the chest-X-ray is unrevealing [21]. Most individuals will recover from the illness after 7–10 days, while others progress quickly and become breathless within the first 48 hours of onset of fever and may present with another syndromic entity that is the ARDS with fever (Figure 15.2, days 3–7).

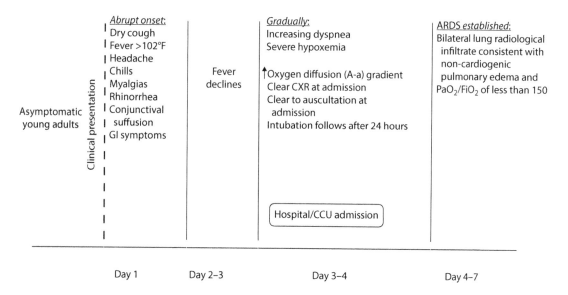

FIGURE 15.2 Clinical onset presentation of severe influenza A and its progression to ARDS. *Abbreviations*: A-a, alveolar arterial gradient; CCU, critical care unit; ARDS, acute respiratory distress syndrome; PaO₂, partial pressure of O₂ in arterial blood; FiO₂, fraction of inspired oxygen; GI, gastrointestinal.

2. Fever with ARDS on admittance: Severe diffuse influenza A pneumonitis on admittance may be suspected in a feverish patient with hypoxic or hypoxic-hypercapnic respiratory failure. Then, ARDS in the form of SaO_2 <90% at room air or frank ARDS with PaO_2/FiO_2 ratio <150 ensues (Figure 15.2). The period between the initial ILIs to the occurrence of the extensive pulmonary failure and the clinical ARDS is typically 6–72 hours [19,22]. The median time from symptoms to hospital admission is usually 3–4 days and to the CCU admission is 1 day. When patient reaches the emergency department at this phase, cough may have become productive with mild blood-stained sputum. Tachypnea is prominent, and the chest radiographic findings are of bilateral interstitial infiltrates, predominantly in the mid-zones. Chest CT scan has greater sensitivity, and mostly, the findings are bilateral alveolar consolidation, followed by either ground glass opacifications or a combination of both (Figure 15.2). These radiologic findings might be explained by the fact that influenza A virus replicated well throughout the lower respiratory tract, inducing alveolar damage with alveolar hemorrhage [23]. Patients admitted at this stage might have conjunctival suffusion [21].

3. Fever with sepsis and multi-organ dysfunction on admittance: Severe diffuse influenza pneumonitis on admittance should also be suspected when sepsis is present. In contrast, with the belief of the solely sepsis association with bacterial agents, viruses can also trigger inflammatory responses. Influenza A virus, by deregulating the innate immune system, leads to endothelial damage and to a growing cause of severe sepsis [24]. Multi-organ failure with shock, acute lung injury, acute liver injury, disseminated intravascular coagulation, and even acute encephalopathy have been described in severe influenza-sepsis [25]. Patients admitted in the CCU might have certain bad prognostic physical signs such as areas of mottled skin and peripheral cyanosis [21]. Influenza-sepsis is often neglected among septic patients.

Fulminant influenza-associated myocarditis with rapid hemodynamic decompensation, although uncommon, could present within 2 weeks of influenza onset symptoms. The most prominent electrocardiogram abnormalities include QT prolongation and other non-specific rhythm disturbances. A high propensity of the influenza A virus toward muscular inflammation is also common. Myositis and rhabdomyolysis may ensue, which rarely cause renal failure.

4. Primary acute febrile encephalopathy/encephalitis on admittance (not attributable to shock): Although influenza-associated encephalopathy has been described mostly in children, it is not unknown to the adults. Acute encephalopathy usually appears in a median of 3 days after the onset of influenza-related symptoms. In a population-based study, neurological complications of patients with severe and fatal influenza A (H1N1) cases were observed in 4% [26]. The CDC has defined the H1N1-associated encephalitis as altered mental status >24 h within 5 days of ILIs' onset in patients with focal neurological signs not explained otherwise [27]. Pleocytosis and protein elevation in the cerebrospinal fluid can be absent [28,29]. Guillain-Barré syndrome and Reye syndrome are also complications associated with primary-influenza brain infection.

Influenza febrile encephalopathy is a missed clinical entity. The intensivists, in order to facilitate mechanical ventilation in patients with severe influenza pneumonia, subjected them to prolonged sedation, making the daily control of the level of consciousness difficult. As a result, elevated intracranial pressure with malignant cerebral edema and seizures, some of the most ominous conditions related to the primary-influenza brain infection, may be missed. Therefore, intensivists who treat influenza-infected patients should be daily vigilant, in any change of the eye pupils with regard to dilation, fixation, and unresponsiveness.

LABORATORY FINDINGS

NON-SPECIFIC LABORATORY DIAGNOSTIC MARKERS

On admission, a presumptive diagnosis of severe influenza infection, based on non-specific laboratory markers, is absolutely necessary to differentiate pneumonia due to influenza from other respiratory viruses. The most common laboratory findings described in patients who had confirmed 2009 H1N1 virus infection are leukopenia (<5000/mm^3) with relative lymphopenia (<1000/mm^3), thrombocytopenia, monocytosis, and severe-refractory hypoxemia, all not explained otherwise. Interestingly, lymphocytes-to-monocytes ratio <2 on admission through day 3 was used as an indicator of influenza A infection [30]. The leukopenia mostly is transient and mild and should not cause alarm for specific hematological tests unless it is prolonged. Severe hypoxemia is indicated by the increase of alveolar-arterial gradient (A-aO_2) of more than 35 or by acute respiratory failure with SaO_2 <90% and PaO_2 <60 mmHg on room air. When a patient is admitted in the CCU, the initial ratio of PaO_2/FiO_2 is usually <150.

Another key laboratory finding is the mildly deranged liver biochemistry after collateral damage in the liver. Serum levels of alanine aminotransferase (ALT), aspartate aminotransferase (AST), alkaline phosphatase (ALP), and gamma-glutamyl transferase (GGT) are increased in the pandemic influenza infection, mostly 2–4 times above the normal ranges. Dissemination of the influenza virus or transient viremia with systematic inflammation that produces perfusion disturbances to the hepatocellular system and hypertransaminemia may be an explanation.

Creatine phosphokinase (CK) increases, and rhabdomyolysis may be present in a critically ill patient with 2009 influenza A(H1N1)-induced respiratory failure. Varying CK levels between 500 U/L and 100 U/L (normal, 13–156 U/L) are noticed. However, in some cases, influenza invasion induces acute myositis or myonecrosis, with a marked elevation of CK up to 10,000 U/L. Acute kidney injury in influenza infection is mainly attributable to shock and not to rhabdomyolysis.

A non-specific laboratory triad identified by the Winthrop-University Hospital Infectious Disease Division allows clinicians to make a rapid, presumptive diagnosis of H1N1 in adults (Table 15.1, A) [31].

TABLE 15.1

Non-Specific Laboratory Diagnostic Triad Identified by the Winthrop-University Hospital Infectious Disease Division Allows Clinicians to Make a Presumptive Diagnosis of H1N1 in Hospitalized Adults

A. Probable H1N1 pneumonia diagnosis

ILIs with temperature >102°F and with severe myalgias, chest-X-ray with no focal or segmental lobar infiltrates and negative rapid influenza test, plus this diagnostic triad:

1. Relative lymphopenia
2. Elevated serum transaminases
3. Elevated CK

B. Definite H1N1 pneumonia diagnosis (laboratory criteria)

ILIs plus one or more of these tests:

1. Rapid influenza A test
2. Respiratory FA viral panel
3. RT-PCR for H1N1

Abbreviations: CK, creatine phosphokinase; ILIs, influenza-like illnesses; RT-PCR, real-time reverse transcriptase polymerase chain reaction; FA, fluorescence antibody.

ACUTE-PHASE PROTEINS AND INFLUENZA PNEUMONIA

The measurement of non-specific inflammation markers, erythrocyte sedimentation rate (ESR), C-reactive protein (CRP), procalcitonin, and fibrinogen may assist in excluding a bacterial coinfection from primary influenza A pneumonia. The CRP and ESR concentrations in serum usually peak during days 2–4 and 4–5 after influenza illness, respectively. Concentrations of procalcitonin greater than 0.5 µg/L support bacterial infection, whereas repeatedly low amounts suggest that bacterial infection is unlikely [32]. Fibrinogen concentrations are mostly low to normal. Measurement of serum ferritin may strongly assist as a diagnostic eliminator toward influenza A and suggests the possibility of an alternate diagnosis (high elevated ferritin levels are identified in *Legionella* infection) [33].

DEFINITIVE LABORATORY DIAGNOSTIC TESTS

A laboratory diagnostic triad identified by the Winthrop-University Hospital Infectious Disease Division allows clinicians to make a definite H1N1 pneumonia diagnosis (Table 15.1, B) [31]. This laboratory confirmation is necessary for the definite diagnosis of the influenza virus infection, the differentiation between epidemic and pandemic viruses, and the management plan of patients.

Important factor that influences influenza laboratory results is the time from illness onset to the collection of respiratory specimens for testing. The highest influenza virus yield is within 4 days of illness onset, and the ideal is to collect respiratory tract specimens within 4 days of illness onset. Another important factor that influences laboratory results is the source of the respiratory specimens tested. Nasopharyngeal aspirates or nose-throat swab samples are considered the specimens of choice in diagnostic testing for influenza virus detection in non-intubated patients [34]. However, for critically ill intubated patients with suspected lower respiratory tract influenza–related disease, lower respiratory tract specimens should be collected and tested. Broncho-alveolar lavage fluid or endotracheal aspirate should be additionally tested by the high-sensitivity and -specificity nucleic acid amplification tests if a high clinical suspicion for influenza exists [35].

Diagnostic tests available for influenza include rapid influenza antigen, viral culture, immunofluorescence antibody, serology, and the real-time reverse transcriptase-polymerase chain reaction (rRT-PCR) assays (Table 15.2). The PCR-based method is the most widely preferred method for detecting influenza virus because of its high sensitivity and specificity. Currently, only the CDC's RT-PCR assay is FDA-cleared for lower respiratory tract specimens [35].

TABLE 15.2

Laboratory Diagnosis of Influenza

Methods	Comments	Sensitivity	Turnaround Time
1. POC rapid influenza test (antigen detection)	• May distinguish Influenza A from B type	10%–70%	15 min–1 h
2. Immunofluorescence direct/indirect antibody testing	• Distinguish Influenza A from B type	25%–93%	technically difficult
3. Serology	• Identifies convalescent stage as compared with acute stage (titers must be ≥ 4) • Valuable in seroepidemiological studies	90%	~24 h
4. Viral cell culture	• Distinguishes 2009 H1N1 Influenza from other Influenza A viruses • Gold standard in Influenza diagnostics	~95%	4–5 days
5. Polymerase chain reaction assays	• Identifies Influenza A and B viral RNA • CDC Human Influenza Virus Real-Time • rRT-PCR Diagnostic Panel (A/B typing Kit) (bronchoalveolar lavages, bronchial washes, tracheal aspirates, lung tissue)	~99%	~3–4 h

Source: Guidance for Clinicians on the Use of RT-PCR and Other Molecular Assays for Diagnosis of Influenza Virus Infection, Available at: https://www.cdc.gov/flu/professionals/diagnosis/molecular-assays.htm.

Abbreviations: POC, point of care; rRT-PCR, real-time reverse transcriptase-polymerase chain reaction; CDC, Centers for Disease Control and Prevention.

DIFFERENTIAL DIAGNOSIS OF SEVERE PRIMARY INFLUENZA

The differential diagnosis of severe primary-influenza pneumonia is wide, since many infectious and non-infectious conditions can cause ILIs. The presence of localized symptoms is important for the differential diagnosis.

INFECTIOUS CAUSES THAT MIMIC PRIMARY-INFLUENZA PNEUMONIA IN CCU

1. *Differential diagnosis of acute onset of high fever with cough and ILI symptoms in the CCU setting*

    Besides influenza A, a variety of respiratory viruses (such as rhinovirus, adenovirus, respiratory syncytial virus, human metapneumonovirus, and parainfluenza viruses) causes ILIs, and it is nearly impossible to differentiate one virus from another. These viruses have been detected in 16%–49% of patients with acute respiratory failure requiring CCU care [36]. Immunocompromised patients with hematological or other malignancies, residents of long-term care facilities, and residents of nursing homes are more vulnerable to respiratory viral infections. People of advanced age are frequently lack of fever and all the protean manifestations of influenza. Also, viral-viral coinfection is not an unusual phenomenon. Table 15.3 presents the differential diagnosis of primary influenza virus pneumonia versus other respiratory viruses in critically ill patients admitted with ILIs.

    Localized symptoms such as the presence of headache and neck pain, nausea, vomiting, and confusion should alert about viral or bacterial meningitis.

Photophobia may be present as well. If a petechial or purpuric rash on hospital presentation exists, this will suggest meningococcemia [37].

The ILIs with fatigue and malaise in the elderly rather than the classical clinical features (abrupt onset of a sore throat, pharyngitis, and cervical lymphadenopathy in the adolescents and young adults) raise the possibility of Epstein–Barr virus (EBV) or mononucleosis infection. Mild to moderately elevated serum transaminases is the predominant laboratory abnormality. A generalized maculopapular or urticarial rash may be noticed when patients are treated for their pharyngitis with ampicillin. Flu-like symptoms in acquired-toxoplasmosis are usually accompanied by swollen non-tender lymph glands and muscle aches that last for a month or more. In acquired toxoplasmosis, a maculopapular/macular rash may rarely appear. Hepatitis B virus can produce a syndrome similar to the ILI syndrome but with fever <102°F, loss of appetite, nausea, vomiting, and polyarthritis. An erythematous or macular/maculopapular rash transiently during the incubation period may be noticed. High fever >104°F, runny nose, swollen eyelids with conjunctivitis, and grayish-white spots (Koplik's spots) in the mouth point toward measles. However, the clinical presentation in immunocompromised hosts is very atypical. A confluent maculopapular or blotchy red spots appear 2–4 days after the onset of illness. *Primary HIV* infection appears like infectious-mononucleosis syndrome that lasts from a few days to 4 weeks. Fever is less than 102°F. A diffuse rash 1–3 weeks after infection, along with the social and sexual history, is helpful in deciding about HIV testing [38]. Most of the previously mentioned

TABLE 15.3

Differential Diagnosis of Respiratory Viruses Causing Primary Pneumonia Among Critically Ill Patients that are Admitted with ILIs

	Pandemic Influenza A	Adenovirus[a]	RSV	Rhinovirus	h-Metapneumovirus	PIVs1-4[b]	Corona virus (MERS-CoV, SARS-CoV)	Pandemic CoVID-19[e]
Incubation	1–3d	7–14d	3–5d	2–4d	3–5d	3–5d	SARS:2–10d MERS: 2–14d other: 2–5d	SARS-CoV-2: 2–14d
Season	winter but also year-round	year-round	winter	fall but also year-round	spring but also year-round	summer but also year-round	winter but also year-round	winter but also year round
Age group	adolescents and adults	all	all	all	all	all (mostly hospitalized, immunosupressed)	adolescents and adults	adolescents and adults
Onset	acute	less acute	less acute	less acute	less acute	less acute	less acute initially	less acute initially
Fever	high (>102.2°F) up to 3d	high (>102°F) prolonged	low-grade (<101°F)	subjective (<102°F)	absence to low grade	low grade	high (>102.2°F)	absence to high (>102.2°F)
Other symptoms/signs besides ILIs	severe prostration severe myalgias forehead ache conjunctivatis cough dry	pharyngo-conjunctivatis	rhinorea cough spastic wheezing/rales hoarseness	asthma or COPD severe exacerbations rhinorea sneezing	cough productive, nasal congestion, asthma or COPD exacerbations, wheezing	croup, hoarseness, sinusitis stridor "pertussoid" cough[c]	shortness of breath, myalgia, diarrhea, Vomiting	dry cough, malaise, severe dyspnea, hypoxemia, oliguria, loss of sense of smell and taste
Primary pneumonia-ARDS	yes	yes	yes (10%)	yes	yes	yes	yes	yes
Encephalitis	yes	yes	yes	yes	seizures	uncommon	yes	uncommon
Myocarditis/pericarditis	yes	uncommon	yes	yes	no	uncommon	no	uncommon
Acute renal failure	yes rarely	acute hemorrhagic cystitis	no	no	no	no	yes	yes
Septic shock-MODs	yes	rarely	no	no	no	no	yes	yes

(Continued)

TABLE 15.3 (Continued)
Differential Diagnosis of Respiratory Viruses Causing Primary Pneumonia Among Critically Ill Patients that are Admitted with ILIs

	Pandemic Influenza A	Adenovirus[a]	RSV	Rhinovirus	h-Metapneumovirus	PIVs1-4[b]	Corona virus (MERS-CoV, SARS-CoV)	Pandemic CoVID-19[e]
Chest X-ray	clear lungs initially, bilateral patchy infiltrates later	bilateral patchy parenchymal opacities	small focal unilateral infiltrates	interstitial or consolidated lesions	ground glass opacity initially, bronchiolitis/bronchitis	no infiltrates or bilateral patchy consolidation	discrete infiltrates	bilateral ground glass opacity
Non-specific laboratory tests	leukopenia, acute thrombocytopenia relative lymphopenia, ↑SGOT/SGPT	leukopenia, acute thrombocytopenia relative lymphopenia, ↑SGOT/SGPT, ↑Cold agglutinin	normal or mildly ↑WBC, ↑% band forms	lymphopenia and ↑C-reactive protein	lymphopenia, neutropenia, ↑SGOT/ SGPT	relative lymphopenia thrombocytopenia lymphocytes/ monocytes ratio <2 on admission through more than 3 days[d]	leukopenia, acute thrombocytopenia relative lymphopenia, ↑SGOT/SGPT	leukopenia, acute thrombocytopenia relative lymphopenia, ↑troponin, ↑ferritin, ↑D-Dimers, ↑SGOT/SGPT

Abbreviations: COPD, chronic obstructive pulmonary disease, CoVID-19, Coronavirus disease 2019, CoVID-19 SARS-CoV-2, severe acute respiratory syndrome coronavirus 2 MERS-CoV, Middle Eastern respiratory syndrome coronavirus, SARS-CoV, Severe acute respiratory syndrome coronavirus, MODs, multiorgan dysfunctions.

a Severe respiratory disease is associated with adenovirus serotypes 5, 7, 14, and 21.

b Parainfluenza type 3 is more commonly associated with pneumonia than other types.

c Cunha B, Mickail N, Schoch P.Human parainfluenza virus type 3 (HPIV 3) community-acquired pneumonia (CAP) mimicking pertussis in an adult: The diagnostic importance of hoarseness and monocytosis. *Heart Lung.* 2011 ;40(6):569–73.

d Cunha BA, Connolly JJ, Irshad N. The clinical usefulness of lymphocyte: monocyte ratios in differentiating influenza from viral non-influenza-like illnesses in hospitalized adults during the 2015 influenza A (H3N2) epidemic: the uniqueness of HPIV-3 mimicking influenza A. *Eur J Clin Microbiol Infect Dis.* 2016 Jan;35(1):155–8.

e The new pandemic SARS-CoV-2 not yet clarified completely as to the natural history, spread patterns, symptoms and complications.

clinical entities are accompanied by a rash on hospital presentation; this is an uncommon feature among adults with influenza A but has been reported mainly in young children [39].

In any patient with recent travel or exposure to mosquitoes, acute onset of ILIs must raise the suspicion about malaria, Zika virus, Chikungunya virus, or dengue virus [38] (please see Table 15.5).

2. *Differential diagnosis of acute onset of fever with ARDS in the CCU setting*

Acute onset of fever with respiratory distress syndrome points mainly toward severe CAP and hospital-associated pneumonia. A differential diagnosis to distinguish primary influenza virus pneumonia versus other respiratory bacteria causing CAP is presented in Table 15.4.

Diffuse pulmonary infiltrates with poor oxygenation at admission (arterial oxygen partial pressure of <60 mmHg or an alveolar-arterial gradient >35 mmHg on room air) suggest *Pneumocystis jirovecii* pneumonia (PJP). HIV patients, cancer patients following organ transplantation or receiving chemotherapy, and rarely immunocompetent adults are infected. Symptoms associated with PJP occur in a subacute fashion, unlike the acute onset of influenza infection [18].

Bacillus anthracis, which causes anthrax, usually begins with non-specific prodromal ILIs that soon escalate into severe respiratory failure and ARDS. The presence of hemorrhagic mediastinal widening with adenopathy in chest radiographs is typical [40].

In the prodromal phase of *hantavirus* infection, the typical findings are fever, myalgias, tachypnea, and tachycardia. Most patients within 24 hours of initial evaluation progress to non-cardiogenic pulmonary edema require mechanical ventilation. Coryza and dry cough are absent. The white blood cell count tends to be raised, with a left-shifted neutrophilia, along with myeloid precursors and atypical lymphocytes. Hematocrit is usually elevated due to hemoconcentration. An initial chest radiograph is usually positive for interstitial and/or alveolar infiltrates with pleural effusions [41].

Malaria-induced ARDS either is the main clinical feature when parasitemia is falling after initiation of treatment or may be seen as part of a severe multisystem malaria-induced illness. Abrupt dyspnea with tachypnea, expiratory wheezes, and frothy sputum are usually the earliest symptoms and signs [37].

3. *Differential diagnosis of acute fever with sepsis and multi-organ dysfunction in the CCU setting*

Infections due to the gram-negative and -positive bacteria and especially the multiresistant ones (*Pseudomonas aeruginosa, Acinetobacter baumannii, Staphylococcus aureus, Enterococci spp*, etc.) are certainly common causes of fever with multi-organ dysfunction in the CCU. Polymorphonuclear leukocytosis and lymphocytopenia, markedly elevated CRP, hypotension, tachycardia, and warm extremities in the early stage of septic shock are the most frequent findings. Patients with bacterial sepsis may also present with vague constitutional symptoms, mild hypotension and tachycardia or fever, and myalgia attributed to "a viral syndrome."

Of great interest are the zoonotic causes of acute fever with organ failures [38,42], as presented in Table 15.5.

Specifically, dengue virus has a huge dynamic with multiple manifestations, from flu-like illnesses with headache, retro-orbital eye pain arthralgia, myalgia, and leukopenia to severe organ (liver, heart, and central

TABLE 15.4

Differential Diagnosis of Primary Influenza Virus Pneumonia Versus Respiratory Bacteria Presenting with ILIs and Causing CAP

Pathogens	CXR Findings	Clinical Signs, Symptoms, Labs
Pandemic influenza A	Initially clear lungs in CXR, bilateral patchy infiltrates later	Severe hypoxemia, relative lymphopenia, ↑SGOT/SGPT, ↓CRP
Streptococcus pneumoniae	Focal/segmental infiltrates	Mild/moderate hypoxemia, leukocytosis, ↑↑↑CRP
Staphylococcus aureus	Focal/segmental infiltrates rapid cavitation in less than 72h	Mild/moderate hypoxemia, leukocytosis, ↑↑↑CRP
Legionella pneumophila	Rapidly progressive bilateral asymmetric infiltrates	Mild/moderate hypoxemia ↑↑ferritin, ↓serum phosphorus, ↑SGOT/SGPT, relative lymphopenia, mental confusion
Klebsiella pneumoniae	Focal/segmental infiltrates cavitation after 3–5 days	mild/moderate hypoxemia leukocytosis, ↑↑↑CRP
Burkholderia pseudomallei	Irregular enlarged (3–15 mm) nodular opacities, bilaterally or segmental or lobar consolidation cavitation	Severe hypoxemia, chest pain, cough (+/−sputum), CRP normal or mildly elevated

Source: Cunha, B., Severe community-acquired pneumonia in critical care, In: Cunha, B. ed., *Infectious Diseases in Critical Care Medicine* (3rd ed.), Informa Healthcare, New York, pp. 168, 2010.

Abbreviations: CAP, community-acquired pneumonia; CXR, chest -X ray; SGOT, Serum Glutamil Oxaloacetic Transaminase; SGPT, Serum Glutamic Pyruvic Transaminase; CRP, C-reactive protein.

TABLE 15.5

Reservoirs, Clinical, and Laboratory Manifestations Among the Usual Zoonotic Infectious Diseases Causing Acute ILI and Multi-Organ Failure Versus Pandemic Influenza A

Pathogens	Usual Reservoirs	Clinical Signs, Symptoms, and Labs
Pandemic influenza A	Human, turkeys, cats, dogs, ferrets	Fever >102°F, pneumonia, myocarditis, hepatitis, encephalitis
Leptospira interrogans Leptospirosis	Brown rat, mice, dogs	Fever >102°F biphasic pattern, headache, renal failure hyperbilirubinemia, coagulation abnormalities, anemia
Rickettsia rickettsii Spotted fever	Dogs, cats	Fever >102°F with relative bradycardia, periorbital, hands and dorsum edema, conjunctival suffusion, acute tubular necrosis, pancreatitis, ARDS, myocarditis, confusion, rash
Coxiella burnetii Acute Q fever	Cattle, sheep, goats, wallabies, cat	Fever >104°F mild transaminitis, hepatomegaly, and/or splenomegaly, ARDS, meningoencephalitis
Yersinia pestis Plague	Squirrels, rock squirrels, chipmunks	Fever >102°F, chills, headache, tachycardia, hypotension malaise, large and edematous lymph nodes (femoral), abdominal pain and gangrene of the extremities, multi-organ failure (septisemic plague)
Francisella tularensis Typhoidal tularemia	Rabbits, hares, and rodents	Fever >102°F chills, sepsis, DIC, ARDS, pericarditis, meningitis and multi-organ failure
Dengue viruses Dengue	Mosquitos (*Aedes aegypti*)	Fever >102°F biphasic pattern, respiratory distress, bleeding, severe organ failure (dengue shock syndrome) transaminase levels > 1000 IU/L, ↑↑↑ferritin, truncal rash
Plasmodium falciparum, Vivax	Mosquitos (*Anopheles*)	Fever >102°F irregular initially. profuse sweeting, impaired consciousness, coma, ARDS, shock, coagulopathy, renal/liver failure, hypoglycemia, metabolic acidosis. ↑↑lactate
Zika virus	Mosquitos (*Aedes albopictus, A. aegypti*), sexual contact, body secretions	Fever <102°F. headache, arthralgias, myalgia, conjunctivitis and maculopapular and pruritic rash (prominent features), mild lymphopenia, mild neutropenia, rarely multi-organ failure
Chikungunya	Mosquito (*Aedes albopictus, A. aegypti*)	Abrupt onset of fever >102°F and peripheral arthralgia, acute cardiac failure septic shock
West Nile virus	Mosquito (*Culex tarsalis, C. pipiens, C. quinquefasciatus*)	Abrupt onset of fever >102°F, headaches, fatigue, myalgias, anorexia, vomiting, maculopapular, non-pruritic rash and rarely hemorrhagic pancreatitis, hepatitis, myocarditis, DIC
Yellow fever	Mosquito (*Aedes aegypti*)	Fever, headache, chills, back pain, fatigue, muscle pain, vomiting, jaundice, transaminitis hemorrhage, renal failure, multisystem organ failure may follow yellow fever vaccination

Source: Simon, E. et al., *J. Emerg. Med.*, 53, 49–65, 2017; Day, M.J. et al., *Emerg. Infect. Dis.*, 18, e1, 2012.

Abbreviations: ARDS, acute respiratory distress syndrome; DIC, disseminated intravascular coagulation.

nervous system) impairment and bleeding. Persistent vomiting, abdominal pain, and mucosal bleeding are important warning symptoms. The biphasic pattern of the fever, the truncal rash, and the elevated serum ferritin are key findings [38]. Typhoidal tularemia resulting from *Francisella tularensis* is characterized by productive cough, pleuritic chest pain, dyspnea, prostration, and frequently gastrointestinal symptoms. Typhoidal and pneumonic tularemia are the most likely forms to lead to sepsis and multi-organ failure [40].

A less familiar tick-borne illness, human *ehrlichiosis*, produces acute ILIs that can progress rapidly to severe multisystem disease with toxic shock-like syndrome, mainly in the elderly, if left untreated.

4. *Differential diagnosis of primary acute febrile encephalopathy*

The season, whether spring or early fall, raises the likelihood of vector-borne infections such as West Nile virus (WNV). The neuroinvasive type

of WNV disease displays fever and headache, meningitis, changes in consciousness, and flaccid limb paralysis (poliomyelitis-like syndrome) [38]. Herpes simplex encephalitis, the most frequent sporadic encephalitis, typically presents with acute onset fever, headache, acute confusional states, personality changes, and seizures, with characteristic electroencephalography lesions [38]. Depending on the geographical area, acute febrile encephalopathy can cause arboviruses (Japanese B encephalitis, La Crosse strain of California) or reovirus (Colorado tick fever virus). Cardinal prodromal symptoms of viral encephalitis are nausea, vomiting, fever, headache, and then confusion with disorientation [43]. Enterovirus 71, a brainstem encephalitis, is frequently accompanied by severe cardiorespiratory symptoms after a prodromal stage of fever, photophobia, vomiting, headache, and abdominal pain [44].

TABLE 15.6

Non-Infectious Mimics of Primary Influenza A Pneumonia

Influenza Pneumonia Mimics	Symptoms, Signs	Clinical, Radiology, or Laboratory Findings
Acute pulmonary edema	Cough, shortness of breath, fatigue	Peripheral edema, orthopnea, S3 or S4 heart sound
Acute eosinophilic pneumonia	Fever, shortness of breath, myalgia, severe respiratory failure	↑↑↑Eosinophils in the bronchoalveolar lavage
Acute respiratory distress bilateral syndrome	Fever, shortness of breath	White-out appearance on chest-X-ray with multiple lungs infiltrates
Diffuse alveolar hemorrhage	Fever, +/− hemoptysis, hypoxemia	Diffuse radiological Infiltrates, ↑↑↑hemosiderin-laden macrophage in the bronchoalveolar lavage, positive autoantibodies
Interstitial lung diseases	Shortness of breath, hypoxemia	Diffuse lung infiltrates on chest X-ray
Pulmonary emboli	Low fever, shortness of breath pleuritic chest pain	Typical findings in CT pulmonary angiography
Atelectasis	Low fever, hypoxemia	Alveolar collapse, bilateral infiltrates on chest X-ray
Transfusion-related ALI	Low fever, hypoxemia	Bilateral opacifications on chest X-ray
Acute lupus	Variable degree respiratory impairment	Focal or diffuse pulmonary consolidation
Acute leukemia/lymphoma	Low fever, difficulty breathing	Focal or diffuse pulmonary consolidation
Engraftment syndrome	Fever, hypoxemia	Skin rash, capillary leak features

NON-INFECTIOUS CAUSES THAT MIMIC PRIMARY INFLUENZA PNEUMONIA IN CCU

In critical care, the common non-infectious mimics of primary influenza A pneumonia are included in Table 15.6.

BACTERIAL INFECTIONS ASSOCIATED WITH SWINE INFLUENZA

Influenza A pneumonia most commonly occurs alone [21]. However, it may be complicated by bacterial coinfection, occurring either simultaneously with onset of influenza illness or as a secondary bacterial infection occurring after influenza illness or clearance of virus. Moreover, bacterial coinfection (either due to gram-negative rods or gram-positive pathogens) may occur in hospital settings, especially when "the patient was getting better, but is now getting worse."

During the 2009 H1N1 influenza pandemic, bacterial pneumonia was present in 4%–33% of hospitalized or critically ill patients [45]. Bacterial pneumonia peaks anywhere from 4–14 days after the primary influenza infection [46].

Streptococcus pneumoniae as well as *Staphylococcus aureus* are the most important pathogens causing secondary bacterial pneumonia after influenza [47]. Especially when *S. pneumoniae* is involved as a secondary bacterial pneumonia, increased morbidity and mortality have been noticed [48]. As far as the methicillin-resistant staphylococcus aureus (MRSA) coinfection is concerned, the US CDC in 2009 reported only one case with MRSA coinfection out of the 272 patients hospitalized with pandemic A(H1N1)2009 influenza virus [19]. However, postmortem lung specimens from 77 cases of fatal A (H1N1) 2009 influenza virus infection demonstrated the evidence of concurrent bacterial infection in 22 (29%) patients, 5 of which were MRSA [49]. In contrast, invasive group A *Streptococcus* (GAS) infection concurrent with either seasonal or 2009 H1N1 influenza

has been less often reported. Concurrent infection influenza A with *Mycoplasma pneumoniae* has been reported among 1060 patients with respiratory tract infections [50].

EMPIRIC THERAPY AND CLINICAL MANAGEMENT OF SEVERE INFLUENZA PNEUMONIA IN CCU

Currently, the approved antiviral influenza medications are oral oseltamivir, intravenous peramivir, and the investigational intravenous zanamivir. They are neuraminidase inhibitors against both influenza A and B viruses, and treatment should be ideally started within 48 hours of symptoms onset but even later in hospitalized patients. Resistance to oseltamivir, zanamivir, and peramivir is currently low, but this can change.

Pharmacokinetically, orally administered oseltamivir has been reported to be adequately absorbed in critically ill adults, with standard doses (75 mg b.i.d) producing therapeutic blood levels [51]. Limited data suggest that higher dosing may not provide an additional clinical benefit [51,52]. Treatment regimens in critically ill patients with respiratory failure can be longer than 5 days because of prolonged influenza viral replication in the lower respiratory tract [53]. Recommended strategies for H1N1-induced severe ARDS patients include low-tidal volume ventilation, prone positioning, nitric oxide inhalation, and finally administration of extracorporeal membrane oxygenation as the rescue therapy.

Antimicrobial co-therapy is not generally recommended in ARDS patients with influenza A (H1N1) [54] but only in cases complicated by bacterial pneumonia. The antimicrobials should show activity against *Staphylococcus aureus*, *Streptococcus pneumonia*, and *Streptococcus pyogenes* and include ampicillin/sulbactam, amoxicillin/clavulanate, third-generation cephalosporins, and respiratory quinolones.

CONCLUSIONS

Influenza A virus is considered a self-limited infection. However, a patient with an ILI can be subjected to severe pneumonia with respiratory failure. Influenza A mainly targets the lower respiratory tract but might present with other distinct clinical syndromic entities in the CCU. Among them, multi-organ failure with ARDS and septic shock are the most prominent. The consideration about the different infectious and non-infectious conditions that mimic influenza pneumonia at admittance must be sufficient. A history of travel and exposures at the earliest possible entry point is essential. In addition, the absence of symptoms of ILIs does not effectively rule out influenza infection, especially in the elderly and immunocompromised people. Knowing the wide spectrum of the presentation and severity of influenza infection, intensivists in the CCU will have to find what they seek to.

REFERENCES

1. Forum of International Respiratory Societies (FIRS). Sheffield (UK): European Respiratory Society; 2013. Available at: http://www.thoracic.org/global-health/firs-report-respiratory-diseases-in-the-world/index.php.
2. Murray CJ, Lopez AD. Measuring the global burden of disease. *N Engl J Med* 2013;369(5):448–457.
3. Sakr Y, Ferrer R, Reinhart K, et al. The intensive care global study on severe acute respiratory infection (IC-GLOSSARI): A multicenter, multinational, 14-day inception cohort study. *Intensive Care Med* 2017;42(5):817–828.
4. Jain S, Self WH, Wunderink RG, et al. Community-acquired pneumonia requiring hospitalization among U.S. Adults. *N Engl J Med* 2015;373:415–427.
5. Rello J, Rodríguez A, Ibañez P, et al. Intensive care adult patients with severe respiratory failure caused by Influenza A (H1N1)v in Spain. *Crit Care* 2009;13(5):R148.
6. Holmes EC, Ghedin E, Miller N, et al. Whole-genome analysis of human influenza A virus reveals multiple persistent lineages and reassortment among recent H3N2 viruses. *PLoS Biol* 2005;3(9):e300.
7. Nicholson KG, Wenster RG, Hay AJ. *Textbook of Influenza*. Oxford: Blackwell Science, 1998:3–18.
8. Guarner J, Falcón-Escobedo R. Comparison of the pathology caused by H1N1, H5N1, and H3N2 influenza viruses. *Arch Med Res* 2009;40:655–661.
9. Ng WF, To KF. Pathology of human H5N1 infection: New findings. *Lancet* 2007;370:1106–1108.
10. Sullivan SG, Chilver MB, Carville KS, et al. Low interim influenza vaccine effectiveness, Australia, 1 May to 24 September 2017. *Euro Surveill* 2017;22(43).
11. Gutiérrez-Pizarraya A, Pérez-Romero P, Alvarez R, et al. Unexpected severity of cases of influenza B infection in patients that required hospitalization during the first postpandemic wave. *J Infect* 2012;65:423–430.
12. Kageyama T, Fujisaki S, Takashita E, et al. Genetic analysis of novel avian A(H7N9) influenza viruses isolated from patients in China, February to April 2013. *Euro Surveill* 2013;18(15):20453.
13. Emergence of avian influenza A(H7N9) virus causing severe human illness—China, February–April 2013. Centers for Disease Control and Prevention (CDC). *Morb Mortal Wkly Rep* 2013;62(18):366–371.
14. Louria D, Blumenfeld H, Ellis J, et al. Studies of influenza in the pandemic of 1957–1958II. Pulmonary complications of influenza. *J Clin Invest* 1959;38(1):213–265.
15. Lessler J, Reich NG, Brookmeyer R, et al. Incubation periods of acute respiratory viral infections: A systematic review. *Lancet Infect Dis* 2009;9:291–300.
16. Harper SA, Bradley JS, Englund JA, et al. Seasonal influenza in adults and children-diagnosis, treatment, chemoprophylaxis, and institutional outbreak management: Clinical practice guidelines of the Infectious Diseases Society of America. *Clin Inf Dis* 2009;48:1003–1032.
17. Taubenberger JK, Morens DM. 1918 Influenza: The mother of all pandemics. *Emerg Infect Dis* 2006;12(1):15–22.
18. Cunha B. Severe community-acquired pneumonia in critical care. In: Cunha B ed. *Infectious Diseases in Critical Care Medicine* (3rd ed.). New York: Informa Healthcare, 2010:168.
19. Jain S, Kamimoto L, Bramley AM, et al. Hospitalized patients with 2009 H1N1influenza in the United States, April–June 2009. *N Engl J Med* 2009;361:1935–1944.
20. Louie JK, Acosta M, Jamieson DJ, Honein MA. Severe 2009 H1N1 influenza in pregnant and postpartum women in California. *N Engl J Med* 2010;362:27–35.
21. Cunha B. Influenza: Historical aspects of epidemics and pandemics. *Infect Dis Clin North Am* 2004;141–155.
22. Kumar A, Zarychanski R, Pinto R, et al. Critically ill patients with 2009 influenza A (H1N1) infection in Canada. *JAMA* 2009;302:1872–1879.
23. Taubenberger JK, Morens DM. The pathology of influenza virus infections. *Annu Rev Pathol* 2008;3:499–522.
24. Steinberg BE, Goldenberg NM, Lee WL. Do viral infections mimic bacterial sepsis? The role of microvascular permeability: A review of mechanisms and methods. *Antiviral Res* 2012;93(1):2–15.
25. Armstrong SM, Mubareka S, Lee WL. The lung microvascular endothelium as a therapeutic target in severe influenza. *Antiviral Res* 2013;99:113–118.
26. Glaser CA, Winter K, DuBray K, et al. A population-based study of neurologic manifestations of severe influenza A (H1N1) pdm09 in California. *Clin Infect Dis* 2012;55:514–520.
27. Center for Disease Control and Prevention (CDC). Neurologic complications associated with novel influenza A (H1N1) virus infection in children. *Morb Mortal Wkly Rep* 2009;58:773–778.
28. Studahl M. Influenza virus and CNS manifestations. *J Clin Virol* 2003;28:225–232.
29. Togashi T, Matsuzono Y, Narita M, et al. Influenza-associated acute encephalopathy in Japanese children in 1994–2002. *Virus Res* 2004;103:75–78.
30. McClain MT, Park LP, Nicholson B, et al. Longitudinal analysis of leukocyte differentials in peripheral blood of patients with acute respiratory viral infections. *J Clin Virol* 20132;58:689–695.
31. Cunha BA, Syed U, Strollo S, Mickail N, Laguerre M. Rapid clinical diagnosis of swine influenza (H1N1) using the Swine influenza diagnostic triad. *Heart Lung* 2010;39(5):461.
32. Ruuskanen O, Lahti E, Jennings LC, Murdoch DR. Viral pneumonia. *Lancet* 2011;377(9773):1264–1275.
33. Cunha BA, Raza M. During influenza season: All influenza-like illnesses are not due to influenza: Dengue mimicking influenza. *J Emerg Med* 2015;48(5):e117–e120.
34. López Roa P, Rodríguez-Sánchez B, Catalán P, et al. Diagnosis of influenza in intensive care units: Lower respiratory tract samples are better than nose-throat swabs. *Am J Respir Crit Care Med* 2012;186(9):929–930.

35. Guidance for Clinicians on the Use of RT-PCR and Other Molecular Assays for Diagnosis of Influenza Virus Infection. Available at: https://www.cdc.gov/flu/professionals/diagnosis/molecular-assays.htm.

36. Karhu J, Ala-Kokko TI, Vuorinen T, et al. Lower respiratory tract virus findings in mechanically ventilated patients with severe community-acquired pneumonia. *Clin Infect Dis* 2014;59(1):62–70.

37. Cunha BA. Rash and fever in the critical care unit. *Crit Care Clin* 1998;14(1):35–53.

38. Simon E, Long B, Koyfman A. Clinical mimics: An emergency medicine-focused review of influenza mimics. *J Emerg Med* 2017;53(1):49–65.

39. Silva ME, Cherry JD, Wilton RJ, et al. Acute fever and petechial rash associated with influenza A virus infection. *Clin Infect Dis* 1999;29:453–454.

40. Cunha BA. Anthrax, tularemia, plague, ebola or smallpox as agents of bioterrorism: Recognition in the emergency room. *Clin Microbiol Infect* 2002;8:489–503.

41. Moolenaar RL, Dalton C, Lipman HB, et al. Clinical features that differentiate hantavirus pulmonary syndrome from three other acute respiratory illnesses. *Clin Infect Dis* 1995;21(3):643–649.

42. Day MJ, Breitschwerdt E, Cleaveland S, et al. Surveillance of zoonotic infectious disease transmitted by small companion animals. *Emerg Infect Dis* 2012;18(12):e1.

43. Curtis S, Stobart K, Vandermeer B. Clinical features suggestive of meningitis in children: A systematic review of prospective data. *Pediatrics* 2010;126:952–960.

44. Ooi MH, Wong SC, Lewthwaite P, et al. Clinical features, diagnosis, and management of enterovirus 71. *Lancet Neurol* 2010;9(11):1097–1105.

45. Rice TW, Rubinson L, Uyeki TM, et al. Critical illness from 2009 pandemic influenza A virus and bacterial coinfection in the United States. *Crit Care Med* 2012;40:1487–1498.

46. Ballinger MN, Standiford TJ. Postinfluenza bacterial pneumonia: Host defenses gone awry. *J Interf Cytok Res* 2010;30(9):643–652.

47. Grabowska K, Högberg L, Penttinen P, et al. Occurrence of invasive pneumococcal disease and number of excess cases due to influenza. *BMC Infect Dis* 2006;6:58.

48. Estenssoro E, Rios FG, Apezteguia C, et al. Pandemic 2009 influenza A in Argentina: A study of 337 patients on mechanical ventilation. *Am J Respir Crit Care Med* 2010;182:41–48.

49. Centers for Disease Control Bacterial co-infections in lung tissue specimens from fatal cases of 2009 pandemic influenza A (H1N1)–United States, May–August 2009. *Morb Mort Wkly Rep* 2009;58:1–4.

50. Renner ED, Helms CM, Johnson W, et al. Coinfections of *Mycoplasma pneumoniae* and *Legionella pneumophila* with influenza A virus. *J Clin Microbiol* 1983;17(1):146–148.

51. Ariano RE, Sitar DS, Zelenitsky SA, et al. Enteric absorption and pharmacokinetics of oseltamivir in critically ill patients with pandemic (H1N1) influenza. *CMAJ* 2010;182(4):357–363.

52. Lee N, Hui DS, Zuo Z, et al. A prospective intervention study on higher-dose oseltamivir treatment in adults hospitalized with influenza A and B infections. *Clin Infect Dis* 2013;57(11):1511–1519.

53. Fiore AE, Fry A, Shay D, Gubareva L, Bresee JS, Uyeki TM. Centers for Disease Control and Prevention (CDC). Antiviral agents for the treatment and chemoprophylaxis of influenza-recommendations of the Advisory Committee on Immunization Practices (ACIP). *MMWR Recomm Rep* 2011;60(1):1–24.

54. Morciano C, Vitale A, De Masi S, et al. Italian evidence-based guidelines for the management of influenza-like syndrome in adults and children. *Ann Ist Super Sanita* 2009;45:185–192.

16 Severe Non-influenza Viral Pneumonia in the Critical Care Unit

David Waldner, Thomas J. Marrie, and Wendy Sligl

CONTENTS

CLINICAL PERSPECTIVE

Respiratory viruses are becoming increasingly recognized as the etiology of severe pneumonia in the critical care unit (CCU). This is due in part to recent advances in diagnostic testing, which have significantly increased our ability to detect respiratory pathogens, many of which are viruses [1,2]. Moreover, the recent emergence of severe acute respiratory syndrome (SARS) and Middle East respiratory syndrome coronavirus (MERS-CoV) has highlighted the importance of non-influenza respiratory viruses as ongoing and evolving causes of severe pneumonia.

EPIDEMIOLOGY AND ETIOLOGY

Community-acquired pneumonia (CAP) results in substantial morbidity and mortality worldwide, with approximately 200 million cases of viral pneumonia occurring annually [3]. It is estimated that of those hospitalized with CAP, 10%–21% require admission to CCUs and approximately 2%–7% die as a result of their infection [1,4,5]. Recent epidemiologic data have implicated non-influenza respiratory viruses in 30%–47% of pneumonia in CCUs, with viruses being the sole etiology in 10%–22% of cases [3,4,6]. Rhinovirus has recently emerged as the most commonly identified respiratory virus in the CCU and has been isolated in approximately 23%–57% of pneumonia cases [4,6]. However, there remains ongoing uncertainty regarding the pathogenicity of rhinovirus and to what extent it contributes to lower respiratory tract infection.

Rhinovirus has historically been isolated as a co-pathogen in mixed infections, with unclear significance [7]. However, more recent studies have implicated rhinovirus as the sole cause of pneumonia in over half of cases, suggesting that rhinovirus should be considered an important and common cause of pneumonia in the critical care setting [6,8]. Bacterial coinfection has been well recognized as a complication of influenza infection, is associated with increased mortality, and was particularly evident during the 2009 H1N1 pandemic [9–11]. However, there is continued controversy regarding the clinical significance of non-influenza respiratory virus isolation concurrently with bacteria from patients with severe pneumonia [4]. Recent studies have estimated that bacterial-viral coinfections account for 9%–39% of cases of severe pneumonia [4,6]. However, unlike influenza-bacterial coinfections, many studies have failed to show any difference in mortality among those with isolated viral (non-influenza) or bacterial pneumonia compared with those with mixed infection [4,6,11].

The most frequent causes of severe viral pneumonia in CCUs include rhinovirus, respiratory syncytial virus (RSV), parainfluenza, human metapneumovirus (hMPV), coronaviruses, and adenovirus (Table 16.1) [1,3,4,6]. Less frequent causes of severe viral pneumonia include cytomegalovirus (CMV), herpes simplex virus (HSV), varicella-zoster virus (VZV), Epstein–Barr virus (EBV), measles, enterovirus, mimivirus, bocavirus, and hantavirus. Additionally, other infectious and non-infectious etiologies need to be considered in the differential diagnosis of severe viral pneumonia (Table 16.1) [12]. Novel viral pathogens continue to emerge as we are now experiencing with pandemic SARS-CoV-2.

RESPIRATORY SYNCYTIAL VIRUS

Respiratory syncytial virus (RSV) is a well-recognized cause of bronchiolitis in children with virtually universal

TABLE 16.1
Etiology and Differential Diagnosis of Severe Viral Pneumonia in the Critical Care Unit

Infectious	Non-Infectious
Viral	Cardiogenic pulmonary edema
Common	Diffuse alveolar hemorrhage
Influenza virus	ARDS (non-infectious)
Rhinovirus	Connective tissue diseases
Parainfluenza virus	Vasculitis
Respiratory syncytial virus	ILD
Human metapneumovirus	Cryptogenic organizing pneumonia
Human coronavirus	Acute exacerbation of IPF
SARS-CoV-2	Hamman-rich syndrome (AIP)
Adenovirus	Acute hypersensitivity pneumonitis
Uncommon	Acute silicosis
Cytomegalovirus	Inhalational injury
Varicella-zoster virus	Near drowning
Herpes simplex virus	Smoke inhalation
Epstein–Barr virus	Chemical
MERS-CoV	Aspiration pneumonitis
Measles	
Hantavirus	**Bioterrorism Agent Inhalation**
Bocavirus	Anthrax
Mimivirus	Ricin
Bacterial	
Fungal	

Abbreviations: MERS-CoV, Middle East respiratory syndrome coronavirus; ARDS, acute respiratory distress syndrome; ILD, interstitial lung disease; IPF, idiopathic pulmonary fibrosis; AIP, acute interstitial pneumonia; SARS- CoV-2, severe acute respiratory syndrome coronavirus 2.

infection before the third year of life. Despite early exposure and development of neutralizing antibodies, immunity is incomplete, and reinfection in adulthood is common [13]. Respiratory syncytial virus accounts for approximately 5%–15% of all cases of CAP and up to 5% of CCU admissions for severe CAP [6,14,15]. While adults of any age are at risk of infection with RSV, those at highest risk for severe disease include patients over the age of 65 years, patients with underlying chronic lung disease, and those with immunosuppressive conditions, especially prior hematopoietic stem cell transplantation (HSCT) and solid organ transplantation (SOT) [14,16]. Increased susceptibility for severe infection among these patients likely reflects waning or suppressed cell mediated immunity [13]. As with other respiratory viruses within the *Paramyxoviridae* family, there is marked seasonal distribution of infection, with annual epidemics in the Northern Hemisphere, primarily occurring in January and February [13].

Acute respiratory infection from RSV typically presents as a self-limited illness in healthy adults; however, in those with underlying comorbidities, severe viral pneumonia as well as acute exacerbation of underlying asthma, chronic

obstructive pulmonary disease (COPD), and cardiac disease can occur [13,14]. The RSV typically causes community-acquired illness, with viral loads peaking early and paralleling symptom severity [17]. Illness typically presents with non-specific upper respiratory tract symptoms. These symptoms include rhinorrhea and cough, as well as wheeze, which appears to be more prevalent in RSV infection compared with other respiratory viruses [18]. Interestingly, in contrast to other respiratory viral infections (including influenza), fever is frequently absent, and infection tends to progress more slowly [13].

Abnormal chest radiography is common, occurring in 31%–49% of hospitalized patients with RSV infection [13]. One study found focal consolidation to be the most common abnormality, with lobar consolidation, multifocal infiltrates, and ground glass opacities also being described [16]. It has been estimated that 10%–21% of patients hospitalized with RSV infection require admission to CCUs, with approximately half of these patients requiring mechanical ventilation [14,16]. The RSV is now recognized as an important cause of acute exacerbation of COPD and has been estimated to account for up to 15% of all exacerbations [19]. Infection in the HSCT population appears to be particularly severe, with high rates of pneumonia [20]. Although not routinely determined, a high viral load, in addition to leukopenia and high-dose steroid use (>2 mg/kg), has been associated with increased mortality in these patients [20].

Mortality associated with RSV infection is highly variable, with approximately 78% of deaths occurring in those over 65 years of age [21]. Among those with RSV pneumonia requiring hospital admission, mortality has been estimated between 15% and 20% [14]. Unfortunately, mortality remains highest among the frail and immunosuppressed, with mortality rates as high as 28% and 39%–47% for patients admitted from long-term care (LTC) facilities and those with prior HSCT, respectively [20,22].

PARAINFLUENZA VIRUSES

Four serotypes of human parainfluenza virus (PIV) have been identified (PIV-1, PIV-2, PIV-3, PIV-4) [23]. Similar to other respiratory viruses belonging to the *Paramyxoviridae* family, their significance as childhood respiratory pathogens has long been recognized; however, their role in causing severe disease in adults has been poorly appreciated. Notable to PIV are the seasonal variations unique to each serotype. PIV-1 accounts for approximately 17%–30% of illnesses and typically circulates biennially, with most cases occurring in the Northern Hemisphere during September and December on odd-numbered years [23,24]. PIV-2 is less frequently encountered, causing only 8%–15% of infections, and like PIV-1, infections tend to peak in September and December; however, seasonal outbreaks occur annually [23,24]. Most clinically significant infections, however, are caused by PIV-3 (52%–71%) [23,24]. PIV-3 causes annual epidemics in the spring and early summer (April to June), with increased activity and longer seasons noted in even years due to the absence of circulating PIV-1 [23,24]. PIV-4 is infrequently encountered, and thus data on seasonality are sparse [23].

Infection with PIV results in a spectrum of disease ranging from mild upper respiratory tract infection to severe pneumonia and exacerbations of underlying cardiopulmonary disease [23,25]. Infection with PIV-3 appears to be associated with a greater risk of lower respiratory tract disease compared with other serotypes, which likely reflects the ability of PIV-3 to infect epithelial cells of the distal airways [26]. The estimated prevalence of hospitalized CAP caused by PIV varies widely from 0.2% to 11.5% [23]. Infections are typically clinically indistinguishable from other respiratory viruses [23]. The PIVs are among the most common respiratory viruses isolated from patients admitted to CCUs with severe CAP, accounting for up to 8% of all cases [6]. Although PIV-3 has previously been associated with more severe disease in adults, a recent study found that while infection with PIV-3 was significantly more common among hospitalized patients, the proportion of patients requiring CCU admission did not differ between serotypes [25]. The overall mortality associated with PIV infection is approximately 5% [25].

Approximately half of patients admitted to hospital with infection from PIV are immunocompromised—most notably those with HSCT and SOT, as well as those with hematologic malignancy [23,25]. The incidence of infection in HSCT recipients and patients with hematology malignancy is approximately 4%, and mortality rates among these patients are estimated at 12% and 7%, respectively [27]. These rates increase significantly to 27% among those who have lower respiratory tract involvement [27]. Most patients with hematologic malignancy or prior HSCT present with isolated upper respiratory tract involvement; however, approximately 20%–39% progress to develop lower respiratory tract disease [27]. Several risk factors have been identified in the progression to lower respiratory tract disease, including lymphopenia, neutropenia at onset of infection, infection within 100 days post-HSCT, and corticosteroid use in a dose-dependent manner [27]. Research pertaining to PIV infection following SOT has primarily focused on lung transplant recipients. Several factors increase the susceptibility to viral infection post lung transplant and include immunosuppressive therapy and the disruption of mucosal immunity, primarily through damage to bronchial lymphoid tissue [28]. Most infections are community-acquired and occur approximately 1 year after transplantation. Infection frequently leads to a reduction in lung function, with a decrease in forced expiratory volume (FEV1) ranging from 13% to 58% [28]. More concerning, however, is the reported association between PIV infection and bronchiolitis obliterans syndrome (BOS), which is a significant cause of morbidity and mortality post lung transplant [28].

Human Metapneumovirus

Human metapneumovirus (hMPV) was first identified in the Netherlands in 2001, causing an acute respiratory illness indistinguishable from RSV [29]. Despite only recent identification, serologic data suggest that hMPV has been circulating for over 50 years [30]. The RSV and hMPV are closely related members of the *Paramyxoviridae* family and have significant clinical overlap. Infection is virtually universal by age 10 years, and reinfection in adulthood likely results from waning immunity or lack of cross-protective antibodies between subtypes [29,30]. Although hMPV continues to primarily cause self-limited acute respiratory illness in children, it has become increasingly recognized as a cause of viral pneumonia in adults, especially among those who are immunosuppressed or have underlying lung disease.

The HMPV has been identified on all continents and has marked seasonal variation, with the majority of cases occurring between January and March in the Northern Hemisphere and between June and July in the Southern Hemisphere [29]. The HMPV has been implicated in 3%–7% of all CAP cases requiring admission to CCUs and accounts for up to 18% of severe viral pneumonia within critical care settings [1,6]. It has been estimated that nearly 30% of patients hospitalized with an acute respiratory illness from hMPV require admission to CCUs, with over half of these patients requiring mechanical ventilator support [31]. The majority of patients with severe hMPV pneumonia have underlying comorbidities, which most commonly include COPD, malignancy, and SOT [31]. Patients with hematologic malignancy or prior HSCT appear to be at particular risk, with up to 7% of patients developing infection and 40% of cases progressing to severe pneumonia [32]. Improved detection methods have also led to hMPV identification in 5%–12% of patients with acute exacerbations of COPD [33]. Additionally, hMPV has been identified as a significant cause of respiratory illness post lung transplant, often leading to graft dysfunction [34]. The HMPV has also been reported to cause outbreaks among elderly patients in long-term care facilities.

The HMPV is often clinically indistinguishable from RSV, presenting with fever, cough, rhinorrhea, and bronchospasm [29,31]. The incubation period is 5–6 days, with viral shedding peaking shortly after symptom onset [29]. Numerous radiographic findings have been reported and include ground glass opacities, scattered nodules, and diffuse alveolar and/or interstitial infiltrates (Figure 16.1); however, none of these findings reliably differentiate hMPV from other pathogens [32]. Among those admitted to CCUs, up to half of patients develop acute respiratory distress syndrome (ARDS) [31].

The HMPV infection in the immunocompetent host primarily results in a self-limiting illness, however, severe disease requiring CCU admission is associated with significant mortality—in fact as high as 18% [6]. Outcomes appear to be closely related to patient age and comorbidity burden, with mortality rates among HSCT recipients and patients with hematologic malignancy as high as 26% [32]. Moreover, during an outbreak of hMPV in an LTC facility in Quebec, Canada, the mortality rate among patients with confirmed infection was 50% [35].

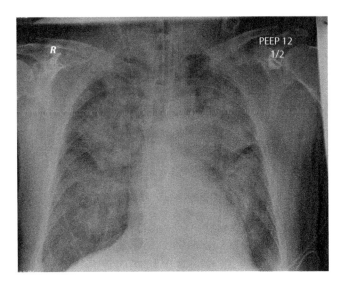

FIGURE 16.1 Pneumonia caused by human metapneumovirus.

CORONAVIRUSES

Since its identification as a cause of upper respiratory tract infection in 1965, four strains of human coronavirus (HCoV-OC43, HCoV-229E, HCoV-NL63, and HCoV-HKU1) have been reported to cause pneumonia [36,37]. Human coronaviruses have been implicated in a minority of severe pneumonia cases requiring CCU admission. Human coronavirus virulence appears to vary by strain, with HCoV-OC43 causing the majority of severe cases [6]. Two additional coronaviruses, MERS-CoV and SARS coronavirus (SARS-CoV), have since emerged from zoonotic origins.

MERS-CoV was first identified in a patient with severe respiratory and multi-organ failure in Saudi Arabia in 2012 [38]. Since then, there have been at least 2040 laboratory-confirmed cases identified in 27 countries, with an overall mortality rate of approximately 35% [39]. It is believed that human infection initially developed as the result of zoonotic transmission from dromedary camels [38]. However, most cases to date have resulted from human-to-human transmission in the health care setting, with little transmission occurring in the community [40]. This is illustrated by the fact that despite 80% of MERS-CoV cases being linked to Saudi Arabia, no confirmed cases to date have occurred as a direct result of attending the annual Hajj pilgrimage [40,41]. This propensity for nosocomial transmission is likely related to the viral kinetics of MERS-CoV, with viral loads reported to peak during the second week of illness, at which point many of those infected are admitted to hospital [42]. Large nosocomial outbreaks originating from a single patient have been reported. These so-called super-spreaders infect a disproportionately large number of patients, perhaps due to breaches in infection control practices as well as increased respiratory secretions and higher viral loads [43,44]. Prompt recognition of befitting travel and exposure history, with subsequent use of contact and droplet precautions, is critical to preventing in-hospital transmission of MERS-CoV. Furthermore, additional airborne precautions should be used when performing aerosol-generating medical procedures (AGMP) on patients with suspected or proven MERS-CoV infection [45].

MERS typically presents with fever, cough, abdominal pain, myalgia, and headache; it is frequently followed by the rapid development of pneumonia and respiratory failure [38,46]. Approximately 53%–89% of patients hospitalized with MERS-CoV require admission to CCUs, with a median duration of 7 days from symptom onset to CCU admission [47]. The majority of patients have abnormal chest radiographs with ground-glass opacities (most common), confluent consolidation, and pleural effusion [48]. Upper lobe involvement is infrequent early in the course of illness; however, radiographic progression appears to be rapid, with involvement of all lung zones, typically during peak radiographic deterioration [48]. Acute renal failure necessitating renal replacement therapy is common, occurring in over half of patients [49]. Despite intensive supportive care, mortality rates in patients with MERS admitted to CCUs remain high, ranging from 58% to 90% [47].

SARS-CoV first emerged in the Guangdong Province in China in November 2002 and by mid-2003 had reached 29 countries, including Canada and the United States, resulting in at least 8069 cases, with 774 confirmed deaths (10% case fatality rate) [50–52]. Similar to MERS-CoV, super-spreader events were reported during the SARS-CoV pandemic, and transmission primarily occurred in the hospital setting, with viral loads typically peaking around the tenth day of illness [52]. Transmission resulted from contact of mucous membranes with infectious respiratory droplets, with airborne transmission also being speculated [52,53]. Approximately, 20%–30% of patients infected with SARS-CoV required admission to CCUs [52]. Coordinated infection-control measures led to a rapid resolution of the SARS outbreak, and no cases have been reported since 2004 [54].

In late December 2019, a small cluster of patients with community-acquired pneumonia of unknown cause were reported in Wuhan, China [55,56]. These cases of pneumonia, now referred to as coronavirus disease 2019 (COVID-19) were later linked to the Huanan Wholesale Seafood Market and is determined to be caused by the novel zoonotic beta-coronavirus, SARS-CoV-2 [55]. It is believed that SARS-CoV-2 originated from a bat coronavirus (bat-SL-CoVZC45) sharing 85% sequence homology [56]. Some of these early cases generated human-to-human transmission with subsequent seeding of secondary community spread. China responded promptly with aggressive case and contact identification, isolation and management, including the unprecedented construction of over 48,000 new hospital beds in Hubei [55]. Extreme social distancing and other suppression strategies were implemented to slow down the transmission and prevent epidemic growth. Despite these measures, infection radiated to other parts of Hubei with a reproduction number (Ro) of approximately 2 to 2.5 [55]. Initially, most cases were believed to be imported from or directly linked to Wuhan; however, studies now show that undocumented cases may have accounted for up to 79% of documented cases within China [57]. Subsequent spread to other countries facilitated by international travel led to large outbreaks in South Korea, Iran, Japan, and onboard the Diamond Princess cruise ship. Continued global spread of SARS-CoV-2 led the World Health Organization (WHO) to declare a pandemic on March 11, 2020.

Containment and transmission interruption of SARS-CoV-2 has proven more challenging than that of SARS-CoV, despite both infections being transmitted via infectious respiratory droplets [55]. This may in part be due to peak viral shedding occurring early at the end of the incubation period when patients are minimally symptomatic [58]. This has raised a global concern for possible asymptomatic transmission which has been documented in case reports, however, the extent to which this has contributed to the spread of COVID-19 is unknown [59]. Following an average incubation period of 5–6 days (ranging from 1 to 14 days), the infected patients most typically experience fever (87.9%), dry cough (67.7%) and fatigue (38.1%), with nasal congestion (4.8%), diarrhea (3.7%), and conjunctivitis (0.8%) reported less frequently [55]. COVID-19 remains asymptomatic to mild in approximately 80% of cases, with more severe disease associated with tachypnea and hypoxia occurring in 13.8% of cases, and critical disease associated with respiratory failure, septic shock, multiorgan failure and ARDS in 6.1% of cases [55]. Advanced age, and underlying comorbidities such as cardiovascular disease, diabetes, hypertension, chronic lung disease, and cancer have been associated with more severe disease [55,60]. Approximately, 2.3% of patients require mechanical ventilation at a median of 14.5 days following the symptom onset [60,61]. Clinical deterioration is commonly observed following the first week of illness with septic shock and ARDS typically developing on day 9 and 12 of illness in 59% and 31% of hospitalized patients, respectively [61]. In contrast to adults, children appear to be less susceptible to infection with those under 10 years accounting for only 1% of cases [62]. Moreover, asymptomatic infection has been reported more frequently in younger individuals, as have atypical presentations including those without fever [62].

Radiographic features of COVID-19 typically progress over weeks beginning with unilateral peripheral ground glass opacities during the preclinical stage that evolve to bilateral diffuse ground-glass opacities (Figure 16.2) predominating within the lower lobes at the time of clinical illness [63,64]. Increasing consolidation and reticulation is frequently observed during the second and third week of symptoms [63,64]. Additional features of septal thickening (35%), air bronchograms (47%), crazy paving pattern (10%), and pleural effusions (10%) have been reported [63]. The diagnosis of COVID-19 relies on virus detection through reverse transcriptase PCR (RT-PCR) primarily from naso- and oropharyngeal specimens; however, early data suggests greater sensitivity with lower respiratory tract specimens (i.e., sputum and bronchial alveolar lavage) [65]. Furthermore, false negative RT-PCR results during early disease have been reported with changes on computed tomography (CT) scan being more sensitive (98% vs. 71%) [66]. Lymphocytopenia is common (83% of cases at admission) and along with elevated alanine aminotransferase, lactose dehydrogenase, troponin, d-dimer, ferritin, and interleukin (IL)-6 levels is associated with increased risk of death [60,61]. Severe disease is associated with immune dysregulation resulting in reduced T-cell counts and a robust innate immune response, including elevated IL-6 levels [61,67,68]. This may contribute to higher viral loads and prolonged viral shedding which is frequently seen in severe cases [69]. Procalcitonin is typically low or normal in COVID-19; however, higher levels have been associated with severe disease and may be in part due to increased IL-6 production [70].

Reported COVID-19 mortality rates have varied greatly from 0.7% to 5.8% in China and up to 7.2% in Italy, likely reflecting the local healthcare systems saturation and the inability to meet demands for intensive care [55,71,72]. The highest mortality rate has been observed in those over 80 years (21.9%) as well as those with cardiovascular disease (13.2%), diabetes (9.2%), hypertension (8.4%), and chronic lung disease (7.6%) [55]. Current treatment is largely limited to supportive care with several studies underway investigating new and repurposed medications. Early data suggests remdesivir, a novel adenosine analogue, which may be effective as it appears to inhibit SARS-CoV-2 in vitro [73,74]. Additionally, older medications such as chloroquine, lopinavir/ritonavir and tocilizumab, a humanized monoclonal antibody against IL-6, have garnered attention with their possible role in treating

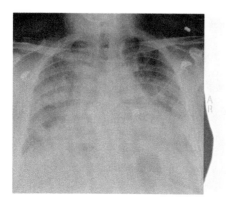
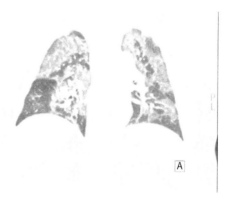

FIGURE 16.2 Extensive bilateral consolidation (left image) on CXR caused by SARS-CoV-2. CT scan (right image) demonstrates diffuse bilateral ground glass opacification.

COVID-19. Unfortunately, an early randomized controlled trial showed lopinavir/ritonavir to have no effect on mortality or SARS-CoV-2 viral clearance in hospitalized patients with severe disease; and however, its effect on less severe or early disease has yet to be established [75].

The total number of cases and fatalities from the COVID-19 pandemic has yet to be determined and will depend on the ability to effectively suppress transmission, identify effective therapies, and develop a vaccine. The capacity of healthcare system will undoubtedly affect the outcomes. It is evident that novel zoonotic coronaviruses possess a unique ability to cause large scale human infection. With a large reservoir of coronaviruses capable of trans-species migration existing in animals such as bats, the world should consider itself on-notice for potential outbreaks in the future.

Adenovirus

Adenovirus (AdV) typically causes a self-limited respiratory, gastrointestinal, or conjunctival illness in both children and adults; however, severe pneumonia is well-described among certain at-risk patient populations and in the setting of emerging serotypes [76]. Over 67 serotypes encompassing seven species (A-G) have been described, with species B (serotypes 3, 7, 11, 14, and 21) being associated with the majority of severe pneumonias [76,77]. Historically, AdV serotypes 4 and 7 have caused severe respiratory illness in crowded settings, primarily among military recruits, and prior to the introduction of a live oral vaccine, these two serotypes infected up to 12% of recruits and accounted for up to 90% of pneumonia cases [78]. Recently, two species, AdV-14 and AdV-55, have emerged as important causes of severe pneumonia among immunocompetent patients [77,79]. Outbreaks of AdV-14 have been reported worldwide in both military recruits and civilians, with up to 17% of patients requiring admission to CCUs and 5% of patients dying from their illness [79]. AdV-55, which appears to have emerged from recombination between AdV-11 and AdV-14, has been associated with more severe pneumonia when compared with other serotypes [77]. While AdV-55 is encountered most frequently in Asia, locally acquired cases have been reported in Europe [80]. Over half of patients with AdV pneumonia have the evidence of consolidation on chest imaging, with patchy infiltrates and ground-glass opacities also described frequently [77,81].

The SOT and HSCT recipients are at particular risk of severe AdV infection with a wide range of presentations, including pneumonia, colitis, hepatitis, hemorrhagic cystitis, and disseminated disease [76]. Infection among HSCT recipients frequently occurs early (<100 days post engraftment) and in those with acute graft-versus-host disease (GVHD) and T-cell-depleted grafts [76]. Latent infection can develop within lympho-epithelial tissue, with most disease post-transplantation resulting from reactivation [82]. Mortality among HSCT recipients with AdV pneumonia and disseminated disease is approximately 50% and 80%, respectively [76]. Cidofovir has been shown to be active against AdV *in vitro* and may

be effective in treating immunocompromised patients with severe disease [83].

Hantavirus

Hantaviruses are enveloped single-stranded RNA viruses within the family *Bunyaviridae* and are capable of causing two distinct illnesses, hemorrhagic fever with renal syndrome (HFRS) and hantavirus cardiopulmonary syndrome (HCPS), which occur primarily in the Old and New Worlds, respectively [84]. These viruses were named after the prototypic Hantaan virus, which was isolated from a striped field mouse near the Hantaan river in South Korea and is now known to have been the causative agent of an outbreak of HFRS among thousands of UN troops during the Korean War [84]. Since this outbreak, several other viruses have been identified as causes of HFRS throughout Europe and Asia and are collectively referred to as Old World hantaviruses [84]. Hantavirus infection was largely unrecognized in the New World prior to an outbreak of HCPS in the Four Corners region of the United States during the spring of 1993 [85]. Sin Nombre virus was the agent responsible for this outbreak and remains the predominant cause of HCPS in North America. In addition to SNV, several other New World hantaviruses have been identified as causes of HCPS, of which Andes virus (ANDV) is the most notable, accounting for most cases in South America [84].

The HCPS remains relatively uncommon in North America, with only 688 and 108 cases reported in the United States and Canada, respectively [86,87]. The majority of these cases occur in the southwestern United States and the western provinces of Canada [86,87]. The geographic distribution of hantaviruses is largely determined by the distribution of their corresponding rodent reservoirs. The common deer mouse (*Peromyscus maniculatus*) serves as the reservoir for SNV. Most infections occur in the spring and early summer when deer mouse breeding occurs [88]. Human infection follows exposure to virus-contaminated aerosols generated from rodent saliva, urine, or feces [84,88]. Activities that increase exposure to infectious aerosolized particles include cleaning or sweeping of barns, sheds, or cellars, especially when ventilation is poor. Additionally, occupational infections have been documented in farmers, trappers, and military personnel [84,88]. Most cases of HCPS are sporadic, with case clusters rarely described and likely resulting from common exposure [89]. Person-to-person transmission of SNV has not been described; however, transmission of ANDV has been documented, albeit rarely [84]. As such, no specific infection control precautions are required for patients with HCPS.

The HCPS is characterized by sequential progression through prodromal, cardiopulmonary, polyuric, and convalescent phases of illness [84]. Symptom onset typically follows an incubation period of 8–20 days [90]. The prodromal phase is characterized by non-specific symptoms, including fever, myalgia, headache, vomiting, and abdominal pain, and typically lasts for 1–6 days. The cardiopulmonary phase is typically heralded by the abrupt onset of

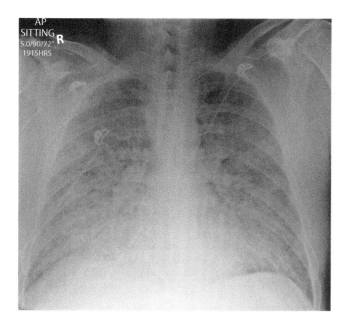

FIGURE 16.3   Bilateral interstitial pneumonia caused by Hantavirus cardiopulmonary syndrome.

non-productive cough [84]. Hantavirus preferentially distributes to the vascular endothelium of the heart and lungs, leading to increased endothelial permeability, and subsequent non-cardiogenic pulmonary edema, which is associated with profound hypoxemia in the majority of cases [85,91]. During this phase, chest radiography typically reveals bilateral interstitial infiltrates (Figure 16.3) and occasionally pleural effusions [84,85]. Up to 84% of patients require intubation and mechanical ventilation, with further deterioration necessitating extracorporeal membrane oxygenation (ECMO) therapy in up to 75% of cases [85,91]. Additional cardinal features of early HCPS include hemoconcentration, which occurs in 26%–81% of cases, and thrombocytopenia, which is invariably present [85,92]. Polyuria follows non-cardiogenic pulmonary edema, signaling illness resolution. This is followed by a period of convalescence, marked by fatigue and generalized weakness, but typically ends in full recovery [84].

Despite intensive supportive therapy, mortality rates from HCPS remain high at 29%–36% [86,87]. The majority of deaths occur during the cardiopulmonary phase as a result of myocardial dysfunction and/or respiratory failure [91]. Prompt recognition of prodromal and early cardiopulmonary symptoms in patients with possible hantavirus exposure is crucial, as patients with suspected HCPS should be rapidly transferred to facilities with advanced critical care capabilities.

Serology and blood polymerase chain reaction (PCR) remain the mainstay of diagnosis; however, results are often delayed. Peripheral blood smear criteria have been used to facilitate timely triaging of suspected HCPS cases [93]. These criteria include hemoconcentration, thrombocytopenia, left shift in the granulocytic lineage, lack of toxic changes in the myeloid lineage, and increased immunoblasts (>10% of lymphoid population). One study found the presence of 5/5

and 4/5 criteria were associated with a specificity of 100% and 93% and a sensitivity of 35% and 89%, respectively, for the diagnosis of HCPS [93]. Moreover, the presence of two or less criteria was associated with a negative predictive value of 100% [93]. As previously mentioned, the diagnosis of hantavirus infection relies on serology or the detection of hantavirus RNA in blood, using reverse transcriptase PCR (RT-PCR). By the time symptoms develop, almost all patients have detectable IgM and most have detectable IgG antibodies.

CONSIDERATIONS IN THE IMMUNOCOMPROMISED PATIENT

As mentioned previously, immunocompromised patients are at particular risk for developing severe viral pneumonia. In addition to the viruses previously discussed, several herpesviruses, including CMV, HSV, and VZV, may cause severe viral pneumonia in the immunocompromised patients. Among these, CMV is most common in HSCT and SOT recipients. In these patients, CMV infection occurs from the reactivation of latent virus remotely acquired by the host, transfer of virus within the allograft, or primary infection following transplantation.

Lung transplant recipients are particularly susceptible to developing CMV pneumonia due to the high viral genomic load harbored by lung tissue during latent infection [94]. The CMV pneumonia can also result from primary infection, which may occur in seronegative recipients who receive seropositive grafts. Despite the implementation of anti-viral prophylaxis among susceptible lung transplant recipients, the reported incidence of CMV pneumonia remains 10%–55% [95,96]. Most disease occurs within 3 months post-transplant and frequently follows the discontinuation of anti-viral prophylaxis [96]. Of particular concern is the reported association between CMV pneumonitis and BOS, which is a significant cause of mortality post lung transplant [97]. In contrast to SOT recipients, the greatest risk of developing CMV pneumonia following HSCT is among seropositive recipients who receive seronegative stem cells [98]. Similarly, there have been significant efforts to reduce CMV pneumonia in this population, and widespread use of prophylactic or pre-emptive treatment strategies has reduced the overall incidence of CMV pneumonia to approximately 5%–8% [98]. The risk remains highest among allogeneic HSCT recipients and generally occurs early (≤100 days) postengraftment. However, the use of prophylactic or pre-emptive treatment strategies has increased the incidence of late (≥100 days post-engraftment) CMV disease [98].

The CMV pneumonia frequently presents with prodromal fever, malaise, and myalgia prior to the development of clinical pneumonitis, which manifests as non-productive cough and dyspnea. Accompanying leukopenia, thrombocytopenia, and elevations of aminotransferases are important findings that should raise suspicion for CMV disease [96]. Chest radiography typically reveals bilateral interstitial infiltrates; however, radiographs may be normal in early disease [98]. Computed tomographic (CT) scan increases the sensitivity

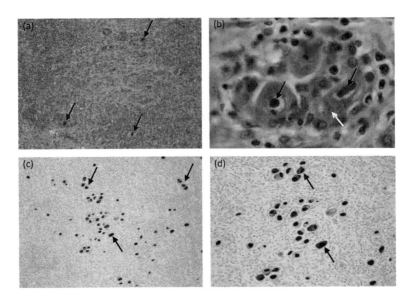

FIGURE 16.4 Photomicrographs of CMV infected cells in a patient with CMV pneumonitis. (a) Multiple CMV infected cells (arrows) (H&E, ×40). (b) Granular cytoplasmic inclusions (white arrow) and large intranuclear inclusion bodies with surrounding halo (black arrows) (H&E, ×1000). (c,d) Immunohistochemistry staining reveals numerous CMV infected cells (arrows) (c, ×40) (d, ×200). (Courtesy of Dr. Lakshmi Puttagunta, University of Alberta, Canada.).

and most often reveals bilateral ground-glass opacities accompanied by multiple small (<10 mm) nodules as well as areas of consolidation [99].

Definitive diagnosis of tissue invasive disease, including pneumonia, requires demonstrating the presence of CMV on tissue biopsy, with the detection of inclusion bodies Figure 16.4 or viral antigens by immunohistochemistry [100]. Detection of CMV on bronchial alveolar lavage (BAL) specimens via rapid shell culture or PCR cannot definitively diagnose CMV pneumonia, as viral shedding can occur with viral reactivation, in the absence of disease [100]. However, the detection of CMV in BAL specimens with PCR has been shown to be a sensitive marker for CMV pneumonitis, and utilization of quantitative PCR appears to increase specificity without compromising sensitivity [101].

More recently, there has been renewed interest in the significance of CMV reactivation among immunocompetent critically ill patients. The reactivation of CMV in critically ill patients is common, with a reported incidence between 10% and 71%, with many studies documenting the presence of CMV in respiratory specimens [102,103]. Multiple observational studies have reported an association between CMV reactivation and CCU length of stay, duration of mechanical ventilation, and mortality [104]. However, causality in this setting remains unclear, with some authors arguing that CMV reactivation merely serves as a marker for underlying disease severity [104]. Interestingly, in a recent phase 2 randomized control trial, ganciclovir did not significantly decrease interleukin (IL)-6 levels, length of stay, or mortality among critically ill CMV seropositive patients, despite a significant reduction in CMV reactivation [105].

Pneumonia caused by VZV is the most common and severe sequela of varicella infection in adults, with pneumonia necessitating hospitalization, complicating approximately 0.25% of cases [106]. Of those requiring admission to the CCU, an underlying immunosuppressive condition is identified in over half of cases—hematologic malignancy, solid organ malignancy, SOT, steroid treatment, and pregnancy are the most common [107]. A typical "chickenpox" rash accompanies and precedes the vast majority (96%) of cases; although rarely, immunocompromised patients may develop VZV pneumonia in the absence of rash [107]. Of those with severe pneumonia, the most frequent radiographic findings are bilateral interstitial infiltrates. Approximately half of patients also display multiple nodules and areas of consolidation on CT scan [107]. Elevated aminotransferases and thrombocytopenia accompany severe pneumonia in 33% and 79% of cases, respectively [107]. Up to half of patients require mechanical ventilation, and as many as one in four develop bacterial pneumonia coinfection [107]. Despite antiviral therapy, the overall mortality of VZV pneumonia among immunocompetent and immunocompromised patients requiring CCU admission is approximately 4% and 42%, respectively [107].

APPROACH TO SEVERE VIRAL PNEUMONIA BY SEASONAL DISTRIBUTION AND EXPOSURE HISTORY

There is significant clinical overlap among most causes of viral pneumonia, and it is often not possible to make reliable diagnoses on clinical findings alone. However, several factors, including seasonal variation, travel, and occupational and environmental exposure history, can help refine diagnostic considerations (Table 16.2). Unfortunately, suboptimal vaccination rates have allowed preventable infections, such as measles, to persist. Infection with measles virus should

TABLE 16.2

Clinical and Epidemiologic Clues to the Diagnosis of Severe Viral Pneumonia

Viral Pathogen	Clinical	Peak Seasonal Distribution[a]	Exposure/Occupation
RSV	↑ Wheeze	January–February	
	↓ Fever		
Parainfluenza virus			
PIV-1		September–December (odd years)	
PIV-2		September–December	
PIV-3		April–June	
HMPV	↑ Wheeze	January–March	Long-term care facility
MERS-CoV	↓ Platelets		Dromedary camel
	AKI		Arabian Peninsula
Hantavirus	↑ HCT	March–August	Deer mouse droppings
	↓ Platelets		Farmer
	Pulmonary edema		Sweeping/cleaning
Adenovirus	↑ Transaminases		Military recruit
	Colitis		
	Hemorrhagic cystitis		
	Conjunctivitis		
CMV	↑ Transaminases		
	↓ WBC		
	↓ Platelets		
VZV	Vesicular rash		Unvaccinated
	↑ Transaminases		Exposure to suspected/known case
	↓ Platelets		
Measles	Koplik's spots		Unvaccinated
	Maculopapular rash		Exposure to suspected/known case

Abbreviations: RSV, respiratory syncytial virus; PIV, parainfluenza virus; HMPV, human metapneumovirus; MERS-CoV, Middle East respiratory syndrome coronavirus; AKI, acute kidney injury; CMV, cytomegalovirus; VZV, varicella-zoster virus; HCT, hematocrit; WBC, white blood cell count; SARS-CoV-2, severe acute respiratory syndrome coronavirus 2.

[a] Northern Hemisphere.

be considered in the setting of pneumonia associated with a maculopapular rash, and a thorough vaccination and exposure history should be obtained.

DIAGNOSIS

Until recently, the detection of respiratory viruses has been limited by insensitive and labor-intensive techniques, with prolonged turn-around time, thus limiting their utility in clinical decision making. These techniques include viral culture, direct fluorescent-antigen (DFA), and direct enzyme-linked immunosorbent assay (ELISA) antigen detection [108]. The recent advent of multiplex real-time RT-PCR (mqRT-PCR) has dramatically increased our ability to detect viral respiratory pathogens and has furthered our understanding of their significance in human disease. Current mqRT-PCR systems, widely referred to as respiratory pathogen panels (RPPs), are enclosed, self-contained assays, thus limiting cross-contamination, human error, and the need for specialized end-user training [108]. Recently, commercialized systems operate on a two-stage PCR assay following the addition of a respiratory specimen into a single-use cartridge [108]. Following specimen lysis and purification, reverse transcription

generates complementary DNA (cDNA) from pathogen-derived RNA. This is followed by multiplex "outer" PCR, which utilizes numerous flanking primers to amplify conserved sequences among various respiratory pathogens. A second PCR reaction follows, which uses primers designed to amplify regions "nested" within specific first stage PCR amplicons.

These second-stage nested PCR reactions occur within individual wells containing specific primers for individual respiratory pathogens and are aided by the addition of fluorescent dye to detect PCR amplification [108]. The implementation of RPPs allows for a "syndromic" approach to the diagnosis of respiratory tract infection. As outlined previously, the majority of viral respiratory pathogens are clinically indistinguishable from one another, and simultaneous testing for multiple respiratory pathogens using mqRT-PCR allows for greater diagnostic ability compared with previous single-pathogen detection methods. The number of pathogens detected by RPPs varies, with some systems able to test for as many as 18 viral (influenza A, influenza A H1N1/2009, influenza A/H3N2, influenza B, PIV-1, PIV-2, PIV-3, PIV-4, enterovirus/ rhinovirus, HCoV-OC43, HCoV-229E, HCoV-NL63, HCoV-HKU1, RSV-A, RSV-B, hMPV, adenovirus, and bocavirus) and two bacterial (*Chlamydophila pneumoniae* and *Mycoplasma pneumoniae*) respiratory pathogens [109].

Initial studies evaluating mqRT-PCR assays have shown them to be highly sensitive, in comparison with previous methods of detection, while maintaining a high level of specificity [108]. The sensitivity of mqRT-PCR using nasopharyngeal swabs and sputum samples has been estimated at 67%–76% and 94%–98%, respectively [110,111]. Additionally, recent data show that performing mqRT-PCR on sputa in addition to nasopharyngeal swabs significantly increases virus detection by approximately 13%–16% [110,111]. Viral pathogens may be absent from the upper respiratory tract in the setting of isolated lower tract infection, and the importance of performing RPP assays on lower tract specimens was highlighted during the 2009 H1N1 pandemic, with one study finding upper respiratory tract specimens to be positive in only 81% of confirmed cases admitted to the CCU [112].

Despite increased ability to detect respiratory viral pathogens in patients with severe pneumonia, the incidence of viral-bacterial coinfection is high, and diagnostics aimed at excluding concomitant bacterial infection are of particular importance. Procalcitonin (PCT), the peptide precursor to calcitonin, has gained significant attention over the past several years as a potential biomarker for distinguishing viral and bacterial pneumonia. The release of PCT has been observed as part of the proinflammatory response of the innate immune system. Synthesis and detection of PCT has been observed *in vitro* following the release of tumor necrosis factor, IL-1, and IL-6 in response to bacteria and bacterial endotoxins [113]. Moreover, PCT secretion appears to be inhibited by the release of interferon gamma, a cytokine that is frequently secreted in response to viral infections [113].

Initial prospective studies utilizing PCT in treatment decision algorithms for CAP have proven to be safe and show potential for reducing antibiotic use in the setting of viral pneumonia [114]. However, prospective trials evaluating the utility of PCT-based treatment algorithms for severe pneumonia in the critical care setting are lacking. The largest study to date evaluating the association between PCT level and pneumonia etiology among patients hospitalized with CAP found PCT to be useful in excluding bacterial infection, with a negative predictive value of 94% using a PCT cut-off of <0.1 ng/mL [115]. Unfortunately, there was neither a PCT cut-off that could completely discriminate between viral and bacterial infection, nor a low PCT level specific for viral infection, as 12% of bacterial pneumonia cases had PCT levels below 0.1 ng/mL [115]. Additionally, it should be noted that few of these patients (22%) were admitted to CCUs [115].

C-reactive protein (CRP) has also been studied, albeit to a lesser extent, as a possible biomarker capable of distinguishing between bacterial and viral causes of pneumonia. However, the reported performance of CRP in identifying a bacterial etiology for lower respiratory tract infections varies widely, with sensitivities ranging from 8% to 99% and specificities ranging from 27% to 95% [116].

TREATMENT

Supportive care is the mainstay of treatment for pneumonia caused by the majority of respiratory viruses. Ribavirin has shown to be effective *in vitro* against many *Paramyxoviridae*, with most studies to date evaluating its role in the treatment and prevention of RSV pneumonia in HSCT recipients [20,23]. Several retrospective studies have shown aerosolized ribavirin to be effective in reducing all-cause and RSV-associated mortality in these patients [20,117]. However, to date, these findings have not been reproduced in any prospective trials, and little is known about the efficacy of ribavirin in other immunosuppressed patient populations [118]. Additionally, no studies have shown ribavirin to be effective in the treatment of pneumonia caused by PIV or hMPV [23,32].

Similarly, there is currently no convincing evidence to support the routine use of anti-viral therapy for the treatment of HCPS or pneumonia caused by coronaviruses, including MERS-CoV and SARS-CoV [45,119]. In contrast, antivirals are imperative for the treatment of severe CMV and VZV pneumonia, especially in the immunocompromised host. Both valganciclovir and intravenous ganciclovir have proven to be effective in the treatment of CMV pneumonia, with ganciclovir being the preferred treatment in severe disease or when gastrointestinal absorption is of concern [100,120,121]. Likewise, acyclovir is effective against VZV, and its use in the treatment of VZV pneumonia is supported by retrospective observational data [107,122–124].

The use of adjunctive corticosteroids in the treatment of CAP has garnered renewed interest recently; however, their role in the treatment of viral pneumonia is less clear [125]. A recent meta-analysis suggested that corticosteroid use in the setting of influenza may increase mortality [126]. Similarly, corticosteroids do not appear to be of benefit in patients hospitalized with RSV pneumonia and may increase the rate of bacterial coinfection [127,128].

Invasive respiratory support is fundamental to the treatment of viral pneumonia complicated by severe respiratory failure. Among mechanically ventilated patients with ARDS, the importance of preventing ventilator-associated lung injury is crucial. Lung protective ventilation using lower tidal volumes (4–8 mL/kg predicted body weight) and lower inspiratory plateau pressures (<30 cm H_2O) is recommended in ARDS patients. based on the results of several trials showing a reduction in mortality when compared with conventional strategies [129,130]. Additionally, venovenous ECMO has proven to be an effective means of respiratory support during severe acute respiratory failure [131]. Among patients with severe ARDS during the 2009 H1N1 pandemic, the use of ECMO was associated with a reduction in mortality compared with conventional therapy [132]. Although prospective trials are lacking, venoarterial ECMO appears to be effective in patients with HCPS, with one case series reporting a survival rate of 67% among patients who failed conventional interventions [91]. However, the optimal timing for initiating ECMO in HCPS is currently unknown [133].

PREVENTION

Appropriate infection control practices are essential in patients with confirmed or suspected respiratory viral illness to prevent nosocomial transmission. Infection-control measures are guided by the presumed route of transmission of individual viruses. The transmission of RSV, hMPV, and PIV is assumed to occur mainly following direct or indirect contact with secretions, while droplet exposure appears to be important in the transmission of influenza, adenovirus, and MERS-CoV [13,45,134,135]. Critical care clinicians should also consider the need for additional precautions (including airborne) while performing AGMP on patients with suspected or proven influenza or MERS-CoV infection [45,134].

CLINICAL SUMMARY

Non-influenza viruses are a common cause of severe pneumonia in the CCU and are associated with significant morbidity and mortality. The availability of advanced PCR-based diagnostics has greatly increased our ability to identify viral pathogens in a timely manner. Clinicians should strongly consider the possibility of viral pneumonia in patients admitted to CCUs with severe respiratory failure and should thoroughly explore patient exposure and travel and medical history. Unlike bacterial pneumonia, the treatment for severe viral pneumonia is largely supportive. Given the significant burden of viral pneumonia in the CCU, further research into the development of effective antivirals is needed.

REFERENCES

1. Jain S, Self WH, Wunderink RG, et al. Community-acquired pneumonia requiring hospitalization among U.S. Adults. *N Engl J Med* 2015;373(5):415–427.
2. Templeton KE, Scheltinga SA, Eeden VD, et al. Improved diagnosis of the etiology of community-acquired pneumonia with real-time polymerase chain reaction. *Clin Infect Dis* 2005;41(3):345–351.
3. Ruuskanen O, Lahti E, Jennings LC, Murdoch DR. Viral pneumonia. *Lancet* 2011;377(9773):1264–1275.
4. Karhu J, Ala-Kokko TI, Vuorinen T, Ohtonen P, Syrjälä H. Lower respiratory tract virus findings in mechanically ventilated patients with severe community-acquired pneumonia. *Clin Infect Dis* 2014;59(1):62–70.
5. Ramirez JA, Wiemken TL, Peyrani P, et al. Adults hospitalized with pneumonia in the United States: Incidence, epidemiology, and mortality. *Clin Infect Dis* 2017;65(11):1806–1812.
6. Choi SH, Hong SB, Ko GB, et al. Viral infection in patients with severe pneumonia requiring intensive care unit admission. *Am J Respir Crit Care Med* 2012;186(4):325–332.
7. Hohenthal U, Vainionpää R, Nikoskelainen J, Kotilainen P. The role of rhinoviruses and enteroviruses in community acquired pneumonia in adults. *Thorax* 2008;63(7):658–659.
8. Jennings LC, Anderson TP, Beynon KA, et al. Incidence and characteristics of viral community-acquired pneumonia in adults. *Thorax* 2008;63(1):42–48.
9. Chertow DS, Memoli MJ. Bacterial coinfection in influenza: A grand rounds review. *JAMA* 2013;309(3):275–282.
10. Morens DM, Taubenberger JK, Fauci AS. Predominant role of bacterial pneumonia as a cause of death in pandemic influenza: Implications for pandemic influenza preparedness. *J Infect Dis* 2008;198(7):962–970.
11. Voiriot G, Visseaux B, Cohen J, et al. Viral-bacterial coinfection affects the presentation and alters the prognosis of severe community-acquired pneumonia. *Crit Care* 2016;20(1):375.
12. Santos E, Talusan A, Brandstetter RD. Roentgenographic mimics of pneumonia in the critical care unit. *Crit Care Clin* 1998;14(1):91–104.
13. Walsh EE. Respiratory syncytial virus infection: An illness for all ages. *Clin Chest Med* 2017;38(1):29–36.
14. Lee N, Lui GCY, Wong KT, et al. High morbidity and mortality in adults Hospitalized for respiratory syncytial virus infections. *Clin Infect Dis* 2013;57(8):1069–1077.
15. Ong DSY, Faber TE, Klouwenberg PMCK, et al. Respiratory syncytial virus in critically ill adult patients with community-acquired respiratory failure: A prospective observational study. *Clin Microbiol Infect* 2014;20(8):O505–O507.
16. Volling C, Hassan K, Mazzulli T, et al. Respiratory syncytial virus infection-associated hospitalization in adults: A retrospective cohort study. *BMC Infect Dis* 2014;14.
17. DeVincenzo JP, Wilkinson T, Vaishnaw A, et al. Viral load drives disease in humans experimentally infected with respiratory syncytial virus. *Am J Respir Crit Care Med* 2010;182(10):1305–1314.
18. Sundaram ME, Meece JK, Sifakis F, Gasser RA, Belongia EA. Medically attended respiratory syncytial virus infections in adults aged ≥50 years: Clinical characteristics and outcomes. *Clin Infect Dis* 2014;58(3):342–349.
19. Ramaswamy M, Groskreutz DJ, Look DC. Recognizing the importance of respiratory syncytial virus in chronic obstructive pulmonary disease. *J Chronic Obstr Pulm Dis* 2009;6(1):64–75.
20. Waghmare A, Campbell AP, Xie H, et al. Respiratory syncytial virus lower respiratory disease in hematopoietic cell transplant recipients: Viral RNA detection in blood, antiviral treatment, and clinical outcomes. *Clin Infect Dis* 2013;57(12):1731–1741.
21. Thompson WW, Shay DK, Weintraub E, et al. Mortality associated with influenza and respiratory syncytial virus in the United States. *JAMA* 2003;289(2):179–186.
22. Falsey AR, Hennessey PA, Formica MA, Cox C, Walsh EE. Respiratory syncytial virus infection in elderly and high-risk adults. *N Engl J Med* 2005;352(17):1749–1759.
23. Russell E, Ison MG. Parainfluenza virus in the hospitalized adult. *Clin Infect Dis* 2017;65(9):1570–1576.
24. Fry AM, Curns AT, Harbour K, Hutwagner L, Holman RC, Anderson LJ. Seasonal trends of human parainfluenza viral infections: United States, 1990–2004. *Clin Infect Dis* 2006;43(8):1016–1022.
25. Russell E, Tardrew S, Ison MG. Parainfluenza virus in hospitalized adults: A 7-year retrospective study. *Open Forum Infect Dis* 2017;4(suppl_1):S578–S579.
26. Porter DD, Prince GA, Hemming VG, Porter HG. Pathogenesis of human parainfluenza virus 3 infection in two species of cotton rats: Sigmodon hispidus develops bronchiolitis, while Sigmodon fulviventer develops interstitial pneumonia. *J Virol* 1991;65(1):103–111.
27. Shah DP, Shah PK, Azzi JM, Chemaly RF. Parainfluenza virus infections in hematopoietic cell transplant recipients and hematologic malignancy patients: A systematic review. *Cancer Lett* 2016;370(2):358–364.

28. Vilchez RA, Dauber J, McCurry K, Iacono A, Kusne S. Parainfluenza virus infection in adult lung transplant recipients: An emergent clinical syndrome with implications on allograft function. *Am J Transplant* 2003;3(2):116–120.

29. Panda S, Mohakud NK, Pena L, Kumar S. Human metapneumovirus: Review of an important respiratory pathogen. *Int J Infect Dis* 2014;25(Supplement C):45–52.

30. Wen SC, Williams JV. New approaches for immunization and therapy against human metapneumovirus. *Clin Vaccine Immunol* 2015;22(8):858–866.

31. Hasvold J, Sjoding M, Pohl K, Cooke CR, Hyzy RC. The role of human metapneumovirus in the critically ill adult patient. *J Crit Care* 2016;31(1):233–237.

32. Shah DP, Shah PK, Azzi JM, El Chaer F, Chemaly RF. Human metapneumovirus infections in hematopoietic cell transplant recipients and hematologic malignancy patients: A systematic review. *Cancer Lett* 2016;379(1):100–106.

33. Martinello RA, Esper F, Weibel C, Ferguson D, Landry ML, Kahn JS. Human metapneumovirus and exacerbations of chronic obstructive pulmonary disease. *J Infect* 2006;53(4):248–254.

34. Hopkins P, McNeil K, Kermeen F, et al. Human metapneumovirus in lung transplant recipients and comparison to respiratory syncytial virus. *Am J Respir Crit Care Med* 2008;178(8):876–881.

35. Boivin G, Serres GD, Hamelin ME, et al. An outbreak of severe respiratory tract infection due to human metapneumovirus in a long-term care facility. *Clin Infect Dis* 2007;44(9):1152–1158.

36. Hamre D, Procknow JJ. A new virus isolated from the human respiratory tract. *Proc Soc Exp Biol Med* 1966;121(1):190–193.

37. Gaunt ER, Hardie A, Claas ECJ, Simmonds P, Templeton KE. Epidemiology and clinical presentations of the four human coronaviruses 229E, HKU1, NL63, and OC43 detected over 3 years using a novel multiplex real-time PCR method. *J Clin Microbiol* 2010;48(8):2940–2947.

38. Arabi YM, Balkhy HH, Hayden FG, et al. Middle East respiratory syndrome. *N Engl J Med* 2017;376(6):584–594.

39. World Health Organization. MERS-CoV global summary and assessment of risk. 2017 [cited October 21, 2017]. Available at: http://www.who.int/csr/disease/coronavirus_infections/archive_updates/en/.

40. Al-Tawfiq JA, Omrani AS, Memish ZA. Middle East respiratory syndrome coronavirus: Current situation and travel-associated concerns. *Front Med* 2016;10(2):111–119.

41. Memish ZA, Almasri M, Turkestani A, Al-Shangiti AM, Yezli S. Etiology of severe community-acquired pneumonia during the 2013 Hajj—part of the MERS-CoV surveillance program. *Int J Infect Dis* 2014;25(Supplement C):186–190.

42. Oh M, Park WB, Choe PG, et al. Viral load kinetics of MERS coronavirus infection. *N Engl J Med* 2016;375(13):1303–1305.

43. Hui DS. Super-spreading events of MERS-CoV infection. *Lancet* 2016;388(10048):942–943.

44. Cho SY, Kang J-M, Ha YE, et al. MERS-CoV outbreak following a single patient exposure in an emergency room in South Korea: An epidemiological outbreak study. *Lancet* 2016;388(10048):994–1001.

45. World Health Organization. Clinical management of severe acute respiratory infection when Middle East respiratory syndrome coronavirus (MERS-CoV) infection is suspected. 2015 [cited December 4, 2017]. Available at: http://www.who.int/csr/disease/coronavirus_infections/case-management-ipc/en/.

46. Assiri A, Al-Tawfiq JA, Al-Rabeeah AA, et al. Epidemiological, demographic, and clinical characteristics of 47 cases of Middle East respiratory syndrome coronavirus disease from Saudi Arabia: A descriptive study. *Lancet Infect Dis* 2013;13(9):752–761.

47. Arabi YM, Al-Omari A, Mandourah Y, et al. Critically ill patients with the Middle East respiratory syndrome: A multicenter retrospective cohort study. *Crit Care Med* 2017;45(10):1683–1695.

48. Das KM, Lee EY, Jawder SEA, et al. Acute Middle East respiratory syndrome coronavirus: Temporal lung changes observed on the chest radiographs of 55 patients. *Am J Roentgenol* 2015;205(3):W267–S274.

49. Arabi YM, Arifi AA, Balkhy HH, et al. Clinical course and outcomes of critically ill patients with Middle East respiratory syndrome coronavirus infection. *Ann Intern Med* 2014;160(6):389–397.

50. Lee N, Hui D, Wu A, et al. A major outbreak of severe acute respiratory syndrome in Hong Kong. *N Engl J Med* 2003;348(20):1986–1994.

51. World Health Organization. Summary of probable SARS cases with onset of illness from 1 November 2002 to 31 July 2003. WHO. 2003 [cited December 13, 2017]. Available at: http://www.who.int/csr/sars/country/table2004_04_21/en/.

52. Peiris JSM, Yuen KY, Osterhaus ADME, Stöhr K. The severe acute respiratory syndrome. *N Engl J Med* 2003;349(25):2431–2441.

53. Yu ITS, Li Y, Wong TW, et al. Evidence of airborne transmission of the severe acute respiratory syndrome virus. *N Engl J Med* 2004;350(17):1731–1739.

54. Pang X, Zhu Z, Xu F, et al. Evaluation of control measures implemented in the severe acute respiratory syndrome outbreak in Beijing, 2003. *JAMA* 2003;290(24):3215–3221.

55. Report of the WHO-China Joint Mission on Coronavirus Disease 2019 (COVID-19) [Internet]. [cited March 21, 2020]. Available at: https://www.who.int/publications-detail/report-of-the-who-china-joint-mission-on-coronavirus-disease-2019-(covid-19).

56. Zhu N, Zhang D, Wang W, et al. A Novel coronavirus from patients with pneumonia in China, 2019. *N Engl J Med* 2020;382(8):727–733.

57. Li R, Pei S, Chen B, et al. Substantial undocumented infection facilitates the rapid dissemination of novel coronavirus (SARS-CoV2). *Science* [Internet]. March 16, 2020 [cited March 19, 2020]. Available at: http://science.sciencemag.org/content/early/2020/03/13/science.abb3221.

58. Anderson RM, Heesterbeek H, Klinkenberg D, Hollingsworth TD. How will country-based mitigation measures influence the course of the COVID-19 epidemic? *The Lancet* 2020;395(10228):931–934.

59. Rothe C, Schunk M, Sothmann P, et al. Transmission of 2019-nCoV Infection from an Asymptomatic Contact in Germany. *N Engl J Med* 2020;382(10):970–971.

60. Guan W, Ni Z, Hu Y, et al. Clinical characteristics of coronavirus disease 2019 in China. *N Engl J Med* [Internet]. February 28, 2020 [cited March 19, 2020]. Available at: http://www.nejm.org/doi/10.1056/NEJMoa2002032.

61. Zhou F, Yu T, Du R, et al. Clinical course and risk factors for mortality of adult inpatients with COVID-19 in Wuhan, China: A retrospective cohort study. *The Lancet* [Internet]. Mar 9, 2020 [cited March 21, 2020]. Available at: https://linkinghub.elsevier.com/retrieve/pii/S0140673620305663.

62. Lu X, Zhang L, Du H, et al. SARS-CoV-2 infection in children. *N Engl J Med* [Internet]. March 18, 2020. Available at: https://www.nejm.org/doi/full/10.1056/NEJMc2005073.

63. Shi H, Han X, Jiang N, et al. Radiological findings from 81 patients with COVID-19 pneumonia in Wuhan, China: A descriptive study. *Lancet Infect Dis* [Internet]. February 24, 2020 [cited March 19, 2020]. Available at: https://linkinghub.elsevier.com/retrieve/pii/S1473309920300864.

64. Salehi S, Abedi A, Balakrishnan S, Gholamrezanezhad A. Coronavirus disease 2019 (COVID-19): A systematic review of imaging findings in 919 patients. *Am J Roentgenol* 2020;1–7.

65. Wang W, Xu Y, Gao R, et al. Detection of SARS-CoV-2 in different types of clinical specimens. *JAMA* [Internet]. March 11, 2020 [cited March 19, 2020]. Available at: https://jamanetwork.com/journals/jama/fullarticle/2762997.

66. Fang Y, Zhang H, Xie J, et al. Sensitivity of chest CT for COVID-19: Comparison to RT-PCR. *Radiology* [Internet]. February 19, 2020 [cited March 19, 2020]. Available at: http://pubs.rsna.org/doi/10.1148/radiol.2020200432.

67. Smits SL, de Lang A, van den Brand JMA, et al. Exacerbated innate host response to SARS-CoV in aged non-human primates. *PLOS Pathog* 2010;6(2):e1000756.

68. Wang Z, Yang B, Li Q, Wen L, Zhang R. Clinical features of 69 cases with coronavirus disease 2019 in Wuhan, China. *Clin Infect Dis* [Internet]. March 16, 2020 [cited March 19, 2020]. Available at: https://academic.oup.com/cid/advance-article/doi/10.1093/cid/ciaa272/5807944.

69. Liu Y, Yan L-M, Wan L, et al. Viral dynamics in mild and severe cases of COVID-19. *Lancet Infect Dis* [Internet]. March 19, 2020 [cited March 21, 2020]. Available at: https://linkinghub.elsevier.com/retrieve/pii/S1473309920302322.

70. Lippi G, Plebani M. Procalcitonin in patients with severe coronavirus disease 2019 (COVID-19): A meta-analysis. *Clin Chim Acta* 2020;505:190–191.

71. Livingston E, Bucher K. Coronavirus disease 2019 (COVID-19) in Italy. *JAMA* [Internet]. March 17, 2020 [cited March 19, 2020]. Available at: http://jamanetwork.com/journals/jama/fullarticle/2763401.

72. Ji Y, Ma Z, Peppelenbosch MP, Pan Q. Potential association between COVID-19 mortality and health-care resource availability. *Lancet Glob Health* 2020;8(4):e480.

73. Wang M, Cao R, Zhang L, et al. Remdesivir and chloroquine effectively inhibit the recently emerged novel coronavirus (2019-nCoV) in vitro. *Cell Res* 2020;30(3):269–271.

74. Ko W-C, Rolain J-M, Lee N-Y, et al. Arguments in favour of remdesivir for treating SARS-CoV-2 infections. *Int J Antimicrob Agents* [Internet]. March 6, 2020 [cited March 19, 2020]. Available at: https://linkinghub.elsevier.com/retrieve/pii/S0924857920300832.

75. Cao B, Wang Y, Wen D, et al. A trial of lopinavir–ritonavir in adults hospitalized with severe Covid-19. *N Engl J Med* [Internet]. March 18, 2020 [cited March 19, 2020]. Available at: http://www.nejm.org/doi/10.1056/NEJMoa2001282.

76. Ison MG, Hayden RT. Adenovirus. *Microbiol Spectr* 2016;4(4). Available at: http://www.asmscience.org/content/journal/microbiolspec/10.1128/microbiolspec. DMIH2-0020-2015.

77. Cao B, Huang GH, Pu ZH, et al. Emergence of community-acquired adenovirus type 55 as a cause of community-onset pneumonia. *Chest* 2014;145(1):79–86.

78. Centers for Disease Control and Prevention (CDC). Two fatal cases of adenovirus-related illness in previously healthy young adults—Illinois, 2000. *Morb Mortal Wkly Rep* 2001;50(26):553–555.

79. Centers for Disease Control and Prevention (CDC). Acute respiratory disease associated with adenovirus serotype 14—four states, 2006–2007. *Morb Mortal Wkly Rep* 2007;56(45):1181–1184.

80. Lafolie J, Mirand A, Salmona M, et al. Severe pneumonia associated with adenovirus type 55 infection, France, 2014. *Emerg Infect Dis* 2016;22(11):2012–2014.

81. Tan D, Fu Y, Xu J, et al. Severe adenovirus community-acquired pneumonia in immunocompetent adults: Chest radiographic and CT findings. *J Thorac Dis* 2016;8(5):848–854.

82. Ison MG. Adenovirus infections in transplant recipients. *Clin Infect Dis* 2006;43(3):331–339.

83. Neofytos D, Ojha A, Mookerjee B, et al. Treatment of adenovirus disease in stem cell transplant recipients with cidofovir. *Biol Blood Marrow Transplant* 2007;13(1):74–81.

84. Avšič-Županc T, Saksida A, Korva M. Hantavirus infections. *Clin Microbiol Infect* 2015.

85. Khan AS, Khabbaz RF, Armstrong LR, et al. Hantavirus pulmonary syndrome: The first 100 US cases. *J Infect Dis* 1996;173(6):1297–14303.

86. Annual U.S. Hantavirus Disease and HPS Case Fatality, 1993–2016 | Hantavirus | DHCPP | CDC. 2017 [cited November 11, 2017]. Available at: https://www.cdc.gov/hantavirus/surveillance/annual-cases.html.

87. Drebot M, Jones S, Grolla A, et al. Hantavirus pulmonary syndrome in Canada: An overview of clinical features, diagnostics, epidemiology and prevention—CCDR: Volume 41-06, June 4, 2015. Canada Communicable Disease Report. 2015 [cited November 11, 2017]. Available at: https://www.canada.ca/en/public-health/services/reports-publications/canada-communicable-disease-report-ccdr/monthly-issue/2015-41/ccdr-volume-41-06-june-4-2015/ccdr-volume-41-06-june-4-2015-1.html.

88. Richardson KS, Kuenzi A, Douglass RJ, Hart J, Carver S. Human exposure to particulate matter potentially contaminated with Sin Nombre virus. *EcoHealth* 2013;10(2):159–165.

89. Webster D, Lee B, Joffe A, et al. Cluster of cases of hantavirus pulmonary syndrome in Alberta, Canada. *Am J Trop Med Hyg* 2007;77(5):914–918.

90. Bharadwaj M, Nofchissey R, Goade D, Koster F, Hjelle B. Humoral immune responses in the hantavirus cardiopulmonary syndrome. *J Infect Dis* 2000;182(1):43–48.

91. Wernly JA, Dietl CA, Tabe CE, et al. Extracorporeal membrane oxygenation support improves survival of patients with Hantavirus cardiopulmonary syndrome refractory to medical treatment. *Eur J Cardiothorac Surg* 2011;40(6):1334–1340.

92. Verity R, Prasad E, Grimsrud K, et al. Hantavirus pulmonary syndrome in Northern Alberta, Canada: Clinical and laboratory findings for 19 cases. *Clin Infect Dis* 2000;31(4):942–946.

93. Dvorscak L, Czuchlewski DR. Successful triage of suspected hantavirus cardiopulmonary syndrome by peripheral blood smear review. *Am J Clin Pathol* 2014;142(2):196–201.

94. Balthesen M, Messerle M, Reddehase MJ. Lungs are a major organ site of cytomegalovirus latency and recurrence. *J Virol* 1993;67(9):5360–5366.

95. Hopkins PM, Aboyoun CL, Chhajed PN, et al. Prospective analysis of 1,235 transbronchial lung biopsies in lung transplant recipients. *J Heart Lung Transplant* 2002;21(10):1062–1067.

96. Kotloff RM, Ahya VN, Crawford SW. Pulmonary complications of solid organ and hematopoietic stem cell transplantation. *Am J Respir Crit Care Med* 2004;170(1):22–48.

97. Snyder LD, Finlen-Copeland CA, Turbyfill WJ, Howell D, Willner DA, Palmer SM. Cytomegalovirus pneumonitis is a risk for bronchiolitis obliterans syndrome in lung transplantation. *Am J Respir Crit Care Med* 2010;181(12):1391–1396.

98. Travi G, Pergam SA. Cytomegalovirus pneumonia in hematopoietic stem cell recipients. *J Intensive Care Med* 2014;29(4):200–212.

99. Franquet T, Lee KS, Müller NL. Thin-section CT findings in 32 immunocompromised patients with cytomegalovirus pneumonia who do not have AIDS. *Am J Roentgenol* 2003;181(4):1059–1063.

100. Kotton CN, Kumar D, Caliendo AM, et al. Updated international consensus guidelines on the management of cytomegalovirus in solid-organ transplantation. *Transplant J* 2013;96(4):333–360.

101. Westall GP, Michaelides A, Williams TJ, Snell GI, Kotsimbos TC. Human cytomegalovirus load in plasma and bronchoalveolar lavage fluid: A longitudinal study of lung transplant recipients. *J Infect Dis* 2004;190(6):1076–1083.

102. Cook CH, Martin LC, Yenchar JK, et al. Occult herpes family viral infections are endemic in critically ill surgical patients. *Crit Care Med* 2003;31(7):1923–1929.

103. Bordes J, Maslin J, Prunet B, et al. Cytomegalovirus infection in severe burn patients monitoring by real-time polymerase chain reaction: A prospective study. *Burns* 2011;37(3):434–439.

104. Papazian L, Hraiech S, Lehingue S, et al. Cytomegalovirus reactivation in ICU patients. *Intensive Care Med* 2016;42(1):28–37.

105. Limaye AP, Stapleton RD, Peng L, et al. Effect of ganciclovir on IL-6 levels among cytomegalovirus-seropositive adults with critical illness: A randomized clinical trial. *JAMA* 2017;318(8):731–740.

106. Guess HA, Broughton DD, Melton LJ, Kurland LT. Population-based studies of varicella complications. *Pediatrics* 1986;78(4):723–727.

107. Mirouse A, Seguin A, Stoclin A, et al. Severe varicella-zoster virus pneumonia: A multicenter cohort study. *Crit Care* 2017;21(1):137.

108. Poritz MA, Blaschke AJ, Byington CL, et al. FilmArray, an automated nested multiplex PCR system for multi-pathogen detection: Development and application to respiratory tract infection. *PLOS ONE* 2011;6(10):e26047.

109. Lee CK, Lee HK, Ng CWS, et al. Comparison of Luminex NxTAG respiratory pathogen panel and xTAG respiratory viral panel FAST version 2 for the detection of respiratory viruses. *Ann Lab Med* 2017;37(3):267–271.

110. Jeong JH, Kim KH, Jeong SH, Park JW, Lee SM, Seo YH. Comparison of sputum and nasopharyngeal swabs for detection of respiratory viruses. *J Med Virol* 2014;86(12):2122–2127.

111. Falsey AR, Formica MA, Walsh EE. Yield of sputum for viral detection by reverse transcriptase PCR in adults hospitalized with respiratory illness. *J Clin Microbiol* 2012;50(1):21–24.

112. Blyth CC, Iredell JR, Dwyer DE. Rapid-test sensitivity for novel swine-origin influenza A (H1N1) virus in humans. *N Engl J Med* 2009;361(25):2493–2493.

113. Gilbert DN. Procalcitonin as a biomarker in respiratory tract infection. *Clin Infect Dis* 2011;52(suppl_4):S346–S3450.

114. Schuetz P, Christ-Crain M, Thomann R, et al. Effect of procalcitonin-based guidelines vs standard guidelines on antibiotic use in lower respiratory tract infections: The ProHOSP randomized controlled trial. *JAMA* 2009;302(10):1059–1066.

115. Self WH, Balk RA, Grijalva CG, et al. Procalcitonin as a marker of etiology in adults hospitalized with community-acquired pneumonia. *Clin Infect Dis* 2017;65(2):183–190.

116. Meer V van der, Neven AK, Broek PJ van den, Assendelft WJJ. Diagnostic value of C reactive protein in infections of the lower respiratory tract: Systematic review. *BMJ* 2005;331(7507):26.

117. Shah DP, Ghantoji SS, Shah JN, et al. Impact of aerosolized ribavirin on mortality in 280 allogeneic haematopoietic stem cell transplant recipients with respiratory syncytial virus infections. *J Antimicrob Chemother* 2013;68(8):1872–1880.

118. Boeckh M, Englund J, Li Y, et al. Randomized controlled multicenter trial of aerosolized ribavirin for respiratory syncytial virus upper respiratory tract infection in hematopoietic cell transplant recipients. *Clin Infect Dis* 2007;44(2):245–249.

119. Mertz GJ, Miedzinski L, Goade D, et al. Placebo-controlled, double-blind trial of intravenous ribavirin for the treatment of hantavirus cardiopulmonary syndrome in North America. *Clin Infect Dis* 2004;39(9):1307–1313.

120. Hecht DW, Snydman DR, Crumpacker CS, Werner BG, Heinze-Lacey B. Ganciclovir for treatment of renal transplant-associated primary cytomegalovirus pneumonia. *J Infect Dis* 1988;157(1):187–190.

121. Erice A, Jordan MC, Chace BA, Fletcher C, Chinnock BJ, Balfour HH. Ganciclovir treatment of cytomegalovirus disease in transplant recipients and other immunocompromised hosts. *JAMA* 1987;257(22):3082–3087.

122. Frangides CY, Pneumatikos I. Varicella-zoster virus pneumonia in adults: Report of 14 cases and review of the literature. *Eur J Intern Med* 2004;15(6):364–370.

123. Wallace MR. Treatment of adult varicella with oral acyclovir: A randomized, placebo-controlled trial. *Ann Intern Med* 1992;117(5):358.

124. Haake DA, Zakowski PC, Haake DL, Bryson YJ. Early treatment with acyclovir for varicella pneumonia in otherwise healthy adults: Retrospective controlled study and review. *Rev Infect Dis* 1990;12(5):788–798.

125. Siemieniuk RAC, Meade MO, Alonso-Coello P, et al. Corticosteroid therapy for patients hospitalized with community-acquired pneumonia: A systematic review and meta-analysis. *Ann Intern Med* 2015;163(7):519.

126. Rodrigo C, Leonardi-Bee J, Nguyen-Van-Tam J, Lim WS. Corticosteroids as adjunctive therapy in the treatment of influenza. *Cochrane Database Syst Rev* 2016;3:CD010406.

127. Lee FEH, Walsh EE, Falsey AR. The effect of steroid use in hospitalized adults with respiratory syncytial virus-related illness. *Chest* 2011;140(5):1155–1161.

128. Lee N, Chan MCW, Lui GCY, et al. High viral load and respiratory failure in adults hospitalized for respiratory syncytial virus infections. *J Infect Dis* 2015;212(8):1237–1240.

129. Fan E, Del Sorbo L, Goligher EC, et al. An official American Thoracic Society/European Society of Intensive Care Medicine/Society of Critical Care Medicine Clinical Practice Guideline: Mechanical ventilation in adult patients with acute respiratory distress syndrome. *Am J Respir Crit Care Med* 2017;195(9):1253–1263.

130. Putensen C. Meta-analysis: Ventilation strategies and outcomes of the acute respiratory distress syndrome and acute lung injury. *Ann Intern Med* 2009;151(8):566.

131. Peek GJ, Mugford M, Tiruvoipati R, et al. Efficacy and economic assessment of conventional ventilatory support versus extracorporeal membrane oxygenation for severe adult respiratory failure (CESAR): A multicentre randomised controlled trial. *Lancet* 2009;374(9698):1351–1363.

132. Noah MA, Peek GJ, Finney SJ, et al. Referral to an extracorporeal membrane oxygenation center and mortality among patients with severe 2009 influenza A(H1N1). *JAMA* 2011;306(15):1659–1668.

133. Arauco Brown R, Murthy J, Manian P, Rumbaoa B, Connolly T. An early aggressive strategy for the treatment of hanta virus cardiopulmonary syndrome: A perspective from an extracorporeal membrane oxygenation center. *Clin Infect Dis* 2014;59(3):458–459.

134. Siegel JD, Rhinehart E, Jackson M, Chiarello L. 2007 Guideline for isolation precautions: Preventing transmission of infectious agents in health care settings. *Am J Infect Control* 2007;35(10, Supplement 2):S65–S164.

135. Centers for Disease Control and Prevention. Guideline for Isolation Precautions: Preventing Transmission of Infectious Agents in Healthcare Settings. 2017 [cited December 5, 2017]. Available at: https://www.cdc.gov/infectioncontrol/guidelines/isolation/appendix/type-duration-precautions.html.

17 Nosocomial Pneumonia in the Critical Care Unit

Burke A. Cunha

CONTENTS

CLINICAL PERSPECTIVE

Nosocomial pneumonia (NP) is a common diagnostic problem in the critical care unit (CCU). Many factors predispose to acquiring bacterial pneumonia in the hospital, e.g., aspiration, intubation, and bacteremia. Underlying cardiopulmonary reserve is an important determinant of severity and prognosis. Elderly patients are particularly predisposed to NP due to lack of mobility, increased likelihood of aspiration, prolonged intubation, and impaired cardiopulmonary function, which contribute to high mortality and morbidity.

Nosocomial pneumonia may be further classified as hospital-acquired pneumonia (HAP) and, in intubated patients, as ventilator-associated pneumonia (VAP). The main clinical challenge with NP/VAP is correct diagnosis, which is the basis for selecting appropriate empiric antibiotic therapy based on predictable NP/VAP pathogens.

DIAGNOSTIC CONSIDERATIONS

Nosocomial pneumonia may be defined as an otherwise-unexplained new pulmonary infiltrate on chest film, with the appearance of a bacterial pneumonia occurring in a patient who has been hospitalized for >1 week [1–6]. Not essential to the diagnosis of NP are non-specific findings that may also be seen in a variety of unrelated infectious or non-infectious disorders, e.g., fever and leukocytosis [7–10].

There are two major diagnostic and therapeutic difficulties in the clinical approach to NP/VAP in the CCU. The critical problem is to establish a clinical syndromic diagnosis of NP/VAP. No other nosocomial infection has so many mimics that present in a similar fashion, causing such diagnostic confusion. In contrast to community-acquired pneumonias (CAPs), in which chest film appearance and sputum Gram stain or culture are useful diagnostically, chest X-ray (CXR) appearance and respiratory secretion cultures are unhelpful in the diagnosis of NP/VAP [1,2,10,11] (Table 17.1).

MIMICS OF NOSOCOMIAL PNEUMONIA

The most difficult diagnostic problems in patients with presumed NP/VAP are related to the non-specific appearance of CXR infiltrates and the interpretation of the clinical relationship of extra-pulmonary findings, if present. Fever and leukocytosis are non-specific findings and may be due to a variety of other infectious or non-infectious disorders. It is important to rule out mimics of NP/VAP with or without fever and leukocytosis that present with pulmonary infiltrates on CXR or chest CT scans. The disorders most likely to mimic the appearance of a NP/VAP on CXR include interstitial lung disease; primary or metastatic bronchogenic carcinomas; pulmonary

TABLE 17.1

Clinical Features of Possible Nosocomial Pneumonia/Ventilator Associated Pneumonia

Chest Radiographs in Possible NP/VAP

Clinical Findings

- Chest film with otherwise-unexplained new infiltrates plus fever and leukocytosis in ventilated/non-ventilated CCU patients.

Comments

- The findings above may also be present with many non-infectious causes, e.g., pulmonary embolism, pulmonary hemorrhage, bronchogenic carcinomas, ARDS, pulmonary, drug reactions, or collagen vascular diseases, SLE, BOOP, or CHF.

Respiratory Secretion Cultures

Clinical Findings

- Single or multiple organisms are reflective of proximal or distal airway colonization and rarely related to the possible pulmonary pathogen in distant lung parenchyma.

Comments

- Common nosocomial pneumonia non-pathogens include *S. maltophilia, B. cepacia, Enterobacter* sp., *Citrobacter* sp., *Flavobacterium* sp., and *Acinetobacter* sp.
- Most aerobic GNB are frequently cultured from respiratory secretions in nosocomial pneumonia.
- Microbial etiology and empiric therapy of nosocomial pneumonia should not be based on respiratory secretion/endotracheal aspirate cultures.
- Potentially pathogenic organisms, e.g., *P. aeruginosa* and *S. aureus*, frequently cultured from respiratory secretions, are common colonizers of respiratory secretions. Unless accompanied by necrotizing pneumonia with rapid cavitation, these organisms should be considered as airway colonizers and not be considered the causative agents of nosocomial pneumonia.
- Culture of multiple organisms is indicative of airway colonization.

Chest Radiographs in Necrotizing Pneumonia

Clinical Findings

- Necrotizing pneumonia with rapid cavitation <72 is a characteristic of only *P. aeruginosa* and *S. aureus.*
- Necrotizing pneumonia with cavitation after 5–7 days is typical of *Klebsiella pneumoniae* pneumonia.

Diagnostic Significance of Blood Cultures

Clinical Findings

- The presentation of MSSA/MRSA necrotizing pneumonia is limited to CAP with simultaneous influenza pneumonia.
- MRSA is rarely, if ever, a cause of NP/VAP.
- Positive BC are most useful in confirming the causative pathogen in CAP due to bacteremic pulmonary pathogens, e.g., *S. pneumoniae* and *H. influenza*e (bacteremia not a feature of M. catarrhalis CAP).
- Blood cultures should be obtained from a peripheral vein (not CVCs) using careful aseptic technique to minimize contaminating blood cultures with skin flora.
- With the exception of bacteremic *P. aeruginosa* NP/VAP, nearly all NP/VAP pathogens are not associated with bacteremia and positive BCs are unhelpful and are often misleading in identifying the cause of NP/VAP. If *bona fide P. aeruginosa* NP/VAP, clinically there should be rapid cavitation as well.
- Elastin fibers (indicating lung necrosis) in respiratory secretions are reflective of a rapidly necrotizing pneumonia due to either *P. aeruginosa* or *S. aureus.* These characteristic clinicopathologic findings are essential in the diagnosis of *P. aeruginosa, Klebsiella pneumoniae* or *S. aureus pneumoniae. S. pneumoniae, H. influenzae, E. coli*, and *Serratia* sp. do not cavitate.

Comments

- Without associated clinical findings, the most common diagnostic error is to consider the blood culture isolate the causative pathogen in potential NP/VAP patients, e.g., *S. aureus, Acinetobacter* sp.
- Since MSSA/MRSA rarely, if ever, causes NP/VAP, blood cultures positive for *S. aureus* are indicative of skin flora or a distinct other source, e.g., osteomyelitis or cutaneous abscess.
- *Acinetobacter* sp. in blood cultures usually indicate skin flora contamination during venipuncture; *Acinetobacter* sp. commonly colonizes urine (CAB), wounds, decubitus ulcers, and skin.
- Positive blood cultures with non-NP/VAP aerobic GNB organisms, e.g., *S. maltophilia, B. cepacia*, and *Enterobacter* sp., are either due to skin flora contamination during venipuncture or may be for a non-pulmonary source, e.g., urine.
- Blood cultures positive for *E. coli* or *S. marcescens* are likely for a distinct non-pulmonary source, e.g., *E. coli* (GI or GU source) and *S. marcescens* (skin or urine source).
- *E. coli* is an uncommon cause of bacteremic CAP but only rarely a cause of NP/VAP.
- *S. marcescens* is very rare cause of NP/VAP and should be suspected with upper lobe infiltrates in pNP/VAP, the only cause of NP/VAP with only upper lobe infiltrates.

(Continued)

TABLE 17.1 (*Continued*)

Clinical Features of Possible Nosocomial Pneumonia/Ventilator Associated Pneumonia

Definitive Diagnosis of Nosocomial Pneumonia

Clinical Findings

- Transbronchial lung biopsy culture.
- Exclusion cultures of skin flora isolates.
- Causative role of pathogen in nosocomial pneumonia proved by showing pathological lung findings and by bacterial pathogen cultures.

Comments

- Pathogenic diagnosis of nosocomial pneumonia is preferred but it is uncommon based on clinical diagnosis, and associated clinical findings are not simply microbiology culture of specimens, which may be contaminated by colonizing organisms in the distal bronchitis.
- Percutaneous or open-lung biopsy.
- Excluding skin colonizers, e.g., *S. aureus* and *Acinetobacter* sp., may contaminate specimen during the procedure; growth of a single *bona fide* NP pathogen is diagnostic.

Autopsy

Clinical Findings

- Autopsy diagnosis is based on lung invasion, e.g., nosocomial pneumonia, by bacteria.

Comments

- Must exclude skin colonizers, e.g., *S. aureus* and *Acinetobacter* sp., that may contaminate the specimen during autopsy.
- *S. aureus* airway colonization is common and a function of CCU length of stay and spectrum/secretion penetration of previous/current antibiotic therapy.

Surveillance Cultures in the CCU

Clinical Findings

- Generally unhelpful in predicting the pathogen in pNP/VAP.

Comments

- Most useful for an infection-control epidemiologic perspective; e.g., when *S. marcescens* prevalence is high, *P. aeruginosa* colonization rates are low and vice versa.

Nasal Swabs

Clinical Findings

- Colonization in the CCU with MRSA is often prolonged and doesn't progress to NP/VAP.

Comments

- Since MSSA/MRSA rarely, if ever, causes NP/VAP, nasal swabs for NPs are clinically irrelevant. For those concerned, a negative nasal swab for MRSA effectively eliminates MRSA for further consideration as colonizer or pulmonary pathogen.
- Empiric therapy, including an anti-MRSA antibiotic, is unnecessary in eliminating MRSA among colonizers (colonization doesn't progress to pneumonia with this organism). Needless to say, regardless of nares culture results (+ or −) for MRSA, empiric therapy is not warranted.

emboli; pulmonary drug reactions; pulmonary hemorrhage; collagen vascular disease affecting the lungs, e.g., systemic lupus erythematous (SLE), pneumonitis, and acute respiratory distress syndrome (ARDS); and, most commonly, congestive heart failure (CHF). Before embarking on a course of empiric antimicrobial therapy for possible NP/VAP, importantly diagnostically, many of the radiologic mimics of NP/VAP have low-grade (<102°F) or no fever. The diagnostic clues to the diagnosis of the mimics of NP/VAP are the disorders characteristic extra-pulmonary findings [1,2,10] (Table 17.2).

MICROBIOLOGIC DATA: COLONIZATION OF SECRETIONS VERSUS CAUSATIVE PATHOGENS

From a clinical standpoint, it is difficult to determine if the patient has NP/VAP. Without invasive diagnostic procedures, it is as difficult to determine the potential lung pathogen in NP/VAP. In contrast to CAP, in which the pneumonia pathogen may be identified in a well-collected uncontaminated sputum sample with alveolar macrophages (AM) which reflects the pathologic process and pathogen in the lung not the airways. In CAP, sputum is unhelpful diagnostically in neutropenic hosts and those with chronic bronchitis. In such patients, sputum is unhelpful, and sputum of patients with exacerbation of chronic bronchitis (AECB) usually grows mixed normal/respiratory flora, reflecting airway colonization. CAPs in patients unable to produce sputum, excluding skin contaminants, e.g., *S. aureus*, vancomycin susceptible enterococci/vancomycin resistant enterococci (VSE/VRE), blood cultures (BCs) may be helpful in identifying the causative organism. In the absence of a non-lung pathogen recovered from the blood, culture is the same organism that is causing CAP. Because *Streptococcus pneumoniae* and *Haemophilus influenzae*

TABLE 17.2

Microbiology of Nosocomial Ventilator Associated Pneumonia in the CCU

Aerobic GNB Potential Nosocomial Pneumonia Pathogens	Clinical Comments
Pseudomonas aeruginosa	• Many cases diagnosed as nosocomial pneumonia (pVAP) are pneumonia mimics
Klebsiella pneumoniae	• *Acinetobacter* is a common colonizer of respiratory tract secretions
Serratia marcescens	• Nosocomial *Acinetobacter* pneumonia occurs in outbreaks or clusters (usually
E. coli	associated with contaminated respiratory support equipment)
Nosocomial Outbreak Pathogens	• Nosocomial *Legionella* pneumonia occurs in outbreaks or clusters usually from a
Acinetobacter sp.	common aerolized water source
Legionella sp.	• Rarely, if ever, a *bona fide* cause of NP/VAP
Non-nosocomial Pneumonia Pathogens	• Without clinical correlation, detection/culture of an organism from respiratory
	secretions (colonization) does not indicate that it is the pathogen
Enterobacter sp.	
Stenotrophomas (formerly *Pseudomonas*) maltophilia	
Burkholderia (formerly *Pseudomonas*) cepacia	
S. aureus (MSSA/MRSA)	

Abbreviation: GNB, Gram-negative bacilli.

are often bacteremic, BCs are important in establishing the etiologic CAP diagnosis in these patients. Blood culture positivity depends on the timing/volume of blood cultures, pre-existing antimicrobial therapy, and the bacteremic propensity of the organism; e.g., bacteremia is uncommon with *Moraxella catarrhalis* [1,2,11–17].

Interpretation of microbiologic culture data requires clinical correlation to determine its site-related relevance (site-pathogen correlation), e.g., respiratory secretion Gram stain/culture in ventilated patients. Definitive diagnostic procedures are percutaneous and/or open-lung biopsies, but these are uncommonly performed. The least sensitive respiratory secretion culture technique is the endotracheal aspiration (ETA) culture to diagnose NP. The recovery of organisms from the distal airways, even semi-quantitative culture techniques obtained by "protected" bronchial brushings (PBB) or bronchoalveolar lavage (BAL), does not differentiate distal airway colonization from the *bona fide* pulmonary infection pathogen. In the CCU, upper and lower airway colonization is the rule. Colonization of the airways is a function of the duration of hospital stay and the spectrum/resistance potential of the antibiotic used. During the first week of hospitalization, the normal respiratory flora of the patient is displaced by nosocomial organisms, i.e., aerobic gram-negative bacilli (GNB) or *S. aureus*. Aside from failing to rule out NP/VAP mimics, the most common clinical error is to assume that respiratory secretion isolates should be treated as lung (NP/VAP) pathogens. Colonization of the proximal and distal airways is not representative of the pathogen causing NP/VAP in lung parenchyma. In intubated patients, airways are rapidly colonized by the CCU flora. If ventilated patients develop new pulmonary infiltrates with fever/leukocytosis, avoid "covering" any or all isolates cultured, if or until the clinical significance of the respiratory secretion isolates is assessed [1–3,5,6].

The recovery of multiple pathogens from respiratory secretion specimens, of ventilated patients regardless of the technique used, is the proof of specimen contamination and not co-pathogenicity (Table 17.3).

Without diagnostic microbiology data, it is difficult for clinicians to devise a rational approach to antibiotic therapy for NPs. Overtreatment, based on respiratory secretion cultures, often results in inappropriate empiric antimicrobial therapy of airway colonizers, not the pathogens in "nosocomial pneumonias" [1,6,18–20]. Because many patients with pulmonary infiltrates and fever do not have NP/VAP, many patients are excessively or needlessly treated after ruling out the mimics of NP/VAP. In the absence of tissue-based diagnostic tests, it is reasonable to treat presumed NP/VAP with a course of appropriate empiric antimicrobial therapy to cover the "usual NP/VAP."

NECROTIZING NOSOCOMIAL PNEUMONIA

Necrotizing pneumonia with rapid cavitation (within 72 hours) is the hallmark of *Pseudomonas aeruginosa* NP/VAP. The NP/VAP with necrosis implies a rapidly invasive destructive process in the lung parenchyma. Aside from rapid cavitation on CXR, an indirect indicator to confirm the diagnosis of a necrotizing pneumonia is by demonstrating elastin fibers in respiratory tract secretions, stained by potassium hydroxide. Elastin fibers are from necrotic lung tissue and are diagnostic of necrotizing pneumonia [1,2]. Multiple cavitary lesions become apparent on CXR <72 hours, and VAP patients with *bona fide S. aureus* (CAP) or *P. aeruginosa* (NP/VAP) pneumonia have elastin fibers in the respiratory secretions [6]. *Klebsiella pneumoniae* also causes a slower and less intense necrotizing pneumonia. The cavitation with necrotizing *K. pneumoniae* pneumonia occurs after 3–5 days rather than in <72 hours [21,22].

TABLE 17.3
Appropriate Empiric Antibiotic Coverage in Nosocomial Pneumonia

Empiric Coverage Should be Directed Against Common Pathogens

Pseudomonas aeruginosa

Klebsiella pneumoniae

Serratia marcescens

E. coli

Coverage Should Not be Added to Cover Non-Pulmonary Pathogens or *S. aureus* (MSSA/MRSA)

Serratia marcescens

Enterobacter cloacae

Stenotrophomas (formerly *Pseudomonas*)
  maltophilia

Burkholderia (formerly *Pseudomonas*)
  cepacia

MSSA/MRSA

- Coverage should be primarily directed against *P. aeruginosa*, which also covers other GNB NP/VAP pathogens
- Do not add vancomycin or linezolid to NP/VAP regimen
- Vancomycin to cover *S. aureus* (MSSA/MRSA) is unnecessary and predisposes to the emergence of VRE
- Vancomycin doesn't eliminate MRSA colonization from respiratory secretions
- MRSA pneumonia may complicate influenza pneumonia is CAP patients
- Negative MRSA nares culture effectively rules out MRSA NP/VAP
- Positive MRSA respiratory secretion of cultures and not predictive MRSA NP/VAP

The differences in cavitation rates are a diagnostic clue to the etiology of the necrotizing pathogen, i.e., *K. pneumoniae* versus *P. aeruginosa* or *S. aureus* [2].

PSEUDOMONAS AERUGINOSA NOSOCOMIAL PNEUMONIA

Although *bona fide P. aeruginosa* NP is characterized by a necrotizing pneumonia, with rapid cavitation within <72 hours, this is uncommon in the clinical setting. Based on respiratory secretion culture data, the incidence of *P. aeruginosa* NP/VAP is overestimated. Nevertheless, *P. aeruginosa*, the most formidable potential NP/VAP pathogen, commonly colonizes respiratory tract secretions but much

less commonly causes NP/VAP. The older literature describes carefully *P. aeruginosa*, correlating its characteristic CXR findings with pathologic data, e.g., elastin fibers and lung biopsy culture [1,2,6].

In contrast with other potential "low virulence" pathogens, e.g., *Enterobacter* sp., *Stenotropomonas* sp., and *Burkholderia* sp., *P. aeruginosa* has a tropism for respiratory tract lining cells and is inherently virulent [3,13,15–17,23]. *P. aeruginosa* adheres to respiratory tract cells more avidly than other aerobic GNB. While *P. aeruginosa* is not the most common NP/VAP pathogen, it is the most virulent pulmonary pathogen causing NP/VAP. Accordingly, empiric therapy of NP/VAP should be directed primarily against *P. aeruginosa*, which also provides coverage against other GNB causes of NP/VAP (Table 17.4).

TABLE 17.4
Optimal Empiric Monotherapy pNP/pVAP

Optimal Empiric Monotherapy	Comments
Meropenem Cefepime	- Avoid monotherapy with ciprofloxacin, ceftazidime, or imipenem because of their high resistance potential in treating aerobic GNB
Optimal Double Drug Regimens for Proven *P. aeruginosa* Necrotizing Nosocomial Pneumonia	- Avoid using ciprofloxacin and ceftazidime in combination regimens, since combination therapy does not eliminate the resistance of these "high resistance potential" antibiotics
- Cefepime *plus either* levofloxacin *or* aztreonam *or* amikacin · - Meropenem *plus either* levofloxacin *or* aztreonam *or* amikacin	- If an aminoglycoside is selected for combination therapy, use "once daily amikacin" (not split dosed) instead of gentamicin or tobramycin to avoid potential *P. aeruginosa* resistance - If you select a quinolone for combination therapy regimen, use levofloxacin, which has excellent anti-*P. aeruginosa* activity equal to ciprofloxacin - Penicillin allergic patients: If the patient by history has had an anaphylactic reaction to penicillin, combination therapy with meropenem plus an aminoglycoside, levofloxacin, or aztreonam provides good anti-*P. aeruginosa* coverage with no cross-reactivity - Ciprofloxacin (not levofloxacin) ceftazidime (not cefepime) or imipenem (not meropenem) predisposes to MRSA colonization or respiratory secretions

Abbreviations: p, presumptive; P, probable.

MULTIPLE PATHOGENS AND CO-INFECTIONS

Excluding polymicrobial abscesses and aspiration pneumonia, it is a cardinal infectious disease principle that one organism is responsible for one infectious disease. This basic principle is true of CAP and NP/VAP. With few exceptions, one pathogen and not co-infection is the rule in CAP as well as NP/VAP [2,3]. In NP/VAP patients, multiple pathogens recovered from respiratory tract secretion cultures are indicative of airway colonization, not polymicrobial lung infection. The recovery of multiple organisms from respiratory tract secretions, regardless of the method of specimen collection employed, is the proof of airway colonization [2,24].

EARLY VERSUS LATE NOSOCOMIAL PNEUMONIA

Some have divided NP into so-called early and late NP patients based on differences in causative organisms and onset of NP after admission. So-called early HAPs are said to occur <5 days after admission, and "late HAP" occur after 5 days in the hospital. The "early group," manifesting pneumonia in the hospital, actually represents incubating CAP that has clinically manifested during the first week of hospitalization. The "early HAP" group is caused by CAP pathogens, i.e., *S. pneumoniae* and *H. influenzae*, and not the usual GNB NP/VAP pathogens. The late HAP group of pathogens represents the traditional nosocomial pathogens (i.e., *P. aeruginosa* as well as other aerobic GNB). Patients developing HAP within 5 days/week of hospitalization should be treated as CAP, and those developing pneumonias after 5 days/week of hospitalization should be treated empirically as NP/VAP [1,2,6,10].

NOSOCOMIAL PNEUMONIA OUTBREAKS

Some aerobic low-virulence GNB cause NPs virtually only in outbreak situations. *Acinetobacter* sp., a common colonizer of respiratory secretions, rarely, if ever, causes NP/VAP and may rarely cause outbreaks or clusters of NP in the CCU. Outbreaks have been caused by *Acinetobacter* sp. from respiratory support equipment, e.g., contaminated respirometers, respiratory tubing, and nebulizers. *Acinetobacter* sp. may also be transferred from patient to patient from contaminated respiratory secretions or the hands of medical personnel. Excluding outbreaks, when *Acinetobacter* sp. cultured from respiratory secretion specimens in the CCU, it invariably represents colonization as isolated cases of *Acinetobacter* sp. pneumonia are very rare [13,15–17,23]. Nosocomial *Legionella* sp. occurs virtually only in outbreak situations and not as isolated cases. The source of *Legionella* sp. is usually related to a source of aerosolized *Legionella* sp.-contaminated water. *Legionella* sp. hospital outbreaks have been related to a variety of sources, e.g., ice cubes and shower heads. In contrast to *Acinetobacter* sp., respiratory secretions of hospital patients are not commonly colonized with *Legionella* sp. in CCUs [2,25–28].

NON-PATHOGENS IN NOSOCOMIAL PNEUMONIAS (NON-FERMENTATIVE AEROBIC GRAM-NEGATIVE BACILLI)

Certain organisms are non-pathogens in NPs, and most of these organisms represent the aerobic gram-negative bacillary flora of the hospital. Most of these organisms also are *water organisms* and survive in an aqueous environment, e.g., respirator secretions, irrigating solutions, and sinks. In the hospital, such aerobic GNB non-fermentative organisms rapidly colonize the patient's respiratory secretions and are often recovered from respiratory secretion cultures (Table 17.5).

TABLE 17.5

Common Problems in the Treatment of Nosocomial Pneumonia

Usual Treatment for Nosocomial Pneumonia	Radiographic and Clinical Non-resolution of pNP/pVAP Comments
• Nosocomial pneumonias may be treated for 7–14 days	• If the patient has a *bona fide* NP/VAP and appropriate empiric therapy was used for therapy, after 3–5 days, there should be considerable improvement in the appearance of pulmonary infiltrates during therapy
MDR GNB Cultured from Respiratory Secretions Comments	• Lack of improvement in pulmonary infiltrates, after 3–5 days, usually indicates that the infiltrates were non-infectious or not due to a bacterial pathogen, e.g., HSV-1 VAP
• Increasing resistance to one or more antibiotics on one of the suggested antibiotic regimens	• Such patients should have a transbronchial, percutaneous, or open-lung biopsy to establish the cause of the non-resolving infiltrates
• Careful to avoid being misled into "chasing" or "covering" MDR GNB in respiratory secretions representing airway colonization	
• Since these organisms are not causes of NP/VAP, it makes no sense to add/change antibiotics	

As mentioned previously, unless an organism can be shown as pathologic by definite lung tissue and histologic diagnosis, isolates should be considered as colonizers and non-pathogens. Aerobic gram-negative bacilli that are common colonizers include *Enterobacter* sp., *Citrobacter* sp., *Flavobacterium* sp, and non-*P. aeruginosa* pseudomonads, i.e., *Burkholderia* (formerly *Pseudomonas*) *cepacia* and *Stenotrophomonas* (formerly *Pseudomonas*) *maltophilia*. *Burkholderia* sp. and *Stenotrophomonas* sp. are potentially pathogenic only in patients with extensive bronchiectasis or cystic fibrosis. In other patients, even in compromised hosts, these non-*P. aeruginosa* pseudomonads have not been proven to cause NPs [1,2,6,10]. The studies describing these organisms as causing NPs are based only on respiratory tract secretion cultures and are clinically invalid. If they are obtained from respiratory secretions of patients with presumed NP/VAP clinicians can dismiss these organisms from therapeutic consideration.

STAPHYLOCOCCUS AUREUS COLONIZATION OF RESPIRATORY SECRETIONS IN VENTILATED PATIENTS

As mentioned previously, among gram-positive organisms, *S. aureus* is a common colonizer of respiratory tract secretions in hospitalized patients. In contrast to CAP patients with influenza, *S. aureus* rarely, if ever, causes NP/VAP. Enterococci commonly colonize the skin and may also colonize respiratory tract secretions. Because enterococci are not NP pathogens, they can be dismissed as colonizers when cultured from respiratory tract secretions with presumed NP and not covered with empiric antimicrobial therapy [1,2,6].

STAPHYLOCOCCUS AUREUS IS NOT A NP/VAP PATHOGEN

Respiratory secretion cultures are not only unhelpful but are nearly always diagnostically misleading in potential NP/VAP patients. Soon after admission, the respiratory flora of a patient begins to change over a few days, and patients become colonized by the hospital's aerobic GNB within a week. If the GNB are aspirated, aspiration NP/VAP may result. Unlike with CAP, blood cultures are usually misleading in patients in establishing a specific microbiologic diagnosis with NP/VAP.

Care must be taken to dismiss blood culture results that are positive for non-NP/VAP pathogens, e.g., *S. aureus*, enterococci, or those from a distant source, e.g., GNB from a urinary source. In a patient with pulmonary infiltrates, fever, and leukocytosis, and *S. aureus* cultured from the respiratory secretions and/or blood cultures is not diagnostic of has *S. aureus* NP/VAP. *S. aureus* in blood cultures are often the result of specimen contamination during blood culture collection or may be related to a central venous catheter (CVC) infections.

Patients with *S. aureus* in their respiratory secretions and/or positive blood cultures without evidence of necrotizing

pneumonia on CXR or tissue biopsy do not have *bona fide S. aureus* NP/VAP. The diagnosis of *S. aureus* NP/VAP depends on the characteristic appearance of the CXR of rapidly necrotizing pneumonia with cavitation in <72 hours and not simply on the presence of *S. aureus* in respiratory secretions or blood cultures. Studies reporting *S. aureus* NP/VAP cases are based on distal airway colonization cultures and not pathologic lung findings or characteristic CXR appearances, and clinicians have been misled into considering *S. aureus* as a nosocomial pathogen. A rare cause of tissue biopsy-proven or autopsy-proven *S. aureus* CP/VAP while no uncommon cause of CAP in influenza patients is rarely, if ever, a *bona fide* cause of NP/VAP. Accordingly, unnecessary empiric *S. aureus* coverage has been unnecessarily included in empiric NP/VAP regimens for decades [2,6,11].

ANAEROBIC ORGANISMS ARE NON-PATHOGENS IN NP/VAP

Aspirated anaerobic organisms, along with the aerobic oral flora in hospitalized patients, are clinically but not therapeutically important in NPs. As in CAP aspiration pneumonia, aspirated oral anaerobes are susceptible to nearly all antibiotics used to treat pneumonias and are therapeutically unimportant in terms of antimicrobial therapy. Specific anti-anaerobic coverage, e.g., *Bacteroides Fragilis*, does not need to be included in community-acquired or NP therapeutic regimens. *Bacteroides fragilis*, the primary anaerobe below the diaphragm, requires specific anti-*B. fragilis* coverage. However, *B. fragilis* are the pathogens in community-acquired and nosocomial aspiration pneumonias [1,2,10].

THERAPEUTIC CONSIDERATIONS IN NP/VAP

APPROPRIATE EMPIRIC COVERAGE FOR *P. AERUGINOSA* AND GNB NP/VAP PATHOGENS

Appropriate empiric antimicrobial therapy is based on coverage of the usual/most likely infecting pathogens, i.e., oral anaerobes not at the infection site. Ideally, a specific diagnosis is desired in each patient, but practically, this is often not possible. Clinicians should ensure direct coverage against *P. aeruginosa* (which includes coverage against other aerobic GNB) in selecting appropriate antimicrobial therapy. It is as important to know what not to cover in empiric antibiotic therapy for NP/VAP. Even if cultured, the following organisms should not be specifically "covered" in the NP/VAP regimen, e.g., *Enterobacter* sp., *Proteus* sp., *Citobacter* sp., *Flavobacterium* sp., *Stenotrophomonas* sp., *Burkholderia* sp., *and Enterococcus* sp. Coverage should be primarily directed against *P. aeruginosa*, which also provide coverage against other aerobic GNB pulmonary pathogens, i.e., *E. coli, Klebsiella* sp., and *Serratia* sp. in patients being empirically treated for NP/VAP. The clinicians should not add antibiotics specifically to "cover" non-pathogenic NP/VAP organisms colonizing respiratory tract secretions, e.g., *Enterobacter* sp., *Stenotrophomonas* sp., and *Burkholderia* sp. [2,6,29,30].

INAPPROPRIATE UNNECESSARY OR EXCESSIVE EMPIRIC COVERAGE

Staphylococcus aureus

S. aureus coverage need not be included in empiric regimens for NP/VAP. In clinical NP trials comparing drugs with anti-*S. aureus* activity, e.g., cefepime, with those without anti-*S. aureus* activity (e.g., ceftazidime), the outcomes are the same. If *S. aureus* was a cause of NP, there would be a significant difference in outcomes between regimens with or without anti-*S. aureus* activity, but outcomes are identical. Similarly, excluding respiratory secretion/blood cultures there are no well-documented reports of MRSA NP with characteristic CXR findings, clinical presentation, or pathologic diagnosis [1,2,6,10].

Anti-*S. aureus* coverage, whether directed against methicillin-sensitive *S. aureus* (MSSA) or MRSA, should not be included in empiric antimicrobial regimens for NP/VAP. Antimicrobial therapy should not be changed or antistaphylococcal coverage added if MSSA or MRSA is recovered from respiratory secretions or peripheral blood cultures. *S. aureus* pneumonia, as mentioned previously, should be diagnosed only if accompanied by the characteristic appearance of necrotizing pneumonia with high spiking fevers, cyanosis, hypotension, and rapid cavitation within 72 hours on chest radiograph with or without elastin fibers in respiratory secretions, as seen with some influenza patients with CAP. The MSSA and MRSA blood cultures from a non-pulmonary source, e.g., intravenous lines, abscesses, or specimen collection contamination, should be appreciated as being unrelated to the patient's pulmonary infiltrates.

The antibiotics recommended for empiric monotherapy (e.g., cefepime and meropenem) have excellent activity against MSSA. Vancomycin should not be added empirically to a single-drug or double-drug regimen, because *S. aureus* is cultured from respiratory secretions or blood. Vancomycin predisposes to vancomycin-resistant *enterococci* (VRE). While a positive nasal swab for MRSA is indicative of airway colonization, a negative swab effectively rules out MSSA/MRSA NP/VAP. Furthermore, vancomycin is ineffective in eradicating MRSA colonization [1,2,6,30].

MONOTHERAPY VERSUS COMBINATION THERAPY

General Principles

Combination therapy is the traditional approach, but the optimal approach to treat NP/VAP is effective monotherapy. For aerobic GNB NP/VAP empiric combination regimens have not been streamlined to equally effective monotherapy regimens. In the past, combination therapy

was used because relative lack of activity of single agents active against *Klebsiella* sp. or *P. aeruginosa*. Clinicians treating *K. pneumoniae* used double-drug therapy because neither antibiotic had sufficient anti-*Klebsiella* activity to be effective alone. At present, antibiotics, e.g., third-generation cephalosporins, fluoroquinolones, and carbapenems have potent anti-*Klebsiella* sp. and anti-*P. aeruginosa* activity, permitting effective empiric monotherapy against *K. pneumoniae* or *P. aeruginosa*. Antibiotics available in past had some but not a high-level antipseudomonal activity, and double-drug therapy was the presumed necessity for empiric *P. aeruginosa* coverage. However, monotherapy is as comparable to combination therapy for empiric *P. aeruginosa* infections. However, for proven *P. aeruginosa* NP/VAP, double-drug therapy may be preferred [1,2,6,31] (Table 17.5).

EMPIRIC MONOTHERAPY ANTIBIOTICS

Antipseudomonal Cephalosporins

The antibiotics that best fulfill the criteria cited earlier include cefepime and meropenem. Cefepime is a fourth-generation cephalosporin and is given less often than ceftazidime, i.e., 2 g (IV) q12h and has not been associated with the emergence of resistant *P. aeruginosa*, as has ceftazidime. High-dose cefepime is also useful against ceftazidime-resistant *P. aeruginosa*. Furthermore, unlike ceftazidime, cefepime does not result in an increase in MRSA colonization. For all these reasons, when a cephalosporin is selected, cefepime is preferred over ceftazidime for empiric monotherapy of NP/VAP [1,2,6,31].

Antipseudomonal Penicillin

Piperacillin/tazobactam is an antipseudomonal penicillin that has been used for empiric monotherapy. However, the addition of tazobactam to piperacillin offers no increase in anti-*P. aeruginosa* activity for the treatment of NP. Piperacillin/tazobactam has only modest *P. aeruginosa* activity. If selected for NP/VAP, piperacillin/tazobactam should be used in "high dose", e.g., 4.5 g (IV) q6h, and given more frequently and furthermore should be used in combination with amikacin 1 g (IV) q24h [1,2,6,31].

Carbapenems

Among the carbapenems, meropenem is preferable to imipenem for empiric monotherapy of NP. Meropenem is highly active against *P. aeruginosa* and does not appreciably result in *P. aeruginosa* resistance. In contrast, imipenem has been associated with *P. aeruginosa* resistance. Imipenem, but not meropenem, may be associated with seizures. Seizures have been associated with high-dose imipenem therapy or its use in renal insufficiency, but imipenem-related seizures may also occur in patients receiving normal doses with normal renal function. Even when given in high doses. Seizures are not an adverse effect of even meningeal-dosed meropenem, e.g., 2 g (IV) q8h. The usual dose of meropenem is 1 g (IV) q8h [1,2,6,31].

COMBINATION THERAPY FOR PROVEN
P. AERUGINOSA NOSOCOMIAL PNEUMONIA

General Principles

If *P. aeruginosa* is the proven pathogen causing NP/VAP, combination therapy with two potent antipseudomonal agents is reasonable. The two antipseudomonal agents selected need not be synergistic but should not predispose to *P. aeruginosa* resistance. Several anti-*Pseudomonas* sp. "high resistance potential" antibiotics without a high degree of inherent activity should not be used in combination regimens because of their *P. aeruginosa* resistance potential. Antibiotics selected should not increase MRSA prevalence. Antibiotics that have problematic side effects should also be avoided. If these criteria are met, the clinician should opt for two antibiotics based on their anti-pseudomonal activity, safety profile, and "low resistance potential." Of these criteria, the use of two agents with the highest activity and low resistance potential is paramount importance in the CCU [1,2,10].

Antipseudomonal Agents for Combination Therapy

Ideal candidates for specific anti-*P. aeruginosa* combination therapy include cefepime and meropenem in combination with levofloxacin, aztreonam, or amikacin. Antibiotics that should not be avoided, if possible, in a combination regimen include ceftazidime, ciprofloxacin, imipenem, and gentamicin. It is a common clinical misconception that resistance can be prevented by using combination antibiotic therapy, but this is not the case. This is true for only a few antibiotics, e.g., TB therapy, but is not a general concept. For example, the addition of "high resistance potential" antibiotic of any anti-pseudomonal drug to a regimen containing ceftazidime, ciprofloxacin, imipenem, or gentamicin does not prevent the emergence of *P. aeruginosa* resistance. The only proven way to prevent the emergence of resistance in the CCU and in the hospital is at the formulary level, by eliminating or restricting from the formulary "high resistance potential" antibiotics that are known to be associated with resistance problems, i.e., ceftazidime, ciprofloxacin, and imipenem. Resistance problems can be minimized, and the clonal spread of resistant strains can be contained by effective infection-control measures [2,6,31].

Quinolones

Levofloxacin is a respiratory quinolone is active against *P. aeruginosa*. Levofloxacin has few side effects. Ciprofloxacin is associated with seizures and should not be used in patients with seizure disorders or central nervous system disorders. In contrast to ciprofloxacin, the use of levofloxacin has not been associated with resistance problems with respect to *S. pneumoniae*, *P. aeruginosa*, or other organisms. Levofloxacin does not predispose to MRSA colonization, as is the case with ciprofloxacin. Levofloxacin does not lower seizure potential or cause seizures vs. ciprofloxacin. If a fluoroquinolone is selected as part of a combination regimen against *P. aeruginosa*, levofloxacin is the preferred quinolone for this purpose [2,31].

Duration of Therapy

Usually, NP/VAP is treated for 2 weeks. If appropriate monotherapy is used, pulmonary infiltrates should be clearing but may not be gone totally during the 2-week treatment period. In such situations, an additional few days of antimicrobial therapy are reasonable, and 3 weeks of therapy are only rarely required. However, if there has been no change in the pulmonary infiltrates, on CXR, despite persistent low-grade fevers and leukocytosis after 2 weeks of appropriate therapy, the patient has, in all probability, a non-antibiotic responsive process caused by a virus or a non-infectious disease entity. Such patients should have a diagnostic procedure, e.g., transbronchial biopsy, percutaneous needle biopsy, or open lung biopsy, to diagnose the cause of the pulmonary infiltrates. Such patients should not receive prolonged courses of empiric antimicrobial therapy or undergo serial changes in antimicrobial therapy in the belief that the wrong spectrum was used or has been selected or the organism has become resistant [2,19].

Patients who have shown no improvement in pulmonary infiltrates and become "failure-to-wean" problems require a different approach. Such patients may also show cytopathogenic effect (CPE) diagnostic of BAL; cytology performed shows herpes simplex virus type 1 (HSV-1). In failure to wean patients with little or no infiltrates on CXR, HSV-1 NP/VAP is not an uncommon problem in the CCU. If HSV-1 CPEs are demonstrated in BAL specimens, the diagnosis of HSV-1 NP/VAP is confirmed. After 3–5 days of acyclovir, patient's pulmonary function is improved and weaning is easily achieved, confirming the diagnosis. Then, a 10-day course of acyclovir is indicated [31–35].

DIAGNOSTIC APPROACH TO PERSISTENT FEVERS, LEUKOCYTOSIS, AND PULMONARY INFILTRATES WHILE ON APPROPRIATE ANTIBIOTIC THERAPY

Persistent infiltrates on CXR or chest CT scan after 2 weeks of appropriate antibiotic therapy are usually due to a mimic of NP, e.g., CHF, or a viral etiology, e.g., HSV-1 VAP. The key determination for all CCU problems is correct diagnosis. If CHF is suggested by radiologic appearance (pulmonary vascular congestion, bilateral pleural effusions, and cardiomegaly) or highly elevated B-type natriuretic peptide (BNP) levels and/or response to diuretics, improvement of CXR infiltrates supports the diagnosis and eliminates the need for further diagnostic tests for NP, and, of course, there is no rationale to add or change antibiotic therapy.

Viral NPs occur but are rare. Infrequent, but not rare, is HSV-1 VAP. HSV-1 VAP presents as "failure to wean" in patients without pre-existing lung disease. Such patients are in the CCU for other reasons and then develop progressive hypoxemia that requires ventilator support. Paradoxically, these patients with normal/near normal appearing CXRs, cannot be weaned. A normal/near-normal CXR with an increased A-a gradient is the clue to the diagnosis. HSV-1 titers or airway vesicles/cultures are not diagnostic. Diagnostic bronchoscopy with BAL fluid cytology is needed for the diagnosis.

Interestingly, CMV, an important cause of viral CAP in normal and compromised hosts, does not cause VAP. If HSV CPEs are demonstrated on BAL cytology, acyclovir therapy results in rapid improvement in a few days and subsequent extubation. If bronchoscopy is not possible if the clinical scenario supports HSV-1, VAP empiric acyclovir is not unreasonable [2,31–35].

There are many causes of new or persistent fever/leukocytosis in the CCU. The most common causes for persistent fever/leukocytosis in the CCU are stress of being in the CCU, hemorrhage, steroids, or drug fever. Non-pulmonary infection /non-infectious disorders should also be considered, e.g., phlebitis, DVT, PE, MI, and pancreatitis (drug or TPN induced). Causes are virtually never urosepsis (without recent urologic instrumentation), even with or without pyuria/bacteriuria. *C. difficile* diarrhea may cause mild leukocytosis without fevers. In contrast, *C. difficile* colitis presents with new high fevers (>102°F) and prominent abdominal pain, often with sudden cessation if antecedent *C. difficile* water diarrhea. In all these scenarios, selecting appropriate therapy depends on accurate clinical syndromic diagnosis. The approach to persistent fever/leukocytosis should be directed at determining the cause, rather than adding or changing antibiotics [2,7,8].

ANTIBIOTIC STEWARDSHIP PROGRAM CONSIDERATIONS IN THE CCU: PREVENTING RESISTANCE AND TREATING COLONIZATION

Optimal antibiotic uses spearheaded by antibiotic stewardship programs (ASPs) are based on selecting appropriate monotherapy (based on predictable pathogens at the site of infection) for the shortest duration to cure the infection. The antibiotics selected should be optimally dosed for effectiveness. In addition, the antibiotic selected should have a "low resistance potential" as well as a "low *C. difficile* potential." Over the years, certain approaches have been tried and failed and have not been proven to be of any benefit, e.g., antibiotic cycling. Antibiotic cycling was purported to limit resistance in the CCU. Without understanding resistance determinants, i.e., the antibiotic resistance potential, simply rotating drugs of varying resistance potentials either worsens resistance or, if there was temporary improvement, vanishes quickly the next drug cycle. De-escalation, i.e., narrowing the spectrum, has no effect on reducing resistance [1,2,36–40].

In treating NP/VAP, de-escalation is often based on narrowing spectrum after respiratory secretion culture/BC data are available. Concept is flawed, but the results of respiratory secretion cultures are not reflective of distal lung pathology, and typically one or more "watery organisms" or *S. aureus* are cultured, and results are often misleading, i.e., colonization needlessly "covering" non-NP/VAP colonizing organisms.

Clinically, it is preferable to initially select well-chosen monotherapy, eliminating the need for polypharmacy and de-escalation. Unfortunately, covering non-NP/VAP organisms is the most common rationale for polypharmacy in the treating of NP/VAP. Unnecessary/excessive antibiotic coverage increases resistance potential, drug adverse effects, drug interactions, and *C. difficile* potential, not to mention unnecessary antibiotic costs. To complicate matters further, in "covering or chasing" *S. aureus* and or "water organisms" colonizing respiratory secretions in the CCU, is not superior to well chosen empiric monotherapy for NP/VAP. Importantly, such an approach does not eliminate the carriage of colonizing water organisms in respiratory secretions. Most antibiotics used to "cover" or "chase" aerobic GNB colonizers have a low V_d that approximates that of body water (V_d –0.5 kg/L). Such antibiotics cannot penetrate into respiratory secretions in sufficient concentration to eliminate organisms' colonization responsible for the respiratory secretions.

Examples of antibiotics commonly used to "treat" GNB colonizers, e.g., cefepime and ceftazidime, have a low V_d, predicting their failure to eliminate GNBs in respiratory secretions. Similarly, vancomycin with a low V_d does not eliminate MSSA/MRSA colonizing respiratory secretion in ventilated patients. Not only are MSSA/MRSA non-pathogens in NP/VAP, empiric vancomycin does not eliminate these organisms from the patient's respiratory secretions. Unlike patients with influenza and MSSA/MRSA CAP, there is no rationale to cover MSSA/MRSA in NP/VAP patients, as these organisms do not cause MSSA/MRSA NP/VAP [2].

SUMMARY

Many CCU patients with possible NP/VAP have new infiltrates on the CXR, fever, and leukocytosis resulting from a variety of non-infectious causes. Because of the high mortality and morbidity associated with NP/VAP, most clinicians treat possible NP/VAP with a 2-week course of empiric antibiotics. Before therapy is initiated, the clinician should rule out other causes of pulmonary infiltrates, fever, and leukocytosis that mimic nosocomial NP/VAP pneumonia, e.g., interstitial bronchogenic disease, primary or metastatic lung carcinomas, pulmonary emboli, pulmonary drug reactions, pulmonary hemorrhage, collagen vascular disease affecting the lungs, ARDS, and BOOP. If these disorders can be eliminated from further diagnostic consideration, then a week course of empiric monotherapy is reasonable. Coverage should be primarily directed against *P. aeruginosa* (not the most common cause of NP), the most virulent NP pulmonary pathogen. Coverage directed against *P. aeruginosa* will also be effective against all other aerobic GNB pathogens causing NP/VAP. The preferred antimicrobials for empiric monotherapy for NP are cefepime or meropenem. Anti-MRSA coverage is unnecessary, since *bona fide S. aureus* NP/VAP, at best, rare.

Selection of antibiotic therapy should not be based on respiratory secretion cultures. Lack of radiographic or clinical response after 2 weeks of appropriate empiric NP monotherapy suggests an alternate diagnosis. In such patients, a lung tissue biopsy diagnosis should be obtained to determine the cause of the persistence of pulmonary infiltrates unresponsive to appropriate antimicrobial therapy.

REFERENCES

1. Cunha BA. Nosocomial pneumonia. Diagnostic and therapeutic considerations. *Med Clin North Am* 2001;85:79–114.
2. Cunha BA. *Pneumonia Essentials* (3rd ed.). Sudbury, MA: Jones & Bartlett, 2010.
3. Koulenti D, Tsigou E, Rello J. Nosocomial pneumonia in 27 ICUs in Europe: Perspectives from the EU-VAP/CAP study. *Eur J Clin Microbiol Infect Dis* 2017;36:1999–2006.
4. Metersky ML, Kalil AC. New guidelines for nosocomial pneumonia. *Curr Opin Pulm Med* 2017;23:211–217.
5. Russell CD, Koch O, Laurenson IF, O'Shea DT, Sutherland R, Mackintosh CL. Diagnosis and features of hospital-acquired pneumonia: A retrospective cohort study. *J Hosp Infect* 2016;92:273–279.
6. Spalding MC, Cripps MW, Minshall CT. Ventilator-associated pneumonia: New definitions. *Crit Care Clin* 2017;33:277–292.
7. Cunha BA. Fever in the critical care unit. *Crit Care Clin* 1998;14:1–14.
8. Cunha BA. Fever in the intensive care unit. *Int Care Med* 1999;25:648–651.
9. DePascale G, Ranzani OT, Nseir S, Chastre J, Welte T, Antonelli M, et al. Intensive care unit patients with lower respiratory tract nosocomial infetions: The ENIRRIs project. *ERJ Open Res* 2017;3:92.
10. O'Horo JC, Kashyap R, Sevilla Berrios R, Herasevch V, Sampathkumar P. Differentiating infectious and noninfectious ventilator-associated complications: A new challenge. *Am J Infect Control* 2016;44:661–664.
11. Agarwal P, Wielandner A. Nosocomial pneumonia from a radiological perspective. *Radiology* 2017;57:13–21.
12. Cunha BA, Klimek JJ, Gracewski J, McLaughlin JC, Quintiliani R. A common source outbreak of Acinetobacter pulmonary infections traced to Wright respirometers. *Postgrad Med* 1980;56:169–172.
13. Pathmanathan A, Waterer GW. Significance of positive Stenotrophomonas maltophilia culture in acute respiratory tract infection. *Eur Respir J* 2005;25:911–914.
14. Razazi K, Mekontso Dessap A, Carteaux G, Jansen C, Decousser JW, de Prost N, Brun-Buisson C. Frequency associated factors and outcome of multidrug resistant intensive care unit acquired pneumonia among patients colonized with extended-spectrum β-lactamase producing enterobacteriaceae. *Ann Intensive Care* 2017;7:61.
15. Ristuccia PA, Cunha BA. Acinetobacter. *Infect Control* 1983;4:226–229.
16. Ristuccia PA, Cunha BA. Enterobacter. *Infect Control* 1985;6:124–128.
17. Scholte JB, Zhou TL, Bergmans DC, Rohde GG, Winkens B, et al. Stenotrophomonas maltophilia ventilator-associated pneumonia. A retrospective matched case-control study. *Infect Dis* 2016;48:738–743.
18. Garnacho-Montero J, Gutierrez-Pizarraya A, Lopez-Garcia I, et al. Pneumonia in mechanically ventilated patients: No diagnostic and prognostic value of different quantitive tracheal aspirates thresholds. *Infect Dis* 2017;4:1–8.
19. Scholze K, Wenke M, Schierholz R, et al. The reduction in antibiotic use in hospitals. *Stsch Arzt Int* 2015;112:714–721.
20. Kwa Al, Low JG, Lee E, Kurup A, Chee HL, Tam VH. The impact of multidrug resistance on the outcomes of critically ill patients with Gram-negative bacterial pneumonia. *Diag Microbiol Infect Dis* 2007;58:99–104.
21. Prince SE, Dominger KA, Cunha BA, Klein NC. Klebsiella pneumoniae pneumonia. *Heart Lung* 1997;26:413–417.
22. Ristuccia PA, Cunha BA. Klebsiella. *Infect Control* 1984;5:343–347.
23. Guyot A, Turton JF, Garner D. Outbreak of Stenotrophomonas maltophilia on an intensive care unit. *J Hosp Infect* 2013;85:303–307.
24. Cawcutt K, Kalil AC. Pneumonia with bacterial and viral coinfection. *Curr Opin Crit Care* 2017;23:385–390.
25. Cunha BA, Thekkel V, Schoch PE. Community-acquired versus nosocomial Legionella pneumonia: Lessons learned from an epidemiologic investigation. *Am J Infect Control* 2011;39:901–903.
26. Agarwal S, Abell V, File TM Jr. Nosocomial (Health Care-Associated) Legionnaire's disease. *Infect Dis Clin North Am* 2017;31:155–165.
27. Cunha BA, Burillo A, Bouza E. Legionnaire's disease. *Lancet* 2016;387:376–385.
28. Cunha BA, Cunha CB. Legionnaire's disease and its mimics: A Clinical perspective. *Infect Dis Clin* 2017;31:95–109.
29. Cunha BA. Antibiotic selection is crucial for optimal empiric monotherapy of ventilator-associated pneumonia. *Crit Care Med* 2007;35:1992–1994.
30. Cunha BA. Ventilator-associated pneumonia: Monotherapy is optimal if chosen wisely. *Crit Care* 2006;10:141.
31. Vacas-Cordoba M, Cardozo-Espinola C, Puerta-Alcalde P, Cilloniz C, Torres A, Garcia-Vidal C. Empirical treatment of adults and hospital acquired pneumonia: Lights and shadows of the 2016 Clinical Practice ATS/IDSA Guidelines. *Rev Esp Quimioter* 2017;1:30–33.
32. Mohan S, Hamid NS, Cunha BA. A cluster of nosocomial herpes simplex virus type 1 pneumonia in a medical intensive care unit. *Infect Control Hosp Epidemiol* 2006;27:1255–1257.
33. Cunha BA, Eisenstein LE, Dillard T, Krol V. Herpes simplex virus (HSV) pneumonia in a heart transplant: Diagnosis and therapy. *Heart Lung* 2007;36:72–78.
34. Salluh JIF, Souza-Dantas VC, Povoa P. The current status of biomarkers for the diagnosis of nosocomial pneumonia. *Curr Opin Crit Care* 2017;23:391–397.
35. Cunha BA, Strollo S, Durie N. Cytomegalovirus reactivation in the intensive care unit: Not a cause of late-onset ventilator-associated pneumonia. *Crit Care Med* 2010;38:341–342.
36. Cunha BA. Strategies to control antibiotic resistance. *Semin Respir Infect* 2002;17:250–258.
37. Cunha BA., Baron J, Cunha CB. Once daily high dose tigecycline-pharmacokinetic/pharmacodynamics based dosing for optimal clinical effectiveness: Dosing matters, revisited. *Expert Rev Anti Infect Ther* 2017;15:257–267.
38. Ismail B, Shafei MN, Harun A, Ali S, Omar M, Deris ZZ. Predictors of polymyxin B treatment failure in Gram-negative healthcare-associated infections among critically ill patients. *J Microbiol Immunol Infect* 2017;17:30113–30115.
39. Cunha BA. Effective antibiotic resistance control strategies. *Lancet* 2001;357:1307–1308.
40. Cunha CB, Cunha BA. (Eds.). *Antibiotic Essentials* (17th ed.). New Delhi, India: Jay Pee Medical Publisher, 2020.

18 Central Venous Catheter Infection in the Critical Care Unit

Emilio Bouza and Almudena Burillo

CONTENTS

Critically ill patients in intensive care units are susceptible to many complications. One of the most serious is central venous catheter (CVC)-related bloodstream infection (CR-BSI).

The use of vascular catheters may give rise to local or systemic infections, such as uncomplicated or complicated bacteremia. Complications of bacteremia include septic thromboembolism, endocarditis, pulmonary or cerebral abscesses, osteomyelitis, or endophthalmitis.

The CR-BSIs show substantial morbidity and non-negligible mortality and are the most frequent reason for catheter withdrawal [1,2]. This has prompted numerous ongoing efforts to reduce the incidence of CR-BSI.

Several excellent reviews have been recently conducted on this topic [3–6]. In this chapter, we review the most important aspects of the diagnosis, management, and prevention of CR-BSIs in patients admitted to critical care units (CCUs).

DEFINITIONS, EPIDEMIOLOGY OF CR-BSI IN CCU PATIENTS, THE EXTENT OF THE PROBLEM

DEFINITIONS

A bloodstream infection (BSI) is diagnosed when a microbial pathogen is recovered from a patient with a clinical infectious syndrome and positive blood culture results (contaminants excluded).

The term CR-BSI is used when the cause of a BSI is an intravascular catheter, as determined through a quantitative culture of the catheter tip or when growth results (time to positivity) obtained in catheter versus peripheral venipuncture blood culture samples are separated long enough (see Diagnosis section).

A CVC is defined as a catheter whose tip is in a central vein. A peripherally inserted central catheter is also a CVC.

A long-term CVC is a catheter anticipated to remain in place for a long (usually >20 days) or indefinite period. These catheters are generally subcutaneously tunneled between the percutaneous exit and vein entry sites or may be fully implanted with a rubber-surfaced subcutaneous chamber that is accessed by a needle.

A short-term CVC is for temporary use and is neither subcutaneously tunneled, nor implanted.

A central line-associated BSI (CLABSI) is defined as a BSI detected in the presence of a CVC or within 48 hours of its removal. The CLABSI cannot be attributed to an infection unrelated to the catheter and have been defined for the *surveillance* of healthcare-associated infection by the National Healthcare Safety Network (NHSN) [7]. This definition is sensitive but relatively unspecific, as it overestimates the true infection incidence and is subjective when determining the infection source.

For purposes of surveillance, a *central-line day* is defined as that experienced by one patient in a healthcare facility with one or more indwelling CVC at a one-time point during a 24-hour period.

EPIDEMIOLOGY

The CR-BSIs are among the most frequent hospital-acquired infections and, in a large proportion, are detected in CCU patients [2,8].

Between 15% and 30% of all hospital-acquired BSIs are related to the use of a percutaneous catheter. Estimates for the United States run at 250,000 episodes over the year

2002, with an associated mortality of 12%–25% (over 30,000 deaths) and an added cost of 3,000–56,167 US dollars for each episode [9,10].

The incidence of CR-BSI varies according to catheter type, the frequency of its use, host underlying disease, and hospitalization ward but mainly depends on the quality of care. Estimates by the National Healthcare Safety Network for the year 2011 range from one episode (in cardiothoracic, medical, surgical, neurosurgical, and surgical CCU) to close to four episodes in burned patients in a CCU for every 1000 days of CVC use [1,11].

According to data collected by Pronovost et al. during the implementation of a prevention bundle, the incidence of infections fell from 2.7 (0.6–4.8) to 1.6 (0–4.4) episodes (median, interquartile range [IQR]) per 1000 catheter-days over 2004–2005 in adult CCUs in Michigan.

Data from 984 adult CCUs in 632 US hospitals indicate that the mean CLABSI rate in 2011 was 0.96 per 1000 central line days (SD, 1.29) [12].

In a recent European study, based on data from 14 CCUs in 11 countries, it was shown that a preventive strategy could decrease CR-BSI from 2.4/1000 to 0.9/1000 CVC-days [13].

In the US CCU patients, CLABSI prevention was associated with estimated net economic benefits for the period 1990–2008, ranging from $640 million to $1.8 billion and corresponding net gains per case from $15,780 to $24,391 [14].

The impact of this problem has also been recently documented in non-CCU patients and linked to other catheter types, such as peripheral venous catheters (PVC) and peripherally inserted CVC (PICC), both widely used outside the CCU settings [15–18].

These data are summarized in Table 18.1.

TABLE 18.1
Frequency of Catheter-Related Bloodstream Infections in Adult CCU Patients

Country	Period	Setting	Frequency	Comments	References
Belgium (Ghent University Hospital)	Jan 1992–Dec 2002	CCU patients	1 episode/1000 cath-days	36,383 admissions Attributable mortality: 1.8% (95% CI −6.4%; −10.0%)	[9]
United States	2002	Entire hospital population (CCU and in-patients)	250,000 episodes	Attributable mortality 12%–25% Cost per episode $25,000 ($30,000–$56,000)	[19,20]
United States	March 2004–Sep 2005	All CCU in Michigan (Keystone project)	Decrease in median 2.7 to 1.6 episodes/1000 cath-days during study	103 CCUs 1981 CCU-months and 375,757 cath-days NNISS definition	[21]
United States	2001–2009	2001–2009	2001: 43,000 CLABSI 2009: 18,000 CLABSI 58% reduction	6000 lives saved $1.8 billion in cumulative excess healthcare costs since 2001	[22]
United States	2011	CCU patients	Cardiac: 1.1 Cardiothoracic: 0.8 Medical: 1.2 Surgical: 0.9 Neurosurgical: 1.0 Surgical: 1.2 Burn: 3.7 (episodes/1000 cath-days)	3854 hospitals in 53 states belonging to the National Healthcare Safety Network	[11]
United States	2011	984 adult CCUs in 632 hospitals	Mean 0.96 (SD, 1.29)/1000 central-line-days	CLABSI episodes	[12]
Europe	Jan 2011–June 2013	14 hospitals in 11 European countries	Fall from 2.4 to 0.9 episodes/1000 cath-days	25,348 patients with 35,831 CVCs Preventive strategy implanted	[13]
United States	March 2004–Dec 2013	All CCU in Michigan (Keystone project)	Fall in mean 2.5 episodes/1000 cath-days in 2004 to 0.76 in 2013	Double the percentage of CCUs with a mean rate of <1 infection/1000 cath-days in 2013, compared with baseline	[23]
Worldwide	Studies published between Jan 1990 and June 2015	A systematic review and meta-analysis	Median CLABSI incidence: 5.7/1000 cath-days in adult CCU	96 articles, 60 in adult CCU patients After prevention bundle implementation, median CLABSI incidence: 2.6/1000 cath-days for all types of CCU	[24]

Abbreviations: CCU, critical care unit; CI, confidence interval; CVC, central venous catheter; cath-days, catheter-days; CLABSI, central line-associated bloodstream infection (see text for explanation).

DIAGNOSIS WITHOUT CATHETER REMOVAL

To make a definite diagnosis of CR-BSI, the catheter has to be implicated as the microbiological source of BSI.

There are two main diagnostic approaches, depending on whether the catheter is removed or left in place [10]. As the positive predictive value of all tests increases significantly with high pre-test clinical probability, rather than performing routine cultures, these should be reserved for when there is clinical suspicion of CR-BSI.

Catheter removal because of clinical suspicion of CR-BSI turns out to be unnecessary in over 70% of cases (i.e., the catheter is sterile) [25]. This is important, as CVC removal will limit vascular access [26], and CR-BSI can often be empirically managed without immediate catheter withdrawal [27,28]. In sections "Paired quantitative cultures, Differential time to positivity and Superficial cultures" we comment on diagnostic procedures not requiring catheter removal.

Conservative methods of diagnosing CR-BSI include superficial cultures (semiquantitative cultures of skin around entry point and catheter hubs), differential paired quantitative blood cultures (comparing colony counts in blood obtained from peripheral veins and catheter hubs), and, more recently, differential time to positivity (DTP). For this last method, time to positivity is compared in blood cultures obtained simultaneously from peripheral veins versus catheter hubs [29–31].

PAIRED QUANTITATIVE CULTURES (CENTRAL AND PERIPHERAL)

To improve the sensitivity of the hub-blood culture, a simultaneous peripheral blood culture sample is obtained and microbial counts compared. When a CR-BSI is present, bacterial overload is observed in the central blood culture. Wing et al. first used differential quantitative blood cultures (in 1979) in a patient with suspected CR-BSI with a permanent indwelling hyperalimentation catheter [32]. Thus, while blood from the peripheral vein showed 25 colonies/mL, blood drawn through the hub displayed more than 10,000 colonies/mL. On CVC catheter removal, it was noted that the tip was infected with the same microorganisms present in the blood.

The CR-BSI is diagnosed when a significantly different colony count of >3:1 is observed for the CVC versus peripheral vein culture. This result has a sensitivity of about 80% and specificity of 90%–100% [26,33].

DIFFERENTIAL TIME TO POSITIVITY

In clinical practice, the time until blood cultures turn positive is measured using automatic devices. In an *in vitro* study, a linear relationship was observed between starting concentrations of various microorganisms and time to culture positivity [34]. The larger the inoculum, the faster a cutoff linked to the metabolic growth and the numbers of microorganisms initially present in the bottle is reached [34]. Using continuous-monitoring blood culture systems, a similar relationship was detected for the diagnosis of CR-BSI due to CNS coagulase-negative

staphylococcus; on average, 1.5 additional hours to positivity were needed for each tenfold increase in concentration [35]. For an accurate interpretation of DTP, a rigorous method is mandatory. The DTP should be calculated before antibiotic administration. The first milliliters of blood drawn through the catheter should be used for culture, and only aerobic bottles are needed [36]. When the catheter has several lumens, blood should be drawn from all lumens [37–39]. A DTP >120 min is highly predictive of CR-BSI [40]. The DTP test shows a sensitivity of 94%, specificity of 89%–91%, positive predictive value of 85%–88%, and negative predictive value of 89%–95%, depending on the type of catheter (short- vs. long-term) and patient [35,41]. It is not a valid diagnostic test for catheter-related candidemia because of the long time needed for blood cultures to become positive [42], and the method seems to perform poorly for most *Candida* spp. [43,44].

SUPERFICIAL CULTURES (COMBINED EXIT-SITE AND HUB CULTURES)

Exit-site cultures mainly give an idea of the extraluminal contamination route, which is predominant for short-term catheters. This diagnostic technique was first proposed by Bjornson et al. in 1982 in patients receiving total parenteral nutrition [45]. These authors noted that the growth of more than 1000 organisms at the catheter entry site was significantly associated with CR-BSI. Catheter hub cultures mostly reflect the endoluminal contamination route as the primary infection route of long-term catheters, such as those used for total parenteral nutrition or in cancer patients [46]. Omitting to test one or more lumens has been linked to failure to detect as many as 37% of colonized lumens [37–39]. The positivity threshold for collected swabs is 15 colony-forming units (CFU) per plate. Gram staining of skin and hub swabs may also be helpful for rapid diagnosis of CR-BSI [47].

Superficial, or "targeted," cultures are only indicated when CR-BSI is suspected. The high sensitivity and high negative predictive values of these cultures mean that they are useful for ruling out CR-BSI [29].

In an article by Bouza et al., superficial cultures, paired quantitative blood cultures, and DTP for a diagnosis of CR-BSI without catheter removal were compared prospectively [48]. The DTP showed a higher sensitivity and negative predictive value for predicting catheter tip colonization than quantitative blood cultures (96.4% and 99.4% vs. 71.4% and 95.6%, respectively). All three tests yielded high negative predictive values. This determined that when a negative result was obtained in any test, catheter colonization and CR-BSI could be reasonably ruled out. The authors claimed that because of their simplicity and low cost, semiquantitative superficial cultures (both catheter exit-site and hubs) and peripheral-vein blood cultures combined could serve to screen for CR-BSI, and differential quantitative blood cultures reserved to confirm results. It is essential that superficial cultures are always accompanied by peripheral blood cultures [4].

VALUE OF A COLONIZED CATHETER TIP WITH CONCOMITANT NEGATIVE BLOOD CULTURE RESULT

In the 2001 guidelines of the Infectious Diseases Society of America (IDSA) on the management of CR-BSI, it was recommended not to treat patients returning a positive tip culture accompanied by a negative blood culture, unless the tip was positive for S. aureus or Candida spp., especially in febrile patients with valvular heart disease or patients with neutropenia (absolute neutrophil count <1000 cells/mL). These microorganisms are more likely to give rise to CR-BSI and its complications than enterococci or gram-negative bacilli [49]. Close follow-up for signs of infection and even a short course of antibiotic therapy (5–7 days) were recommended.

Since then, new data have emerged on the outcome of patients with positive tip cultures and concomitant negative blood cultures.

Two retrospective studies concluded that an intravascular catheter colonized by S. aureus was a strong predictor of later CR-BSI by this microorganism. Antibiotic treatment initiated within 24 hours of catheter removal significantly reduced the risk of subsequent S. aureus bacteremia (SAB) [50,51]. This was confirmed in a later study examining data from patients acquired over the period 2003–2008 [52]. In a meta-analysis of their data and of data from three previous studies, the authors concluded that antibiotic therapy led to an absolute risk reduction of 13.6% for subsequent bacteremia by S. aureus. The number needed to treat to prevent one episode of BSI was 7.4 patients. Hence, early initiation of antibiotic therapy for catheters colonized by S. aureus prevented subsequent bacteremia.

In the 2009 IDSA guidelines, it was therefore recommended to treat patients with tip cultures positive for S. aureus [49].

In a similar retrospective study, a lower incidence of SAB after removal of a colonized catheter was found in patients given early antibiotic treatment (13% vs. 4%) (OR 4.2, 95% CI = 1.1–15, 6) [52]. This study also included a meta-analysis of other four retrospective studies, which yielded an OR of 5.8 (95% CI: 2.6–13.2) for SAB when antibiotic therapy was not initiated [52].

Our group has also examined this issue. Patients returning a positive catheter tip culture result for methicillin-resistant S. aureus had a 4.1% risk of developing a late CR-BSI episode, also associated with a higher crude mortality rate [53]. Accordingly, we would also recommend therapy in this situation.

In another retrospective study examining Candida spp. tip colonization (2003–2007), we noted an incidence of subsequent candidemia of only 1.7%. Further, in this context, multivariate analysis of risk factors for a poor prognosis showed that antifungal therapy was not protective (OR = 0.82; 95%: 0.27–2.47) [54]. This conclusion was also reported by López-Medrano et al. [55]. These authors found that, in patients with a catheter tip colonized with Candida spp., the incidence of a later candidemia was 2.5% and that antifungals were not protective in over half (55%) of patients. They also noted that

the potential benefits of preemptive treatment (with a number necessary to treat to prevent 1 episode of Candida-related complication estimated at 36) were scarce, and they therefore only recommended a close patient follow-up.

In a study by Park et al., the risk of infectious complications after catheter removal was higher when the tip was colonized by Candida spp. (7.7%) than by bacteria (1.8%). Consequently, these authors recommended antifungal therapy for all patients with positive catheter tip cultures and negative blood cultures [56].

The 2018 Optimal Practices for the Management of CR-BSI in CCU Patients, issued by a panel of world experts, include recommendations for the management of tip colonization by other microorganisms [3]. It is not clear that a similar anticipative treatment is required for other microorganisms.

In summary, the decision to treat a patient in whom the catheter tip is colonized must be individualized. In patients with a tip positive for S. aureus and in those in septic shock with no other obvious explanation for their clinical picture, antimicrobial therapy is justified.

It should be mentioned that catheter tips should not be routinely sent for culture; this is necessary only if there is clinical suspicion of infection [57].

EMPIRICAL ANTIBIOTIC TREATMENT

The antimicrobial treatment of systemic CR-BSI should be based on identifying the etiologic agent in blood cultures and antimicrobial susceptibility testing. Patient characteristics must always be taken into account. If the CCU patient is not stable, empirical antibiotic treatment should be given, covering both the gram-positive and gram-negative organisms that most often cause these infections. The predominant hospital or unit flora and knowledge of previous colonization by multi-resistant microorganisms may condition the choice of empirical therapy.

General considerations include source control, namely catheter removal (which depends on the pathogen and catheter type) and the intravenous administration of a rapid bactericidal agent [3]. Recent guidelines on the management of these infections in critically ill patients do not either recommend the use of lock therapy (instilling high concentrations of antibiotics into the catheter lumen for extended periods as a valid option for both prevention and treatment of CR-BSI) or attempts to salvage the catheter [3].

As a universal rule, a glycopeptide (vancomycin, 15 mg/kg every 12 h) or lipopeptide (daptomycin, 10 mg/kg every 24 h) is recommended to cover gram-positive organisms, together with a fourth-generation cephalosporin, carbapenem, or beta-lactam/beta-lactamase inhibitor, with or without an aminoglycoside to cover gram-negative microorganisms.

Risk factors for infection with gram-positive microorganisms are cirrhosis, diabetes mellitus, and previous quinolones [4].

Risk factors for infection with a gram-negative bacillus include the existence of an outbreak (of CR-BSI), spinal cord injury, femoral location of the catheter, hematological malignancy with neutropenia, previous colonization of the gastrointestinal tract with multi-resistant gram-negative bacilli, prolonged CCU stay, postoperative status, and diabetes mellitus [4].

Empirical antifungals for *Candida* spp. should only be administered in exceptional circumstances, including severe sepsis or septic shock in a critical patient with previous multiple colonized sites, or in patients with hematological malignancies and associated neutropenia. Other risk factors to be considered for empirical antifungal treatment include femoral catheter location, solid tumors, total parenteral nutrition, and long-standing therapy with anti-anaerobic agents or broad-spectrum antibiotics [3,4].

It should be kept in mind that, when designating the duration of antimicrobial therapy, day 1 is the first day on which negative blood culture results are obtained [49].

Local infections that are not accompanied by systemic symptoms in patients not under immunosuppression should be treated with topical antimicrobials based on exit site culture results after catheter removal [49]. In immunosuppressed patients, if the infection does not resolve or if a purulent exudate appears, antimicrobial therapy should be similar to that for systemic infections.

Catheter removal is mandatory in patients with severe sepsis, hemodynamic instability, endocarditis or evidence of metastatic infection, erythema of the insertion site, or local exudate due to suppurative thrombophlebitis. The catheter should also be removed if bacteremia persists after 72 h of antimicrobial therapy to which the isolated pathogen from blood cultures is susceptible. Further, if the isolated pathogen is *S. aureus* or another difficult-to-eradicate microorganism such as *Bacillus* spp., *Candida* spp., and mycobacteria, the catheter should also be removed (Table 18.2). To maintain a catheter, *all* the requirements included in Table 18.3 must be fulfilled.

TABLE 18.2
Criteria for Catheter Removal (Any of the Following)

Easily replaceable catheter

Hemodynamic instability

Severe sepsis

Bacteremia that persists despite >72 hours of effective antibiotics

Endocarditis, or evidence of metastatic infection

Erythema of the insertion site or local exudate due to suppurative thrombophlebitis

CR-BSI caused by *Staphylococcus aureus*, *Pseudomonas aeruginosa*, enterococci, fungi, or mycobacteria[a]

Source: Mermel, L.A. et al. *Clin. Infect. Dis.*, 49, 1–45, 2009.

Abbreviations: CR-BSI, catheter-related bloodstream infection.

[a] Unless there are unusual extenuating circumstances (e.g., no alternative catheter insertion site); with a persisting catheter, antibiotic lock therapy should also be prescribed during this same period (see Targeted Antibiotic Therapy section).

TABLE 18.3
Criteria for Catheter Maintenance (All of the Following)

Difficult-to-replace catheter

No signs of tunnel infection

Sterile blood cultures within 72 h of the initiation of appropriate antibiotic treatment

No signs of endocarditis, embolism or metastatic infection

Microorganisms that may be treated with both lock therapy and systemic antibiotics without catheter removal

Hemodynamic stability

Source: Mermel, L.A. et al. *Clin. Infect. Dis.*, 49, 1–45, 2009.

TARGETED ANTIBIOTIC THERAPY

COAGULASE-NEGATIVE SPECIES OF *STAPHYLOCOCCI*

Coagulase-negative *staphylococci* are the most common cause of CR-BSI.

Vancomycin is the drug of choice. Alternative drugs are teicoplanin and daptomycin. In immunocompetent patients without prosthetic materials other than the catheter, catheter withdrawal leads to cure rates close to 100%, even in the absence of systemic antimicrobial treatment. Catheter removal is always recommended to avoid the recurrence of the BSI, and systemic antibiotics should be administered for periods probably not inferior to 3–5 days to cover for these microorganisms [4].

If the catheter is maintained or if inflammatory markers persist after catheter withdrawal, antibiotic therapy should be extended to 10–14 days. If the catheter is maintained in place, antibiotic lock therapy should also be prescribed during this same period.

In the case of immunosuppression, neutropenia, or patients with orthopedic prostheses, systemic antibiotic therapy is always recommended, even after the vascular catheter has been removed.

It should be noted that the coagulase-negative *S. lugdunensis* behaves very much like *S. aureus* (it can also cause endocarditis and metastatic infections), and treatment for this microorganism should always be administered for at least 14 days.

Staphylococcus aureus

In patients with a CR-BSI due to *S. aureus*, catheter withdrawal is mandatory.

The choice of systemic antibiotics depends on the susceptibility of the microorganism and whether the patient is allergic or not to beta-lactams.

For methicillin-susceptible strains, cloxacillin (2 g IV every 4 h) or cefazolin (1–2 g IV every 8 h) are the drugs of choice. In infections caused by methicillin-resistant *S. aureus* (MRSA) or in patients allergic to beta-lactams, therapy can be vancomycin or daptomycin.

Intravenous antibiotics must be administered for 14 days. In cases of metastatic complications, intravenous therapy should be extended to 4–6 weeks.

It is recommended to perform control blood cultures at 72 h for *all* patients with SAB since up to half (54%) of those without fever have persistent bacteremia [58].

It should be considered that *S. aureus* is the most frequent causative agent of BSI. *S. aureus* is the cause of 23% of all BSI episodes [59]; 54% of nosocomial BSI, 18% of non-nosocomial health-care related BSI and 26% of CA-BSI [60]. Further, 6% to 26% of all CR-BSI episodes are caused by *S. aureus* [60–62,64].

The frequency of infective endocarditis (IE) in patients with SAB is not negligible. The rate varies, depending on whether a TEE is performed at the time of diagnosis of the BSI, or during follow-up [63]. In CA-SAB, up to 21% of patients are present with IE [60]. When SAB is hospital-acquired, the frequency of IE is 4%–9% [60,62]. In patients with nosocomial and health-care related SAB, IE is present in up to 18%–39% [61].

Recent guidelines recommend a transesophageal echocardiogram (TEE) in all patients with *S. aureus* bacteremia (SAB) [4]. However, some authors limit this test to patients with valvular heart disease, a prosthetic material, injection drug use, or when the CR-SAB persists after catheter removal and adequate antibiotic therapy [64]. In the case of a negative TEE with persistent positive blood cultures 72 h later, suppurative thrombophlebitis of the veins where the catheter was inserted, or another source of intravascular infection need to be ruled out by radiographic testing.

In the 2018 Spanish guidelines, in patients with SAB, echocardiography is recommended in the following situations: prolonged BSI, catheter used for hemodialysis, community-acquired BSI (CA-BSI), metastatic foci of infection, injection drug abuse, permanent CVC, intracardiac device, cardiac structural abnormality or previous infective endocarditis [4].

Since TEE is not always available, it can lead to complications, and is an expensive diagnostic tool, some studies have identified the risk factors for IE to preselect patients for TEE.

Patients with SAB and a *low-risk* of IE are as follows:

1. Those with a known SAB focus
2. Those without the classical risk factors for IE by *S. aureus* (see later)
3. Those in whom SAB clears within 72 hours of the start of the antibiotic treatment

Patients with SAB and a *high-risk* of IE are as follows [61,64]:

1. Those with CA-BSI
2. Those with intravenous drug abuse
3. Those in which SAB persists 72 hours after the start of appropriate antibiotic treatment and catheter removal (which should be as soon as possible)
4. Those with permanent intracardiac devices (prosthetic heart valve, pacemaker, cardioverter-defibrillator, or vascular graft)

5. Cardiac transplant patients
6. Those with congenital heart disease
7. Those with a ventriculoatrial shunt
8. Those with a previous IE episode
9. Those on hemodialysis
10. Those with spinal infection
11. Those with non-vertebral osteomyelitis

In a retrospective chart review study (N = 678), Palraj et al. designed a score ("PREDICT") to guide the use of TEE in patients with SAB [65]. The TEE was performed in the first 2 weeks of SAB onset and at week 12 in 68% and 71% of patients, respectively. The authors proposed a two-stage screening strategy, which combines the predictive values of risk scores for days 1 (21% sensitivity, 96% specificity, 89% negative predictive value) and 5 (99% sensitivity and 98.5% negative predictive value). Using this strategy to select candidates for TEE, only three IE episodes would have been missed in their cohort of 678 patients. The authors concluded that this is a simple score that uses the type of SAB (onset), the presence of a cardiovascular implantable electronic device, and duration of BSI to guide the optimal use of TEE. Based on high-risk factors, or PREDICT score, the number of TEE indications can be reduced by one-third. The preselection of patients who undergo TEE based on the presence of these risk factors leads to underdiagnosis of IE in only 0.5% of patients [65, Soriano, 2011 # 572].

Notably, TEE should also be performed when there is high clinical suspicion of IE, regardless of the existence or not of risk factors, when SAB recurs or relapses, or in cases of an abnormal TEE. International societies recommended a repeat TEE after 5–7 days in patients with a high suspicion of IE if the initial examination was negative [66,67].

It is also important to remember that up to 40% of patients with SAB and IE have no risk factors [60].

The CR-BSIs caused by *S. lugdunensis* must be managed in the same way as CR-SAB.

Enterococcus spp.

The mainstay treatment of enterococcal CR-BSI (ECR-BSI) with proven absence of IE is, in our opinion, monotherapy with ampicillin if the strain is susceptible [4]. This absence would be suggested by a NOVA score <4 (see later). If the strain is ampicillin resistant, then vancomycin is the second choice. If strains are both ampicillin- and vancomycin-resistant, linezolid or daptomycin can be used, depending on the susceptibility profile. The role of combination therapy has yet to be established.

Given the importance of BSI duration as a risk factor for IE due to any microorganism, including *enterococci* [68,69], control blood cultures are recommended 72 h after the start of antibacterial therapy.

Enterococci are a common cause of BSI [1]. They are currently the fourth leading cause of CR-BSI and represent 4%–6% of all CR-BSI at our hospital [68,70]; 76% of these catheters were CVC. Further, ECR-BSI was present in 23% of cases of a catheter tip colonized with *Enterococcus* spp. From

January 2003–December 2010, the incidence of ECR-BSI due to *E. faecalis* increased annually by 20%. Most episodes were caused by *E. faecalis* (85%), and 19% of all episodes were polymicrobial. IE was present in 4% of ECR-BSI.

Enterococcal endocarditis represents 10% of all cases of IE [71,72].

Given the recent rise in BSI due to enterococci, our group tried to identify patients with ECR-BSI with a low risk of IE to obviate the need for costly and time-consuming TEE. Over the period of September 2003 to October 2012, we performed a prospective cohort study (all patients with E-BSI) and a case-control study (patients with/without enterococcal IE) at our center. We developed a score for enterococcal IE designated NOVA based on the variables: Number of positive blood cultures (3/3 blood cultures or the majority >3, 5 points; unknown Origin of bacteremia, 4 points; prior heart Valve disease, 2 points; and Auscultation of a heart murmur, 1 point. A score <4 points suggested a low risk of enterococcal IE. Our score showed a sensitivity of 100% and a specificity of 35%, and the number needed to screen to find a case of IE was 7. This score was later validated by a Danish group [72].

In summary, as in the case of CR-SAB, *E. faecalis* CR-BSI requires a thorough investigation to search for complicated infection [3].

Nonetheless, it should be borne in mind that scores are created to *assist* clinical judgment and never to replace it.

GRAM-NEGATIVE BACILLI

In the majority of published series, CR-BSIs caused by these pathogens require catheter removal for a definitive cure. Catheter maintenance has been linked to high recurrence rates, even after a prolonged course of systemic antibiotics. The antibiotics administered should be those to which the microorganism is susceptible *in vitro*. Cephalosporins, with or without beta-lactamase inhibitors, monobactams, carbapenems, or aminoglycosides, are the most widely used antimicrobials.

The duration of therapy should be of a minimum of 7 days [4] or, preferably, of 14 days [3].

If catheter maintenance is attempted, systemic therapy should be accompanied by antibiotic lock therapy, and antibiotics should be extended to 10–14 days [4]. In these patients, echocardiography is not mandatory [4]. The TEE is, however, required in patients with valvular heart disease and persistent BSI despite adequate therapy.

Candida Species

In patients with a catheter-related *Candida* infection, catheter removal is mandatory.

Antifungals should be continued for fourteen days after the first negative blood culture. The choice of drug depends on the clinical situation of the patient, previous azole use, and whether the patient is colonized by an azole-resistant species. In severely immunosuppressed patients, an echinocandin is recommended. In these cases, an ophthalmologic exam should be negative for the fungus, since these molecules do not cross the blood-brain barrier.

Targeted therapy will be later adjusted based on species identification and susceptibility results [4]. As with *S. aureus*, in candidemic patients, a TEE is also mandatory. When negative initially, TEE and fundus exams should be repeated after 5–7 days if high suspicion of infectious endocarditis persists [67].

The main risk factors for IE in adult patients with candidemia, or CR-candidemia, are as follows:

1. Prosthetic heart valves or another valve disease
2. Injection drug abuse
3. Indwelling central venous catheter
4. Cancer chemotherapy
5. Prior bacterial endocarditis

For more recommendations on how to manage patients with CR-candidemia, the reader is referred to the 2016 Infectious Diseases Society of America (IDSA) Candidiasis Guidelines and the 2015 American Heart Association Infective Endocarditis Guidelines [73,74].

DURATION OF ANTIBIOTIC TREATMENT

The duration of antibiotic treatment depends on many factors, e.g., the causative microorganism, catheter, patient, and the presence or not of complications. Most authors recommend a 10- to 14-day course in a largely empirical and opinion-guided basis [3].

The length of therapy depends on whether a clinical and microbiological (negative follow-up blood cultures) response is achieved in less than 72 hours after the catheter is removed and adequate systemic antibiotics have been initiated.

The duration of systemic antibiotics is conditioned by negativization of blood cultures in all patients, catheter removal, guidewire exchange, or antibiotic lock therapy added to systemic treatment. Hence, new blood cultures should be obtained 72 hours after the start of treatment to check for blood sterilization. If cultures remain positive, serial blood cultures should be performed every 48–72 hours until blood sterilization.

No strong evidence exists to support current recommendations regarding duration of the antibiotic treatment.

A 5-day antibiotic course is accepted for coagulase-negative staphylococci if the catheter is removed. In the case of catheter maintenance, treatment should be given for 7–14 days.

Exceptions to this general recommendation are CR-BSIs by *S. aureus*, which need a minimum of 14 days or even 4–6 weeks of antibiotics in the case of complications, and CR-candidemia, which also requires an additional 14 days of treatment after the first negative follow-up blood culture.

Sequential oral therapy may be considered in patients who are clinically stable, lack metastatic complications, and whose blood cultures turn negative after the start of antibiotic treatment and catheter removal.

RULING OUT COMPLICATIONS

As already mentioned, follow-up blood cultures are mandatory for all patients. In the case of *S. aureus*, *S. lugdunensis*, or *Candida* spp., these should be performed every 72 h, until they become sterile.

PREVENTION DURING CATHETER IMPLANTATION

Surveillance programs for the prevention of CR-BSI consist of bundles of simple and effective preventive measures implemented both during catheter insertion and maintenance, in association with staff training. Such programs have had a significant impact on BCR-BSI rates in CCUs [75].

Strict adherence to these recommendations has enabled a 60% reduction in the frequency of episodes in North American CCUs. In 2009, the estimated number of episodes of CR-BSI was 18,000, representing a decrease of 58% since 2001 [22].

In Spain, a program (Estudio nacional de vigilancia de infección nosocomial en Unidades de Cuidados Intensivos [ENVIN-UCI]) for the surveillance of infections associated with devices in CCU patients with more than 100 participating hospitals was started in 1994 [76,77]. This program offers annual rates of CR-BSI adjusted by different denominators, such as days of catheter-use, days of CCU hospitalization, and number of patients admitted to CCUs. These data have enabled the comparisons and the design of prevention programs and assessment of their included measures.

The most recent American guidelines for the prevention of intravascular catheter-related infections were issued in 2011 by the IDSA, the Centers for Disease Control and Prevention (CDC), and the Healthcare Infection Control Practices Advisory Committee of the CDC [78]. Primary areas of emphasis are as follows: (a) Training healthcare workers to insert and maintain catheters; (b) implementing sterile barrier precautions during CVC placement; (c) applying >0.5% chlorhexidine with alcohol to the skin for preparation; (d) avoiding regular CVC replacement as a preventive strategy; and (e) the choice of short-term CVCs impregnated with antiseptics/antibiotics or sponge dressings impregnated with chlorhexidine if there is no decline in infection rate despite compliance with other strategies (e.g., training, sterile barrier precautions, and chlorhexidine >0.5% with alcohol for skin antisepsis).

These guidelines also stress that measures should be implemented as bundles, and compliance rates of all bundle components documented and reported as benchmarks to improve quality and performance.

As in many other CCUs, we have combined the recommendations of each bundle (catheter insertion and maintenance) and new contributions from the literature to generate two charts in a pocket guide to help compliance (Tables 18.4 and 18.5) [6,79,80].

Since the start of the CR-BIS prevention project in Michigan's CCUs by Pronovost et al., dramatic reductions in the incidence of this nosocomial infection have been reported in a multitude of articles.

TABLE 18.4
Precautions for CVC Insertion: Hospital General Universitario Gregorio Marañón, Madrid, Spain

Hand hygiene using conventional soap and water, and preferably, alcohol-based hand-rub products.

Maximal sterile barrier precautions: Cap, mask, sterile gown, sterile gloves, and a sterile full body drape.

Skin preparation with alcoholic chlorhexidine 2%. Let dry for 30 s to 2 min.

Catheter kit: standard supply carts or kits (e.g., assembled by healthcare organizations) containing all recommended supplies.

Subclavian vein > jugular vein > femoral vein.

Consider echocardiographic guidance for catheter placement. This is mandatory for femoral insertion.

Choose a catheter made of polyurethane or silicone.

Follow the insertion protocol strictly. Any staff member can interrupt the insertion procedure when a recommendation is not met during the process.

Cover insertion site with sterile gauze or transparent dressing.

If the procedure was performed in an emergency, switch the catheter (even through a guidewire) for an impregnated catheter with antibiotics in under 48 h.

Use a checklist to verify and document all the above steps.

TABLE 18.5
Precautions for CVC Maintenance: Hospital General Universitario Gregorio Marañón, Madrid

Use alcohol solutions before catheter manipulation and sterile gloves except for palpation through the dressing to discern tenderness.

Monitor insertion site daily by inspection if a transparent dressing is used and by palpation for a gauze dressing.

Change gauze dressings every 2 days and transparent dressings every 7 days (except if the dressing is soiled or moistened; then it should be changed immediately).

Disinfect skin with 2% alcoholic chlorhexidine and the connectors with alcohol wipes before each manipulation.

Do not use povidone-iodine antiseptic ointment or bacitracin/gramicidin/polymyxin B ointment at the insertion site (except for hemodialysis catheters).

Use dressings impregnated with chlorhexidine for CVC. Change every 7 d.

Use closed connectors (split septum) on all catheter lumens. Change every 7 d.

Change administration sets every 7 d (coinciding with connectors). Aseptic technique. If propofol, change the administration set every 6–12 h.

Ask the responsible physician on a daily basis for the need to continue using the catheter.

Do not replace the catheter through a guide wire when there is suspicion of infection. If this was unavoidable, submit catheter tip for microbiological culture and insert a new catheter coated with antibiotics.

When catheter-related infection is suspected, submit the catheter tip or complete reservoir for microbiological culture.

The most recent recommendations for prevention have been compiled in guidelines, systematic reviews, and meta-analyses [3,5,6,78,81–95].

To mention just a few of these recommendations: Intensive care should be practiced in closed-units, bedside ultrasonography should be used for catheter insertion in all instances, needleless securement devices are recommended, and disinfection caps for passive hub decontamination are effective in reducing hub colonization and BSI rates [6]. Our group has analyzed the efficacy of the use of ethanol locks for the prevention and treatment of these infections [96,97]. In an *in vitro* model, we observed that an ethanol-based lock solution with 40% ethanol + 60 IU heparin administered daily for 72 hours is sufficient to almost eradicate the metabolic activity of bacterial and fungal biofilms. While we do not recommend this precaution for prevention, we do think that it is effective in the treatment of a CR-BSI [97].

SUCCESS OF CONTROL PROGRAMS

In response to the Keystone Initiative proposed by Pronovost et al. (2003) and put into practice by a series of Michigan hospitals and health organizations, the median rate of infections at a typical CCU dropped from median 2.7 per 1000 patients to zero after 3 months. The Keystone Initiative published its results in the December 2006 *New England Journal of Medicine* [21]. In the first 3 months of the program, infection rates in Michigan's CCUs diminished by 60%. In the first 18 months, an estimated 1500 lives and $100 million were saved. For almost 4 years, these improvements continued [98]. Bundles are unquestionably effective.

In a systematic review and meta-analysis, Ista et al. identified 96 suitable studies addressing the efficacy of catheter insertion and maintenance bundles to prevent CR-BSI in CCU patients of all ages [24]. In adult CCUs, the incidence of CLABSI fell from a baseline value of 1.2 to 46.3 per 1000 catheter-days (median 5.7, IQR 3.1–9.5) to 0.33 to 19.5 per 1000 catheter-days (median 2.0, IQR 1.1–3.7). Study duration ranged from 6 to 108 months (median 32; IQR 22–39). In 25% of the studies, it was reported that impacts were sustained. In 12% of the studies, compliance with the full catheter insertion bundle improved from 7% to 45% after bundle implementation compared with the median of 82% before measurement. In 11 studies, compliance enhanced after bundle implementation from 65% to 100% for maximal barrier precaution and from 30% to 100% for hand hygiene. Absolute compliance for the maintenance bundle improved by 14%–24% after implementation. In the accompanying editorial, it was stated that bundles are unquestionable effective but not easy to implement. Their success often relies on a multimodal adaptation of the bundle strategy to the local context. Continuous monitoring is essential.

In conclusion, while on the worldwide scale the incidence of CR-BSI is falling, the more developed countries complying with all the items of prevention bundles have seen a more significant reduction in infection rates.

CONCLUSIONS

Rates of CR-BSI are declining. Reasonably effective diagnostic methods are available to rule out a CVC as the origin of a BSI. Risk scores designed to avoid a TEE are helpful tools but should never replace clinical assessment of patients, their close follow up and the expert opinion of the responsible physician. Treatment should be guided and consist of reduced spectrum antimicrobials once the cause of infection is known. So far, no randomized control trial has served to determine the best duration of antibiotic treatment. Perhaps in the future, biomarkers will help tailor antimicrobial treatment.

There are several unresolved issues. For instance, the most novel management procedure for the treatment and prevention of CR-BSI. For antibiotic-lock therapy, we lack uniform recommendations on the pharmacological agents or concentrations to use. There are no commercial preparations available; solutions need to be prepared by dilution from intravenous drugs. It is not known whether anticoagulants should be added and at what dose or the minimum time they should be left to act. Neither has it been established if antimicrobials or molecules such as ethanol are better. Finally, there is a need for more human resources to efficiently implement existing prevention bundles.

REFERENCES

1. Wisplinghoff H, Bischoff T, Tallent SM, Seifert H, Wenzel RP, Edmond MB. Nosocomial bloodstream infections in US hospitals: Analysis of 24,179 cases from a prospective nationwide surveillance study. *Clin Infect Dis* 2004;39:309–317.
2. Beekmann SE, Henderson DK. Chapter 302: Infections caused by percutaneous intravascular devices. In: Bennett JE, Dolin R, Blaser MJ eds. *Mandell, Douglas, and Bennett's Principles and Practice of Infectious Diseases* (8th ed.). Philadelphia, PA: Elsevier Saunders, 2015:3310–3324.
3. Timsit JF, Rupp M, Bouza E, et al. A state of the art review on optimal practices to prevent, recognize, and manage complications associated with intravascular devices in the critically ill. *Intensive Care Med* 2018;44:742–759.
4. Chaves F, Garnacho-Montero J, Del Pozo JL, et al. Diagnosis and treatment of catheter-related bloodstream infection: Clinical guidelines of the Spanish Society of Infectious Diseases and Clinical Microbiology and (SEIMC) and the Spanish Society of Spanish Society of Intensive and Critical Care Medicine and Coronary Units (SEMICYUC). *Med Intensiva* 2018;42:5–36.
5. Rupp ME, Karnatak R. Intravascular catheter-related bloodstream Infections. *Infect Dis Clin North Am* 2018;32:765–787.
6. Bell T, O'Grady NP. Prevention of central line-associated bloodstream infections. *Infect Dis Clin North Am* 2017;31:551–559.
7. Horan TC, Andrus M, Dudeck MA. CDC/NHSN surveillance definition of health care-associated infection and criteria for specific types of infections in the acute care setting. *Am J Infect Control* 2008;36:309–332.
8. Fagan RP, Edwards JR, Park BJ, Fridkin SK, Magill SS. Incidence trends in pathogen-specific central line-associated bloodstream infections in US intensive care units, 1990–2010. *Infect Control Hosp Epidemiol* 2013;34:893–899.

9. Blot SI, Depuydt P, Annemans L, et al. Clinical and economic outcomes in critically ill patients with nosocomial catheter-related bloodstream infections. *Clin Infect Dis* 2005;41:1591–1598.

10. Raad I, Hanna H, Maki D. Intravascular catheter-related infections: Advances in diagnosis, prevention, and management. *Lancet Infect Dis* 2007;7:645–657.

11. Dudeck MA, Horan TC, Peterson KD, et al. National Healthcare Safety Network report, data summary for 2011, device-associated module. *Am J Infect Control* 2013;41:286–300.

12. Furuya EY, Dick AW, Herzig CT, Pogorzelska-Maziarz M, Larson EL, Stone PW. Central line-Associated bloodstream infection reduction and bundle compliance in intensive care units: A national study. *Infect Control Hosp Epidemiol* 2016;37:805–810.

13. van der Kooi T, Sax H, Pittet D, et al. Prevention of hospital infections by intervention and training (PROHIBIT): Results of a pan-European cluster-randomized multicentre study to reduce central venous catheter-related bloodstream infections. *Intensive Care Med* 2018;44:48–60.

14. Scott RD, Sinkowitz-Cochran R, Wise ME, et al. CDC central-line bloodstream infection prevention efforts produced net benefits of at least $640 Million during 1990–2008. *Health Aff (Millwood)* 2014;33:1040–1047.

15. Marschall J. Catheter-associated bloodstream infections: Looking outside of the ICU. *Am J Infect Control* 2008;36:S172. e5–e8.

16. Freixas N, Bella F, Limon E, Pujol M, Almirante B, Gudiol F. Impact of a multimodal intervention to reduce bloodstream infections related to vascular catheters in non-ICU wards: A multicentre study. *Clin Microbiol Infect* 2013;19:838–844.

17. Zingg W, Cartier V, Inan C, et al. Hospital-wide multidisciplinary, multimodal intervention programme to reduce central venous catheter-associated bloodstream infection. *PLOS ONE* 2014;9:e93898.

18. Guembe M, Perez-Granda MJ, Capdevila JA, et al. Nationwide study on the use of intravascular catheters in internal medicine departments. *J Hosp Infect* 2015;90:135–141.

19. Dimick JB, Pelz RK, Consunji R, Swoboda SM, Hendrix CW, Lipsett PA. Increased resource use associated with catheter-related bloodstream infection in the surgical intensive care unit. *Arch Surg* 2001;136:229–234.

20. O'Grady NP, Alexander M, Dellinger EP, et al. Guidelines for the prevention of intravascular catheter-related infections. Centers for Disease Control and Prevention. *MMWR Recomm Rep* 2002;51:1–29.

21. Pronovost P, Needham D, Berenholtz S, et al. An intervention to decrease catheter-related bloodstream infections in the ICU. *N Engl J Med* 2006;355:2725–2732.

22. Centers for Disease C, Prevention. Vital signs: Central line-associated blood stream infections—United States, 2001, 2008, and 2009. *Morb Mortal Wkly Rep* 2011;60:243–248.

23. Pronovost PJ, Watson SR, Goeschel CA, Hyzy RC, Berenholtz SM. Sustaining reductions in central line-associated bloodstream infections in Michigan intensive care units: A 10-year analysis. *Am J Med Qual* 2016;31:197–202.

24. Ista E, van der Hoven B, Kornelisse RF, et al. Effectiveness of insertion and maintenance bundles to prevent central-line-associated bloodstream infections in critically ill patients of all ages: A systematic review and meta-analysis. *Lancet Infect Dis* 2016;16:724–734.

25. Mermel LA, Farr BM, Sherertz RJ, et al. Guidelines for the management of intravascular catheter-related infections. *Clin Infect Dis* 2001;32:1249–1272.

26. Safdar N, Fine JP, Maki DG. Meta-analysis: Methods for diagnosing intravascular device-related bloodstream infection. *Ann Intern Med* 2005;142:451–466.

27. Benezra D, Kiehn TE, Gold JW, Brown AE, Turnbull AD, Armstrong D. Prospective study of infections in indwelling central venous catheters using quantitative blood cultures. *Am J Med* 1988;85:495–498.

28. Rijnders BJ, Peetermans WE, Verwaest C, Wilmer A, Van Wijngaerden E. Watchful waiting versus immediate catheter removal in ICU patients with suspected catheter-related infection: A randomized trial. *Intensive Care Med* 2004;30:1073–1080.

29. Cercenado E, Ena J, Rodriguez-Creixems M, Romero I, Bouza E. A conservative procedure for the diagnosis of catheter-related infections. *Arch Intern Med* 1990;150:1417–1420.

30. Fortun J, Perez-Molina JA, Asensio A, et al. Semiquantitative culture of subcutaneous segment for conservative diagnosis of intravascular catheter-related infection. *J Parenter Enteral Nutr* 2000;24:210–214.

31. Bouza E, Munoz P, Burillo A, et al. The challenge of anticipating catheter tip colonization in major heart surgery patients in the intensive care unit: Are surface cultures useful? *Crit Care Med* 2005;33:1953–1960.

32. Wing EJ, Norden CW, Shadduck RK, Winkelstein A. Use of quantitative bacteriologic techniques to diagnose catheter-related sepsis. *Arch Intern Med* 1979;139:482–483.

33. Blot F. Diagnosis of catheter-related infections. In: Seifert H, Jansen B, Farr B eds. *Catheter-Related Infections*. New York: Marcel Dekker, 2005:37–76.

34. Blot F, Schmidt E, Nitenberg G, et al. Earlier positivity of central-venous-versus peripheral-blood cultures is highly predictive of catheter-related sepsis. *J Clin Microbiol* 1998;36:105–109.

35. Blot F, Nitenberg G, Chachaty E, et al. Diagnosis of catheter-related bacteraemia: A prospective comparison of the time to positivity of hub-blood versus peripheral-blood cultures. *Lancet* 1999;354:1071–1077.

36. Blot F. Diagnosis of catheter-related infections. In: Seifert H, Jansen B, Farr BM eds. *Catheter-Related Infections* (2nd ed.). New York: Marcel Dekker, 2005:60.

37. Robinson JL. Sensitivity of a blood culture drawn through a single lumen of a multilumen, long-term, indwelling, central venous catheter in pediatric oncology patients. *J Pediatr Hematol Oncol* 2002;24:72–74.

38. Guembe M, Rodriguez-Creixems M, Sanchez-Carrillo C, Perez-Parra A, Martin-Rabadan P, Bouza E. How many lumens should be cultured in the conservative diagnosis of catheter-related bloodstream infections? *Clin Infect Dis* 2010;50:1575–1579.

39. Cuellar-Rodriguez J, Connor D, Murray P, Gea-Banacloche J, National Institutes of Health BMDUSA. Discrepant results from sampling different lumens of multilumen catheters: The case for sampling all lumens. *Eur J Clin Microbiol Infect Dis* 2014;33:831–835.

40. Raad I, Hanna HA, Alakech B, Chatzinikolaou I, Johnson MM, Tarrand J. Differential time to positivity: A useful method for diagnosing catheter-related bloodstream infections. *Ann Intern Med* 2004;140:18–25.

41. Bouza E, Alvarado N, Alcala L, et al. A prospective, randomized, and comparative study of 3 different methods for the diagnosis of intravascular catheter colonization. *Clin Infect Dis* 2005;40:1096–1100.

42. Park KH, Lee MS, Lee SO, et al. Diagnostic usefulness of differential time to positivity for catheter-related candidemia. *J Clin Microbiol* 2014;52:2566–2572.

43. Bouza E, Alcala L, Munoz P, Martin-Rabadan P, Guembe M, Rodriguez-Creixems M. Can microbiologists help to assess catheter involvement in candidaemic patients before removal? *Clin Microbiol Infect* 2013;19:E129–E135.

44. Bouza E, Martin-Rabadan P, Echenagusia A, et al. Diagnosis of venous access port colonization requires cultures from multiple sites: Should guidelines be amended? *Diagn Microbiol Infect Dis* 2014;78:162–167.

45. Bjornson HS, Colley R, Bower RH, Duty VP, Schwartz-Fulton JT, Fischer JE. Association between microorganism growth at the catheter insertion site and colonization of the catheter in patients receiving total parenteral nutrition. *Surgery* 1982;92:720–727.

46. Segura M, Llado L, Guirao X, et al. A prospective study of a new protocol for 'in situ' diagnosis of central venous catheter related bacteraemia. *Clin Nutr* 1993;12:103–107.

47. Leon M, Garcia M, Herranz MA, et al. [Diagnostic value of Gram staining of peri-catheter skin and the connection in the prediction of intravascular-catheter-related bacteremia]. *Enferm Infecc Microbiol Clin* 1998;16:214–2148.

48. Bouza E, Alvarado N, Alcala L, Perez MJ, Rincon C, Munoz P. A randomized and prospective study of 3 procedures for the diagnosis of catheter-related bloodstream infection without catheter withdrawal. *Clin Infect Dis* 2007;44:820–826.

49. Mermel LA, Allon M, Bouza E, et al. Clinical practice guidelines for the diagnosis and management of intravascular catheter-related infection: 2009 update by the Infectious Diseases Society of America. *Clin Infect Dis* 2009;49:1–45.

50. Ruhe JJ, Menon A. Clinical significance of isolated *Staphylococcus aureus* central venous catheter tip cultures. *Clin Microbiol Infect* 2006;12:933–936.

51. Ekkelenkamp MB, van der Bruggen T, van de Vijver DA, Wolfs TF, Bonten MJ. Bacteremic complications of intravascular catheters colonized with *Staphylococcus aureus*. *Clin Infect Dis* 2008;46:114–118.

52. Hetem DJ, de Ruiter SC, Buiting AG, et al. Preventing *Staphylococcus aureus* bacteremia and sepsis in patients with *Staphylococcus aureus* colonization of intravascular catheters: A retrospective multicenter study and meta-analysis. *Medicine (Baltimore)* 2011;90:284–288.

53. Guembe M, Rodriguez-Creixems M, Martin-Rabadan P, Alcala L, Munoz P, Bouza E. The risk of catheter-related bloodstream infection after withdrawal of colonized catheters is low. *Eur J Clin Microbiol Infect Dis* 2014;33:729–734.

54. Perez-Parra A, Munoz P, Guinea J, Martin-Rabadan P, Guembe M, Bouza E. Is Candida colonization of central vascular catheters in non-candidemic, non-neutropenic patients an indication for antifungals? *Intensive Care Med* 2009;35:707–712.

55. Lopez-Medrano F, Fernandez-Ruiz M, Origuen J, et al. Clinical significance of Candida colonization of intravascular catheters in the absence of documented candidemia. *Diagn Microbiol Infect Dis* 2012;73:157–161.

56. Park KH, Kim SH, Song EH, et al. Development of bacteraemia or fungaemia after removal of colonized central venous catheters in patients with negative concomitant blood cultures. *Clin Microbiol Infect* 2010;16:742–746.

57. Rello J, Valles J, Fontanals D, Jubert P, Segura F. Antimicrobial use in patients with positive intravascular catheter cultures: A six-month prospective survey in a teaching hospital. *Infect Control Hosp Epidemiol* 1996;17:668–669.

58. Khatib R, Johnson LB, Fakih MG, et al. Persistence in *Staphylococcus aureus* bacteremia: Incidence, characteristics of patients and outcome. *Scand J Infect Dis* 2006;38:7–14.

59. Shorr AF, Tabak YP, Killian AD, Gupta V, Liu LZ, Kollef MH. Healthcare-associated bloodstream infection: A distinct entity? Insights from a large U.S. database. *Crit Care Med* 2006;34:2588–2595.

60. Le Moing V, Alla F, Doco-Lecompte T, et al. *Staphylococcus aureus* bloodstream infection and Endocarditis—a prospective cohort study. *PLOS ONE* 2015;10:e0127385.

61. Soriano A, Mensa J. Is transesophageal echocardiography dispensable in hospital-acquired *Staphylococcus aureus* bacteremia? *Clin Infect Dis* 2011;53:10–12.

62. Kaasch AJ, Barlow G, Edgeworth JD, et al. *Staphylococcus aureus* bloodstream infection: A pooled analysis of five prospective, observational studies. *J Infect* 2014;68: 242–251.

63. Wong D, Keynan Y, Rubinstein E. Comparison between transthoracic and transesophageal echocardiography in screening for infective endocarditis in patients with *Staphylococcus aureus* bacteremia. *Eur J Clin Microbiol Infect Dis* 2014;33:2053–2059.

64. Mirrakhimov AE, Jesinger ME, Ayach T, Gray A. When does S aureus bacteremia require transesophageal echocardiography? *Cleve Clin J Med* 2018;85:517–520.

65. Palraj BR, Baddour LM, Hess EP, et al. Predicting Risk of Endocarditis Using a Clinical Tool (PREDICT): Scoring system to guide use of echocardiography in the management of *Staphylococcus aureus* bacteremia. *Clin Infect Dis* 2015;61:18–28.

66. Nishimura RA, Otto CM, Bonow RO, et al. 2014 AHA/ACC guideline for the management of patients with valvular heart disease: A report of the American College of Cardiology/ American Heart Association Task Force on Practice Guidelines. *J Am Coll Cardiol* 2014;63:e57–e185.

67. Habib G, Lancellotti P, Antunes MJ, et al. 2015 ESC Guidelines for the management of infective endocarditis: The Task Force for the Management of Infective Endocarditis of the European Society of Cardiology (ESC). Endorsed by: European Association for Cardio-Thoracic Surgery (EACTS), the European Association of Nuclear Medicine (EANM). *Eur Heart J* 2015;36:3075–3128.

68. Bouza E, Kestler M, Beca T, et al. The NOVA score: A proposal to reduce the need for transesophageal echocardiography in patients with enterococcal bacteremia. *Clin Infect Dis* 2015;60:528–535.

69. Berge A, Krantz A, Ostlund H, Naucler P, Rasmussen M. The DENOVA score efficiently identifies patients with monomicrobial Enterococcus faecalis bacteremia where echocardiography is not necessary. *Infection* 2018.

70. Reigadas E, Rodriguez-Creixems M, Sanchez-Carrillo C, Martin-Rabadan P, Bouza E. Uncommon aetiological agents of catheter-related bloodstream infections. *Epidemiol Infect* 2015;143:741–744.

71. Stryjewski ME, Corey GR. Editorial commentary: NOVA score to predict endocarditis in patients with enterococcal bacteremia: Sticking to valves or to scores? *Clin Infect Dis* 2015;60:536–538.

72. Dahl A, Lauridsen TK, Arpi M, et al. Risk factors of endocarditis in patients with *Enterococcus faecalis* bacteremia: External validation of the NOVA score. *Clin Infect Dis* 2016;63:771–775.

73. Baddour LM, Wilson WR, Bayer AS, et al. Infective endocarditis in adults: Diagnosis, antimicrobial therapy, and management of complications: A scientific statement for healthcare professionals from the American Heart Association. *Circulation* 2015;132:1435–1486.

74. Pappas PG, Kauffman CA, Andes DR, et al. Clinical Practice Guideline for the Management of Candidiasis: 2016 Update by the Infectious Diseases Society of America. *Clin Infect Dis* 2016;62:e1–e50.

75. Pronovost PJ, Weaver SJ, Berenholtz SM, et al. Reducing preventable harm: Observations on minimizing bloodstream infections. *J Health Organ Manag* 2017;31:2–9.

76. Palomar M, Alvarez-Lerma F, Riera A, et al. Impact of a national multimodal intervention to prevent catheter-related bloodstream infection in the ICU: The Spanish experience. *Crit Care Med* 2013;41:2364–2372.

77. ENVIN-HELICS [database on the Internet] 2018 [cited September 22nd, 2018]. Available at: http://hws.vhebron.net/envin-helics/.

78. O'Grady NP, Alexander M, Burns LA, et al. Guidelines for the prevention of intravascular catheter-related infections. *Clin Infect Dis* 2011;52:e162–e193.

79. Bouza E, Guembe M, Pérez-Granda MJ. Innovative strategies for preventing central-line associated infections. *Curr Treat Options Infect Dis* 2014;6:1–16.

80. Lorente L. What is new for the prevention of catheter-related bloodstream infections? *Ann Transl Med* 2016;4:119.

81. Zhang P, Lei JH, Su XJ, Wang XH. Ethanol locks for the prevention of catheter-related bloodstream infection: A meta-analysis of randomized control trials. *BMC Anesthesiol* 2018;18:93.

82. Kuo SH, Lin WR, Lin JY, et al. The epidemiology, antibiograms and predictors of mortality among critically-ill patients with central line-associated bloodstream infections. *J Microbiol Immunol Infect* 2018;51:401–410.

83. Norris LB, Kablaoui F, Brilhart MK, Bookstaver PB. Systematic review of antimicrobial lock therapy for prevention of central-line-associated bloodstream infections in adult and pediatric cancer patients. *Int J Antimicrob Agents* 2017;50:308–317.

84. Labriola L, Pochet JM. Any use for alternative lock solutions in the prevention of catheter-related blood stream infections? *J Vasc Access* 2017;18:34–38.

85. Hina HR, McDowell JRS. Minimising central line-associated bloodstream infection rate in inserting central venous catheters in the adult intensive care units. *J Clin Nurs* 2017;26:3962–3973.

86. Chong HY, Lai NM, Apisarnthanarak A, Chaiyakunapruk N. Comparative efficacy of antimicrobial central venous catheters in reducing catheter-related bloodstream infections in adults: Abridged cochrane systematic review and network meta-analysis. *Clin Infect Dis* 2017;64:S131–S40.

87. Lai NM, Lai NA, O'Riordan E, Chaiyakunapruk N, Taylor JE, Tan K. Skin antisepsis for reducing central venous catheter-related infections. *Cochrane Database Syst Rev* 2016;7:Cd010140.

88. Lai NM, Chaiyakunapruk N, Lai NA, O'Riordan E, Pau WS, Saint S. Catheter impregnation, coating or bonding for reducing central venous catheter-related infections in adults. *Cochrane Database Syst Rev* 2016;3:Cd007878.

89. Ullman AJ, Cooke ML, Mitchell M, et al. Dressings and securement devices for central venous catheters (CVC). *Cochrane Database Syst Rev* 2015;Cd010367.

90. Marschall J, Mermel LA, Fakih M, et al. Strategies to prevent central line-associated bloodstream infections in acute care hospitals: 2014 update. *Infect Control Hosp Epidemiol* 2014;35 Suppl 2:S89–S107.

91. Flodgren G, Conterno LO, Mayhew A, Omar O, Pereira CR, Shepperd S. Interventions to improve professional adherence to guidelines for prevention of device-related infections. *Cochrane Database Syst Rev* 2013;Cd006559.

92. Parienti JJ, du Cheyron D, Timsit JF, et al. Meta-analysis of subclavian insertion and nontunneled central venous catheter-associated infection risk reduction in critically ill adults. *Crit Care Med* 2012;40:1627–1634.

93. O'Horo JC, Silva GL, Munoz-Price LS, Safdar N. The efficacy of daily bathing with chlorhexidine for reducing healthcare-associated bloodstream infections: A meta-analysis. *Infect Control Hosp Epidemiol* 2012;33:257–267.

94. Marik PE, Flemmer M, Harrison W. The risk of catheter-related bloodstream infection with femoral venous catheters as compared to subclavian and internal jugular venous catheters: A systematic review of the literature and meta-analysis. *Crit Care Med* 2012;40:2479–2485.

95. Ge X, Cavallazzi R, Li C, Pan SM, Wang YW, Wang FL. Central venous access sites for the prevention of venous thrombosis, stenosis and infection. *Cochrane Database Syst Rev* 2012;Cd004084.

96. Perez-Granda MJ, Barrio JM, Munoz P, et al. Ethanol lock therapy (E-Lock) in the prevention of catheter-related bloodstream infections (CR-BSI) after major heart surgery (MHS): A randomized clinical trial. *PLOS ONE* 2014;9:e91838.

97. Alonso B, Perez-Granda MJ, Rodriguez-Huerta A, Rodriguez C, Bouza E, Guembe M. The optimal ethanol lock therapy regimen for treatment of biofilm-associated catheter infections: An in-vitro study. *J Hosp Infect* 2018.

98. Pronovost PJ, Goeschel CA, Colantuoni E, et al. Sustaining reductions in catheter related bloodstream infections in Michigan intensive care units: Observational study. *BMJ* 2010;340:c309.

19 Acute Infective Endocarditis and Its Mimics in the Critical Care Unit

John L. Brusch

CONTENTS

Over the last 30 years, there has been a significant change in the nature of infective endocarditis (IE) This is due to the rise of *S. aureus* valvular infections that have been brought about by the development of various intravascular devices, prosthetic heart valves, the aging of the population, and the epidemic of intravenous drug abuse (IVDA). In addition, there has been a corresponding increase in the immunosuppressed population caused by a variety of diseases and their treatments. Nowhere are these changes better reflected than in the patients cared for in the critical care unit (CCU). Many, if not most, cases of acute CCU IE (ACCUIE) should be classified as nosocomial IE (NIE) or healthcare-associated IE (HCIE). This term describes the cases of IE in individuals who have been admitted to a hospital at least 72 hours prior to the onset of symptoms (NIE) or who have had a history of an invasive procedure, with potential for producing a bloodstream infection (BSI) during a hospitalization of less than 8 weeks prior. Healthcare-associated IE (HCIE) may be preferable to NIE, since it applies to all sites that care for patients, such as infusion centers [1,2].

It is important to remember that patients are admitted to the CCU for a wide variety of valvular infections but that they may also acquire IE in the CCU. This is especially true for people who are admitted for postoperative care after major cardiac surgery such as implantation of a prosthetic valve. They are especially susceptible to NIE because of the wide variety of invasive monitoring, therapeutic lines, and urinary catheters. There is a variety of reasons for admission, including congestive heart failure (64%), septic shock (21%), neurological deterioration (15%), and cardiopulmonary arrest (9%). While in the CCU, multi-organ failure developed in 64% of patients; prosthetic valve endocarditis (PVE) occurred in 21%; transthoracic echocardiography (TTE) was found to be useful in only 33%; and 91% of patients ultimately underwent a TEE. Inpatient mortality was 84% for those treated medically and 35% for those undergoing surgical approaches [3].

The diagnosis of NIE that is acquired within the CCU is quite challenging because of the absence of many of the classic signs and symptoms of valvular infection.

To a great deal, the profile of organisms, involved in ACCUIE, is dependent on the services that a given hospital provides. Clearly, tertiary care centers will have a higher rate of immunosuppressed patients and those who have received prosthetic heart valves and intracardiac devices. Community hospitals may well have a large population of IVDA. There is limited information concerning the causative organisms of ACCUIE. The available data indicate that the most common pathogens are Staphylococcal species, including methicillin-sensitive *S. aureus* (MSSA), methicillin-resistant *S. aureus* (MRSA), and coagulase-negative staphylococci (CoNS), which account for 45%. *Streptococcus* species constituted approximately 25% of cases. Somewhat surprising, only 3%–4% were due to *Candida* and *Aspergillus* spp., with a smaller amount of gram-negative endocarditis (Table 19.1).

DIFFERENTIAL DIAGNOSIS OF ACCUIE

To be included in the differential diagnosis of ACCUIE, the clinical picture must include the presence of bacteremia without a valvular vegetation or a valvular vegetation without the bacteremia. Of course, if both factors are present, the diagnosis of IE has already been achieved.

TABLE 19.1

Pathogens of ACCUIE

Organism	Comments
S. *aureus*	The most common cause of acute IE, including PVE, IVDA, and IE, related to intravascular infections. Approximately 35% of cases of S. *aureus* bacteremia are complicated by IE.
S. *lugdunensis*	A coagulase-negative *Staphylococcus* that is as aggressive as S. *aureus*.
S. *milleri* group (S. *anginosus*, S. *intermedius*, S. *constellatus*)	Unlike other *Streptococci*, they can invade tissues and produce suppurative complications.
Group D *streptococci*	Third most common cause of IE. They may produce alpha, beta, or gamma hemolysis. Source is GI or GU tracts. They are approximately 25% of cases. Somewhat surprising, only 3%–4% were due to *Candida* and *Aspergillus* spp., with a smaller amount of gram-negative endocarditis. Associated with a high rate of relapse. Growing problem of antimicrobial resistance. Most cases are subacute.
Group B *streptococci*	Seen in alcoholics, cancer patients, and diabetics, as well as in pregnancy. Forty percent mortality rate. Complications include CHF, thrombi, and metastatic infection.
Groups A, C, G *Streptococci*	More frequently seen in the elderly and diabetics. Mortality rate is 30%–70%. Commonly complicated by the development of myocardial abscesses.
S. *pneumonia*	Currently cause <5% of cases; follows acute course. Usually a complication of pneumoniae (1% of cases complicated by IE).
P. *aeruginosa*, S. *marcescens*	Most common causes of ABE in left-sided IVDAIE.
Fungal IE	*C. albicans* is the most common isolate (especially in PVE) and *C. parapsilosis* or *C. tropicalis* in IVDA. *Aspergillus* species recovered in 33% of fungal IE.
Polymicrobial IE	*Pseudomonas, enterococci,* and S. *aureus*. Seen in IVDA and cardiac surgery.

Abbreviations: ACCUIE, acute infective endocarditis.

NON-INFECTIOUS MIMICS

The most effective mimics of ACCUIE are the following: Marantic endocarditis or non-bacterial thrombotic endocarditis (NBTE), viral myocarditis, systemic lupus erythematosus (SLE), and atrial myxoma. These processes are included in this discussion of ACCUIE, because they may closely resemble NIE.

Individuals with NBTE are usually afebrile. If fever is present, it is most likely due to an underlying malignancy. Significant vegetations, which frequently embolize, may be present. There are no associated bacteremias. The most common causes of NBTE are various neoplasms, followed in frequency by SLE.

Patients with viral myocarditis may present with a fever, murmur, and peripheral emboli. The murmur is the result of febrile tachycardia, combined with ventricular dilatation. Valvular vegetations and bacteremias are absent.

Flare-ups of SLE are often marked with a fever greater than 102°F. Libman-Sacks verrucous valvular vegetations are present. They do no embolize. However, the cerebritis of SLE may resemble the effects of cerebral emboli.

Patients with left atrial myxomas have murmurs and often are febrile. Myxomatous material may embolize in a manner closely resembling that of subacute bacterial endocarditis. The erythrocyte sedimentation rate (ESR) is quite elevated. Both atrial myxomas and SLE produce a polyclonal gammopathy. Blood cultures are negative [4,5].

INFECTIOUS MIMICS

The most challenging infectious mimics to rule out the ACCUIE are S. *aureus* BSIs, especially when they meet the criteria of a continuous bacteremia. Intravenous catheters are the most common underlying source [6].

CLINICAL SYNDROMIC DIAGNOSIS

Arriving at a working diagnosis and appropriate therapeutic approach are dependent on formulating a clinical syndromic diagnosis, which is based on recognizing the key clues that are provided by the history, physical examination, non-specific laboratory tests, and imaging studies.

HISTORICAL CLUES

The possibility of IE has to be raised in those febrile CCU patients with a history of IVDA, prosthetic valve, or other intracardiac devices.

Fungal IE, especially that caused by *Candida* spp., should be considered in the presence of a prosthetic valve or a central venous catheter present in 44.6% and 30.4% of fungal IE patients, respectively. A total of 20.3% of patients had received prolonged courses of wide-spectrum endocarditis [7].

It is important to recognize that chronic forms of IE culture-negative infective endocarditis may be admitted to the CCU because of acute clinical deterioration. They may well be misdiagnosed as mimics of IE or as a variant of NIE. A well-obtained epidemiological history is the first step in arriving at the correct diagnosis. For example, *Bartonella* spp. IE infects those exposed to cats (*B. henselae*) or the homeless with lice infection (*Bartonella quintana*). *Legionella* IE primarily infects prosthetic valves implanted in facilities with a history of outbreaks of *Legionalla* [7]. The NIE or HCIE has to be considered in older patients whose symptoms developed after 72 hours of hospitalization or that developed within 60 days of hospitalization, during which a procedure was performed with significant potential for producing a BSI [8,9].

SIGNS AND SYMPTOMS CLUES

As compared with subacute IE (SBE), acute IE is a far more aggressive process. Whereas the manifestations of SBE are immunologically mediated, those of acute IE are due to direct infectious cardiac damage. In *S. aureus* acute IE, the diagnosis is classically arrived at within 10 days of onset of symptoms as compared with 6 weeks in the case of SBE [9]. There is a sudden onset of high fever and chills. Often, there is no previous history of valvular disease. In total, 30%–40% of patients will develop severe congestive heart failure due to destruction of the leaflets, detachment of leaflets from the annulus, or rupture of the chordae tendinae or of the papillary muscles of the aortic valve. The presentation of acute aortic insufficiency differs from chronic aortic regurgitation in that the mean pulse and left ventricular end-diastolic pressure and stroke volume markedly reduced there is early closure of the mitral valve, which is preceded by the appearance of an Austin Flint murmur. Occasionally, only resting tachycardia may be indicative of this heart failure. The patient may suffer from a variety of neuropsychiatric symptoms brought about by septic cerebral emboli. Other extra-cardiac complications of acute IE include spinal cord emboli and abscesses, splenic abscess. and other systemic emboli. Renal complications occur in 40%–50% of *S. aureus* IE. These include infarction, acute glomerulonephritis, interstitial nephritis, and acute cortical necrosis.

Osteomyelitis and septic arthritis are not common features of acute IE.

Less than 5% of native valve endocarditis are right sided. Tricuspid valve infection results in septic emboli to the lung. Symptoms include fever, cough, hemoptysis, and pleuritic pain. Empyema may complicate these infections. Only 5% of patients with right-sided disease have a murmur [10].

Clinical signs and symptoms of PVE in general are very similar to those of native valve IE. The exception is PVE that begins within a few weeks of valve implantation. In this case, the signs and symptoms may be obscured by common surgical complications such as pneumonia and wound infections. PVE caused by *S. aureus* may produce septic shock because of massive extension of paravalvular abscess. Because it is implanted in a previously damaged heart, congestive heart

failure (CHF) develops earlier more severely in PVE than in NVE. The rest of the intracardiac complications are quite similar to those of native valve IE [11].

However, these distinctions between acute and subacte IE have become less distinct. Use of antibiotics to treat signs and symptoms of IE that are erroneously attributed to other infections results in suppressing but not eradicating the valvular infection. This process leads to the development of NIE or HCIE. These categories represent valvular infections due to the increasing use of intravascular devices such as central or peripheral intravenous catheters, pacemakers, defibrillators, hemodialysis catheters, and shunts hyperalimentation lines. Intravascular-related BSIs (CRBSIs) have increased well over 100% since the 1980s and have become the most frequent cause of NIE (60%), with pyelonephritis and GU procedures accounting for 20%–30% of cases. Central venous catheters present the greatest risk of causing NIE. Catheter-related BSIs significantly increase 3–4 days after their insertion. NIE may involve both sides of the heart. The right-sided type involves valves that have been damaged by an intravascular line (i.e., Swan-Ganz catheter), which are then infected by a nosocomial bacteremia. In the left-sided type, a previously damaged or a prosthetic valve is infected by a transient bacteremia.

The presenting symptoms and signs of NIE differ considerably from that of acute acquired ones in the community. Patients with NIE or HCIE are significantly older. This may explain their blunted response to the infection. There is a lower rate of splenomegaly or peripheral stigmata. Only 25% are able to mount a significant fever, and only 62% exhibit a leukocytosis. The tricuspid valve is involved more than the aortic valve. There is a greater incidence of pulmonary edema and sepsis. All these factors delay the diagnosis of NIE [6,11]. Common presentations of NIE or HCIE in the CCU include fever of unknown source; peripheral thromboembolisms; CNS complications; hypotension; new or changing murmur; CHF; tachycardia; increase in inflammatory markers such as sedimentation rate; anemia; and acute kidney injury [1]. Prosthetic valves appear to be at a significantly greater risk of developing NIE even during a transient bacteremia (Table 19.2) [12].

TABLE 19.2

Challenges to Diagnosing NIE/HCIE

1. Less likely to be febrile than in community-acquired disease
2. May resemble a vasculitis or drug reaction
3. Other sites (e.g., chest and urine) are erroneously diagnosed as the cause of the patient's deterioration
4. Frequently inadequate number of blood culture are obtained because of the severity of illness

Abbreviation: NIE/HCIE, nosocomial infective endocarditis/healthcare associated infective endocarditis.

FASTIDIOUS ORGANISMS

In total, 90% of *Coxiella burnetii* IE present with intermittent low-grade fevers and diffuse purpuric rashes caused by immune complex vasculitis. The CHF develops later in its course. Arterial emboli are seen in 20% of patients, with significant splenomegaly in 50%.

Signs and symptoms of *Bartonella* IE are quite nonspecific, including low-grade fever, malaise, and weight loss. Eventually, CHF will develop in 90%.

Legionella IE may present as pericarditis or myocarditis. Cardiac tamponade or constrictive pericarditis may occur. The myocarditis may progress to the point of frank heart failure. Often, there are findings of concurrent *Legionella* pneumonia.

Culture-negative endocarditis (CNIE) is a valvular infection in "which aerobic and anaerobic blood cultures of three sufficient samples drawn over 24–48 hours remain negative." Improved microbiological methods, techniques and the use the modified Duke's criteria have decreased the incidence of CNIE from almost 30% to 5%. In the United States, the most common cause of CNIE of centimeters a year he is the administration of antibiotics prior to obtaining blood cultures, up to 70% of cases. This practice is usually prompted by concern that the patient's rapid clinical deterioration precludes holding off on antibiotics for the 10–15 minutes required to draw three sets of blood cultures [13].

In *S. aureus* IVDA, tricuspid valve infection and septic emboli to the lung produce symptoms of cough pleuritic pain and hemoptysis. At the time of presentation, empyema may be present in 5% of tricuspid valve infections.

Only 5% of patients with right-sided disease have a murmur. Abdominal pain may be due to splenic infarcts or abscesses or ischemic colitis. Neurological involvement of IVDAIE has two distinct CNS features due to gram-negative infection. These include panophthalmitis and cerebral mycotic aneurysms. Septic arthritis is seen in 10%–20% of *S. aureus* cases.

CLINICAL PRESENTATION OF PACEMAKER IE

Pacemaker IE may present as localized to the generator pocket or as a bacteremia or as right-sided IE. The absence of fever does not rule out the presence of bacteremia in this situation. Early pacemaker pocket infections present as wound infections with erosions of the overlying skin. Pacemaker IE is subacute in nature. Radiologic changes of pneumonia, abscess, or septic emboli complicate 30%–45% of cases. *S. aureus* is again the most common pathogen seen in patients who have both bacteremia and vegetations. It is important to remember that the pacemaker system infections may occur without associated valvular infection. The opposite is also true that the pacemaker system may be uninvolved in the face of active valvular infection.

KEY NON-SPECIFIC LABORATORY CLUES

The most commonly abnormal non-specific laboratory tests are anemia, elevated sedimentation rate, microscopic hematuria, proteinuria, elevated serum creatinine, elevated C-reactive protein, and elevated troponins. These types of abnormal values are not very helpful in diagnosing ACCUIE. However, more recent measures of inflammation, such as procalcitonin (PCT), hold out some promise in identifying ACCUIE pathogens and when to discontinue antibiotic therapy. Serum levels of PCT can distinguish between gram-positive and gram-negative BSIs as well between sites of infection and bacterial pathogens. In addition, changes in PCT levels are an early indicator of prognosis and survival, as well as reducing the length of antimicrobial therapy in treating bacteremias [14,15].

Electrocardiograms are most useful in detecting conduction abnormalities and PVCs that are caused by septal abscesses or myocarditis seen in 9% of patients. These may manifest as a prolonged PR interval or by AV dissociation or left bundle branch block developed during the course of IE.

Abscesses that involve the upper septum are silent electrocardiographically. Those that are secondary to mitral involvement come on more slowly, as compared with the complete heart block that can appears suddenly with aortic valve involvement [16].

Nuclear scans have not been found to be useful for the diagnosis or management of IE. Cardiac CT, single-photon emission CT fused with conventional CT (Spect/ST), and F-FDG Pet CT scans and MRI imaging appear to contribute to echocardiography in detecting suppurative complications such as aortic root abscesses [16]. A CT scan of the spleen should be obtained in cases of persistent or relapsing ACCUIE to rule out the presence of splenic abscesses. Cardiac catheterization plate is little if any role in the diagnosis of ACCUIE. The indications for echocardiography in managing ACCUIE include the following:

1. Patients with the clinical syndrome of CNIE.
2. To rule out valvular infection in those with a continuous or non-continuous BSI or fungemia in the setting of vascular catheters.
3. To detect intracardiac complications of ACCUIE.
4. To detect infections of intracardiac devices.
5. To monitor response of IE to antibiotic therapy, especially in the setting of vegetations greater than 1 cm. These large vegetations are associated with increased risk of cerebral emboli.
6. For follow-up of intracardiac complications status post surgery.
7. Re-evaluation of those with known valvular infection and persistent BSI fever or worsening valvular function (Table 19.3).

The diagnosis of IE should never be based solely on echocardiographic findings in the setting of negative blood cultures. There must be a compatible history findings and physical examination or other imaging studies that support this diagnosis. The TEE is generally more sensitive than TTE for detecting valvular vegetations. However, state-of-the-art TTE equipment is the equal of TEEs, except in the setting of prosthetic valves. In evaluation of tricuspid valve vegetations, both types of echocardiogram are equivalent. The TTE should be used initially in all cases, except for in the setting of a prosthetic valve. The TEE

TABLE 19.3

Role of Echocardiography in the Diagnosis of ACCUIE

1. In suspected CNIE
2. In patients with severe bacteremia in setting of an intravascular catheter
3. To detect vascular changes and paravalvular abscess
4. To monitor response to therapy of large (>1 cm) vegetations with or without cerebral emboli to determine the need for "vegectomy" or valve replacement
5. Reevaluation of individuals not responding to therapy

Abbreviation: ACCUIE, acute infective endocarditis.

TABLE 19.4

Indications for Initial Use of TEE for Evaluation of ACCUIE

1. Presence of prosthetic valves
2. Presence of lung disease
3. Presence of morbid obesity
4. Presence of clinical emboli
5. Presence of intracardiac devcies

Abbreviation: ACCUIE, acute infective endocarditis.

should always be used to assess this type of valve. Table 19.4 presents other conditions in which a TEE may yield better images. A TEE should be performed if the results of the TTE are equivocal. A TEE may still be preferred in the evaluation of intracardiac devices (pacemaker, defibrillators, and left ventricular assistive devices [LVADS]) [17,18] (Table 19.4).

MANAGEMENT OF INTRAVASCULAR-ASSOCIATED *S. AUREUS* BACTEREMIA

In the past, management of *S. aureus* bacteremia in the presence of an intravascular catheter required promptly removing the catheter, initiating appropriate antibiotic therapy, and monitoring of blood culture results in 4–5 days, as well as performing TTE. If follow-up blood cultures were negative and there was no evidence of metastatic infection, a total of 2 weeks of anti-staphylococcal therapy was believed to be sufficient. If follow-up blood culture findings were positive, a TEE should be performed. In the event that the TEE demonstrates findings of IE, the patient is treated for 4–6 weeks of antistaphylococcal antibiotics. This approach excludes patients with prosthetic valves or vascular grafts

Although resorting immediately to TEE is becoming more common place, often, it is not necessary. A scoring system has been developed to help differentiate patients with valvular infection from those with *S. aureus* BSIs originating from sites such as splenic abscesses associated with osteomyelitis. Patients with underlying implantable cardiac device, whose *S. aureus* BSI developed in the community, have the highest risk of IE and should undergo immediate TEE. If the TEE findings are negative, they should be repeated in 5 days. It is important to recognize that in up to 30% of cases of persistent

BSI associated with an intravascular device, the cause is not identified. In some cases, it may be due to persistent endotheliosis. This is a process in which *S. aureus* infection of an intravascular catheter invades and multiplies within the adjacent endothelial cells. Eventually, the Staphylococci leave the cells and perpetuates BSI. Currently, the duration of antibiotic therapy for each case of *S. aureus*-related BSI must be individualized.

Documenting the presence of a continuous bacteremia along with a valvular vegetation that is consistent with valvular infection is the keystone for diagnosing ACCUIE. Essentially, these are the two major criteria of the Modified Duke Criteria. These criteria define a continuous bacteremia as two sets of blood cultures drawn at least 12 hours apart or three or four blood cultures, with the first and last sets separated by at least 1 hour, which grows out the same organism, which is compatible with valvular infection. The minor criteria are dropped because they are not relevant for the diagnosis of ACCUIE. It is important to remember that the Duke Criteria were developed in respect to left-sided native valve endocarditis They do not necessarily pertain to the complexities of NIE or HCIE [20,21].

BLOOD CULTURE TECHNIQUES

It is essential to avoid contaminating blood culture draws. One false-positive culture can result in 4 days of unnecessary hospitalization. The most common cause of false-positive blood cultures is inadequate skin preparation. Isopropyl alcohol (70%) should be applied and followed by 2% tincture of iodine or chlorhexidine.

The skin should be allowed to dry before the puncture is performed. Blood should always be drawn from separate sites and not be drawn from intravascular lines, except for the purpose of determining line infection. Ten milliliters should be added to each bottle to achieve a 1/10 dilution of blood. Such a ratio decreases the inhibitory effect on bacterial growth by antibiotics that may be present. The volume of blood is the most important factor in retrieving the pathogen. There is no need to change needles between the blood draw and injecting it into the culture bottle. The addition of resins and other substances to neutralize antibiotics as well as interfering with the inhibitory effects of leukocytes, lysozyme, and complement on bacterial growth are of dubious value [22,23].

Never draw one set of blood cultures because contamination cannot be ruled out, and it is impossible to establish a state of continuous bacteremia. One set of blood cultures is often worse than not drawing any at all.

The significance of a positive blood culture correlates with the following:

1. The organism retrieved-CoNS is significant in the setting of a prosthetic valve but really so in individuals with native valves.
2. Multiple blood cultures that are positive for the same organism. In native valve endocarditis, there is no

advantage in drawing more than three sets of blood cultures. Possible exceptions are in those patients who have received antibiotics. In general, the shorter the incubation time, the more severe the clinical illness.

Techniques such as Melki and matrix-assisted laser desorption/ionization-time of flight (MALDI-TOF) have been developed to allow quicker identification within the same day of the bacteria growth on agar. However, the minimum inhibitory concentration (MIC) susceptibilities for gram-negative and gram-positive isolates will require another 24 hours. Technique does not identify resistant pathogens such as MRSA and extended spectrum beta-lactamase (ESBL) [24].

EMPIRIC THERAPY

Choosing the most appropriate empiric antibiotic therapy of ACCUIE is dependent on making the correct syndromic diagnosis.

Caveats: It is important to distinguish between true acute valvular infection subacute and chronic diseases, which are admitted to the CCU, because of rapid clinical decline.

Vancomycin is regarded by many as clinically inferior to daptomycin or linezolid. Its potential for nephrotoxicity makes it achieve therapeutic levels in patients with fluctuating renal function.

1. Acute IE in normal hosts
   - Usual pathogens: MRSA and MSSA
   - Suggested treatment: Daptomycin 12 mg/kg (IV) every 24 hours or linezolid 600 mg (IV) every 12 hours
2. Intravenous drug abuser IE
   - Usual pathogens: MRSA and MSSA
   - Suggested treatment: Daptomycin 12 mg/kg (IV) every 24 hours or Linezolid 600 mg (IV) every 12 hours.
   - *Pseudomonas aeruginosa*, *Serratia marcescens*, and other gram-negative bacilli. Because valvular infection is much less aggressive with these organisms than that produced by *S. aureus*, one could certainly withhold coverage unless definitively identified by blood cultures.
   - Meropenem 1 g (IV) every 8 hours
3. Early prosthetic valve endocarditis (PVE) (developing within 60 days of implantation)
   - Usual bacterial pathogens: *S. aureus*, coagulase-negative staphylococci
   - Usual pathogens: MRSA and MSSA
4. Late prosthetic valve endocarditis (greater than 60 days after implantation)
   - Usual organisms: *S. viridans* and coagulase-negative staphylococci
   - Usual pathogens: MRSA and MSSA
   - Suggested treatment: Daptomycin 12 mg/kg (IV) every 24 hours or linezolid 600 mg (IV) every

12 hours plus gentamicin 120 mg or 2.5 mg/kg every 24 hours.
5. Nosocomial IE
   - Usual organisms: *S. aureus*, coagulase-negative staphylococci, enterococci, *Streptococcal* spp., and gram-negative bacilli
   - Usual pathogens: MRSA and MSSA
   - Suggested treatment: Daptomycin 12 mg/kg (IV) every 24 hours or linezolid 600 mg (IV) every 12 hours
   - Gram-negative bacilli: Meropenem 1 g (IV) every 8 hours
   - Consider coverage of *Candida* spp: Micafungin 150 or 3 mg/kg (IV) every 24 hours [21]

COMMON COMPLICATIONS OF ACUTE IE

1. Native valve
   Left-sided endocarditis
   a. Intracardiac
      - Refractory CHF: 35%–40%
      - Myocardial septal abscesses
      - Paravalvular abscesses: 35%
   b. Extracardiac
      - Neurological stroke and cerebral abscesses, mycotic aneurysms, spinal cord abscesses
      - Non-neurological infections of prosthetic joints, splenic abscesses
      - Renal kidney infarcts, acute glomerulonephritis, interstitial nephritis, acute cortical necrosis
      - Musculoskeletal: Vertebral osteomyelitis
      - Right-sided endocarditis refer to IVDA IE
2. Intravenous drug abuser ACCUIE
   - Right-sided disease
   - Complications primarily intracardiac, which include right-sided vegetations and septic pulmonary emboli
   - Left-sided disease is similar to that of native valve IE of normal individuals.

PROGNOSIS

Left-sided native valve acute native valve ACCU IE has an all-cause mortality of 25% at 6 months. This is often associated with marked abnormal mental status. Medical therapy, by itself, is a very high failure rate. The rate of mortality determined mainly by the amount of comorbid conditions. It ranges from 7% with one condition to 69% with four underlying conditions.

IVDA IE

Essentially, 100% of uncomplicated infections survive. In those with tricuspid vegetations >2 cm, mortality approximates 33%. It is higher in patients with HIV and with CD4 counts of 200 or less, and in *S. aureus* left-sided endocarditis.

Acute CCU NIE mortality rate over time has decreased for all pathogens from 80% to 35%–56%, except for *S. aureus* infections. The failure to perform indicated cardiac surgery results in a high rate of in hospital stroke, and CHF.

Acute CCU-Associated PVE

Approximately 30% of PVE case do not require surgery. However, surgical intervention is absolutely necessary for *S. aureus* PVE. Major indications for surgery include severe CHF paravalvular abscess and its complications, especially recurrent embolization. Delaying indicated surgery to allow valvular infections to "cool down" only. This leads to worsening infection and poorer outcomes. Such delays are never warranted [25–27].

SUMMARY

During the last 30 years, the nature of IE has markedly changed. *S. aureus* has become the most common cause of IE due to many factors: An aging population; a growing immuno-suppressed population, the epidemic of IVDA, and especially the increasing use of intracardiac and intravascular devices. The primary source of BSI that leads to IE has become the *S. aureus*-infected intravenous catheter (60% of cases). Most cases of ACCUIE are either NIE or HCIE. The diagnosis of these two types of valvular infection is quite challenging. Up to 40% of cases are not properly diagnosed until the end stages of life or after death. They may mimic non-infectious processes. There is a low rate of peripheral manifestations. The tricuspid valve is more frequently involved than the aortic valve. Because valvular infection may have been erroneously attributed to other processes such as pneumonia and urinary tract infections, antibiotics are begun before appropriate blood cultures are drawn.

This discussion has been formulated on syndromic approach to the diagnosis of the patient. It is important for the CCU provider to re-assess patients for NIE or HCIE when they fail to respond to appropriate antibiotic therapy.

REFERENCES

1. Sharma V, Candilio L, Hausenloy DJ. Infective endocarditis: In intensive care perspective. *Trends Anesth Crit Care* 2012;2:36.
2. Martin-Davila P, Fortun J, Navas E, et al. Nosocomial endocarditis in a tertiary hospital: An increasing trend in native valve cases. *Chest* 2005;128:772.
3. Karth GD, Koreny M, Binder T, et al. Complicated infective endocarditis necessitating ICU admission: Clinical course and prognosis. *Critical Care* 2002;6:149.
4. El-Shami K, Griffiths E, Streiff M. Nonbacterial thrombotic endocarditis in cancer patients: Pathogenesis, diagnosis and treatment. *Oncologist* 2007;12:518.
5. Cunha BA. The mimics of endocarditis. In: Brusch JL ed. *Infective Endocarditis: Management in the Era of Intravascular Devices.* New York: InformaHealthcare, 2007.
6. Fernandez–Hildalgo N, Almirante B, Tomos P, et al. Contemporary epidemiology and prognosis of heath care-associated infective endocarditis. *Clin Infect Dis* 2008;47:1287.
7. Pierrotti LC, Baddoural M. Fungal endocarditis, 1995–2000. *Chest* 2002;122:302.
8. Brusch JL. Legionnaire's disease: Cardiac manifestations. *Infect Dis Clin North Am* 2017;31:95.
9. Valles J, Ferrer R. Bloodstream infections in the ICU. *Infect Dis Clin North Am* 2009;23:557.
10. Cahill TJ, Pendegrast BD. Infective endocarditis. *Lancet* 2016;387:882.
11. Wang A, Athan E, PappasPA, et al. Contemporary clinical profile and outcomes of prosthetic valve endocarditis. *JAMA* 2007;2297:1354.
12. Brusch JL. Nosocomial and healthcare–associated infective endocarditis (iatrogenic infective endocarditis) In Brusch JL ed. *Infective Endocarditis: Management in the Era of Intravascular Devices.* New York: InformaHealthcare, 2007.
13. Lepidi H, Durack DT, Raoult D. Diagnostic methods: Current best practices and guidelines for histologic evaluation in infective endocarditis. *Infect Dis Clin North Am* 2002;16:339.
14. Yan ST, Sun LC, JiaB, et al. Procalcitonin levels in blood-stream infections caused by different sources and species of bacteria. *Am J Emer Med* 2017;35:579.
15. Pantelidou IM. Can procalcitonin monitoring reduce the length of antibiotic treatment in bloodstream infections? *Int J Antimicrob Agents* 2015;46 Suppl1:S10.
16. Dinubile M, Calderwood S, Steinhaus DA, et al. Conduction abnormalities complicating native valve endocarditis. *Am J Cardiol* 1986;58;1213.
17. Bruun NE, Habi BG, Thuny F, Sogaard P. Cardiac imaging in infectious endocarditis. *Eur Heart J* 2014;35:624.
18. Jassal DS, Picard MH. Echocardiography. In: Brusch JL ed. *Infective Endocarditis: Management in the Era of Intravascular Devices.* New York: Informa Healthcare, 2007.
19. Kaasch AJ, Jung N. Editorial commentary: Transesophageal echocardiographynin Staphylococcus bloodstream infection-always needed? *Clin Infect Dis* 2015;61:29.
20. Li JS, Sexton DJ, Mick N, et al. Proposed modifications to the Duke criteria for the diagnosis of infective endocarditis. *Clin Infect Dis* 2000;30:633.
21. Baddour LM, Epstein AE, Erickson CC, et al. Update on cardiovascular implantable electronic device infections and their management: A scientific statement from the American Heart Association. *Circulation* 2010;121:458.
22. Bates DW, Lee TH. Rapid classification of positive blood cultures: Prospective validation of a multivariate algorithm. *JAMA* 1992;2607:1962.
23. Prendergast BD. Diagnostic criteria and problems in infective endocarditis. *Heart* 2004;90:611.
24. Shingal N, Kumari M, Virdi JS. MALDI-TOF mass spectrometry: An emerging technology for microbial identification and diagnosis. *Front Microbiol* 2015:791.
25. Leroy O, Georges H, Devos P, et al. Infective endocarditis requiring ICU admission: Epidemiology and prognosis. *Ann Intensive Care* 2015;5(1):45.
26. Grubitzsch H, Christ T, Melzer C, et al. Surgery for prosthetic valve endocarditis associations between morbidity, mortality and costs. *Eur J Cardio Thorac Surg* 2016;22:784.
27. Park LP, Chu VH, Peterson G, et al. Validated risk score or predicting 6-month mortality in infective endocarditis. *J Am Heart Assoc* 2016;18:2016.

20 Diagnostic Approach to Myocarditis in the Critical Care Unit

Shabnam Seydafkan and Jason M. Lazar

CONTENTS

CLINICAL PERSPECTIVE

Acute myocarditis refers to inflammation of the myocardium that can result from multiple infectious and non-infectious etiologies, including viral infection, bacterial infections, tick-borne diseases, and systemic inflammatory disorders, such as acute kidney injury, sarcoidosis, and systemic lupus erythematosus. Although the prevalence of myocarditis in critically ill patients has not been specifically studied in the critical care setting, conditions that predispose to myocarditis are common in such patients, and acute myocarditis likely occurs far more commonly than recognized. Studies evaluating myocarditis from other settings would support a high prevalence of myocarditis in the intensive care and coronary care units. The incidence of myocarditis, reported by the *International Classification of Diseases*, 9th Revision, diagnoses was 22 per 100,000 people or approximately 1.5 million cases in the 2013 world population [1]. Myocarditis is estimated to occur in 5%–15% of common infections. While the majority of cases are presumed to be subclinical, as patients are asymptomatic, acute myocarditis can progress to left ventricular (LV) failure, congestive heart failure, and death. It may also present with ventricular arrhythmias manifesting as sudden cardiac death or even resemble acute myocardial infraction.

CLINICAL PRESENTATION

The majority of cases of acute infectious myocarditis are presumed to be asymptomatic, leaving its true overall incidence and course ill-defined. Alternatively, acute myocarditis may result in congestive heart failure, chest pain syndromes mimicking acute myocardial infarction, and/or arrhythmias. Clinical manifestations are likely variable because viral myocarditis, which accounts for the majority of cases in the United States, is currently viewed to progress in three stages: Acute, which involves direct invasion of an infectious agent into the myocardium, causing myonecrosis; subacute, in which further injury is mediated by autoimmune mechanisms; and chronic, involving diffuse myocardial fibrosis and cardiac dysfunction, leading to dilated cardiomyopathy [2]. Also, because these conditions are more commonly associated with primary myocardial disease, the diagnosis of acute myocarditis poses a challenge in the cardiac care unit.

While the overall prevalence of myocarditis in each of the settings, namely acutely decompensated heart failure, acute chest pain syndromes, and arrhythmias, is unknown, patients with myocarditis likely present with a predominant heart failure presentation most commonly. In the European Study of Epidemiology and Treatment of Cardiac Inflammatory Diseases, the symptoms of myocarditis included dyspnea in 72%, chest pain in 32%, and arrhythmias in 18% of cases [3]. Moreover, myocarditis has been reported to accompany 4%–80% of cases of acute and chronic cardiomyopathy collectively, particularly in those with symptoms of shorter duration [4]. Summary of clinical presentations and course in myocarditis are displayed in Figure 20.1.

Clinical features prompting suspicion of myocarditis in acute heart failure include younger patient age, lack of prior cardiac history, and symptom onset during or immediately following a systemic or viral illness. The illness may present with flu-like symptoms of respiratory or gastrointestinal nature including fever, chills, cough, coryza, myalgia, pharyngitis, anorexia, and diarrhea. In general,

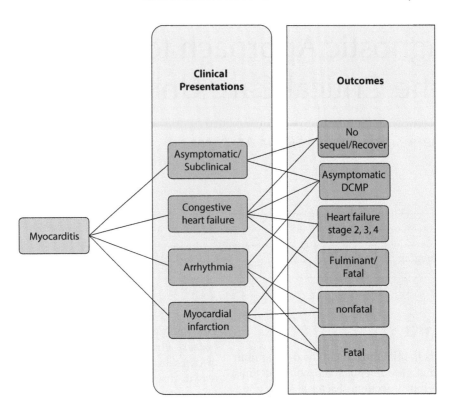

FIGURE 20.1   Clinical presentation and outcome.

patients reporting myalgias during the prodromal illness of a viral syndrome are more likely to have accompanying cardiac involvement [5]. The signs and symptoms of heart failure due to myocarditis are otherwise indistinguishable from other causes of LV dysfunction and include dyspnea, orthopnea, paroxysmal nocturnal dyspnea, and fatigue. Abdominal discomfort related to hepatomegaly and peripheral edema result from right ventricular failure. The duration of symptoms is brief (less than 3 months) in over two-thirds of patients with biopsy-proven myocarditis [4]. Other physical findings include tachycardia disproportionate to the degree of fever, tachypnea, and narrowed pulse pressure from a low cardiac output. Left ventricular failure results in leftward displacement of the apical impulse, the presence of a third and/or fourth heart sound, a systolic murmur of mitral regurgitation, and rales on pulmonary auscultation. Elevation of jugular venous pressure and peripheral edema arise from right-sided failure. In addition, substernal or precordial chest pain occurs in approximately one-third of patients and is likely related to contiguous involvement of the pericardium (myopericarditis). The presence of a pericardial rub supports contiguous pericarditis and along with chest pain is an important clue as to pericardial involvement, which is predictive of future recurrences of myocarditis [6]. Myocarditis can become a chronic progressive disease and is estimated to account for 10%–20% of cases of dilated cardiomyopathy [7]. In 2015, there were approximately 354,000 deaths from myocarditis and cardiomyopathy, with a death rate of 4.8 per 100,000 people [8].

The North American experience in myocarditis has reported more than 50% of patients to experience chronic cardiomyopathy, transplantation, or death more than 5 years following myocarditis [1]. Accordingly, a high index of clinical suspicion is required to pursue and make the diagnosis of myocarditis.

Myocarditis may also present with a variety of supraventricular and ventricular arrhythmias that can be fatal. While post-mortem examination of patients presenting with sudden death has often identified myocarditis as an unexpected cause, the diagnosis is rarely considered in the setting of out of hospital cardiac arrest [9]. It is notable that non-cardiac causes account for 15% of out-of-hospital cardiac arrests, one-third of which have positive blood cultures [9]. Acute myocarditis can also present with chest pain and electrocardiographic changes that mimic acute myocardial infarction. Importantly, myocarditis should be considered in patients presenting with acute coronary syndromes who fulfill the diagnosis of acute myocardial infarction with normal or nonobstructive coronary arteries on coronary angiography. In a meta-analysis including 556 such patients who then went on to undergo cardiac magnetic resonance imaging, 33% had myocarditis. Young age and high C-reactive protein (CRP) levels along with younger age were associated with myocarditis, whereas male sex, hyperlipidemia, high troponin level, and low CRP levels were associated with "true" myocardial infarction [10]. As this clinical scenario is commonly encountered in cardiac care unit patients, acute myocarditis is under-recognized.

ELECTROCARDIOGRAM

The electrocardiogram (ECG) is almost always abnormal in active myocarditis [5,11]. ST-segment and T-wave changes are the most frequent electrocardiographic findings and may be diffuse or focal. ST segment deviation may be depressed or elevated. ST elevations are associated with elevation of troponin and CPK levels, thereby prompting suspicion of recent myocardial infarction. The presence of ST elevation without reciprocal ST depression has been proposed to be useful in differentiating myocarditis [12]. The presence of pathological Q waves may further mimic myocardial infarction. Other ECG findings include conduction abnormalities such as atrioventricular block and bundle branch block. A QTc prolongation 440 ms, an abnormal QRS axis, and ventricular ectopic beats have been associated with poor clinical outcome. A prolonged QRS duration of $\geq$120 ms reflects intraventricular electrical dyssynchrony and is an independent predictor for cardiac death or heart transplantation. Signs of ischemia have no prognostic value for risk stratification [6,13]. Overall, ECG findings are rather non-specific in suspected myocarditis. The chest X-ray may reveal cardiomegaly and pulmonary edema, although myocardial dysfunction may not be apparent on portable films that are taken in the critical care setting.

POTENTIAL CAUSES AND VIRAL SEROLOGY

The causes of acute myocarditis are diverse and include infections (viral, bacterial, and protozoal), toxins, drugs, hypersensitivity, chemical, and physical agents. In Europe and North America, viral infections are the most common causes of myocarditis, and it is estimated that 1%–5% of all patients with acute viral infections may involve the myocardium.

The clinical syndrome of myocarditis was first described in the mid-1800s in patients with mumps and epidemic pleurodynia. Myocarditis was encountered during the influenza A pandemic during the first part of the century. Subsequently, poliovirus became a leading cause of myocarditis; however, its incidence has markedly declined after widespread vaccination efforts. Over the past several decades, the relative frequency of infectious agents causing myocarditis has changed. In the past, the group B Coxsackieviruses were responsible for most cases of documented human disease. Other enteroviruses, including the Coxsackie A and echoviruses, were also important causes of myocarditis as well [14]. While other viruses have been identified through molecular methods, the spectrum of viruses causing disease has changed during recent years. After 1995, the prevalence of enterovirus appears to have decreased while that of adenovirus has increased. In the early-2000s, cases related to Parvovirus-B (PVB19) and Human Herpes Virus-6 (HHV6) spiked, and later in 2007, Hepatitis C Virus (HCV) and Epstein–Barr Virus (EBV) were the most common [15]. In subjects with more chronic symptoms and "inflammatory cardiomyopathy," parvovirus B19 and human herpes virus 6 genomes were predominant [8].

Over the last several decades, HIV and tick-borne (non-viral) infections have emerged as the leading cause of myocarditis. Anti-retroviral therapy has altered the clinical course of HIV-related cardiomyopathy, as most patients exhibit heart failure symptoms, with an only mild reduction of LV ejection fraction [16].

Acute viral infection is typically diagnosed by serological detection of IgM or IgA in the initial sample or recent IgG seroconversion in immuno-enzyme or immunofluorescence assays. In general, serologic proof of acute infection requires a fourfold rise in antibody titer or the detection of virus-specific IgM. However, the interpretation of serologic findings is complicated by the delay from actual infection to clinical presentation when serological determination is made. High background prevalence of viruses such as the Coxsackie B virus IgM is particularly in patients with dilated cardiomyopathy [17] and the lack of correlation between serology findings and detection of viral genome upon endomyocardial biopsy [18,19]. Therefore, determination of viral serology is not routinely recommended, but it is still used with frequency in clinical practice.

Bacterial pathogens are responsible for some cases of myocarditis and reach the myocardium by direct hematogenous spread of microorganisms or by contiguous spread from an infected heart valve. Gonococci, meningococci, *Brucella*, *Salmonella*, staphylococci, and streptococci have all been reported to cause bacterial myocarditis [20]. Bacteria such as *Corynebacterium diphtheriae* and *Clostridium perfringens* elaborate toxins that are directly cytotoxic to myocytes [21]. Other organisms known to cause atypical pneumonias, such as *Mycoplasma pneumoniae*, *Legionella pneumophila*, *Chlamydia pneumoniae*, and *Chlamydia psittaci*, are unusual but known causes of myocarditis. It is underappreciated that isolated myocardial involvement in tuberculosis is rare, but there are reports of sudden cardiac death, atrioventricular block, ventricular arrhythmias, and congestive cardiac failure secondary to tuberculosis [22].

A number of tick-borne diseases have been associated with myocarditis. Lyme disease, which is caused by the spirochete *Borrelia burgdorferi*, is known to cause myocarditis, which usually manifests as conduction disturbances. Infections with rickettsia commonly cause myocarditis as well, e.g., Rocky Mountain spotted fever and scrub typhus [23]. In South America, myocarditis secondary to Chagas disease caused by *Trypanosoma cruzi* is fairly common. The other trypanosome species, *T. gambiense* and *T. rhodesiense*, that cause African sleeping sickness can infect the heart as well. *Trichinella spiralis*, *Toxoplasma gondii*, and *Echinococcus* are causes of myocarditis in developing nations.

Disseminated fungal infections such as aspergillosis, cryptococcosis, and candidiasis have all been reported to result in myocarditis, with the majority occurring in immunocompromised individuals [24]. The infectious causes of myocarditis and the associated clinical and laboratory features are listed in Table 20.1.

In addition to infection, systemic inflammatory disorders such as sarcoidosis, systemic lupus erythematosus (SLE),

TABLE 20.1
The Most Common Etiologies of Acute Myocarditis

Infectious

Viral

Adenoviruses, Echoviruses, Enteroviruses (e.g., Coxsackieviruses), Cytomegalovirus, Epstein–Barr virus, Human Herpesvirus 6, Hepatitis C Virus, Human Immunodeficiency Virus (HIV), Influenza A virus, Parvovirus B19

Bacterial

Chlamydia, Corynebacterium diphtheria, Legionella, Mycobacterium tuberculosis, Mycoplasma, Staphylococcus, Streptococcus A, Streptoccocus pneumoniae

Fungal

Actinomyces, Aspergillus, Candida, Cryptococcus

Parasitic

Toxoplasma gondii, Trypanosoma cruzi

Helminthic

Echinococcus granulosus, Trichinella spiralis

Rickettsial

Coxiella burnetti, Rickettsia typhi

Spirochetal

Borrelia burgdorferi, Leptospira, Treponema pallidum

Non-Infectious

Autoimmune pericarditis

Celiac disease, Churg-Strauss syndrome, Crohn's disease, dermatomyositis, giant cell myocarditis, hypereosinophilic syndrome, Kawasaki disease, lupus erythematodes, lymphofollicular myocarditis, rheumatoid arthritis, sarcoidosis, scleroderma, ulcerative colitis

Drug/toxin-related

Penicillin, ampicillin, cephalosporins, tetracyclines, sulfonamides, antiphlogistics, benzodiazepines, clozapine, loop and thiazide diuretics, methyldopa, smallpox vaccine, tetanus toxoid, tricyclic antidepressants, Amphetamines, anthracyclines, catecholamines, cocaine, cyclophosphamide, 5-fluorouracil, phenytoin, trastuzumab

Toxin: Ethanol

Other substances: Arsenic, copper, iron

Others: Radiotherapy, thyrotoxicosis

and rheumatoid arthritis can induce myocardial inflammation and are also well known to increase the risk for coronary artery disease. Of note, as immune checkpoint inhibitors have emerged as an important treatment modality for various cancers, this class of drug has been reported to cause acute myocarditis in up to 1% of cases [25]. While the exact mechanism is uncertain, cardiotoxicity is felt to be related to activation and infiltration of cytotoxic T-cells into the myocardium and patients with underlying autoimmune disease and diabetes mellitus may be especially prone [25]. A history of checkpoint inhibitor use is important, as such cases may be responsive to steroid therapy.

BIOMARKERS OF INFLAMMATION AND MYOCARDIAL INJURY

Non-specific markers of inflammation, including erythrocyte sedimentation rate and white blood cell count, are neither sensitive nor specific for myocarditis. In the Myocarditis Treatment Trial for acute and subacute forms of myocarditis, leukocytosis was present in one of five patients, and about half had elevated erythrocyte sedimentation rates [26]. Increased white blood cell count and other markers of stronger immune response were associated with more profound cardiac dysfunction presentation. In recent years, CRP determination has been increasingly used to refine cardiovascular risk stratification, as CRP has been identified in coronary atherosclerotic plaque. Levels of CRP, an acute-phase reactant, increase dramatically in response to severe bacterial infection, trauma, and other inflammatory conditions. Although CRP levels are commonly elevated in patients with viral myocarditis [27,28], they are also increased in numerous chronic conditions, thereby limiting specificity. Determination of CRP levels may be advantageous in patients presenting with fulfilling the diagnosis of acute myocardial infarction with normal or non-obstructive coronary arteries on coronary angiography. Among 556 such patients who then underwent cardiac MRI, a high CRP level along with younger age was associated with myocarditis, whereas male sex, treated hyperlipidemia, high troponin ratio, and low CRP were associated with "true" myocardial infarction [10]. In the setting of dilated cardiomyopathy, consideration of CRP raises more questions than answers. Among 66 patients diagnosed with dilated cardiomyopathy that were referred for endomyocardial biopsy, CRP was present in the myocardium in 27% of cases [29]. Myocardial but not serum levels of CRP correlated with other histological markers of inflammation.

Creatine phosphokinase myocardial band (CPK-MB) isoenzyme, a more specific marker of myocyte injury, is quite insensitive in active myocarditis, as only 6% of patients have elevated serum levels [30]. However, the frequency of CPK-MB elevation is higher (approximately 75%) in patients with ST segment elevation on ECG. By comparison, one-third of patients had elevated serum levels of troponin I, another biochemical marker of myocardial injury [30]. Cardiac troponins I and T, regulatory components of the contractile apparatus, are considered sensitive indicators of myocardial injury. Superior sensitivity and specificity of troponins over creatinine phosphokinase led the European Society of Cardiology and American College of Cardiology to long ago redefine acute myocardial infarction based on elevated troponin I or troponin T levels rather than creatinine phosphokinase MB levels [31]. Troponin elevation without the classical peaking pattern of acute myocardial infarction is often the inciting event that prompts suspicion of myocarditis. However, increased use of troponin assays in settings other than acute coronary syndromes has led to the realization that elevated levels reflect myocyte injury and have been associated with adverse outcomes in a variety of disease states, including pulmonary embolism, sepsis, myocarditis, chronic kidney disease, and acute stroke. Elevated troponins in these conditions are felt to reflect myocardial necrosis. Moreover, highly sensitive Tn assays can detect myocardial injury substantially earlier than the previous generation of assays but limit specificity even further. Of note, a recent study reported greater diagnostic accuracy using high-sensitivity troponin T assay with an area under curve of 0.88, a sensitivity of 83%, and specificity of 80%, using a cutoff of 50 ng/L [32]. Given uncertainty as to the clinical course relative to symptom onset, troponin T levels were markedly lower in patients with a history of symptoms longer than 13 days. Also, troponin determination in the setting of myocarditis is further limited in lacking prognostic value [33,34].

ECHOCARDIOGRAPHY

Cardiac imaging modalities such as transthoracic echocardiography and cardiac blood pool imaging may show both diffuse and regional wall motion abnormalities during active myocarditis. Echocardiography has evolved into one of the most commonly used tests in the field of cardiovascular medicine. Its utility, portability, and widespread applicability have led to its routine use in the cardiac care and critical care unit settings. Echocardiography is a non-specific but important component of the diagnostic workup for acute myocarditis and is helpful in suggesting a diagnosis, guiding the acute management, and determining prognosis, as well as differentiating the underlying causes of heart failure such as valvular, congenital, and amyloid heart disease of myocarditis. Classic findings of myocarditis include global hypokinesis with or without pericardial effusion. Segmental wall motion abnormalities can be seen both in myocardial infarction and in myocarditis. In one study, LV dysfunction was found in 69% of patients with biopsy-proven myocarditis and in 88% of patients presenting with congestive heart failure [35]. In most cases of LV dysfunction, the LV was normal in size and not dilated, as expected in other types of cardiomyopathy. Failure of the LV to dilate might be related to decreased ventricular compliance associated with LV hypertrophy, a common echocardiographic and pathological finding in myocarditis. Nevertheless, reduced LV systolic function with normal LV chamber size in the setting of congestive heart failure provides another clue as to the possibility of myocarditis [36]. Left ventricular dysfunction occurs in one-fourth of patients with the right ventricle also normal in size in most cases. Also, echocardiography is highly sensitive in detecting pericardial effusions, which have been reported in as many as 57% of patients with myocarditis [37]. Echocardiography can distinguish fulminant vs. acute myocarditis, using the Felker criteria, as there is usually near-normal LV diastolic dimensions and increased septal thickness secondary to acute myocardial edema in fulminant myocarditis, whereas in acute myocarditis, there is increased diastolic dimension [38]. The LV

function improved significantly in patients with fulminant myocarditis at 6 months as compared with patients with acute myocarditis. Echocardiography can be helpful in predicting prognosis. Presence of right ventricular systolic dysfunction is a powerful independent predictor of death or need for heart transplantation in patients with myocarditis [3,39].

The development of speckle (ultrasound bright spots within the myocardium) tracking software has been a major advancement in echocardiography that allows for the measurement of global longitudinal strain (GLS), an integrated measure of LV myocardial deformation along the longitudinal axis that is more sensitive than LV ejection fraction. Assessment of GLS has shown incremental prognostic value in primary cardiovascular disease states and is clinically used to detect earlier chemotherapy-induced cardiac dysfunction with greater sensitivity. In the setting of myocarditis, several studies have supported GLS measurement in cases of suspected myocarditis. One study found lowered GLS in patients presenting with acute myocarditis and normal LV ejection fraction [40]. Other studies have found the magnitude of regional shortening to correlate with magnetic resonance image findings of necrosis, fibrosis, and myocardial edema [41,42]. In addition to identifying subclinical LV dysfunction, LV longitudinal strain appears to be useful for predicting functional recovery of the left ventricle on follow-up [43].

MAGNETIC RESONANCE IMAGING

Cardiac magnetic resonance imaging (MRI) has emerged as an important non-invasive technique to visualize the inflammatory tissue changes of acute myocarditis, including edema, hyperemia and capillary leakage, necrosis, and fibrosis. Myocardial edema results from cellular inflammation and appears as a regional or global area of high signal intensity in T2-weighted images within the myocardium, relative to that of skeletal muscle. Hyperemia and capillary leakage are detected by contrast images, showing early gadolinium contrast enhancement of the myocardium during the early washout period, and require quantitative analytic techniques. Early gadolinium enhancement results from myocyte membranes damage, allowing for the intravenously administered gadolinium to diffuse into the cells. Necrosis and fibrosis appear as late gadolinium enhancements, particularly in the sub-epicardial region of the left ventricle. The International Consensus Group on Cardiac Magnetic Resonance Diagnosis of Myocarditis developed specific recommendations known as the Lake-Louise criteria for diagnosing myocarditis, which included the use of all three imaging markers [44]. The presence of at least two of the three tissue-based criteria provides a diagnostic accuracy of 78% for the detection of myocardial inflammation. In contrast to echocardiography, MRI can discriminate myocarditis from myocardial infarction. Myocarditis is characterized by mid-wall involvement, sparing the sub-endocardium, whereas in infarction, the sub-endocardium is involved first. Also, the addition of early and late gadolinium enhancement helps distinguish myocarditis from myocardial infarction [45]. Myocarditis exhibits normal first pass perfusion imaging and non-segmental non-subendocardial delayed enhancement (focal or diffuse) predominantly in the inferolateral location. Early segmental subendocardial defects with corresponding segmental subendocardial or transmural delayed high enhancement are characteristic of patients with myocardial infarction. While various sequencing protocols have been developed in order to optimize image acquisition and quality, cardiac MRI also allows for tissue characterization by mapping the myocardium with T1-weighted images for scar and T2-weighted images for edema. T1 and T2 mapping along with evaluation of the extracellular volume fraction has been shown to significantly improve the diagnostic accuracy of cardiac MRI compared with standard Lake-Louise criteria [45,46]. Therefore, a combined MRI approach using T2-weighted imaging, early and late gadolinium enhancement, provides a high diagnostic accuracy that is comparable to endomyocardial biopsy. It has been increasingly relied upon as a useful "go-to" tool in the diagnosis and assessment of patients with suspected acute myocarditis but is limited in patients with acute and chronic kidney disease, for those who are unstable for transport and require continuous hemodynamic monitoring, for patients unable to cooperate, and for those with metal implants.

ENDOMYOCARDIAL BIOPSY

Non-invasive imaging techniques are limited by their inability to distinguish between vial and other subtypes of the immune response. In 2013, the Position Statement of the European Society of Cardiology Working Group on Myocardial and Pericardial Diseases emphasized that endomyocardial biopsy (EMB) is necessary for the final confirmation and accurate classification of myocarditis based on infiltrating cells or histological character of lesions such as lymphocytic or eosinophilic infiltration, giant cell myocarditis (GCM), granulomatous or necrotizing process, and autoimmune features because of the prognostic and therapeutic implications on these categories [47]. The Dallas criteria, proposed in 1986, established that the diagnosis of myocarditis required an inflammatory infiltrate and evidence of myocyte damage and provided the basis for histopathological categorization. However, the Dallas criteria were limited due to sampling errors, variation in expert interpretation, variance with other markers of viral infection and immune activation in the heart, as well as the lack of relevance for management and clinical outcome. In the Myocarditis Treatment Trial, only 64% of cases had the diagnosis of myocarditis confirmed by the expert pathology panel who reviewed the histopathology findings, and there was considerable variability in expert interpretation of myocardial biopsy [26,48]. Moreover, the Dallas criteria did not predict responsiveness to immunosuppression. Accordingly, the

Dallas criteria are currently viewed to be no longer adequate for diagnosis of acute myocarditis. Guidelines suggest the use of EMB to be limited to patients with new-onset heart failure of less than 2 weeks' duration, associated with a normal sized or dilated left ventricle with hemodynamic compromise; to patients with new-onset heart failure of 2 weeks to 3 months' duration with a dilated left ventricle, ventricular arrhythmia, or high-degree atrioventricular blockade; or to patients whose condition fails to respond to treatment in 1–2 weeks [49,50]. Also, the patchy nature of acute inflammation provided high false negatives rates, which makes the yield directly related to the number of biopsy specimens obtained. Using the Dallas criteria, one biopsy specimen provided a 25% yield and five specimens provided a 66% yield [51]. Therefore, the biopsy sampling is now considered adequate if eight or more samples are obtained, but each sampling increases the risk of complications. A recent MRI study used focal imaging abnormalities to guide heart biopsy investigation of possible myocarditis. The authors showed that the earliest myocardial inflammatory abnormalities were evident in the lateral wall of the left ventricle, and only these sites revealed myocarditis by histological examination [52]. At present, parvovirus B19 and adenoviruses are most frequently identified in endomyocardial biopsies [15]. These limitations and the emergence of cardiac MRI have led to the declining use of EMB tissue biopsy at present. Since the treatment of acute myocarditis is still mainly supportive, EMB is presently reserved for when GCM is suspected, as immunotherapy has been shown to improve the survival for patients who deteriorate despite supportive treatment.

In conclusion, the clinical manifestations of acute myocarditis are quite variable, ranging from lack of symptoms to fulminant heart failure, arrhythmias, and sudden cardiac death. This condition is difficult to distinguish from other conditions causing cardiac symptoms, electrocardiographic changes, myocardial enzyme release, and LV dysfunction. While its overall prevalence in critically ill patients is unknown, acute myocarditis likely occurs far more commonly than recognized. The diagnosis can be difficult due to the lack of specificity of test findings, particularly in the cardiac care setting. Cardiac magnetic resonance imaging has emerged as an important imaging modality, as endomyocardial biopsy has been used less commonly because of relatively high complication rates, sampling error, and wide interobserver variability in the interpretation of histology findings.

REFERENCES

1. Cooper LT, Jr., Keren A, Sliwa K, Matsumori A, Mensah GA. The global burden of myocarditis: Part 1: A systematic literature review for the global burden of diseases, injuries, and risk factors 2010 study. *Global Heart* 2014;9:121–129.
2. Caforio AL, Marcolongo R, Basso C, Iliceto S. Clinical presentation and diagnosis of myocarditis. *Heart* 2015; 101(16):1332–1344.
3. Schultz JC, Hilliard AA, Cooper LT, Jr., Rihal CS. Diagnosis and treatment of viral myocarditis. *Mayo Clin Proc* 2009;84:1001–1009.

4. Chow LC, Dittrich HC, Shabetai R. Endocardial biopsy in patients with unexplained congestive heart failure. *Ann Intern Med* 1988;109:535–539.

5. Lewes D, Rainford DJ, Lane WF. Symptomless myocarditis and myalgia in viral and mycoplasma pneumonia infections. *Br Heart J* 1974;36:924–932.

6. Johnson RA, Palacios I. Dilated cardiomyopathies of the adult. *N Engl J Med* 1982;307:1119–1126.

7. Sole MJ, Liu P. Viral myocarditis: A paradigm for understanding the pathogenesis and treatment of dilated cardiomyopathy. *J Am Coll Cardiol* 1993;22:99A–105A.

8. Heymans S, Eriksson U, Lehtonen J, Cooper LT, Jr. The quest for new approaches in myocarditis and inflammatory cardiomyopathy. *J Am Coll Cardiol* 2016;68:2348–2364.

9. Leoni D, Rello J. Cardiac arrest among patients with infections: Causes, clinical practice, and research implications. *Clin Microbiol Infect* 2017;23(10):730–735.

10. Tornvall P, Gerbaud E, Behaghel A, et al. Myocarditis or "true" infarction by cardiac magnetic resonance in patients with a clinical diagnosis of myocardial infarction without obstructive coronary disease: A meta-analysis of individual patient data. *Atherosclerosis* 2015;241(1):87–91.

11. Karjalainen J, Heikkila J. Acute pericarditis: Myocardial enzyme release as evidence for myocarditis. *Am Heart J* 1986;111:546–552.

12. Nakashima H, Honda Y, Katayama T. Serial electrocardiographic findings in acute myocarditis. *Intern Med* 1994;3659–3666.

13. Karjalainen J. Functional and myocarditis-induced T-wave abnormalities. Effect of orthostasis, beta blockade, and epinephrine. *Chest* 1983;83(6):868–874.

14. See DM, Tilles JG. Viral myocarditis. *Rev Infect Dis* 1991;13:951–956.

15. Shauer A, Gotsman I, Keren A, Zwas DR, Hellman Y, Durst R, Admon D. Acute viral myocarditis: Current concepts in diagnosis and treatment. *IMAJ* 2013;15:180–185.

16. Kaplan RC, Hanna DB, Kizer JR. Recent insights into cardiovascular disease (CVD) risk among HIV-infected adults. *Curr HIV/AIDS Rep* 2016;13(1):44–52.

17. Keeling PJ, Lukaszyk A, Poloniecki J, Caforio AL, Davies MJ, Booth JC, McKenna WJ. A prospective case-control study of antibodies to coxsackie B virus in idiopathic dilated cardiomyopathy. *J Am Coll Cardiol* 1994;(23):593–598.

18. Calabrese F, Thiene G. Myocarditis and inflammatory cardiomyopathy: Microbiological and molecular biological aspects. *Cardiovasc Res* 2003;(60):11–25.

19. Mahfoud F, Gärtner B, Kindermann M, et al. Virus serology in patients with suspected myocarditis: Utility or futility? *Eur Heart J* 2011;32(7):897–903.

20. Knowlton KU, Savoia MC, Oxman MN. Myocarditis, Pericarditis. In: Mandell GL, Bennett JE, Dolin R eds. *Principles and practice of infectious diseases*. Cambridge, MA, 2009:1153–1172.

21. Gore I. Myocardial changes in fatal diphtheria: A summary of observations in 221 cases. *Am J Med Sci* 1948;215:257–266.

22. Cowley A, Dobson L, Kurian J, Saunderson C. Acute myocarditis secondary to cardiac tuberculosis: A case report. *Echo Res Pract* 2017;4:K25–K29.

23. Nontrowitz NE, Smith RH. Myocarditis update. *Emerg Med* 1993;25:69–74.

24. Atkinson JB, Connor DH, Robinowitz M, McAllister HA, Virmani R. Cardiac fungal infections: Review of autopsy findings in 60 patients. *Hum Pathol* 1984;15:935–942.

25. Ganatra S, Neilan TG. Immune checkpoint inhibitor-associated myocarditis. *Oncologist* 2018;23(8):879–886.

26. Mason JW, O'Connell JB, Hershkowitz A, Rose NR, McManus BM, Billingham ME, Moon TE. A clinical trial of immunosuppressive therapy for myocarditis. *N Eng J Med* 1995;333:269–275.

27. Guo JG. Detection of cardiac troponin and high-sensitivity C reactive protein in children with viral myocarditis. *Nan Fang Yi Ke Da Xue Xue Bao* 2008;28(6):1076–1077.

28. Kawamura K, Kitaura Y, Morita H, Deguchi H, Kotaka M. Viral and idiopathic myocarditis in Japan: A questionnaire survey. *Heart Vessels Suppl* 1985;1:18–22.

29. Zimmermann O, Bienek-Ziolkowski M, Wolf B, Vetter M, Baur R, Mailänder V, Hombach V, Torzewski J. Myocardial inflammation and non-ischaemic heart failure: Is there a role for C-reactive protein? *Basic Res Cardiol* 2009;104(5):591–599.

30. Smith SC, Ladenson JH, Mason JW, Jaffe AS. Elevations of cardiac Troponin I associated with myocarditis. *Circulation* 1997;95:163–168.

31. Korff S, Katus HA, Giannitsis E. Differential diagnosis of elevated troponins. *Heart* 2006;92(7):987–993.

32. Ukena C, Kindermann M, Mahfoud F, et al. Diagnostic and prognostic validity of different biomarkers in patients with suspected myocarditis. *Clin Res Cardiol* 2014;103:743–751.

33. Imazio M, Brucato A, Barbieri A, et al. Good prognosis for pericarditis with and without myocardial involvement: Results from a multicenter, prospective cohort study. *Circulation* 2013;128:42–49.

34. Gilotra NA, Minkove N, Bennett MK, Tedford RJ, Steenbergen C, Judge DP, Halushka MK, Russell SD. Lack of relationship between serum cardiac troponin I level and giant cell myocarditis diagnosis and outcomes. *J Card Fail* 2016;22(7):583–585.

35. Pinamonti B, Alberti E, Cigalotto A, Dreas L, Salvi A, Silvestri F, Camerini F. Echocardiographic findings in myocarditis. *Am J Cardiol* 1988;62:285–291.

36. Laissey JP, Hyafil F, Juliard JM, Schouman-Claeys E, Steg PG, Faraggi M. Differentiating acute myocardial infarction from myocarditis: Diagnostic value of early-and delayed-perfusion cardiac MR imaging. *Radiology* 2005;237:75–82.

37. Carniel E, Sinagra G, Bussani R, Di Lenarda A, Pinamonti B, Lardieri G, Silvestri F. Fatal myocarditis: Morphologic and clinical features. *Ital Heart J* 2004;5:702–706.

38. Felker GM, Boehmer JP, Hruban RH, Hutchins GM, Kasper EK, Baughman KL, Hare JM. Echocardiographic findings in fulminant and acute myocarditis. *J Am Coll Card* 2000;36:227–232.

39. Dominguez F, Kuhl U, Pieske B, Garcia-Pavia P, Tschope C. Update on myocarditis and inflammatory cardiomyopathy: Reemergence of endomyocardial biopsy. *Revista Espanola de Cardiologia* 2016;69:178–187.

40. Di Bella G, Carerj S, Recupero A, et al. Left ventricular endocardial longitudinal dysfunction persists after acute myocarditis with preserved ejection fraction. *Echocardiography* 2018;35(12):1966–1973.

41. Leitman M, Vered Z, Tyomkin V, Macogon B, Moravsky G, Peleg E, Copel L. Speckle tracking imaging in inflammatory heart diseases. *Int J Cardiovasc Imaging* 2018;34(5):787–792.

42. Logstrup BB, Nielsen JM, Kim WY, Poulsen SH. Myocardial edema in acute myocarditis detected by echocardiographic 2D myocardial deformation analysis. *Eur Heart J Cardiovasc Imaging* 2016;17(9):1018–1026.

43. Luetkens JA, Petry P, Kuetting D, Dabir D, Schmeel FC, Homsi R, Schild HH, Thomas D. Left and right ventricular strain in the course of acute myocarditis: A cardiovascular magnetic resonance study. *RöFo* 2018;190(8):722–732.

44. Friedrich MG, Sechtem U, Schulz-Menger J, et al. International Consensus Group on Cardiovascular Magnetic Resonance in Myocarditis: A JACC White Paper. *J Am Coll Cardiol* 2009;(53):1475–1487.

45. Roller FC, Harth S, Schneider C, Krombach GA. T1, T2 mapping and extracellular volume fraction (ECV): Application, value and further perspectives in myocardial inflammation and cardiomyopathies. *RöFo* 2015;187(9):760–770.

46. Radunski UK, Lund GK, Stehning C, Schnackenburg B, Bohnen S, Adam G, Blankenberg S, Muellerleile K. CMR in patients with severe myocarditis: Diagnostic value of quantitative tissue markers including extracellular volume imaging. *JACC Cardiovasc Imaging* 2014;7(7):667–675.

47. Krejci J, Mlejnek D, Sochorova D, Nemec P. Inflammatory cardiomyopathy: A current view on the pathophysiology, diagnosis, and treatment. *BioMed Res Int* 2016;2016:4087632.

48. Shanes JG, Ghali J, Billingham ME, et al. Interobserver variability in the pathologic interpretation of endomyocardial biopsy results. *Circulation* 1987;75:401–405.

49. Kuhl U, Schultheiss HP. Viral myocarditis. *Swiss Med Wkly* 2014;144:W14010.

50. Cooper LT, Baughman KL, Feldman AM, et al. The role of endomyocardial biopsy in the management of cardiovascular disease: A scientific statement from the American Heart Association, the American College of Cardiology, and the European Society of Cardiology endorsed by the Heart Failure Society of America and the Heart Failure Association of the European Society of Cardiology. *Eur Heart J* 2007;28:3076–3093.

51. Chow LH, Radio SJ, Sears TD, McManus BM. Insensitivity of right ventricular endomyocardial biopsy in the diagnosis of myocarditis. *J Am Coll Cardiol* 1989;14:915–920.

52. Hauck AJ, Kearney DL, Edwards WD. Evaluation of postmortem endomyocardial biopsy specimens from 38 patients with lymphocytic myocarditis: Implications for role of sampling error. *Mayo Clin Proc* 1989;64:1235–1245.

21 Intra-Abdominal Surgical Infections and Their Mimics in the Critical Care Unit

Donald E. Fry

CONTENTS

Severe intra-abdominal infection (IAI) is a common diagnosis for patients in the critical care unit (CCU). The typical patient will have had a perforated viscus and will have been to the operating room, where the source of the infection has been managed by resection, plication, or exteriorization. Drainage and debridement will have been a likely requirement in the operation. Antibiotics will have been started. Because of the severity of the infection, or because of the presence of co-morbid conditions that represent major risk factors for patient survival, management of the patient will require critical care management by qualified intensivists for recovery. Effective CCU management will require effective antibiotic selection, appropriate supportive care of the physiologic changes associated with IAI, and timely decisions about abscess or failure of suture lines.

A less common scenario is the surgical patient that has not had IAI but is in the CCU for management of other major surgical interventions. These patients may then have a spontaneous perforation as a complication from the original procedure that leads to hospital-acquired IAI. This unanticipated IAI is not suspected and requires an astute intensivist to recognize that IAI is present. Hospital-acquired IAI becomes especially challenging for source control of the offending event and also because of the unique challenges of antimicrobial therapy.

PATHOPHYSIOLOGY AND DIFFERENTIAL DIAGNOSES OF IAI

Intra-abdominal infection customarily begins with peritonitis. The peritoneum covers the parietal surface of abdominal cavity and the visceral surface of most abdominal organs. The peritoneal surface has been measured to be 1.4 m^2 and approximates the equivalent of 80% of the skin area of the adult [1]. The peritoneal sac is typically sterile and has a small volume of peritoneal fluid, which is an ultrafiltrate of human plasma from hydrostatic tissue pressure of visceral perfusion.

The peritoneal fluid is cleared by lymphatic fenestrations on the abdominal surface of the diaphragm [2]. The piston-like actions of the diaphragm with normal ventilation creates a negative pressure, which results in movement of fluid toward the upper abdominal for clearance into the lymphatic system of the thoracic duct [3]. With perforation of an abdominal viscus, the natural movement of this fluid results in the dissemination of microbial infection throughout the peritoneal space and creates movement of pathogens toward the diaphragm. Infection occurs with microbial dissemination, adherence of pathogens to the peritoneal mesenchymal cells, and activation of the inflammatory response. The sequelae of the inflammatory response in community-acquired IAI results in the physical findings of rebound abdominal tenderness, gastrointestinal ileus, fever, leukocytosis, tachycardia, tachypnea, and fluid redistribution from inflammation, with associated volume depletion. In the setting of hospital-acquired IAI, painful abdominal incisions will masquerade newly identified abdominal pain, and narcotic analgesia or sedation will make these new-onset events in the CCU setting less apparent.

Intra-abdominal infection is a constellation of many different diseases that arise from different anatomic areas and with different pathogenic microbes [4]. Intra-abdominal infection is either intra- or extra-peritoneal in domain. Intra-peritoneal infection may uncommonly arise as *primary peritonitis*, where patients with abnormal volumes of intraperitoneal fluid (e.g., ascites) have seeding of the peritoneal space by hematogenous or lymphatic-borne bacteria from a remote site [5]. Primary peritonitis is managed with medical therapy only. Primary peritonitis may result in an exploratory laparotomy and will result in post-operative CCU management. Rarely, primary peritonitis may occur in surgical patients as a hospital-acquired event following other surgical interventions and should be kept in mind for the patient that has ascites from pre-existent liver disease. *Secondary peritonitis* is the most common IAI for surgical patients and occurs from perforation of a primary gastrointestinal disease process (e.g., diverticulitis) and resultant infection in the peritoneal space [6]. Secondary peritonitis is usually the cause of admission to the CCU for IAI patients but, as stated earlier, can occur as a complication among both surgical and medical patients who did not have any infection present at admission. *Tertiary peritonitis* is failed management of secondary peritonitis with complex intra-abdominal abscess or a persistent infection with a thick fibrino-purulent process that extends across the surface of the parietal and visceral peritoneum [7]. Tertiary peritonitis is commonly managed with an open abdomen. Other sources of IAI include those secondary to pathogens, introduced from either peritoneal dialysis catheters [8] or surgical drains that have provided conduits for environmental microbes to access the peritoneal cavity. Finally, extra-peritoneal IAI may be identified in the peri-pancreatic or peri-nephric area and can prove difficult to diagnose and manage.

Any one of these different sources of IAI will present with the usual non-specific symptoms. For the intensivist or infectious disease consultant, the diagnosis of postoperative secondary peritonitis is known from the operating room findings. Medical management of the infection and monitoring the progress of the patient become the principal objectives of care. The diagnostic dilemma in these patients evolves when patients have continued fever and leukocytosis and a failure to promptly resolve the IAI after operation and appropriate antibiotics. Abscess formation or technical failures of the surgical intervention require a sophisticated approach for effective management.

When leaking anastomoses or abdominal abscess is suspected, conventional physical examination is of limited value. Most of these patients will have a recent abdominal incision that makes the recognition of localized or rebound tenderness problematic. Most of these patients will be on narcotic pain control, or sedation for ventilator-dependent patients will further compromise the abdominal examination. Elderly patients, those with chronic illnesses, and those on immunosuppressive medications will also have a blunted host response. C-reactive protein, erythrocyte sedimentation rates, and procalcitonin concentrations are biomarkers that can identify the presence of severe inflammation but lack the specificity to differentiate the source of IAI or whether IAI is the actual cause [9]. All patients will usually have leukocytosis and varying degrees of hypoalbuminemia. Blood cultures for likely pathogens are useful when positive, but pyogenic infections infrequently lead to bacteremia, especially in patients receiving broad-spectrum antibiotics in the CCU [10]. Evolving organ dysfunction from pulmonary failure, renal failure, elevated liver enzymes, and coagulopathy may indicate that presence of sepsis but will not differentiate IAI from other non-abdominal sources of infection.

The mainstay of diagnosis for the IAI patient is computerized tomography (CT) with contrast. Intravenous and intraluminal contrast permits differentiation of fluid collections from intraluminal air-fluid levels. Intravenous contrast may provide enhancement of the inflammatory margin about the abscess collection (Figure 21.1). The anatomic precision and timeliness of the CT scan have made it the diagnostic method

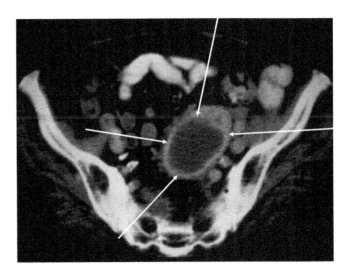

FIGURE 21.1   A CT scan of a postoperative abscess. The use of intravenous contrast demonstrates the enhancement of the inflammatory perimeter (arrows) about the abscess collection.

of choice for the patient suspected of abscess or technical failure of abdominal suture lines [11]. The CT scan permits the use of percutaneous drainage methods to manage many of the identified abscess collections. Other imaging techniques, including ultrasound and radioscintigraphy (gallium-67), have been used in the past but do not have the accuracy of the CT scan [12]. Magnetic resonance imaging has also been used but generally does not have better results that the CT scan.

INFECTION MIMICS OF IAI

The CCU patients have multiple different potential hospital-acquired infections, and the post-laparotomy patients with IAI are particularly vulnerable for these additional sites. Intercurrent infectious "mimics" may give the impression that abdominal infection is not resolving when the clinical syndrome of persistent infection is due to a second cause. Non-laparotomy surgical patients in the CCU may have these other infectious complications that give the impression that new IAI is developing by presenting symptoms that are deceiving. *Ventilator-associated pneumonia* (VAP) is a common secondary infection in the IAI patient because of the environmental contamination of the airway, barotrauma that increases lung vulnerability to secondary infection, and the pulmonary dysfunction and edema associated with the systemic consequences of the IAI process itself. The VAP results in a clinical syndrome of septicemia that is not unlike the underlying IAI process [13], and chest roentgenograms will have changes in the patient on the ventilator that cannot be visually differentiated from pneumonia. Abdominal distention and intestinal ileus commonly accompany VAP, and uncertainty about continued IAI or infection in the lung will be a clinical conundrum. High-pressure ventilatory support has been associated with pneumoperitoneum and may mislead the clinician that an intra-abdominal perforation is present [14]. Also, both VAP and IAI can be present synchronously in the patient.

The presence of VAP requires bronchoalveolar lavage both for diagnosis of ≥10^4 organisms/mL and for the identification of the pathogen [15]. *Urinary tract infection* may lead to pyelonephritis and even perinephric abscess as complications of urinary catheter drainage in IAI patients. *Intravenous central catheter-associated bloodstream infections* are risks for the CCU patient with an indwelling subclavian or peripheral indwelling central catheter who is being treated for IAI. Also, when abdominal incisions have been primarily closed, the intensivist cannot overlook *deep surgical site infections* as a cause of a continued septic syndrome, especially in the obese patient. Careful clinical evaluation of the surgical site is always warranted in the surgical patient with infection that has not been defined.

Finally, the infection mimic of IAI of considerable concern is *Clostridium difficile* infection. Endogenous or environmentally transmitted spores of this pathogen, when provided the altered microbiome of the colon under conditions of critical illness and extensive antibiotic administration, will result in non-specific signs and symptoms in the CCU patient [16]. Abdominal distention with cramping abdominal pain is common. Elderly patients and those on extensive opioid treatment for pain may not manifest the characteristic diarrhea symptoms of this infectious complication. The abdomen will be distended, and tenderness may or may not be present. A high index of suspicion for this complication requires studies of stool toxin assays or diagnostic polymerase chain reaction studies for implementation of specific antibiotic therapy [17]. Failure to identify and treat this infection will lead to colonic necrosis and perforation.

NON-INFECTIOUS MIMICS OF IAI

Abdominal pain and distention are common observations in postoperative surgical patients in the CCU who may or may not represent poorly responsive and persistent infection or in patients with new hospital-acquired IAI. Ileus following laparotomy management may persist and intensify, as volume resuscitation increases the edema in the intestinal tissues and coordinated peristalsis has not returned after surgical manipulation. The abdominal distention increases the tangential stress on the abdominal wall and the pain that is experienced by the patient. The tense postoperative abdomen will have rebound tenderness not because of infection but due to the tension on the incision. The increased abdominal pressure may evolve into an *abdominal compartment syndrome* that creates respiratory distress and may even impair kidney function, especially in those patients who have had a large volume of resuscitation fluids [18]. In these circumstances, it is the abdominal compartment syndrome that is the cause of the organ-failure syndromes and not invasive infection. Decompression of the abdomen may be necessary to manage the compartment syndrome that is associated with the increased pressure that has developed in the closed abdomen with severe inflammation [19]. Similarly, elderly surgical patients may experience *acute colonic pseudo-obstruction* (Ogilvie's syndrome) with the presence

of massive distention of the colon because of severe illness and opioids for pain management. The clinician can easily become concerned that surgically treatable IAI is present because of the pain and tenderness from tension on the recent incision. Neostigmine has been successfully used in the treatment of these patients [20]. Mechanical decompression or cecostomy may occasionally be necessary to avoid cecal perforation from the distended colon.

Ischemic injuries to abdominal contents may be associated with abdominal pain and distention. Hypovolemia and anemia can result in ischemic injury and transmural necrosis of colonic structures that will lead to IAI, if not recognized and managed. Embolic and non-occlusive ischemic injury can affect large and small bowel. Embolic events require a high index of suspicion for the elderly patient, usually with generalized vascular disease. The diagnosis of embolic occlusion will usually require CT angiography [21]. If peritoneal signs are present, the mesenteric ischemia from emboli may require prompt surgical intervention without further diagnostic efforts if success is to be achieved.

While debate continues about the genesis of *acalculous cholecystitis*, it is likely to be an ischemic injury of the gallbladder wall that is the combination of splanchnic vascular disease and increased intraluminal pressure within the gallbladder lumen from poor bile transport. It is associated with right upper quadrant pain but no gallstones. Physical findings of rebound tenderness may be present, but most patients have altered sensorium, are on ventilatory support, and have sedation/opioids that suppress responsiveness. These patients are recognized with gallbladder distention on ultrasound examination of the right upper quadrant but without the presence of calculi. A high index of suspicion is necessary to promptly identify non-calculous cholecystitis. Either percutaneous decompression or removal of the gallbladder is necessary for management to avoid the sustained ischemia and gallbladder perforation from increased intraluminal pressure [22]. Medical management alone is not sufficient. Failure to recognize acalculous cholecystitis leads to transmural gangrenous changes and perforation into the abdomen cavity.

Postoperative *acute pancreatitis* causes abdominal pain, distention, and rebound tenderness that might be interpreted as acute IAI. This complication is most commonly seen following biliary, pancreatic, and gastric surgical procedures. Drug-associated pancreatitis and idiopathic episodes of pancreatitis can occur following any procedure. The severe inflammation of the retroperitoneal space will result in the systemic inflammatory response syndrome without infection. Tachypnea, tachycardia, fever, leukocytosis, lactic acidosis, acute respiratory failure, oliguria, and hypotension are identified and have the appearances of a septic syndrome but without infection. Aggressive volume replacement, with maintenance of systemic perfusion and oxygenation, is essential, but antibiotics are not part of the management [23]. Severe acute pancreatitis will have secondary microbial contamination of the inflamed retroperitoneum, and a necrotizing infectious pancreatitis and abscess can be the result. Selected cases of severe pancreatitis with an associated systemic inflammatory response may require percutaneous aspiration of peripancreatic fluid to determine whether infection is present and if antibiotics are needed. Severe necrotizing infection of the pancreas and associated lesser sac space comprise a severe illness with dense purulent material and sloughed pancreatic tissue that will require a carefully timed open surgical debridement [24].

FAILED INITIAL TREATMENT OF IAI

The usual scenario of IAI in the surgical patient in the CCU begins with the diagnosis of secondary peritonitis, and the patient undergoes an abdominal operation for control of the source of infection. Especially with fecal peritonitis, the patient is then transferred to the CCU for continued care. Volume resuscitation is essential to maintain systemic perfusion and oxygenation. Many of these patients will require ventilator support to achieve adequate oxygenation.

Empirical antibiotic selections are made to cover the likely pathogens to be participating in the infection. Antibiotic selections should be consistent with recent guidelines by the Surgical Infection Society [25] and the World Society of Emergency Surgery [26], both of which provide very similar recommendations for specific selections (Table 21.1). For community-acquired colonic perforations, the enteric gram-negative rods (e.g., *E. coli*) and anaerobic species (e.g., *Bacteroides fragilis*) must be covered with a single antibiotic choice (piperacillin-tazobactam) or a combination therapy with a broad-spectrum cephalosporin (e.g., ceftriaxone) and metronidazole as a reasonable choice. Some have recommended empirical coverage of *Enterococcus* sp., but evidence to support this addition is limited for the initial management of community-acquired IAI. Dosing strategies should be aggressive, since these patients will have an expanded volume of distribution, and a hyperdynamic circulation that may make conventional dosing inadequate because of rapid drug elimination. Confirmation of the pathogens by cultures when gross fecal peritonitis is present is not necessary, since failure to recover anaerobic species in such a circumstance is common and does not justify discontinuation of anaerobic coverage [27].

While there is a general agreement about which antibiotics should be selected for empirical treatment, there continues to be a debate about the *duration* of therapy of community-acquired IAI. A recent prospective, randomized trial (STOP-IT) demonstrated that 4 days of appropriate antibiotics are sufficient when compared with longer courses [28]. The clinical evidence demonstrates that progressive clinical improvement at this point justifies discontinuation of antibiotic therapy. When patients have not responded to normalization of vital signs, fever, and leukocytosis at 4 days, then patients need to be evaluated for abdominal abscess as the cause for continued infection. Deterioration of the patient's clinical condition even earlier than the 4-day postoperative threshold indicates that source control may have been inadequate and imaging studies are needed.

As noted earlier, CT scanning of the abdomen with contrast is the reliable method for the establishment of abscess and undrained infection. Abscesses tend to be identified in the physiologic drainage basins of the abdominal cavity, which are the sub-diaphragmatic space, the sub-hepatic space, the lateral pericolic gutters, and the pelvis [29]. Purulent collections

---

TABLE 21.1

The Recommendations for Antibiotic Choices in the Treatment of Community-Acquired Intra-Abdominal Infections by the Surgical Infection Society of North America

Drug Choice	Comments
Ertapenem	Recommended for low-risk patients; long elimination half-life favors twice-daily dosing
Moxifloxacin	Recommended for low-risk patients; fluoroquinolones are recommended for patients with hypersensitivity to β-lactam drugs
Piperacillin/tazobactam	Recommended for higher-risk patients; long record of use in IAI; requires 6-hour dosing schedule
Doripenem	Recommended for higher-risk patients; addition of ampicillin or vancomycin for severe sepsis or septic shock should be considered
Imipenem-cilastatin	Recommended for higher-risk patients
Meropenem	Recommended for higher-risk patients; addition of ampicillin or vancomycin for severe sepsis or septic shock should be considered
Cefotaxime plus metronidazole	Recommended for low-risk patients; cefuroxime has been substituted for cefotaxime but has less supportive data
Ceftriaxone plus metronidazole	Recommended for low-risk patients; long half-life of ceftriaxone favors twice-daily dosing
Ciprofloxacin plus metronidazole	Recommended for low-risk patients; fluoroquinolones are recommended for patients with hypersensitivity to β-lactam drugs
Cefepime plus metronidazole	Recommended for higher-risk patients; addition of ampicillin or vancomycin for severe sepsis or septic shock should be considered
Aztreonam plus metronidazole plus vancomycin	Recommended for higher-risk patients; this is an option for patients with hypersensitivity to β-lactams but is less well supported by data

Source: Mazuski, J.E. et al., *Surg. Infect.*, 18, 1–76, 2017.

are identified in the dependent areas of the abdominal cavity and are influenced by the forces of gravity. Exceptions will be the abdomen that has had multiple previous operations, where false dependencies are created from adhesion formation. In these latter circumstances, abscess can be identified in virtually any location, including sub-fascial and interloop collections. Effective contrast permits resolution of all anatomic structures and greatly facilitates percutaneous drainage methods. The accuracy of CT-directed drainage has greatly reduced the need for open reoperation and its attendant complications of intestinal fistula and surgical wound morbidity.

Patients may still require an open surgical reoperation for abscess, even in the era of CT-directed percutaneous drainage [30]. Abscesses may be in locations that cannot be accessed without transgressing other anatomic structures. Abscesses may be in multiple locations and logistically cannot be drained. Percutaneous drainage may not be followed by clinical resolution of the infection, in which case a failed suture line, non-dependency of the drain, or loculations within the abscess cavity requires an open approach. The open exploration may require management of the abdominal cavity by leaving the fascia open and local management of the open abdominal cavity in the days and weeks that follow. This open abdomen will often have a thick fibrinopurulent exudate across the surface of the abdominal contents, is commonly described as tertiary peritonitis, and requires frequent local debridement and carefully performed dressing changes to avoid intestinal fistula as a complication.

Drainage of abscess, whether by open or percutaneous methods, requires that culture and sensitivity data be obtained from the infection site [31]. The effects of resistant pathogens persisting in the IAI may be an effect, and the consequences of hospital-acquired pathogens from drains and other sources may account for resistant or unusual pathogens that will require alternative antibiotic choices to accompany source control. Pathogens that are seen in failed treatment of IAI include resistant gram-negative pathogens, *Enterococcus* sp., methicillin-resistant *Staphylococcus aureus* or *epidermidis*, *Pseudomonas aeruginosa*, and even *Candida* sp. These resistant pathogens are particularly prevalent in the patient who requires multiple drainage episodes and in the patient with tertiary peritonitis. Expanded-spectrum carbapenem and vancomycin are commonly used in these circumstances, but antibiotic selection needs to be tailored to culture and sensitivity results, including the use of antifungal therapy if needed.

CCU-ACQUIRED IAI

Intra-abdominal infection in the CCU is usually from an infection that was the cause of patient admission. However, patients will have events that result in the occurrence of a new IAI as a complication during the CCU admission. These patients may have been elective gastrointestinal operations that had a suture line leak during the CCU stay, with subsequent infection. These CCU-acquired infections may have been the result of spontaneous perforations or ischemic events that resulted in secondary infections.

In the CCU-acquired IAI, patients may have major risk factors that included shock, hypoxia, extended surgical procedures, and comorbid conditions that have led to critical care management. The aggregate effect of these risk factors, combined with the surgical stress of a major operation, can lead to perforation and IAI, even in those patients without abdominal surgery. The superimposition of acute bacterial peritonitis as a complication of care in the CCU is a very morbid event with a high-risk of fatal outcome.

Failed suture lines with gastrointestinal leaks are reported to occur in 3%–6% of cases following resections [32]. Colonic suture line leaks are more common than other locations in the intestinal tract. Rectosigmoid suture lines are more likely to leak than elsewhere in the colon because of poorer pelvic blood supply from the inferior mesenteric artery, greater risks of suture line tension for anastomoses in the pelvis, and the greater number of intraluminal bacteria resulting in infection of the suture line [33]. All patients in the CCU with recent surgical suture lines in the abdomen should have an index of suspicion for this complication.

When patients have had recent laparotomy, the abdominal examination is infrequently helpful in the diagnosis of a leak because of the recent abdominal incision. The acute onset of fever and leukocytosis and the new onset of gastrointestinal ileus following a seemingly uneventful early postoperative course suggest that an untoward event has occurred. Abdominal CT imaging with contrast is essential to identify leaks in the intestinal track. Suture line leaks that are not loculated but are free into the peritoneal cavity require immediate reoperation. Extravasation from a suture line that is wall-off may be amenable to percutaneous drainage in selected cases, depending on the severity of the patient's response to the infection.

Another case of IAI in the postoperative laparotomy patient is the perforation of an injured dissection site on the intestine. Adhesions of the intestine are common among patients with prior laparotomy, and unappreciated transmural injury of serosal injury with delayed perforation does occur as an unexplained cause of IAI. As with other causes, CT scanning with contrast will provide the best information with free-air or extravasated contrast to confirm perforation and the need for surgical intervention.

Spontaneous perforations of the gastrointestinal tract with new-onset IAI among CCU patients are uncommon. Perforations of acute stress-induced gastroduodenal ulcer were more common in the era prior to the perioperative use of histamine-antagonists and proton-pump inhibitors. It is likely that contemporary critical care management with improved oxygenation and perfusion has also diminished the role of ischemia in the so-called stress ulceration and acute perforation of past decades. While uncommon, acute gastroduodenal perforation from acute ulceration may be the cause, with acute abdominal pain and distention in the surgical patient following major procedures. The patients will usually have fever and leukocytosis, but these findings may be obscured in the setting of corticosteroid or other immunosuppressive treatments. The classic finding was the identification of free-air under the diaphragm on the upright chest roentgenogram. Plain abdominal radiographic studies are uncommon in current management, but free-air and/or extravasation of contrast with the abdominal CT scan confirms the diagnosis. Surgical intervention is necessary for source control of the perforation.

An uncommon spontaneous intestinal perforation is secondary to cytomegalovirus infection in patients with advanced HIV disease who have undergone operation [34]. Symptoms are similar to those of perforated ulcers, but the immunosuppressed condition of these patients will obscure clinical findings. Acute clinical deterioration and abdominal distention with or without rebound tenderness will lead to a CT scan and the diagnosis of perforation. Prompt surgical repair is necessary in this highly morbid complication.

Complications of the mimics of the IAIs discussed previously are a cause of new infection in the abdominal cavity that must be identified and managed. Toxic megacolon from advanced *C. difficile* infection can result in ischemic perforation if the primary infection is not recognized and promptly treated. Ogilvie's syndrome can lead to perforation of the cecum from increased intraluminal pressure when not preemptively managed. Gangrenous cholecystitis with perforation and IAI can result when acalculous cholecystitis is not identified and transmural ischemia of the gallbladder wall leads to perforation. In all these circumstances, the surgical patient in the CCU will have a common clinical pathway of acute deterioration, abdominal distention, and tenderness, as well as characteristic findings of fever and leukocytosis. Immediate open surgical intervention is necessary to avoid deaths from these complications. Clinical awareness and vigilance for these "mimics" of IAI can lead to prompt management and avoidance of the perforative events.

In summary, IAI is a common reason for patients to be admitted to the CCU for sustained management until the infection has resolved. Failure of these patients to respond to appropriate initial source control and systemic antibiotics indicates that a search for abscess or technical failures of the initial operation must be pursued. Abscess collections can be percutaneously drained in most cases with CT imaging. Unfortunately, IAI can occur as a new event among surgical and medical CCU patients. The CCU-acquired perforations require open surgical intervention. The mimics of IAI must be remembered, and their appropriate management is required for the desired patient outcomes. Antibiotic therapy for the patient with community-acquired IAI must target aerobic gram-negative rods and enteric anaerobic bacteria. Patients with abscess or tertiary peritonitis following the treatment of secondary peritonitis and those patients with a hospital-acquired perforation as the cause of IAI will have hospital-acquired microflora. Antibiotic selection must have quality culture and sensitivity information to direct appropriate management in the era of highly resistant-organisms from the healthcare environment.

REFERENCES

1. Albanese AM, Albanese EF, Miño JH, et al. Peritoneal surface area: Measurements of 40 structures covered by peritoneum: Correlation between total peritoneal surface area and the surface calculated by formulas. *Surg Radiol Anat* 2009;31:369–377.
2. Tsilibary EC, Wissig SL. Absorption from the peritoneal cavity: SEM study of the mesothelium covering the peritoneal surface of the muscular portion of the diaphragm. *Am J Anat* 1977;149:127–132.
3. Autio V. The spread of intraperitoneal infection: Studies with roentgen contrast medium. *Acta Chir Scand* 1964;36 (Suppl): 321:1–31.
4. Lopez N, Kobayashi L, Coimbra R. A comprehensive review of abdominal infections. *World J Emerg Surg* 2011;6:7.
5. Sheer TA, Runyon BA. Spontaneous bacterial peritonitis. *Dig Dis* 2005;23:39–46.
6. Mazuski JE. Intraabdomial infections. In: Fry DE ed. *Surgical Infections.* London, UK: JP Medical Publication, Chapter 6, 2013:75–88.
7. Chromik AM, Meiser A, Hölling J, et al. Identification of patients at risk for development of tertiary peritonitis on a surgical intensive care unit. *J Gastrointest Surg* 2009;13:1358–1367.
8. Htay H, Cho Y, Pascoe EM, et al. Center effects and peritoneal dialysis peritonitis outcomes: Analysis of a national registry. *Am J Kidney Dis* 2018;71:814–821.
9. Suarez-de-la-Rica A, Maseda E, Anillo V, et al. Biomarkers (procalcitonin, C reactive protein, and lactate) as predictors of mortality in surgical patients with complicated intra-abdominal infection. *Surg Infect* 2015;16:346–351.
10. Schermer CR, Sanchez DP, Qualls CR, et al. Blood culturing practices in a trauma intensive care unit: Does concurrent antibiotic use make a difference? *J Trauma* 2002;52:463–468.
11. Roberts BW. CT-guided intra-abdominal abscess drainage. *Radiol Technol* 2015;87:187CT–203CT.
12. Fry DE. Peritonitis. In: Fry DE ed. *Surgical Infections.* Boston, MA: Little, Brown and Co (Publ), Chapter 22, 1995: 227–240.
13. Cohen J, Brun-Buisson C, Torres A, Jorgensen J. Diagnosis of infection in sepsis: An evidence-based review. *Crit Care Med* 2004;32(11 Suppl):S466–S494.
14. Madura MJ, Craig RM, Shields TW. Unusual causes of spontaneous pneumoperitoneum. *Surg Gynecol Obstet* 1982;154:417–420.
15. American Thoracic Society: Guidelines for the management of adults with hospital-acquired, ventilator-associated, and healthcare-associated pneumonia. *Am J Respir Crit Care Med* 2005;171:388–416.
16. Napolitano LM, Edmiston CE Jr. *Clostridium difficile* disease: Diagnosis, pathogenesis, and treatment update. *Surgery* 2017;162:325–348.
17. Sartelli M, Malangoni MA, Abu-Zidan FM, et al. WSES guidelines for management of *Clostridium difficile* infection in surgical patients. *World J Emerg Surg* 2015;10:38.
18. Maluso P, Olson J, Sarani B. Abdominal compartment hypertension and abdominal compartment syndrome. *Crit Care Clin* 2016;32:213–222.
19. Chiara O, Cimbanassi S, Biffl W, et al. International consensus conference on open abdomen in trauma. *J Trauma Acute Care Surg* 2016;80:173–183.
20. Valle RG, Godoy FL. Neostigmine for acute colonic pseudo-obstruction: A meta-analysis. *Ann Med Surg (Lond)* 2014;3:60–64.

21. Bala M, Kashuk J, Moore EE, et al. Acute mesenteric ischemia: Guidelines of the World Society of Emergency Surgery. *World J Emerg Surg* 2017;12:38.

22. Treinen C, Lomelin D, Krause C, et al. Acute acalculous cholecystitis in the critically ill: Risk factors and surgical strategies. *Langenbecks Arch Surg* 2015;400:421–427.

23. Tenner S, Baillie J, DeWitt J, et al. American College of Gastroenterology guideline: Management of acute pancreatitis. *Am J Gastroenterol* 2013;108:1400–1415;1416.

24. Mowery NT, Bruns BR, MacNew HG, et al. Surgical management of pancreatic necrosis: A practice management guideline from the Eastern Association for the Surgery of Trauma. *J Trauma Acute Care Surg* 2017;83:316–327.

25. Mazuski JE, Tessier JM, May AK, et al. The Surgical Infection Society revised guidelines on the management of intra-abdominal infection. *Surg Infect* 2017;18:1–76.

26. Sartelli M, Catena F, Abu-Zidan FM et al. Management of intra-abdominal infections: Recommendations by the WSES 2106 consensus conference. *World J Emerg Surg* 2017;12:22.

27. Mosdell DM, Morris DM, Voltura A, et al. Antibiotic treatment for surgical peritonitis. *Ann Surg* 1991;214:543–549.

28. Sawyer RG, Claridge JA, Nathens AB, et al. Trial of short-course antimicrobial therapy for intraabdominal infection. *N Engl J Med* 2015;372:1996–2005.

29. Fry DE, Garrison RN, Heitsch RC, et al. Determinants of death in patients with intra-abdominal abscess. *Surgery* 1980;89:517–523.

30. Fry DE. Reoperative Surgery for Abdominal Wall Infection and Intraabdominal Abscess. In: Mizrahi S, Polk HC Jr, Reissman P eds. *Reoperative Abdominal Surgery*. London, UK: JP Medical Publishers, Chapter 5, 2014:29–36.

31. Snydman DR. Empiric antibiotic selection strategies for healthcare-associated pneumonia, intra-abdominal infections, and catheter-associated bacteremia. *J Hosp Med* 2012;7 (Suppl 1): S2–S12.

32. Kingham TP, Pachter HL. Colonic anastomotic leak: Risk factors, diagnosis, and treatment. *J Am Coll Surg* 2009;208:269–278.

33. Shogan BD, Belogortseva N, Luong PM, et al. Collagen degradation and MMP9 activation by Enterococcus faecalis contribute to intestinal anastomotic leak. *Sci Transl Med* 2015;7:286ra68.

34. Michalopoulos N, Triantafillopoulou K, Beretouli E, et al. Small bowel perforation due to CMV enteritis infection in an HIV-positive patient. *BMC Res Notes* 2013;6:45.

22 *Clostridium difficile* and Its Mimics in the Critical Care Unit

Burke A. Cunha

CONTENTS

CLINICAL PERSPECTIVE

Clostridium difficile is a gram-positive aerobic bacillus that is found in colon flora. The fecal carriage of *C. difficile* is asymptomatic. Sensitive stool detection methods may be positive in *C. difficile* carriers without diarrhea. *C. difficile* may be induced to produce two exotoxins (A/B) that are responsible for symptomatic disease, i.e., diarrhea/colitis. *C. difficile* strains vary in their virulence (amount of toxin produced), resulting in a spectrum of disease ranging from watery diarrhea to pancolitis [1–5].

C. DIFFICILE DIARRHEA VS. C. DIFFICILE COLITIS

The spectrum of clinical manifestation of *C. difficile* ranges from profuse watery diarrhea (resembling cholera and other secretory diarrheas) to pancolitis (resembling *Shigella* dysentery). There are critical differences in pathophysiology, i.e., a toxigenic mucosal disorder (*C. difficile* diarrhea) vs. an invasive transmural process (*C. difficile* colitis). Usually, the patient presents with either diarrhea or colitis, and occasionally, *C. difficile* colitis patients have a diarrhea component. These differences are analogous to comparing ulcerative colitis (UC) (a mucosal process without colon wall invasion) with Crohn's disease, i.e., regional enteritis (RE) (a transmural process extending into the intestinal wall) [6–8].

These critical differences in pathophysiology have important therapeutic implications. Just as UC is treated differently than RE, similarly, the treatment of *C. difficile* diarrhea differs markedly from that of *C. difficile* colitis. In recent *C. difficile* studies, all too often, treatment covers both entities and the relative efficacy of each component; i.e., oral vancomycin is difficult to evaluate [9–11].

THERAPEUTIC IMPLICATIONS OF C. DIFFICILE DIARRHEA VS. C. DIFFICILE COLITIS

The therapeutic aim of *C. difficile* diarrhea therapy is to provide high intraluminal concentrations of an *C. difficile* antibiotic, e.g., oral vancomycin. Oral vancomycin does not penetrate into the colon wall important since the process is mucosal and not invasive. The usual explanation given for vancomycin use in *C. difficile* colitis is that it won't hurt when the patient is ill [2,12,13]. In contrast, *C. difficile* colitis is an invasive process primarily involving the colon wall. Anti-*C. difficile* drugs for *C. difficile* colitis must penetrate the colon wall to treat colitis. Vancomycin given orally/intravenously doesn't penetrate the colon wall. Clearly, unless there is a diarrhea component, adding oral vancomycin in *C. difficile* colitis makes little sense [11]. Preferred antibiotics that are highly effective against *C. difficile* and penetrate the infected colon wall effectively are metronidazole, nitazoxanide, and tigecycline [9,14,15].

C. DIFFICILE DIARRHEA IN THE CCU

In the CCU, otherwise-unexplained acute onset of profuse watery diarrhea (20–30 watery movements/day) should be considered as due to *C. difficile* until proven otherwise. *C. difficile* diarrhea is not accompanied by fever >102°F and includes marked leukocytosis, abdominal pain/tenderness, and usually no diarrhea. In contrast, *C. difficile* colitis with the clinical features described previously may present abruptly with abdominal pain and findings of colitis and no preceding watery diarrhea. Alternately, a patient with *C. difficile* diarrhea may suddenly experience a decrease cessation of watery movements.

Accurate diagnosis is key in selecting optimal empiric therapy [16–20]. Diagnosis is based on a positive stool test for *C. difficile* toxins A/B plus pancolitis on abdominal CT scan [6,19]. The critical care unit (CCU) dilemma is that patients with *C. difficile* positive stool test may be reflective of *C. difficile* carriage. Residents of chronic care facilities are frequently asymptomatic *C. difficile* carriers, as are recently discharged hospitalized patients. Commonly, watery stools due to stool softners, laxatives, contrast media, etc. may test positive for *C. difficile*. Such patients are readily differentiated from true *C. difficile* diarrhea by the low number of watery stools per day. In contrast, with true *C. difficile* diarrhea, the watery diarrhea is profuse (20–30 movements/day) vs. 2–3 soft stools/day in a patient on laxatives and positive *C. difficile* carriage [2,6].

DIFFERENTIAL DIAGNOSTIC APPROACH

C. DIFFICILE DIARRHEA

In the CCU, diarrhea may be caused in a variety of ways. First, many medications may cause increased intestinal motility, e.g., macrolides, laxatives, and stool softeners. Additionally, enteral feeds in the CCU may result in diarrhea via two mechanisms. First, some enteral feeds cause diarrhea in some patients, not others (if suspected, change to another eternal feed product). Second, enteral feeds, if given in high volume, may result in watery diarrhea, e.g., 80–100 mL/hour. If enteral feed high volume is suspected, cut back on the infusion to 20–40 mL/hour, and diarrhea will decrease markedly or stop. Importantly, enteral feeds are protective against *C. difficile* [21]. If stools test positive for *C. difficile* in someone receiving an enteral feed, suspect *C. difficile* carriage, i.e., not true *C. difficile* diarrhea [15,16,20].

While it is assumed that antibiotics are always the cause of *C. difficile* diarrhea, this is actually not the case. However, if due to antibiotics, *C. difficile* may occur as long as 8 weeks after antibiotic exposure. Of the many antibiotics in several antibiotic classes, only β-lactams and clindamycin are most commonly associated with *C. difficile*. Antibiotics may cause non-*C. difficile* diarrhea by altering the colon flora, e.g., ceftriaxone, or by increasing intestinal notity, e.g., erythromycin, or as an irritative diarrhea due to poor oral absorption, e.g., ampicillin (vs. amoxicillin) [15,16]. In CCU patients with acute-onset watery *C. difficile* diarrhea, medications known to be associated with *C. difficile* diarrhea include proton pump inhibitors (PPIs), some psychiatric drugs, and cancer chemotherapy drugs [15,22,23]. Importantly, the only nosocomial infectious cause of acute-onset watery diarrhea is *C. difficile*. If a polymerase chain reaction (PCR) stool test is negative for *C. difficile*, there is no need for repeating the testing [24,25]. Cessation of diarrhea indicates resolution of *C. difficile* diarrhea. Repeat testing is not a test of cure and may remain positive for 8 weeks after infection. Unless there is a break in hand washing (from a hospital water problem) or a contaminated food-borne outbreak, community-acquired diarrheal pathogens,

Salmonella sp., *Shigella* sp., *Campylobacter* sp., *Yersinia* sp., and *E. coli*, should not be considered. Stool cultures for these community acquired pathogens need not be done in nosocomial diarrhea.

C. DIFFICILE COLITIS

As mentioned, the clinical presentation of *C. difficile* colitis differs fundamentally from *C. difficile* diarrhea. The onset of colitis may abrupt with high fevers >102°F, abdominal pain and tenderness, marked leukocytosis, and no diarrhea. Usually, the entire colon is involved, i.e., of *C. difficile* pancolitis. Less commonly, early presentation of *C. difficile* colitis will be that of segmental colitis rather than pancolitis [6,11,16].

Alternately, if a patient with *C. difficile* diarrhea (on appropriate therapy) abruptly ceases, then progression to colitis should be the working diagnosis, and an abdominal CT scan should done to confirm the presence of *C. difficile* colitis. In contrast, *C. difficile* diarrhea responds to therapy, demonstrating a gradual decrease in number of watery stools per day, e.g., 30/day to 27/day to 23/day to 19/day to 15/day to 8/day to 2–3/day, etc., before stools become soft/semiformed [2,15,16].

The differential diagnostic approach involves ruling out other causes of segmental colitis and pancolitis. If the abdominal CT scan shows segmental colitis, a non-*C. difficile* etiology is most likely. Alternately, differential diagnostic approach to pancolitis involves considering UC and mesenteric ischemia, but these patients are *C. difficile* negative, excluding carriers [16–18,26].

THERAPEUTIC CONSIDERATIONS C. DIFFICILE DIARRHEA VS. C. DIFFICILE COLITIS

C. DIFFICILE DIARRHEA

Because with *C. difficile* diarrhea the process is intraluminal and limited to colon mucosa, the aim of therapy is to deliver high intraluminal concentrations of effective anti-*C. difficile* drugs, e.g., oral vancomycin. Intraluminal concentrations of oral vancomycin are 1000–3000 μg/mL. Vancomycin resistance is not an issue, nor is systemic absorption [15,27]. In contrast, intraluminal colon levels with oral or IV metronidazole are very low (subtherapeutic). Furthermore, metronidazole resistance to *C. difficile* is high and increasing over time [10,28–30].

The efficiency of oral vancomycin therapy is dose/time dependent, i.e., dosing matters. The minimally effective oral vancomycin dose is 125 mg (PO) q6h. However, 250 mg (PO) q6h is more regularly effective. The speed of resolution of *C. difficile* diarrhea is also dose dependent and has important infection control implications, i.e., impacts on CCU/hospital length of stay.

An effective approach to begin treatment of *C. difficile* diarrhea is to begin with vancomycin 250 mg (PO) q6h and evaluate the response (decrease in stools/day) after 3 days of treatment. If there has been a marked decrease in liquid stools/day, e.g., 16/day or 18/day, then complete 10–14 days of therapy with the same dose of oral vancomycin [15].

If there is little/no decrease in stools/day with vancomycin 250 mg (PO) q6h, increase the dose to 500 mg (PO) q6h and again reevaluate the response, i.e., decrease in stools/day after 3 days. At 500 mg (PO) q6h, virtually, all patients rapidly respond to this dose. Since resistance is not an issue, if there is no response (after 3 days) to vancomycin 500 mg (PO) q6h, obtain an abdominal CT scan to rule out colitis [15,16].

Metronidazole (IV/PO) has an important role in *C. difficile* colitis therapy, but its efficacy is questionable in *C. difficile* diarrhea [10]. Unlike oral vancomycin, oral metronidazole is well-absorbed from the mucosa of the colon, resulting in very low/subtherapeutic intraluminal concentrations [28–30]. Importantly, while metronidazole is highly effective in *C. difficile* colitis (penetrates the colon wall), it is suboptimal for *C. difficile* diarrhea. The only other *C. difficile* antibiotic comparable to oral vancomycin and superior to metronidazole is nitazoxanide.

Therapy for *C. difficile* diarrhea should not be tapered in response to clinical improvement. The patient should receive a full course of oral vancomycin therapy, with the optimal effective dose (500 or 250 mg) for the patient [15] (Table 22.1).

C. difficile Colitis

With *C. difficile* pancolitis, the aim of therapy is two-fold. First, the drug(s) used should have a high degree of anti-*C. difficile* activity. Second, these antibodies should achieve therapeutic colon wall levels. High intraluminal levels are of no benefit in a transmural colon wall process. Third, pancolitis is often accompanied by microscopic translocation of colon flora from the wall into the peritoneum, i.e., causing microscopic peritonitis. Furthermore, pancolitis may result in colon perforation or toxic megacolon/perforation [31].

It is prudent to primarily treat the *C. difficile* colitis and secondarily to give an antibiotic with little or no *C. difficile* potential that is effective against colon flora that may be involved in potential peritonis/perforation.

TABLE 22.1

C. difficile Diarrhea: Therapeutic Approach

Preferred Therapy	Alternate Therapy
C. difficile Diarrhea[a–e]	*C. difficile* Diarrhea
• Vancomycin 250 mg (PO) q6h × 7–10 days[a] (If no improvement in 3 days, ↑ dose to 500 mg (PO) q6h x7 days)[b]	• Nitazoxanide 500 mg (PO) q12h × 7–10 days **or** • Metronidazole 250 mg (PO) q6h × 7–10 days[a]

[a] With *C. difficile* diarrhea (not colitis), **treatment failure common with vancomycin 125 mg (PO) q6h and with metronidazole at any dose**. (Flagyl frequently fails!)

[b] If no improvement after 3 days with vancomycin 500 mg (PO) q6h, **rule out colitis with abdominal CT scan**. If abdominal CT scan shows **colitis**, treat as *C. difficile* **colitis**.

[c] When treating *C. difficile* diarrhea or colitis, **discontinue antibiotics with a high *C. difficile* potential**, e.g., **clindamycin, ciprofloxacin, and β-lactams** (excluding ceftriaxone). Patients being treating with levofloxacin or moxifloxacin should not be concurrently taking proton pump inhibitors (PPIs). Either discontinue the PPI or switch to a H_2 blocker during quinolone therapy.

[d] **Avoid *C. difficile* "prophylaxis."** Do not treat "history of *C. difficile*." Instead, repeat *C. difficile* stool PCR to verify current diagnosis. **Treat *C. difficile* diarrhea only if PCR + for *C. difficile*. Even if stool + for *C. difficile*, do not treat minimal loose stools (*C. difficile* carrier) and consider other causes of loose stools, e.g., stool softeners and laxatives.**

[e] **Avoid anti-spasmatics in *C. difficile* diarrhea**, which may result in *C. difficile* colitis.

	Therapeutic Principles			
	IV Vancomycin	Oral Vancomycin	IV/PO Metronidazole	Nitazoxanide
• **High intra-luminal levels**	0	+	0	+
• **Resistance potential**	0	0	+	0

Source: Cunha, C.B. and Cunha, B.A., *Antibiotic Essentials* (16th ed.), Jay Pee Medical Publishers, New Delhi, India, 2018.

TABLE 22.2
***C. difficile* Colitis: Therapeutic Approach**

Preferred Therapy	Alternate Therapy
***C. difficile* Colitis**	***C. difficile* Colitis**
Mild/Moderately Severe[a]:	**Mild/Moderately Severe[a]:**
• Metronidazole 1 g (IV) q24h until cured	• Metronidazole 500 mg (PO) q6h until cured
plus	**plus either**
• Ertapenem 1 gm (IV) q24h (until colitis improves or associated peritonitis resolves)	• Tigecycline 200 mg (IV) × 1 dose, then 100 mg (IV) q24h until cured
	or
	• Nitazoxanide 500 mg (PO) q12h until cured
	±
	• Vancomycin 500 mg (PO) q6h until cured[a]
Severe Pancolitis[b]	
• Tigecycline 200 mg (IV) × 1 dose, then, 100 mg (IV) q24h until cured	
plus	
• Metronidazole 500 mg (IV/PO) q6h–8h until cured	
plus	
• Nitazoxanide 500 mg (PO) q12h × until cured	

[a] In *C. difficile* colitis *without* associated diarrhea, oral vancomycin is of no benefit.

[b] Colectomy may be lifesaving in severe *C. difficile* pancolitis.

Therapeutic Principles

	PO/IV Vancomycin	PO/IV Metronidazole	Nitazoxanide	Tigecycline
• **Effective colon wall levels**	0	+	+	+
• **Coverage against colon flora (microscopic peritonitis)**	0	0	0	+

Source: Cunha, C.B., and Cunha, B.A., *Antibiotic Essentials*, 16th ed., Jay Pee Medical Publishers, New Delhi, India, 2018.

The cornerstone of treatment for *C. difficile* pancolitis has been metronidazole (IV/PO). Alternately, nitazoxanide is highly efficacious in both *C. difficile* diarrhea (superior to metronidazole) and *C. difficile* colitis (comparable to metronidazole). Oral or parental vancomycin has a limited role in the therapy of *C. difficile* colitis and is usually added out of habit or desperation. In those cases of *C. difficile* colitis with a diarrhea component, it is not unreasonable to add oral vancomycin to the colitis regimen. Certainly, vancomycin should not be administered by enema, because it may result in colon perforation, since the colon in colitis is inflamed and friable.

Early preemptive therapy for potential microbial translocation of bacteria (microscopic peritonitis) or colon perforation is prudent. Therefore, with severe pancolitis, an antibiotic effective against coliforms and *B. fragilis* is reasonable. It doesn't matter which agent is selected, but preferably select one that doesn't cause *C. difficile*, e.g., piperacillin/tazobactam. Aside from nitazoxanide, alternate effective in *C. difficile* colitis is tigecycline [32–34]. Tigecycline has several advantages. First, the use of tigecycline is protective against *C. difficile*. Second, by itself, it is highly effective against *C. difficile*. Third, and importantly, it also provides preemptive therapy of microscopic/gross peritonitis [35–39]. Optimal therapy for *C. difficile* pancolitis is metronidazole plus tigecycline. In severe cases of pancolitis, nitazoxanide may be given orally via NG or PEG tube [15]. Treatment of *C. difficile* colitis should be continued until clinical resolution on abdominal CT scan. Transition to oral therapy for completion of *C. difficile* colitis treatment is best done with nitazoxanide (Table 22.2). *C. difficile* colitis accompanied by colon toxic megasolon or perforation may require surgical intervention. Should surgery become necessary, tigecycline provides optimal therapy for colon surgery due to toxic megacolon/colon perforation [13,40].

REFERENCES

1. Bartlett JG, Chang TW, Gurwith M, et al. Antibiotic-associated pseudomembranous colitis due to toxin-producing clostridia. *N Engl J Med* 1978;298:531–534.
2. Gerding DN, Johnson S, Peterson LR, et al. *Clostridium difficile*-associated diarrhea and colitis. *Infect Control Hosp Epidemiol* 1995;16:459–477.
3. Tedesco FJ, Barton RW, Alpers DH. Clindamycin-associated colitis. A prospective study. *Ann Intern Med* 1974;81:429–433.
4. Mylonakis E, Ryan ET, Calderwood SB. *Clostridium difficile*—associated diarrhea: A review. *Arch Intern Med* 2001;161:525–533.
5. Prechter F, Katzer K, Bauer M, Stallmach A. Sleeping with the enemy: Clostridium difficile infection in the intensive care unit. *Crit Care* 2017;21:260.
6. Hurley BW, Nguyen CC. The spectrum of pseudomembranous enterocolitis and antibiotic-associated diarrhea. *Arch Intern Med* 2002; 162:2177–2184.
7. Larson HE, Price AB, Honour P, et al. *Clostridium difficile* and the aetiology of pseudomembranous colitis. *Lancet* 1978;1:1063–1066.
8. Bartlett JG, Gerding DN. Clinical recognition and diagnosis of *Clostridium difficile* infection. *Clin Infect Dis* 2008;46:S12–S18.
9. Bouza E, Burillo A, Munoz P. Antimicrobial Therapy of *C. difficile*-associated Diarrhea. *Med Clin North Am* 2006;90:1141–1163.
10. Barkin JA, Sussman DA, Fifadara N, Barkin JS. *Clostridium difficile* infection and patient-specific antimicrobial resistance testing reveals a high metronidazole resistance rate. *Dig Dis Sci* 2017;62:1035–1042.
11. Napolitano LM, Edmiston CE Jr. *C. Difficile* disease: Diagnosis, pathogenesis, and treatment update. *Surgery* 2017;162:325–348.
12. Yassin SF, Young-Fadok TM, Zein NN, et al. *Clostridium difficile* associated diarrhea and colitis. *Mayo Clin Proc* 2001;76:725–730.
13. Dallal RM, Harbrecht BG, Boujoukas AJ, et al. Fulminant *Clostridium difficile*: An underappreciated and increasing cause of death and complications. *Ann Surg* 2002;235:363–72.
14. Nelson RL, Suda KJ, Evans CT. Antibiotic treatment for *C. difficile*-associated diarrhea in adults. *Cochrane Database Syst Rev* 2017;3:CD004610.
15. Cunha CB, Cunha BA. *Antibiotic Essentials* (15th ed). Jay Pee Medical Publishers: New Delhi, India, 2017.
16. Siegal D, Syed F, Hamid N, Cunha BA. Campylobacter jejuni pancolitis mimicking idiopathic ulcerative colitis. *Heart Lung* 2005;34:288–290.
17. Siegel DS, Hamid N, Cunha BA. Cytomegalovirus colitis mimicking ischemic colitis in an immunocompetent host. *Heart Lung* 2005;34:291–294.
18. Tang DM, Urrunaga NH, von Rosenvinge EC. Pseudomembranous colitis: Not always *C. difficile*. *Clev Clin J Med* 2016;83:361–366.
19. Chandrasekaran R, Lacy DB. The role of toxins in *C. difficile* Infection. *FEMS Micro Rev* 2017;41:723–750.
20. Caines C, Gill MV, Cunha BA. Non-*Clostridium difficile* nosocomial diarrhea in the intensive care unit. *Heart Lung* 1997;26:83–84.
21. Shim JK, Johnson S, Samore MH, et al. Primary symptomless colonisation by *Clostridium difficile* and decreased risk of subsequent diarrhoea. *Lancet* 1998;351:633–636.
22. Dial S, Alrasadi K, Manoukian C, et al. Risk of *Clostridium difficile* diarrhea among hospital inpatients prescribed proton pump inhibitors: Cohort and case-control studies. *CMAJ* 2004;171:33–38.
23. Lowe DO, Mamdani MM, Kopp A, et al. Proton pump inhibitors and hospitalization for *Clostridium difficile*-associated disease: A population-based study. *Clin Infect Dis* 2006;43:1272–1276.
24. Nistico JA, Hage JE, Schoch PE, Cunha BA. Unnecessary repeat *Clostridium difficile* PCR testing in hospitalized adults with *C. difficile*-negative diarrhea. *Eur J Clin Micro Infect Dis* 2013;32:97–99.
25. Mohan SS, McDermott BP, Parchuri S, Cunha BA. Lack of value of repeat stool testing for *C. difficile* toxin. *Am J Med* 2006;119:e7–e8.
26. Cunha BA, Thekkel V, Eisenstein L. Community-acquired norovirus diarrhea outbreak mimicking a community-acquired *C. difficile* diarrhea outbreak. *J Hosp Infect* 2008;70:98–100.
27. Cunha BA. Vancomycin. *Med Clin North Am* 1995;79:817–831.
28. Bolton RP, Culshaw MA. Faecal metronidazole concentrations during oral and intravenous therapy for antibiotic associated colitis due to *Clostridium difficile*. *Gut* 1986; 27:1169–1172.
29. Teasley DG, Gerding DN, Olson MM, et al. Prospective randomised trial of metronidazoleversus vancomycin for *Clostridium difficile*-associated diarrhoea and colitis. *Lancet* 1983;2:1043–1046.
30. Pelaez T, Alcala L, Alonso R, et al. Reassessment of *Clostridium difficile* susceptibility to metronidazole and vancomycin. *Antimicrob Agents Chemother* 2002;46:1647–1650.
31. Pepin J, Valiquette L, Cossette B. Mortality attributable to nosocomial *Clostridium difficile*-associated disease during an epidemic caused by a hypervirulent strain in Quebec. *CMAJ* 2005;173:1037–1042.
32. McVay CS, Rolfe RD. In vitro and in vivo activities of nitazoxanide against *C. Difficile*. *Antimicrob Agents Chemother* 2000;44:2254–2258.
33. Musher DM, Logan N, Hamill RJ, Dupont HL, Lentnek A, Gupta A, Rossignol JF. Nitazoxanide for the treatment of *C. difficile* colitis. *Clin Infect Dis* 2006;43:421–427.
34. Musher DM, Logan N, Mehendiratta V, Melgarejo NA, Garud S, Hamill RJ. *C. difficile* colitis that fails conventional metronidazole therapy: Response to nitazoxanide. *J Anti Chemother* 2007;59:705–710.
35. DiBella S, Nisii C, Petrosillo N. Is tigecycline a suitable option for *C. difficile* infection? Evidence from the literature. *Int J Anti Agents* 2015;46:8–12.
36. Gergely Szabo B, Kadar B, Szidonia Lenart K, et al. Use of intravenous tigecycline in patients with severe *C. difficile* infection: A retrospective observational cohort study. *Clin Microbiol Infect* 2016;20:476–481.
37. Hung YP, Lee JC, Lin HJ, Liu HC, Wu YH, Tsai PJ, Ko WC. Doxycycline and tigecycline: Two friendly drugs with a low association with *C. difficile* infection. *Antibiotics* 2015;4:216–229.

38. Kundrapu S, Hurless K, Sunkesula VC, Tomas M, Donskey CJ. Tigecycline exhibits inhibitory activity against *C. difficile* in the intestinal tract of hospitalized patients. *Int J Anti Agents* 2015;45:424–426.

39. Manea E, Sojo-Dorado J, Jipa RE, Banea SN, Rodriguez-Bano J, Hristea A. The role of tigecycline in the management of *C. difficile* infection: A retrospective cohort study. *Clin Micro Infect* 2017;S1198–S1743X.

40. McDonald LC, Killgore GE, Thompson A, et al. An epidemic, toxin gene-variant strain of *Clostridium difficile*. *N Engl J Med* 2005;353(23):2433–2441.

41. Cunha CB, Cunha BA. *Antibiotic Essentials* (16th ed.). New Delhi, India: Jay Pee Medical Publishers, 2018.

23 Diagnostic Approach to Fulminant Hepatitis in the Critical Care Unit

Huei-Wen Lim and David Bernstein

CONTENTS

BACKGROUND

Fulminant hepatitis (FH) or acute liver failure (ALF) is defined as the sudden loss of hepatic function resulting in hepatic encephalopathy and coagulopathy. Without timely intervention, FH can lead to multi-organ failure and significant mortality risk. Based on the data received from the US Acute Liver Failure Study Group (ALFSG) Registry over a 10-year period (1998–2007), acetaminophen toxicity was the most common cause of ALF in the United States, accounting for almost half of the ALF cases during this period [1]. Viral causes of FH, especially A, B, and E, on the other hand, are more prevalent in developing countries [2]. Despite improved survival over the decades, ALF remains a burgeoning health epidemic due to the increased incidence of viral hepatitis and increased mortality associated with ALF, even when emergency liver transplantation is available.

In this chapter, we expand on the aforementioned causes of FH/ALF and summarize the current diagnostic approach to FH in the CCU.

HEPATITIS A VIRUS

Hepatitis A infection is caused by the hepatitis A virus (HAV), an RNA virus that is fecal-orally transmitted. Its spread has been associated with risk factors such as poor sanitation, exposure to contaminated food or water, sexual intercourse with an HAV-positive person, or sex among men who have sex with men. The HAV infection has an incubation period of 28 days, after which symptoms begin abruptly with nausea, vomiting, abdominal pain, fever, and malaise [3]. Individuals infected with HAV can have alanine aminotransferase (ALT) and aspartate aminotransferase (AST) levels greater than 1000 IU/mL (ALT > AST), serum bilirubin more than 10 mg/dL, alkaline phosphatase (ALP) up to 400U/L, and a prolonged prothrombin time (PT) or international normalization ration (INR). The presence of at least two of the following components predicts an increased risk for transplant or death: (1) day 1 serum creatinine level >2.0 mg/dL, (2) day 1 serum ALT <2600 IU/mL, (3) need for intubation, and (4) need for intravenous pressors [4]. Specific diagnosis can be made by detection of serum IgM anti-HAV antibodies at the time of symptom onset, which peaks during the acute phase of the illness and remains in the serum for 6 months. The HAV-RNA by reverse transcription-polymerase chain reaction (RT-PCR) may be detected in the serum prior to anti-HAV antibody development, although it is not readily available in practice [5]. There is no HAV-specific therapy, and treatment includes fluids and supportive care.

HEPATITIS B VIRUS

Hepatitis B infection is caused by the hepatitis B virus (HBV), a DNA virus transmitted primarily through sexual contact in the United States and perinatally in southeast Asia. Its incubation period is 1–4 months, after which a serum sickness-like syndrome manifests as a prodromal phase, followed by constitutional symptoms such as nausea, vomiting, abdominal pain, and jaundice [3]. The ALF affects <1% of HBV-infected persons, yet HBV remains the main cause of ALF in Asia [6]. The PT and INR are prognostic markers of infection, and both ALT and AST may be greater than 1000 IU/mL in ALF (ALT > AST). The ALF may develop *de novo*, in the setting of existing chronic HBV infection, by reactivation of previously inactive hepatitis B especially during chemotherapy for malignancy, with the use of biological therapy or during/after successful hepatitis C treatment, or with hepatitis D virus superinfection [3]. The diagnosis is made by the detection of hepatitis B surface antigen (HBsAg) and/or anti-hepatitis B core IgM (IgM anti-HBc), with markers of HBV replication, hepatitis B e-antigen (HBeAg), and HBV DNA also present in the serum. In the fulminant phase, HBV DNA and HBsAg levels drop rapidly as ALF develops secondary to the massive immune-mediated lysis of infected hepatocytes, and IgM anti-HBc may be the sole marker of acute HBV infection. There is no specific therapy for HBV, and treatment includes fluids and supportive care. Antivirals such as tenofovir and entecavir can be used in ALF, although their efficacy remains unclear.

HEPATITIS C VIRUS

Hepatitis C virus (HCV) is an RNA virus transmitted predominantly through blood-to-blood exposure such as intravenous drug use, intranasal cocaine use, transfusion of contaminated blood products, and healthcare-associated accidental needle stick exposure. The HCV has been rarely reported to cause ALF. Acute HCV infection develops 2–26 weeks after exposure, with symptoms similar to that of other acute viral hepatitides, if symptomatic. Acute hepatitis C is diagnosed via detection of HCV RNA in the serum, as HCV antibody may take 3 months to become positive following exposure [7]. According to the Centers for Disease Control and Prevention (CDC), the current opioid epidemic has led to triple the number of cases of hepatitis C among

people aged 20–29 years and more than double the cases in people aged 30–39 years from 2009 to 2015. There is no specific therapy for HCV, and treatment includes fluids and supportive care.

HEPATITIS D VIRUS

Hepatitis D virus (HDV) is a RNA virus considered as a sub-viral satellite, because it requires HBsAg to propagate its own genome. Approximately 15 million individuals are infected with HDV worldwide, with endemic regions being the Mediterranean basin and East Asia. Transmission occurs via mucosal or percutaneous routes [8]. The HDV is associated with hepatitis B. Both infections may be acquired simultaneously (acute HBV/HDV), or HDV acute infection may occur in chronic hepatitis B (superinfection). Clinically, symptoms mimic that of other viral hepatitides, with serum ALT and AST levels at presentation dependent on the degree of liver necrosis. The incubation period ranges from 3 to 7 weeks. A subset of acute HDV patients presents with ALF within 2–10 days of exposure [3]. The HDV infection is diagnosed by detection of total (IgM and IgG) anti-HDV antibodies via enzyme immunoassays (EIA) and the presence of HBsAg indicating HBV infection. IgM anti-HBc is seen in patients with an acute HBV/HDV coinfection. A negative total anti-HDV test does not rule out an acute infection, as positive results appear 4 weeks after an acute infection. The HDV RNA by molecular hybridization or RT-PCR has been shown to be an early and sensitive marker of HDV replication in acute hepatitis. There is no specific therapy for HDV, and treatment includes fluids and supportive care.

HEPATITIS E VIRUS

Hepatitis E virus (HEV) is an RNA virus that is transmitted fecal-orally. The HEV infection is a major cause of ALF in developing countries, comprising 20%–40% of all ALF cases. In pregnancy, especially in the third trimester, the disease is more severe and has a mortality rate of 20% [9,10]. The incubation period ranges from 15–60 days, and symptoms are similar to that of other viral hepatitides. Symptoms generally coincide with an acute elevation of ALT and AST levels in the 1000s, along with elevated serum bilirubin and INR. The diagnosis is based on the detection of IgM anti-HEV antibodies, HEV RNA, or the development of IgG anti-HEV antibodies within 6–12 months in a previously seronegative individual. IgM anti-HEV appears during the early phase of an acute infection and disappears over 4–5 months, while IgG anti-HEV appears shortly after IgM and persists through the convalescent phase. The HEV RNA is not readily available and needs to be sent to specialized laboratories or to the CDC to obtain results. There is no specific therapy for HEV, and treatment includes fluids and supportive care (Table 23.1).

TABLE 23.1
Characteristics of Hepatitis Viruses

	Transmission	Endemic Areas	Diagnosis of Acute Disease
HAV	Fecal-oral, sexual, poor sanitation, exposure to contaminated food/water	Developing countries	HAV IgM, HAV RNA
HBV	Blood transfusion, needle sticks, sexual, perinatal	Asia, sub-Saharan Africa, Amazon basin, Eastern Europe	HbsAg, IgM anti-HBc, HbeAg and HBV DNA IgM anti-Hbc may be sole marker for acute infection
HCV	Blood transfusion, needle sticks, perinatal	Worldwide	HCV RNA
HDV	Blood transfusion, needle sticks, sexual, perinatal	Mediterranean, East Asia	HBsAg and IgM anti-HBc must be present, IgG and IgM anti-HDV, HDVRNA
HEV	Fecal-oral	Worldwide	IgM HEV, HEV RNA

HERPES SIMPLEX VIRUS

Herpes simplex virus 1 and 2 (HSV) are double-stranded DNA viruses that belong to the herpesvirus family, *Herpesviridae*, and can be contracted through direct contact with an active lesion or body fluid of an infected person. The HSV is an uncommon cause of ALF that typically occurs in immunosuppressed patients [3]. The HSV hepatitis accounts for less than 1% of all cases of ALF and carries a mortality rate of 80% secondary to delayed diagnosis [11]. Patients who are male, older than 40 years, immunosuppressed, and/or with other liver diseases are more likely to progress to death and need liver transplantation [12]. Clinical symptoms of HSV infection include fever, anorexia, abdominal pain, leukopenia, and coagulopathy. The absence of mucocutaneous lesions seen in half of patients leads to a high frequency of delayed diagnosis [13]. Laboratory abnormalities include low to normal bilirubin, resulting in anicteric hepatitis, transaminase levels 100- to 1000-fold above baseline (AST > ALT), and a prolonged INR. Diagnosis is made through the detection of antibodies against HSV (IgM and IgG anti-HSV) in serum and confirmatory testing of PCR in blood or tissues [11]. HSV DNA by PCR is the most sensitive test for the diagnosis of HSV hepatitis [14]. Rapid initiation of acyclovir increases the rates of transplant-free survival.

CYTOMEGALOVIRUS

Cytomegalovirus (CMV), a member of the herpesvirus family, is a double-stranded DNA virus. Transmission occurs via sexual or perinatal exposure, close contact with infected individuals, or contact with infected blood and tissue. The CMV infection is typically a latent asymptomatic disease in otherwise-healthy people, while CMV-related ALF is common in immunocompromised patients. In the absence of preventative therapy, CMV infection develops in 30%–70% of transplant recipients; its incidence depends on the serostatus of the donor and recipient [15]. The CMV-presenting symptoms include a syndrome resembling that of infectious mononucleosis characterized by fever, sore throat, fatigue, and lymphadenopathy. Diagnostic modalities for CMV infection include serological testing, PCR, culture, and histopathology [16,17]. Laboratory testing must be interpreted in the appropriate clinical context, given its high false-positive rate in patients who do not have active disease. In immunocompromised patients, CMV PCR and CMV pp65 antigenemia assay are diagnostic of CMV infection, while in immunocompetent patients, positive IgM anti-CMV (detectable within the first 2 weeks after symptom onset) or fourfold increase of IgG anti-CMV (detectable 4–6 months after symptom onset) and plasma PCR are usually diagnostic [18]. Serological testing has no role in diagnosing CMV infection in the immunocompromised host. The CMV presenting with hypoalbumenia, hyperbilirubinemia, and high titers of CMV by PCR is associated with a poor prognosis [15]. Treatment of CMV hepatitis is oral ganciclovir, although oral valganciclovir may be used in selected mild to moderate cases [19].

EPSTEIN–BARR VIRUS

The Epstein–Barr virus (EBV), also called human herpesvirus-4 (HHV-4), belongs to the herpesvirus family and is one of the most common human viruses. It causes infectious mononucleosis, which results in fever, sore throat, enlarged lymph nodes in the neck, vomiting, and fatigue. Symptoms of mild hepatitis and cholestasis occur in approximately 90% of infected individuals [20]. It is often spread through contact with saliva and rarely through semen or blood. In a study of ALF patients enrolled into the US ALFSG, 0.21% of the participants were found to have EBV-related ALF, reflecting the rare occurrence of ALF in EBV [20]. These cases of ALF, however, were associated with a high fatality rate. Although clinically significant hepatic damage usually occurs in immunosuppressed patients, acute severe hepatitis in young, immunocompetent patients has been reported [21]. The diagnosis is made by the presence of positive EBV viral capsid antigen (VCA) IgM with or without positive EBV VCA IgG antibody titers or serum measurements of EBV DNA through PCR [20]. Compared with other viruses, ALF caused by EBV typically presents with a cholestatic enzyme pattern, with variable serum aminotransferase levels and jaundice [22].

TABLE 23.2

Interpretation of EBV Virus Serological Profiles

VCA IgM	VCA IgG	EBNA IgG	Interpretation
−	−	−	Negative EBV status
+	−	−	Early primary infection
+	+	−	Acute primary infection
−	+	+	Past infection
−	−	+	Isolated EBNA IgG
−	+	−	Isolated VCA IgG
+	+	+	Indeterminate

Abbreviation: EBNA IgG, Epstein–Barr nuclear antigen IgG.

Patients may or may not have the classical symptoms of infectious mononucleosis at presentation. The small number of EBV-related ALF cases makes potential ALF risk factors difficult to identify (Table 23.2).

HUMAN HERPESVIRUS-6

Human herpesvirus-6 (HHV-6) consists of a set of two closely related herpesviruses known as HHV-6A and HHV-6B that almost invariably have humans as their primary host. The seroprevalence of HHV-6 among the adult population is as high as 82%–100%, even though primary infection is rare [23]. The virus is a common cause of liver dysfunction and ALF, especially in the immunosuppressed transplant patient. The HHV-6 infection often causes exanthema subitum in infants and a mononucleosis-like syndrome in adults. Pretransplant HHV-6 infection and concurrent CMV infection are identified risk factors associated with liver dysfunction following hepatic transplantation [24]. The diagnosis of HHV-6 infection can be made based on a positive HHV-6 serum antigen test (monoclonal antibodies against specific HHV-6A and -B antigens as well as a polyclonal antibody against HHV-6 U90 protein), which detects the presence of the virus in peripheral blood mononuclear cells, the presence of HHV-6 antigens on liver biopsy, or the demonstration of HHV-6 serology (IgG or IgM anti-HHV-6) by means of indirect EIA. A greater than fourfold rise in IgG titers is considered diagnostic, as most people are seropositive for HHV-6 IgG. While anti-HHV-6 develops within 4–7 days of infection, it may be unreliable, as IgM can be falsely positive in healthy adults [23]. Foscarnet, ganciclovir, and cidofovir may be used to treat acute disease [25].

VARICELLA-ZOSTER VIRUS

Varicella-zoster virus (VZV) is a herpesvirus well-known to be contagious in childhood; it can affect both immunosuppressed and immunocompetent adults. The predisposition of immunosuppressed adults, especially post organ transplant or HIV patients, to contract VZV infection and develop ALF is well-known [26]. These patients have a high incidence of other visceral involvement, such as pneumonitis

and meningoencephalitis. The VZV infection begins with a vague abdominal or back pain, followed by fever, cutaneous rash, acute hepatitis, and coagulation impairment, leading to disseminated intravascular coagulation and gastrointestinal hemorrhage. The rash of VZV begins as erythematous papules that may precede, coincide with, or follow the onset of hepatitis, making the diagnosis of this complication difficult [26] Diagnosis can be made via viral culture, the presence of detectable VZV DNA by PCR in the serum, or direct immunofluorescence on liver biopsy. Serologic testing is generally not helpful to diagnose VZV in ALF but can be used to determine susceptibility and the need for immunization [27]. Treatment of VZV hepatitis is intravenous acyclovir.

EBOLA VIRUS

Ebola, also called Ebola hemorrhagic fever, is a viral hemorrhagic fever of humans caused by the Ebola virus, a member of the *Filoviridae* family. It is spread by direct contact with body fluids, such as blood, stool, and vomitus of an infected human. Ebola is characterized by fever, fatigue, vomiting, diarrhea, rash, kidney, liver failure, and occasionally bleeding. It is associated with a high case fatality rate of 54.7%, with fatality rates reported to increase with age and high viral load [28]. Patients with Ebola virus disease were found to have AST/ALT levels of more than five times the upper limit of normal and, in severe cases, levels of more than 15 times the upper limit of normal [29]. Diagnosis of Ebola can be made by serum PCR on blood drawn within 3 days of the onset of symptoms. A rapid chromatographic immunoassay (ReEBOV) that detects Ebola virus antigen can provide results within 15 minutes; however, this has been associated with false-positive results in 10% of patients who tested negative by PCR [30]. On postmortem liver biopsy, hepatocellular necrosis with minimal inflammation is the primary histological finding. There is no specific therapy for Ebola, and treatment includes fluids and supportive care.

DENGUE FEVER

Dengue fever (DF) is a febrile illness endemic in tropical countries; it is caused by the infection of one of four dengue viruses spread by the *Aedes aegypti* or *Aedes albopictus* mosquitoes. Dengue-related ALF has been well-described in the literature and occurs more commonly among children, with few incidences in adults. The incubation period is 3–14 days. Clinical features include fever, abdominal pain, nausea/vomiting, skin rash, and anorexia. Liver involvement in DF includes hepatomegaly and transient variable liver test abnormalities (AST > ALT) [31]. Hypoproteinemia, hypoalbuminemia, and coagulation abnormalities have been reported [32,33]. Diagnosis is based on the detection of viral nucleic acid in serum by RT-PCR assay or via detection of viral antigen nonstructural protein 1 with enzyme-linked immunosorbent assay (ELISA). Immunoglobulin IgM is also widely used for definitive diagnosis [34]. There is no specific therapy for DF, and treatment includes fluids and supportive care.

YELLOW FEVER

Yellow fever (YF) is a viral disease endemic to the tropical regions of Africa and South America; it is spread primarily by *Aedes aegypti*. It has a high case fatality rate and can manifest with life-threatening disease associated with fever, jaundice, renal failure, and hemorrhage. In severe cases, hepatic coma and death may develop. Laboratory abnormalities include marked transaminase elevations (AST > ALT), with mildly elevated ALP, direct bilirubin levels, and a prolonged INR [35]. Diagnosis is made by ELISA for IgM and is confirmed by a rise in titer between paired acute and convalescent samples. Rapid diagnostic test using PCR to detect virus in the blood and viral culture can also be used. Liver biopsy should be avoided in the acute phase of yellow fever, as fatal hemorrhage may occur [36]. There is no specific therapy for YF, and treatment includes fluids and supportive care.

COXSACKIE B VIRUS

Coxsackie B virus (COX B) belongs to a family of RNA viruses, *Picornaviridae*, that infects the heart, pleura, pancreas, and liver of early infancy, causing pleurodynia, myocarditis, pericarditis, and hepatitis. Coxsackie hepatitis is frequently associated with myocarditis [37]. The ALF develops as part of a disseminated viral infection, where fever, jaundice, and petechiae are the most consistent findings on admission. A biphasic fever pattern has also been reported. Jaundice and coagulopathy are poor prognostic indicators. Laboratory abnormalities include anemia, thrombocytopenia, prolongation of PT and activated thromboplastin time, marked transaminases elevation (AST > ALT), and elevated fibrin degradation product levels [38]. Diagnosis can be made by serological paired complement fixation antibody (IgG and IgM) titers for COX B, with at least a fourfold rise in titer between acute and convalescent phased [37]. The RT-PCR is diagnostic of infection, and cell cultures are useful when isolate serotyping is important. There is no specific therapy for COX B, and treatment includes fluids and supportive care.

ADENOVIRUS

Adenovirus is a ubiquitous double-stranded DNA virus that is an important cause of febrile illness in childhood. Rarely, adenovirus may disseminate and cause severe hepatic necrosis and fulminant hepatic failure, especially in immunocompromised hosts. Adenovirus hepatitis is a concern in pediatric liver transplant recipients, as it may be fatal. Transmission occurs through aerosolized droplets, fecal-oral exposure, or swimming pool water. The clinical features of ALF caused by adenovirus include high fevers, rapid rise in transaminases, hemodynamic instability, and a bleeding diathesis [39]. Detection of adenoviral infections in patients can be made through PCR, viral culture, or direct antigen assays [40]. Definitive diagnosis requires a liver biopsy. Immunohistochemically, adenovirus is characterized by intranuclear inclusion bodies in the biopsy material [41].

There is no specific therapy for adenovirus, and treatment includes fluids and supportive care.

ECHOVIRUS

Echovirus is an RNA virus that belongs to the genus *Enterovirus* and is transmitted fecal-orally. It is the leading cause of acute febrile illness and the most common cause of aseptic meningitis in infants and young children. The ALF and systemic infection caused by echovirus-18 have been reported in adult hematopoietic stem cell transplant recipient and are associated with fever, nausea, vomiting, and diarrhea. Laboratory abnormalities include elevated AST and ALT levels 10 times above the upper limit of normal, hyperbilirubinemia, elevated ALP, and thrombocytopenia. Detection can be made via a reverse transcriptase-seminested PCR (RT-snPCR) assay in plasma, cerebrospinal fluid, and liver biopsy specimen and is currently the gold standard for diagnosis. Viral culture is proven to be useful; however, diagnosis can be delayed. Treatment with plasmapheresis, intravenous immunoglobulin (IVIG), and antiviral agents have been attempted with variable success [42].

PARAMYXOVIRUS

Paramyxoviridae is a family of RNA viruses that is associated with diseases such as measles, mumps, and respiratory tract infections (respiratory syncytial virus). Giant cell hepatitis, a relatively common pathological finding in neonates, is a cholestatic disorder caused by a virus in the Paramyxovirus family that is associated with symptoms of cholestatic jaundice, dark urine, light/acholic stools, and hepatomegaly. In adults, the viral course is typically rapid. Laboratory abnormalities resemble that of other viral hepatitides [43,44]. On liver biopsy, numerous enlarged multinucleated hepatocytes with abundant cytoplasm can be seen. Specific ELISA and RT-PCR testing can be performed, although the diagnosis is usually based on clinical findings [43]. Its occurrence has been reported in post-liver transplantation patients and is treated effectively with ribavirin [44].

PARVOVIRUS B19

Parvovirus B19 is a DNA virus belonging to the *Parvoviridae* family. Parvovirus B19 occurs commonly in children and manifests as erythema infectiosum or aplastic anemia. In adults, arthropathy or hydrop fetalis during pregnancy can occur [45]. Parvovirus B19 has been associated with ALF in solid-organ transplantation and hematopoietic stem cell transplantation. Clinical manifestation is atypical and can include fever, rash, arthralgia, anemia and organ-invasive disease such as hepatitis and myocarditis. Liver function abnormalities resemble that of other viral hepatitides [46]. Diagnosis can be made via serology (IgM and IgG) and serum PCR for parvovirus B19, although serology is unreliable in the context of immunosuppression, as patients may mount a delayed immune response. Direct viral detection in blood or, in the case of hepatitis, liver biopsy specimen should be performed if both serology and PCR are negative but suspicion remains high. Treatment of parvovirus B19 is with intravenous immunoglobulins [45,46].

AUTOIMMUNE HEPATITIS

Autoimmune hepatitis (AIH) can present acutely as a spontaneous flare of a pre-existing chronic disease, acute disease, chronic disease with superimposed acute injury, or after treatment of a pre-existing liver disease with immunomodulators and liver transplantation. Acute presentations of AIH account for 25% of all cases and may be confused with acute viral disease [47]. The clinical presentation of acute AIH is indistinguishable from that of other acute viral hepatitides and requires specific antibody testing for accurate diagnosis. Autoimmune hepatitis is more common in women than in men, and there may be a history of significant childhood acne, hirsutism, and amenorrhea [48]. On acute presentation, as many as 50% may already have cirrhosis. The diagnosis of acute AIH is made by a combination of elevated serum globulins, predominantly serum IgG, and a positive anti-smooth muscle antibody with or without a positive antinuclear antibody. Liver biopsy typically will reveal plasma cells, rosette formation with or without the presence of fibrosis, or cirrhosis. Acute AIH is treated with either oral or intravenous steroids [47].

REFERENCES

1. Lee WM, Squires RH, Jr., Nyberg SL, Doo E, Hoofnagle JH. Acute liver failure: Summary of a workshop. *Hepatology* 2008;47(4):1401–1415.
2. Lee WM. Etiologies of acute liver failure. *Semin Liver Dis* 2008;28(2):142–152.
3. Jayakumar S, Chowdhury R, Ye C, Karvellas CJ. Fulminant viral hepatitis. *Crit Care Clin* 2013;29(3):677–697.
4. Taylor RM, Davern T, Munoz S, et al. Fulminant hepatitis A virus infection in the United States: Incidence, prognosis, and outcomes. *Hepatology* 2006;44(6):1589–1597.
5. Rezende G, Roque-Afonso AM, Samuel D, et al. Viral and clinical factors associated with the fulminant course of hepatitis A infection. *Hepatology* 2003;38(3):613–618.
6. Lavanchy D. Hepatitis B virus epidemiology, disease burden, treatment, and current and emerging prevention and control measures. *J Viral Hepat* 2004;11(2):97–107.
7. Loomba R, Rivera MM, McBurney R, et al. The natural history of acute hepatitis C: Clinical presentation, laboratory findings and treatment outcomes. *Aliment Pharmacol Ther* 2011;33(5):559–565.
8. Gaeta GB, Stroffolini T, Chiaramonte M, et al. Chronic hepatitis D: A vanishing Disease? An Italian multicenter study. *Hepatology* 2000;32(4 Pt 1):824–827.
9. Aggarwal R. Hepatitis E: Clinical presentation in disease-endemic areas and diagnosis. *Semin Liver Dis* 2013;33(1):30–40.
10. Patra S, Kumar A, Trivedi SS, Puri M, Sarin SK. Maternal and fetal outcomes in pregnant women with acute hepatitis E virus infection. *Ann Intern Med* 2007;147(1):28–33.
11. Riediger C, Sauer P, Matevossian E, Muller MW, Buchler P, Friess H. Herpes simplex virus sepsis and acute liver failure. *Clin Transplant* 2009;23(Suppl 21):37–41.
12. Norvell JP, Blei AT, Jovanovic BD, Levitsky J. Herpes simplex virus hepatitis: An analysis of the published literature and institutional cases. *Liver Transpl* 2007;13(10):1428–1434.
13. Kaufman B, Gandhi SA, Louie E, Rizzi R, Illei P. Herpes simplex virus hepatitis: Case report and review. *Clin Infect Dis* 1997;24(3):334–338.
14. Levitsky J, Duddempudi AT, Lakeman FD, et al. Detection and diagnosis of herpes simplex virus infection in adults with acute liver failure. *Liver Transpl* 2008;14(10):1498–1504.
15. Kim JM, Kim SJ, Joh JW, et al. The risk factors for cytomegalovirus syndrome and tissue-invasive cytomegalovirus disease in liver transplant recipients who have cytomegalovirus antigenemia. *Transplant Proc* 2010;42(3):890–894.
16. Chou S. Newer methods for diagnosis of cytomegalovirus infection. *Rev Infect Dis* 1990;12(Suppl 7):S727–S736.
17. Kotton CN, Kumar D, Caliendo AM, et al. Updated international consensus guidelines on the management of cytomegalovirus in solid-organ transplantation. *Transplantation* 2013;96(4):333–360.
18. Ross SA, Novak Z, Pati S, Boppana SB. Overview of the diagnosis of cytomegalovirus infection. *Infect Disord Drug Targets* 2011;11(5):466–474.
19. Razonable RR, Humar A, Practice ASTIDCo. Cytomegalovirus in solid organ transplantation. *Am J Transplant* 2013;13(Suppl 4):93–106.
20. Mellinger JL, Rossaro L, Naugler WE, et al. Epstein–Barr virus (EBV) related acute liver failure: A case series from the US acute liver failure study group. *Dig Dis Sci* 2014;59(7):1630–1637.
21. Pagidipati N, Obstein KL, Rucker-Schmidt R, Odze RD, Thompson CC. Acute hepatitis due to Epstein–Barr virus in an immunocompetent patient. *Dig Dis Sci* 2010;55(4):1182–1185.
22. Vine LJ, Shepherd K, Hunter JG, et al. Characteristics of Epstein–Barr virus hepatitis among patients with jaundice or acute hepatitis. *Aliment Pharmacol Ther* 2012;36(1):16–21.
23. Harma M, Hockerstedt K, Lautenschlager I. Human herpesvirus-6 and acute liver failure. *Transplantation* 2003;76(3):536–539.
24. Harma M, Hockerstedt K, Krogerus L, Lautenschlager I. Pretransplant human herpesvirus 6 infection of patients with acute liver failure is a risk factor for posttransplant human herpesvirus 6 infection of the liver. *Transplantation* 2006;81(3):367–372.
25. Lautenschlager I, Razonable RR. Human herpesvirus-6 infections in kidney, liver, lung, and heart transplantation: Review. *Transpl Int* 2012;25(5):493–502.
26. Kusne S, Pappo O, Manez R, et al. Varicella-zoster virus hepatitis and a suggested management plan for prevention of VZV infection in adult liver transplant recipients. *Transplantation* 1995;60(6):619–621.
27. Maggi U, Russo R, Conte G, et al. Fulminant multiorgan failure due to varicella zoster virus and HHV6 in an immunocompetent adult patient, and anhepatia. *Transplant Proc* 2011;43(4):1184–1186.
28. Xu Z, Jin B, Teng G, et al. Epidemiologic characteristics, clinical manifestations, and risk factors of 139 patients with Ebola virus disease in western Sierra Leone. *Am J Infect Control* 2016;44(11):1285–1290.
29. Hunt L, Gupta-Wright A, Simms V, et al. Clinical presentation, biochemical, and haematological parameters and their association with outcome in patients with Ebola virus disease: An observational cohort study. *Lancet Infect Dis* 2015;15(11):1292–1299.

30. Boisen ML, Cross RW, Hartnett JN, et al. Field validation of the ReEBOV antigen rapid test for point-of-care diagnosis of Ebola virus infection. *J Infect Dis* 2016;214(suppl 3):S203–S209.

31. Samanta J, Sharma V. Dengue and its effects on liver. *World J Clin Cases* 2015;3(2):125–131.

32. Saha AK, Maitra S, Hazra S. Spectrum of hepatic dysfunction in 2012 dengue epidemic in Kolkata, West Bengal. *Indian J Gastroenterol* 2013;32(6):400–403.

33. Karoli R, Fatima J, Siddiqi Z, Kazmi KI, Sultania AR. Clinical profile of dengue infection at a teaching hospital in North India. *J Infect Dev Ctries* 2012;6(7):551–554.

34. Hunsperger EA, Munoz-Jordan J, Beltran M, et al. Performance of dengue diagnostic tests in a single-specimen diagnostic algorithm. *J Infect Dis* 2016;214(6):836–844.

35. Monath TP, Vasconcelos PF. Yellow fever. *J Clin Virol* 2015;64:160–173.

36. Gardner CL, Ryman KD. Yellow fever: A reemerging threat. *Clin Lab Med* 2010;30(1):237–260.

37. Persichino J, Garrison R, Krishnan R, Sutjita M. Effusive-constrictive pericarditis, hepatitis, and pancreatitis in a patient with possible coxsackievirus B infection: A case report. *BMC Infect Dis* 2016;16:375.

38. Wang SM, Liu CC, Yang YJ, Yang HB, Lin CH, Wang JR. Fatal coxsackievirus B infection in early infancy characterized by fulminant hepatitis. *J Infect* 1998;37(3):270–273.

39. Vyas JM, Marasco WA. Fatal fulminant hepatic failure from adenovirus in allogeneic bone marrow transplant patients. *Case Rep Infect Dis* 2012;2012:463569.

40. Haura EB, Winden MA, Proia AD, Trotter JE. Fulminant hepatic failure due to disseminated adenovirus infection in a patient with chronic lymphocytic leukemia. *Cancer Control* 2002;9(3):248–253.

41. Ronan BA, Agrwal N, Carey EJ, et al. Fulminant hepatitis due to human adenovirus. *Infection* 2014;42(1):105–111.

42. Lefterova MI, Rivetta C, George TI, Pinsky BA. Severe hepatitis associated with an echovirus 18 infection in an immune-compromised adult. *J Clin Microbiol* 2013;51(2):684–687.

43. Phillips MJ, Blendis LM, Poucell S, et al. Syncytial giant-cell hepatitis. Sporadic hepatitis with distinctive pathological features, a severe clinical course, and paramyxoviral features. *N Engl J Med* 1991;324(7):455–460.

44. Hassoun Z, N'Guyen B, Cote J, et al. A case of giant cell hepatitis recurring after liver transplantation and treated with ribavirin. *Can J Gastroenterol* 2000;14(8):729–731.

45. Eid AJ, Brown RA, Patel R, Razonable RR. Parvovirus B19 infection after transplantation: A review of 98 cases. *Clin Infect Dis* 2006;43(1):40–48.

46. Eid AJ, Chen SF, Practice ASTIDCo. Human parvovirus B19 in solid organ transplantation. *Am J Transplant* 2013;13(Suppl 4):201–205.

47. Czaja AJ. Acute and acute severe (fulminant) autoimmune hepatitis. *Dig Dis Sci* 2013;58(4):897–914.

48. Makol A, Watt KD, Chowdhary VR. Autoimmune hepatitis: A review of current diagnosis and treatment. *Hepat Res Treat* 2011;2011:390916.

24 Diagnostic Approach to Acute Kidney Injury in the Critical Care Unit

Sonali Gupta, Divyansh Bajaj, Sana Idrees, and Joseph Mattana

CONTENTS

CLINICAL PERSPECTIVE

Acute kidney injury (AKI) is a common cause of morbidity and mortality in the critical care setting. Recent studies have demonstrated that there has been a progressive rise in the incidence of dialysis-requiring AKI [1]. It constitutes a major financial burden and entails increased utilization of resources and prolongation of the length of hospital stay. Patients admitted in these settings frequently have multiple comorbidities, and the occurrence of AKI in patients can further complicates their hospital course. Management of AKI often requires multidisciplinary team action, with a focus on timely identification of risk factors, early diagnosis, and targeted interventions. In this chapter, we will focus on the etiology of AKI, the syndromic approach to AKI, its clinical workup, and strategies for management, including fluid resuscitation and renal replacement therapy.

ETIOLOGY OF AKI IN THE CRITICAL CARE SETTING

Acute kidney injury is a broad category that includes various etiologies, pathogenic mechanisms, and risk factors. Some of the well-known risk factors for the development of AKI in the critical care setting include infections, shock, need for intubation and mechanical ventilation, exposures to nephrotoxic agents including antibiotics, non-steroidal anti-inflammatory drugs (NSAIDs) and radiocontrast, advanced age, presence of heart failure, liver failure, chronic kidney disease, anemia, and immunosuppression [2].

The traditional classification of AKI into three groups, including prerenal azotemia, intrinsic renal diseases, and postrenal (urinary obstruction), provides a basic framework by which pathophysiological mechanisms can be grouped. However, AKI can also be regarded as a syndrome associated with various clinical conditions.

PRERENAL AKI

Prerenal AKI accounts for 60%–70% of all AKI cases in critically ill patients [2]. Renal autoregulation helps to maintain a constant renal blood flow (RBF) and glomerular filtration rate (GFR) within a wide range of mean arterial blood pressure (80–180 mmHg) [3]. However, conditions associated with decreased effective arterial volume resulting in blood pressure below the lower limit of the autoregulatory range can result in sufficient reduction in GFR to lead to the development of AKI. A characteristic feature of prerenal AKI is that it is transient, being reversible, with prompt restoration of normal effective arterial volume.

ISCHEMIC AND NEPHROTOXIC AKI

Acute kidney injury often results from prolonged and protracted ischemia, hypoxia, or exposure to nephrotoxic medications or other agents such as radiocontrast and endogenous substances such as myoglobin. Historically, this condition has been termed acute tubular necrosis, given its histological findings. The mechanisms by which ischemic and nephrotoxic AKI reduces the GFR appear to include tubular obstruction by necrotic renal tubular epithelial cells, which have become swollen and aggregated via formation of intercellular adhesions as well as intense and persistent renal vasoconstriction with altered tubular dynamics [4]. In contrast to prerenal azotemia, acute tubular necrosis is characterized by delayed reversibility in those cases in which renal recovery takes place.

AKI AND SEPSIS

Sepsis and septic shock remain very common causes of AKI in critically ill patients and account for more than 50% of cases of AKI in the critical care unit [5–7]. While previously regarded as mainly the result of ischemia from hypotension, sepsis-mediated AKI is now known to be a severe and multifactorial process, with renal injury arising not only from hypotension but also additional factors, including renal vasoconstriction, microcirculatory flow abnormalities, cytokine-mediated cell injury, oxygen radical-mediated damage, and others. Hence, in addition to the mechanisms by which acute tubular necrosis is believed to lead to a reduction in GFR with ischemic and nephrotoxic insults, additional mechanisms appear to play a role in the reduction in GFR in sepsis. Sepsis-related AKI is strongly associated with a worse prognosis [7,8]. Younger age, early initiation of appropriate antimicrobials, low APACHE II scores, and community-acquired rather than hospital-acquired infection are variables associated with a better prognosis and earlier recovery from AKI [8]. The timing of the development of AKI is also important, with occurrences later in the course of sepsis being associated with a worse clinical outcome and increased mortality rates [8].

AKI AND RHABDOMYOLYSIS

Acute kidney injury associated with rhabdomyolysis is another important category and is typically seen after major trauma or crush injuries, extreme physical activity, vascular ischemia, endocrine disorders, or with pressure necrosis, as may occur with drug intoxication. Kidney injury is mainly triggered by myoglobin release and filtration resulting in direct tubular toxicity, renal vasoconstriction, and formation of intratubular casts [9].

HEART-KIDNEY INTERACTIONS AND AKI: CARDIORENAL SYNDROMES

The presence of numerous connectors between the kidney and heart predisposes patients with heart disease to developing AKI. Common risk factors for development of AKI in cardiovascular patients include advanced age, myocardial infarction, stroke, heart failure, hypertension, diabetes mellitus, advanced New York Heart Association heart failure functional class, and previous hospitalizations for heart failure [10]. Acute kidney injury in the setting of acute decompensated heart failure, a form of Type 1 cardiorenal syndrome, is characterized by a hemodynamically mediated decrease in RBF, compounded by increased sympathetic output, renin-angiotensin system activation, and increased release of inflammatory mediators among various mechanisms [11,12]. Cardiac interventions themselves may predispose to AKI through mechanisms, including exposure to iodinated radiocontrast. Patients undergoing such procedures often have pre-existing comorbidities, including diabetes, hypertension, and use of medications such as diuretics that may make them especially vulnerable to contrast induced AKI. Acute kidney injury has been reported to occur in about 10% of patients after percutaneous coronary angiography and has been associated with increased cardiovascular morbidity and mortality [13].

While AKI following percutaneous coronary angiography is usually due to radiocontrast nephrotoxicity, other cases may be due to development of atheroembolic renal injury, with livedo reticularis and hypocomplementemia being additional clues to this disorder. Patients undergoing cardiac surgery are also at increased risk of developing AKI, and even small rises in serum creatinine have been associated with increased mortality and have been shown to be an independent risk factor for subsequent development of chronic kidney disease [14–17].

AKI IN THE SETTING OF LIVER DISEASE

Hepatorenal syndrome (HRS) is a potentially reversible functional renal impairment seen in patients with advanced liver cirrhosis or fulminant hepatic failure. It is characterized by marked reduction in GFR and renal plasma flow (RPF) in the absence of other cause of renal failure. The pathogenesis includes splanchnic vasodilation resulting in portal hypertension, decreased effective arterial volume and blood pressure resulting in renal vasoconstriction, and activation of the renin-angiotensin-aldosterone system, which fails to remit despite infusion of albumin. Tubular function is preserved with the absence of proteinuria or histologic changes in the kidney. There are two subtypes of HRS: Type 1 HRS is a rapidly progressive form of AKI, often triggered by bacterial infection such as spontaneous bacterial peritonitis, and is defined by doubling of initial serum creatinine to a level >2.5 mg/dL or by a 50% reduction in creatinine clearance to a level of <20 mL/min in less than 2 weeks. Type 2 HRS refers to a less severe form of HRS with a moderate, steadily progressive decline in renal function. Urinary findings in patients with HRS mimic those of patients with prerenal conditions, and it is important to distinguish HRS from such states as well as from acute tubular necrosis, which may result from ischemia, nephrotoxic agents, and infection [18–24].

AKI AND MALIGNANCY

Acute kidney injury in the setting of malignancy may result from the malignancy itself and or the therapies that are used to treat it [25]. Malignancy may cause AKI via the development of urinary tract obstruction and paraneoplastic syndromes such as hypercalcemia and glomerular disease. For example, nearly 50% of patients with multiple myeloma can develop AKI secondary to cast nephropathy, which is caused by intratubular obstruction by filtered free light chains and is associated with a worse 1-year survival [26]. The key factor in treatment is rapid lowering of filtered light chains with chemotherapeutic agents and in some cases plasmapheresis.

A number of commonly used chemotherapeutic agents are associated with renal side effects, and the etiologic spectrum continues to broaden with the introduction of new agents. Cisplatin has a well-known association with the development of tubular toxicity and acute tubular necrosis along with magnesium wasting [27]. An additional mechanism of AKI is via vascular damage, resulting in the development of thrombotic microangiopathy, as seen with gemcitabine and inhibitors of vascular endothelial growth factor [28]. Various drugs associated with cancer therapy may also result in AKI by causing interstitial nephritis [29].

Another form of AKI in the setting of malignancy occurs with tumor lysis syndrome with the induction phase of treatment of hematological malignancies being a classic scenario for development of this disorder. It is associated with characteristic findings of hyperuricemia, hyperkalemia, hyperphosphatemia, and secondary hypocalcemia that can lead not only to AKI but also to other serious clinical complications, including cardiac dysrhythmias and pulmonary edema. Approximately 50%–70% of patients with tumor lysis syndrome may require renal replacement therapy [30]. Early collaboration between the oncologist and nephrologist is important to anticipate the occurrence of tumor lysis syndrome and assure timely management.

AKI AND AUTOIMMUNE DISEASES

Various autoimmune disorders such as antineutrophil cytoplasmic antibody (ANCA) vasculitis and systemic lupus erythematous are associated with AKI. The pathogenesis includes the production of autoantibodies, with a consequent inflammatory environment resulting in tissue damage and blood vessel injury. Presence of volume overload, hematuria, proteinuria, and systemic manifestations help point toward vasculitis and glomerulonephritis, though renal biopsy is generally needed to provide a definitive diagnosis to optimally guide management.

AKI AND THROMBOTIC MICROANGIOPATHY

Thrombotic microangiopathies are rare causes of AKI and require prompt recognition and treatment. Well-described etiologies include thrombotic thrombocytopenic purpura, hemolytic uremic syndrome (which can be subdivided into typical and atypical forms), disseminated intravascular coagulation, malignant hypertension (referred to now as hypertensive emergency), scleroderma renal crisis, and drug toxicity such as can occur with calcineurin inhibitors. The pathogenesis includes thrombosis of capillaries and arterioles due to endothelial damage. Determining the cause of the thrombotic microangiopathy is essential, as this will guide the appropriate therapy [31].

AKI AND INTRA-ABDOMINAL HYPERTENSION/ ABDOMINAL COMPARTMENT SYNDROME

Intra-abdominal hypertension is an important and increasingly recognized cause of AKI, especially in the critical care setting. A variety of factors, including recent abdominal surgery, increased intra-abdominal pressure from ascites, ileus or intestinal obstruction, decreased abdominal wall compliance (obesity, mechanical ventilation), and factors resulting

in increased capillary permeability (burns, trauma, sepsis, acidosis, pancreatitis, coagulopathy), are associated with this condition. The pathogenesis appears to be related to compression of the intra-abdominal and intrathoracic blood vessels, venous congestion, and renal interstitial edema, along with elevation of renal parenchymal and renal vein pressures, with the net effect being a compromise of the renal microcirculation and renal function [32].

CLINICAL SYNDROMIC APPROACH TO THE PATIENT WITH AKI

The goal of the initial evaluation of the patient with AKI is to determine whether the problem is most likely prerenal in origin, a postrenal problem, or an intrinsic renal disorder to avoid delays in recognizing serious diagnoses as well as missed opportunities to address readily correctable conditions. It is important that diagnoses of prerenal states and obstruction are not delayed, as these are generally very treatable conditions, and premature anchoring on potential intrinsic renal diagnoses may distract attention from these possibilities. Similarly, the presence of what appears to be a prerenal state based on clinical findings does not preclude the possibility of a serious intrinsic renal disorder. In order to classify the renal problem accurately early in the evaluation, it is important to take a stepwise approach, as outlined in Figure 24.1.

HISTORY AND PHYSICAL EXAMINATION

The initial workup, outlined in Table 24.1, includes a detailed history to identify risk factors that can increase the susceptibility of patient to suffer AKI. A thorough review of all medications with particular attention to potentially nephrotoxic medications and agents and those with a known predisposition to causing interstitial nephritis is essential. The history must include a careful review of potential risk factors and precipitants for AKI and their timing, including exposure to intravenous radiocontrast, liver disease, heart failure, fluid loss and/or poor intake, bleeding, infection, trauma with significant muscle injury, malignancy with risk for tumor lysis syndrome, and recent surgery with a careful review of the operative record, looking for episodes of significant hypotension. A detailed physical examination with assessment of intravascular volume status is crucial. Fluid status should be assessed by looking at skin turgor, testing for orthostasis, and evaluating for signs of volume overload (such as pedal edema, raised jugular venous distension, S_3, pulmonary rales, and ascites). Intravascular volume cannot be measured directly but can be inferred by the presence or absence of fluid responsiveness. Respiratory variation of the inferior vena cava diameter on ultrasound and dynamic changes of central venous pressure (CVP) or arterial pulse pressure is often utilized in critical care settings to assess volume status. Finally, urine output (UO) with assessment of oliguria (generally considered to be present with UO of less than 0.3 mL/kg/h or about 500 mL/d) is one of the most important bedside measures to

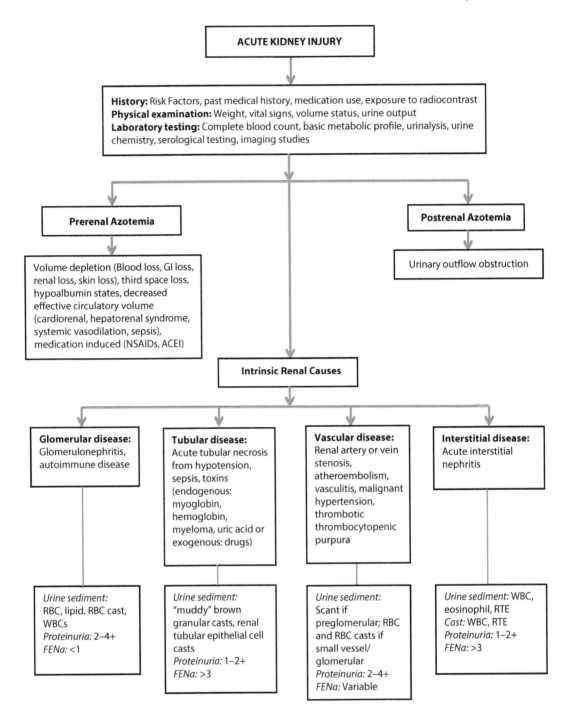

FIGURE 24.1　Approach to the patient with acute kidney injury.

assess kidney function, though it is important to remember that the majority of cases of AKI are nonoliguric.

MECHANISTIC CATEGORIZATION OF AKI

Based on the history and physical examination, the goal is to try to begin to categorize the AKI into a prerenal etiology, an intrinsic etiology, or a postrenal etiology, so that proper selection of laboratory, imaging, and other testing can be carried out, and rapid identification of conditions requiring urgent treatment can be achieved.

PRERENAL STATES

Prerenal states can often be identified through a careful history and physical examination, with attention to findings related to volume status, cardiopulmonary function, and systemic disorders, which can help point to decreased effective arterial volume as the mechanism causing AKI. Laboratory findings consistent with these states include a bland urinalysis and a low urine sodium (generally less than 20 mEq/L) (Table 24.2). Of note, similar laboratory findings will be obtained in the presence of either hypovolemia or heart

TABLE 24.1

Using the History and Physical Examination to Differentiate Likely Causes of AKI

	Prenatal Etiology	Intrinsic Renal Disease	Postrenal Etiology
History	History of hemorrhage, diarrhea, vomiting, increased nasogastric tube suction, burns, leg swelling, shortness of breath, yellowing of skin	Recent use of nephrotoxic medication, recent contrast dye exposure, recent vascular surgery, vascular catheterization, foamy urine, hematuria, fever, rash, arthralgia, toxin exposure	History of benign prostate enlargement or cancer, pelvic cancer, pelvic radiation, prior urinary retention, urinary stones, poor urinary stream, urinary hesitancy
Physical Examination	**Signs of volume loss:** tachycardia, low blood pressure, orthostatic hypotension, poor skin turgor, dry mucous membranes, weak peripheral pulses, delayed capillary refill **Sign of heart failure:** elevated jugular venous pressure, S_3, pulmonary rales, peripheral edema, hepatomegaly **Sign of liver disease:** Icterus, ascites, caput medusae, spider angiomata, palmar erythema, gynecomastia, testicular atrophy	Hypertension, fever, oral/nasal ulcers (SLE, vasculitis), rash (SLE, acute interstitial nephritis), joint swelling (autoimmune disease, SLE), petechiae (vasculitis, TTP), livedo reticularis (atheroembolic event), fundoscopic findings in malignant hypertension, bruit (vascular etiology), pulmonary findings (ANCA-vasculitis, anti-GBM disease)	Enlarged prostate, palpable bladder, enlarged kidneys, abnormal pelvic examination

TABLE 24.2

Differentiating Prerenal Azotemia from Intrinsic Renal Causes of AKI

Indices	Prerenal Etiology	Intrinsic Renal Etiology
Blood urea nitrogen to creatinine ratio	>20	<20
Urine osmolality (mOsm/L)	>500	<400
Urine specific gravity	>1.020	1.010
Fractional excretion of sodium (%)	<1	>1
Fractional excretion of urea (%)	<25	>50
Urine sodium (mEq/L)	<20	>40
Urine to serum creatinine	>40	<20
Renal failure index (urine sodium × plasma creatinine/urine creatinine)	<1	>1
Urine sediment	Bland, perhaps hyaline casts	Granular, muddy brown

failure, e.g., in both instances, low effective arterial volume and not overall volume status per se is the cause of the AKI and associated laboratory abnormalities.

POSTRENAL CAUSES

There are many conditions that may result in urinary tract obstruction, with prostatic disease being a common etiology in older men. While a review of all causes of urinary tract obstruction is beyond the scope of this review, there are several important clinical caveats to keep in mind. One is that prompt diagnosis followed by early relief of obstruction is associated with improvement in renal function in most and that delayed recognition may result in permanent renal damage. Fortunately, obstruction can usually be readily diagnosed by ultrasonography or computed tomography.

However, some cases of obstruction may not be associated with a dilated urinary tract, such as with retroperitoneal hemorrhage or lymphoma involving the retroperitoneum, and hence, in the appropriate setting when there is a high index of suspicion for obstruction, a negative renal ultrasound should not preclude further investigation. Another important point to remember is that while complete obstructions will cause anuria, most obstructions are partial, and urine output may be preserved, and hence, the absence of oliguria or anuria should not by itself be considered sufficient to rule out urinary tract obstruction.

INTRINSIC RENAL CAUSES AND HOW TO DIFFERENTIATE THEM

A useful way to categorize intrinsic AKI is based on what part of the kidney is affected (i.e., tubules, glomeruli, interstitium, and vasculature). Acute tubular necrosis is the most common type of intrinsic AKI in hospitalized patients and typically results from ischemia, exposure to exogenous and endogenous nephrotoxins, and sepsis, as discussed earlier. Identification of a precipitating event is a key component of the diagnosis of this disorder. In contrast to a prerenal etiology, its clinical course is characterized by delayed recovery (when recovery takes place) despite appropriate fluid resuscitation. Laboratory findings also differ between the two conditions; as in contrast to prerenal states, acute tubular necrosis is characterized by an elevated urine sodium, isosthenuria, and a urine sediment, which typically contains "muddy brown" granular casts. An approach to differentiating prerenal states from acute tubular necrosis is outlined in Table 24.2. Differentiating prerenal states from acute tubular necrosis as a cause of AKI can be challenging, as pre-existing chronic renal disease or diuretic use may result in elevated urine sodium in prerenal patients, and some patients with acute tubular necrosis have a low urine sodium, and hence, clinical judgment is extremely important in the interpretation of laboratory findings.

Glomerular causes of AKI include glomerulonephritis, such as in the setting of lupus, infection, or pulmonary renal syndromes (e.g., Goodpasture syndrome and ANCA-associated vasculitides). Urinary findings of hematuria (typically dysmorphic hematuria) with proteinuria are strongly suggestive of a glomerular/small vessel vascular etiology of AKI. Further testing, including serology and biopsy, is usually required to make a specific diagnosis.

Acute interstitial nephritis can be secondary to many conditions, most commonly resulting from medication use [29]. In about one-third of cases, there is a history of maculopapular erythematous rash, fever, and arthralgia. Sterile pyuria with eosinophiluria and peripheral eosinophilia are classical findings, but as with some of the physical examination findings, they may be absent, and kidney biopsy may be needed to distinguish between acute interstitial nephritis and other causes of AKI. Acute events involving the renal arteries or veins can also lead to intrinsic AKI, such as with embolic events from atrial fibrillation and a mural cardiac thrombus, as well as in situ thrombosis, as can occur with severe hypotension and stasis in a patient with underlying renovascular atherosclerotic disease. A more common cause of vascular disease-causing AKI is renal atheroembolic disease as may occur following arterial catheterization, vascular surgery, or anticoagulation. A detailed review of these disorders is beyond the scope of this chapter.

DIAGNOSTIC TESTING IN THE APPROACH TO AKI

BLOOD TESTING

Basic blood testing should include a complete blood count, serum electrolytes and creatinine and blood urea nitrogen (BUN). The rise in serum creatinine is commonly delayed after kidney function decline in the critical care setting, and hence, it is important to remember that creatinine can be a suboptimal marker for AKI in such settings. Other blood testing will depend on the clinical scenario and may include examination of the peripheral smear for the presence of schistocytes, tear cells and rouleaux phenomenon, myoglobin and free hemoglobin levels, creatine kinase levels, serum uric acid, lactate dehydrogenase (LDH), complement levels, antinuclear antibody (ANA), ANCA including anti-myeloperoxidase antibodies and anti-proteinase-3 antibodies, anti-glomerular basement membrane antibodies (anti-GBM), hepatitis B and C virus studies, antistreptolysin (ASO), serum immunofixation, serum free light chains, and prostate-specific antigen (PSA) levels. If sepsis is suspected, a basic septic screen should be performed. A summary of selected laboratory testing used in the assessment of AKI is provided in Table 24.3.

URINE STUDIES

Urinalysis is an important noninvasive test in the initial workup of AKI. It should be studied in detail as each of its parameters can give important clues regarding diagnosis.

TABLE 24.3

Selected Laboratory Testing to Differentiate Causes of Intrinsic AKI

Test	Etiology of AKI
Positive ANA, ds DNA	Autoimmune, SLE
Positive urine culture, blood culture, septic screen	Sepsis
Elevated uric acid	Malignancy/tumor lysis syndrome
Elevated prostate specific antigen	BPH, prostate cancer
Elevated antistreptolysin O titer	Post streptococcal glomerulonephritis
Elevated antineutrophil cytoplasmic antibody (ANCA)	Vasculitis
Elevated anti-glomerular basement membrane antibody (anti GBM Ab)	Goodpasture syndrome
Low complement levels	Lupus nephritis, atheroembolic disease, membranoproliferative glomerulonephritis, postinfectious glomerulonephritis, hepatitis B and related disease, cryoglobulinemia
Elevated creatine kinase, myoglobin	Rhabdomyolysis
Increased anion gap metabolic acidosis with osmolar gap	Drug toxicity/poisoning (ethylene glycol)
Signs of intravascular hemolysis (elevated LDH, indirect bilirubin, elevated reticulocyte count, schistocytes on peripheral smear, decreased haptoglobin)	Hemolytic uremic syndrome (HUS), thrombotic thrombocytopenic purpura (TTP), SLE, autoimmune disease

Urine color, pH, specific gravity and testing for glucose, protein, ketones, leukocyte esterase, nitrites, RBCs, WBCs, eosinophils, casts, and crystals can help greatly in differentiating the general cause of AKI (Table 24.4). Spot urine protein-to-creatinine ratio can be used to assess the extent of proteinuria, though in the setting of AKI, it may be less reliable. In some cases where there is proteinuria and or hematuria, it may represent underlying chronic kidney disease, which itself is a risk factor for AKI.

Measurement of urine electrolytes is a valuable tool in assessing function of the renal tubules. Commonly used variables are fractional excretion of sodium (FENa) and urea (FEUrea). FENa is helpful in distinguishing prerenal from intrinsic renal causes of AKI but can be misleading in nonoliguric states and in patients on diuretics. In patients receiving diuretics, measurement of FEUrea may be useful as an alternative to FENa and may also be helpful in predicting development of AKI, when measured after surgery [33].

NEWER BIOMARKERS OF AKI

The US Food and Drug Administration (FDA) approved NephroCheck® in 2014 to evaluate the risk of developing moderate to severe AKI in hospitalized, critically ill patients.

TABLE 24.4

Urinalysis Findings as Clues to the Cause of AKI

Urinalysis Findings	Etiology
Pyuria	Infection
Sterile pyuria	Interstitial nephritis
Hematuria	Glomerulonephritis, infection, stone, obstruction, malignancy
Eosinophiluria	Interstitial nephritis, atheroembolic disease
RBC cast/dysmorphic RBCs	Glomerulonephritis, vasculitis, malignant hypertension
WBC casts	Acute pyelonephritis, acute interstitial nephritis
Hyaline casts	Prerenal azotemia/post renal cause
Broad granular casts	Chronic kidney disease
Muddy brown casts	Acute tubular necrosis
Waxy cast	Tubular/interstitial disease
Crystalluria	Calcium oxalate (ethylene glycol), uric acid (tumor lysis syndrome), medications (acyclovir, indinavir)
Hemoglobin/myoglobin casts (red-brown cast)	Intravascular hemolysis, rhabdomyolysis

It is a urine test that detects two biomarkers, insulin-like growth factor binding protein 7 (IGFBP-7) and tissue inhibitor of metalloproteinase 2 (TIMP-2). Based on their levels, a score is derived that indicates the likelihood of developing moderate-severe AKI within the next 12 hours. However, it should not be used alone, and the FDA recommends it is to be used in conjunction with other clinical and laboratory tests [2,34].

IMAGING STUDIES

Renal ultrasonography is particularly helpful to rule out the underlying existing structural renal disease and diagnosing obstruction of the urinary collecting system. Loss of corticomedullary differentiation and decreased kidney size are findings suggestive of chronic kidney disease, which can help in cases when the diagnosis of AKI is uncertain, such as in a patient presenting to the hospital with an elevated serum creatinine but without any prior available laboratory testing or any helpful medical history. In cases where ultrasound is not available or if there is concern about potential disease of the retroperitoneum such as tumor, fibrosis, and hemorrhage, then non-contrast computed tomography can be done. Renal Doppler ultrasound and contrast-enhanced ultrasound have recently emerged as potential tools for bedside assessment of renal perfusion and renal microcirculation, respectively, and for predicting the reversibility of AKI, especially in the critical care setting [35,36]. Beyond being a convenient bedside tool to assess renal perfusion, it offers the advantage of providing noninvasive real-time imaging with the ability to perform dynamic and repeated assessment. It can detect early renal insults and

help distinguish transient from persistent AKI as well as the impact of vasopressors and fluid challenges on renal perfusion. However, Doppler-based resistive index (RI) needs to be interpreted carefully, taking into account patient age, pre-existing subclinical vascular stiffness, and intra-abdominal pressure [37].

BLADDER PRESSURE

Bladder pressure should be measured in patients presenting with AKI when abdominal compartment syndrome is being considered, such as in patients following abdominal surgery, as discussed previously. An intra-abdominal pressure of less than 10 mmHg rules out abdominal compartment syndrome as the cause of AKI. Patients with bladder pressures of 15–25 mmHg are at risk for abdominal compartment syndrome, and bladder pressures above 25 mmHg often points to abdominal compartment syndrome as the cause of AKI [32,38].

RENAL BIOPSY

Most patients with AKI, such as those with clinical and laboratory findings suggestive of acute tubular necrosis, will not require renal biopsy. While beyond the scope of this review, it should be noted that renal biopsy has an important role in evaluating patients, with findings suggestive of conditions such as glomerulonephritis, vasculitis, and interstitial nephritis, both for diagnostic purposes and to guide therapy. For example, renal biopsy findings are important in guiding decisions regarding immunosuppressive therapy in patients with ANCA-associated vasculitis and lupus nephritis. Confirmation of a diagnosis of interstitial nephritis can help prompt early discontinuation of a drug and perhaps institution of glucocorticoid therapy, which may help improve renal function. Many of the therapies used to treat these conditions entail risk of substantial toxicity and renal biopsy and, therefore, play a critical role in such decision making.

CLINICAL PEARLS IN INTERPRETING TEST RESULTS IN THE CRITICAL CARE SETTING

Patients in the critical care setting often have conditions that may interfere with the interpretation of various laboratory tests. For example, while serum creatinine is used as a marker of renal function, its rate of rise may be misleading in the setting of fluid overload. This is because the creatinine, which is being produced is accumulating in a larger volume of distribution, and hence, its rate of rise may be blunted, leading the clinician to underestimate the severity of the reduction in GFR. Patients with low muscle mass produce creatinine at a lower rate, and hence, the rise in serum creatinine in a patient with AKI with low muscle mass may be further blunted. It should also be remembered that serum creatinine lags behind the reduction in GFR, which can further delay the recognition of AKI in the critical care setting. In addition, some drugs such as trimethoprim may interfere with tubular secretion of creatinine, which could thereby result in a rise in serum creatinine without a reduction in GFR, hence leading to an incorrect diagnosis of AKI. It is also important to remember that in AKI, the patient is not in a steady state, and therefore, serum creatinine levels cannot be used to calculate an estimated GFR, therefore assuming a GFR of less than 10 mL/min is prudent. Other tests may be challenging to interpret as well. Recent urinary catheterization may result in hematuria and may falsely suggest the presence of glomerulonephritis. Certain serological tests such as ANA testing may yield false-positive results in the presence of infection, for example. Hence, it is very important that the clinician always interprets the laboratory findings in the context of the patient's clinical condition.

MANAGEMENT OF AKI

There are some basic principles that apply to the treatment of all patients with AKI, with additional interventions depending on the type of AKI and clinical context. Therapy must be directed toward the underlying pathophysiological factor, and interventions must be taken to avoid further renal injury (such as avoiding exposure to nephrotoxic agents) and modify other therapies for the reduction in GFR, the most common example being adjusting the dosing of renally cleared medications while remembering the caveat that serum creatinine cannot be used to estimate the GFR in the setting of AKI. Management of fluid and electrolyte balance and nutrition are extremely important in all patients in the critical care setting, though AKI can make this challenging, as outlined in later sections.

FLUID RESUSCITATION

If prerenal factors are suspected, immediate hemodynamic resuscitation should be started. Central volume status should be monitored clinically (physical examination, neck vein inspection, measurement of blood pressure, and heart rate) or through invasive hemodynamic monitoring as needed (central venous catheter and arterial cannula), both to avoid excessive fluid accumulation and undertreatment of hypovolemia. In general, crystalloid solutions will be the optimal choice to help expand the extracellular volume, with one exception being HRS, where albumin infusions have a well-defined role [39,40].

VASOPRESSORS

Some patients may remain hypotensive (mean arterial pressure <65–70 mmHg) even after restoring intravascular volume or may have a low cardiac output state. These patients can benefit from inotropic drugs such as the use of norepinephrine in septic shock, where it is the vasopressor of choice. Vasopressors are also used in the HRS, and when used, they should be given concurrently with albumin [40].

DIURETICS

Diuretics have been used in AKI for many years to help manage volume overload such as in patients with cardiorenal syndromes in the setting of decompensated heart failure. There are theoretical reasons why diuretics might be helpful in AKI, but studies have yielded conflicting results regarding the effects of loop diuretics in AKI, with some showing benefit and others showing harm. More recently, an analysis of post-AKI fluid balance and mortality was carried out using data from the Fluid and Catheter Treatment Trial (FACTT), a multicenter, randomized controlled trial evaluating a conservative versus liberal fluid-management strategy [41]. Positive fluid balance after AKI was associated with increased mortality. As for the effects of diuretic therapy, mortality was reduced, but this effect was not independent of its effect on fluid balance, and hence, it was concluded that the favorable effect of diuretic therapy on survival is likely due to its effect on improving fluid balance. Hence, in the setting of AKI, diuretic therapy can serve as an aid in helping avoid extensive fluid accumulation, which may thereby improve outcomes.

RENAL REPLACEMENT THERAPY

The optimal timing of initiating renal replacement therapy (RRT) for AKI in the critical care setting requires careful consideration of the overall clinical picture, the patient's severity of illness, presence of oliguria, presence of fluid overload, severity of electrolyte and acid-base disturbances, and associated non-renal organ failure rather than specific serum creatinine or urea values alone, keeping in mind the precautions that must be taken in interpreting serum creatinine levels in the critical care setting. Different modalities for RRT in the critical care setting are available and include intermittent hemodialysis (IHD), hybrid therapies (prolonged intermittent RRT [PIRRT], sustained low efficiency dialysis [SLED], extended daily dialysis [EDD]), continuous RRT (CRRT), and peritoneal dialysis (PD). Selection of the optimal RRT modality should be individualized based on both patient-specific and critical care unit-specific operational characteristics [42,43].

The gradual removal of solute, water, and electrolytes, offered by CRRT, may make it the preferred therapy in certain circumstances where the patient is more susceptible to volume and osmotic/metabolic fluctuations. It may offer better hemodynamic and volume homeostasis in hemodynamically unstable patients with considerable volume overload and is generally a preferable option in patients with acute brain or liver injury, where rapid shifts in blood osmolality may contribute to an iatrogenic increase in intracranial pressure. The CRRT is also recommended in situations where extracorporeal life support therapies are applied. It can be performed using diffusive clearance (continuous venovenous hemodialysis [CVVHD]), convective clearance (continuous venovenous hemofiltration [CVVH]), or a combination of both (continuous venovenous hemodiafiltration [CVVHDF]). Although convective modalities offer greater clearance of middle molecules compared with diffusive clearance, this has not been shown

TABLE 24.5

Comparison Between Intermittent Hemodialysis and Continuous Renal Replacement Therapy for AKI

Intermittent Hemodialysis	Continuous Renal Replacement
Advantages:	**Advantages:**
• Relatively inexpensive	• Can be done in the less hemodynamically stable patient
• Less labor intensive	
• Short duration	• Technically less difficult
• Less anticoagulant use	• Does not require dialysis personnel: CCU staff can be trained
• Better in the setting of severe hyperkalemia	
	• Ongoing control of solute, electrolytes, acid base and volume
Disadvantages:	**Disadvantages:**
• Technical difficulties	• Less widely available than hemodialysis
• Require hemodialysis personnel to perform	
• Require fresh supply of water	• Requires continuous use of anticoagulation
• Potential for more hemodynamic instability and electrolyte imbalance from rapid solute shifts and fluid removal	• Not as effective in state of severe hyperkalemia
	• May not have local nursing staff who are credentialed to perform

to affect clinical outcomes in the AKI setting, and the choice between modalities should be determined by local expertise. A comparison of RRT modalities is provided in Table 24.5.

Intermittent hemodialysis may be considered when more rapid mobilization of fluid is a priority, provided the patient can be expected to tolerate metabolic fluctuations and fluid shifts. It provides the most rapid solute clearance and is the initial preferred option in the setting of life-threatening hyperkalemia or drug poisonings. For those patients who are hemodynamically unstable and would typically be best treated with CRRT but have severe hyperkalemia or another life-threatening condition related to their AKI, an initial period of HD with pressor support may be attempted with a subsequent change to CRRT. Specific strategies can be applied to improve hemodynamic tolerance of IHD such as using conservative initial ultrafiltration rates, reduced dialysate temperature, and sodium profiling. Of note, studies to date have not supported an overall survival benefit of CRRT compared with intermittent therapies [44].

The PIRRT represents a hybrid therapy between IHD and CRRT, performed over 6–12 hours either daily or between 3 and 6 days per week. It includes approaches such as extended daily dialysis with filtration, SLED, and accelerated venovenous hemofiltration [45]. It provides the advantage of a dialysis-free period, allowing physical rehabilitation without compromising hemodynamics and adequacy of dialysis.

The literature pertaining to the best timing for discontinuation of RRT in the setting of apparent recovery from AKI is limited. Several variables such as 24-h urine creatinine excretion, daily urea excretion, and 2-h creatinine clearance have been studied as predictors of successful weaning from RRT, though urine output appears to have the greatest predictive value [46]. As for the identification of AKI, novel biomarkers could be of great potential value in aiding decision making regarding when to discontinue RRT.

COMPLICATIONS

There are many complications which can arise in AKI and these can be organized into several categories. First, the decrease in GFR may lead to fluid overload, acid-base and electrolyte disturbances, and uremic sequelae such as pericarditis, platelet dysfunction predisposing to bleeding, and neurological changes. Second, the disorder causing AKI may itself lead to major complications such as with sepsis, malignancy, and toxicity from certain drugs. Third, the therapies used to treat and manage AKI may also lead to complications, including vascular events related to central venous access for HD or CRRT and adverse effects of immunosuppressive therapies, plasmapheresis, and other treatments. There is also an emerging body of scientific literature demonstrating that damage to the renal parenchyma, even in the absence of a major reduction in GFR, may lead to substantial changes in the expression of various cytokines and other mediators of inflammation and damage in multiple organs [47]. Acute kidney injury also predisposes patients to prolonged length of hospital stay and its attendant risk of hospital-acquired infections, deconditioning, and other adverse sequelae. It should also be noted that substantial psychological stress for the patient and family often results from AKI and its subsequent course. A summary of complications in AKI is provided in Table 24.6.

PROGNOSIS

The incidence of AKI in the critical care unit can range from 20% to 50%, with a higher incidence in septic patients [48], and an overall mortality in this group approaching 50%–55% [49]. Studies of critically ill patients with severe AKI requiring RRT have reported at least 33% of the patients to be RRT-dependent on discharge, with 5%–12.5% having a long-term requirement for RRT [50]. Although mortality in AKI in critically ill patients has historically been thought to be principally the consequence of underlying comorbidity rather than the AKI itself,

TABLE 24.6
Complications of AKI

Neurological	Asterixis, seizure, irritability, uremic encephalopathy
Cardiovascular	Volume overload, arrhythmia, pericarditis, pericardial effusion, myocardial infarction
Pulmonary	Pulmonary edema, pulmonary embolism
Gastrointestinal	Nausea, vomiting
Hematological	Platelet dysfunction, anemia
Metabolic	Hyperkalemia, hyponatremia, hypocalcemia, hyperphosphatemia, hypermagnesemia, metabolic acidosis
Dialysis-related	Dialysis disequilibrium
	Dialysis catheter-associated complications

there is increasing evidence to suggest AKI is an independent predictor of increased mortality [51]. The prognosis often depends on severity of AKI as well as the underlying cause. Prerenal and postrenal causes are generally easier to treat and tend to be associated with better prognoses. Sepsis-related AKI, especially in critical care units, is associated with the worst prognosis [7,8]. In addition, an episode of AKI is not only associated with short-term morbidity and mortality, but it has significant long-term effects as well. A graph of mortality demonstrates a biphasic pattern, with a high incidence in the initial diagnostic phase, followed by the immediate post-critical care unit phase [52]. A long-term need for RRT has a major adverse effect on quality of life, incurs a substantial financial burden, and confers increased odds of being transferred to a long-term care facility. In those who experience an apparent resolution of the acute phase of AKI, abnormal renal function may persist. For example, microalbuminuria has been observed to persist for several years afterward. In those patients who appear to have fully recovered from an episode of AKI, there is an increased subsequent risk of developing chronic kidney disease, and long-term follow-up of renal function in the patient with apparently resolved AKI is warranted.

CONCLUSION

Acute kidney injury is a common problem encountered in the critical care setting and continues to entail substantial morbidity and mortality. The most common causes include low effective arterial volume states and acute tubular necrosis secondary to hypotension, sepsis, or nephrotoxic medications. Other causes merit consideration and a logical, systematic approach beginning with a thorough history and physical examination, and selective use of laboratory testing and imaging studies can help optimize rapid identification of AKI and its likely cause and avoid delayed recognition of a serious etiology requiring urgent intervention. Early recognition and timely targeted intervention are the key to reducing the morbidity and mortality associated with this disorder. Ongoing research on biomarkers for early detection of AKI as well as therapies to promote renal repair hold promise to transform the management of this important disorder in the critical care setting over the coming years.

REFERENCES

1. Hsu RK, McCulloch CE, Dudley RA, Lo LJ, Hsu CY. Temporal changes in incidence of dialysis-requiring AKI. *J Am Soc Nephrol* 2013;24(1):37–42.
2. Mohsenin V. Practical approach to detection and management of acute kidney injury in critically ill patient. *J Intensive Care* 2017;5:57.
3. Loutzenhiser R, Griffin K, Williamson G, Bidani A. Renal autoregulation: New perspectives regarding the protective and regulatory roles of the underlying mechanisms. *Am J Physiol Regul Integr Comp Physiol* 2006;290(5):R1153–R1167.
4. Bonventre JV, Yang L. Cellular pathophysiology of ischemic acute kidney injury. *J Clin Invest* 2011;121(11):4210–4221.
5. Bagshaw SM, Uchino S, Bellomo R, et al. Septic acute kidney injury in critically ill patients: Clinical characteristics and outcomes. *Clin J Am Soc Nephrol* 2007;2(3):431–439.
6. Oppert M, Engel C, Brunkhorst FM, et al. Acute renal failure in patients with severe sepsis and septic shock—A significant independent risk factor for mortality: Results from the German prevalence study. *Nephrol Dial Transplant* 2008;23(3):904–909.
7. Zarbock A, Gomez H, Kellum JA. Sepsis-induced acute kidney injury revisited: Pathophysiology, prevention and future therapies. *Curr Opin Crit Care* 2014;20(6):588–595.
8. Alobaidi R, Basu RK, Goldstein SL, Bagshaw SM. Sepsis-associated acute kidney injury. *Semin Nephrol* 2015;35(1):2–11.
9. Malinoski DJ, Slater MS, Mullins RJ. Crush injury and rhabdomyolysis. *Crit Care Clin* 2004;20(1):171–192.
10. Lekawanvijit S, Krum H. Cardiorenal syndrome: Acute kidney injury secondary to cardiovascular disease and role of protein-bound uraemic toxins. *J Physiol* 2014;592(18):3969–3983.
11. Ronco C, McCullough P, Anker SD, et al. Cardio-renal syndromes: Report from the consensus conference of the acute dialysis quality initiative. *Eur Heart J* 2010;31(6):703–711.
12. Salleck D, John S. Cardiorenal syndrome. *Med Klin Intensivmed Notfmed* 2017;114:439–443.
13. Ohno Y, Maekawa Y, Miyata H, et al. Impact of periprocedural bleeding on incidence of contrast-induced acute kidney injury in patients treated with percutaneous coronary intervention. *J Am Coll Cardiol* 2013;62(14):1260–1266.
14. Scabbia EV, Scabbia L. The cardio-renal syndrome (CRS). *IJC Metabolic & Endocrine* 2015;9(Supplement C):1–4.
15. Cruz DN. Cardiorenal syndrome in critical care: The acute cardiorenal and renocardiac syndromes. *Adv Chronic Kidney Dis* 2013;20(1):56–66.
16. Gnanaraj J, Radhakrishnan J. Cardio-renal syndrome [version 1; referees: 3 approved] 2016;5:2123.
17. Bock JS, Gottlieb SS. Cardiorenal syndrome: New perspectives. *Circulation* 2010;121(23):2592–2600.
18. Low G, Alexander GJ, Lomas DJ. Hepatorenal syndrome: Aetiology, diagnosis, and treatment. *Gastroenterol Res Pract* 2015;2015:207012.
19. Erly B, Carey WD, Kapoor B, McKinney JM, Tam M, Wang W. Hepatorenal syndrome: A review of pathophysiology and current treatment options. *Semin Intervent Radiol* 2015;32(4):445–454.
20. Sandhu BS, Sanyal AJ. Hepatorenal syndrome. *Curr Treat Options Gastroenterol* 2005;8(6):443–450.
21. Salerno F, Gerbes A, Gines P, Wong F, Arroyo V. Diagnosis, prevention and treatment of hepatorenal syndrome in cirrhosis. *Postgrad Med J* 2008;84(998):662–670.
22. Venkat D, Venkat KK. Hepatorenal syndrome. *South Med J* 2010;103(7):654–661.
23. Munoz SJ. The hepatorenal syndrome. *Med Clin North Am* 2008;92(4):813–837, viii–ix.
24. Angeli P. Hepatorenal syndrome. In: Vincent J-L ed. *Intensive Care Medicine: Annual Update 2006*. New York: Springer New York, 2006:661–670.
25. Rosner MH, Perazella MA. Acute kidney injury in patients with cancer. *N Engl J Med* 2017;377(5):500–501.
26. Walther C, Podoll AS, Finkel KW. Treatment of acute kidney injury with cast nephropathy. *Clin Nephrol* 2014;82(1):1–6.
27. Goldstein RS, Mayor GH. Minireview. The nephrotoxicity of cisplatin. *Life Sci* 1983;32(7):685–690.
28. Humphreys BD, Sharman JP, Henderson JM, et al. Gemcitabine-associated thrombotic microangiopathy. *Cancer.* 2004;100(12):2664–2670.

29. Rossert J. Drug-induced acute interstitial nephritis. *Kidney Int.* 2001;60(2):804–817.

30. Abu-Alfa AK, Younes A. Tumor lysis syndrome and acute kidney injury: Evaluation, prevention, and management. *Am J Kidney Dis* 2010;55(5 Suppl 3):S1–S13, quiz S4-9.

31. Brocklebank V, Wood KM, Kavanagh D. Thrombotic microangiopathy and the kidney. *Clin J Am Soc Nephrol* 2017;13:300–317.

32. Mohmand H, Goldfarb S. Renal dysfunction associated with intra-abdominal hypertension and the abdominal compartment syndrome. *J Am Soc Nephrol* 2011;22(4):615–621.

33. Darmon M, Vincent F, Dellamonica J, et al. Diagnostic performance of fractional excretion of urea in the evaluation of critically ill patients with acute kidney injury: A multicenter cohort study. *Crit Care* 2011;15(4):R178.

34. Coca SG, Yalavarthy R, Concato J, Parikh CR. Biomarkers for the diagnosis and risk stratification of acute kidney injury: A systematic review. *Kidney Int* 2008;73(9):1008–1016.

35. Wang L, Mohan C. Contrast-enhanced ultrasound: A promising method for renal microvascular perfusion evaluation. *J Transl Int Med* 2016;4(3):104–108.

36. Schnell D, Darmon M. Bedside doppler ultrasound for the assessment of renal perfusion in the ICU: Advantages and limitations of the available techniques. *Crit Ultrasound J* 2015;7(1):24.

37. Ninet S, Schnell D, Dewitte A, Zeni F, Meziani F, Darmon M. Doppler-based renal resistive index for prediction of renal dysfunction reversibility: A systematic review and meta-analysis. *J Crit Care.* 2015;30(3):629–635.

38. Papavramidis TS, Marinis AD, Pliakos I, Kesisoglou I, Papavramidou N. Abdominal compartment syndrome—Intra-abdominal hypertension: Defining, diagnosing, and managing. *J Emerg Trauma Shock.* 2011;4(2):279–291.

39. Ding X, Cheng Z, Qian Q. Intravenous fluids and acute kidney injury. *Blood Purif* 2017;43(1–3):163–172.

40. Lenz K, Buder R, Kapun L, Voglmayr M. Treatment and management of ascites and hepatorenal syndrome: An update. *Therap Adv Gastroenterol* 2015;8(2):83–100.

41. Grams ME, Estrella MM, Coresh J, Brower RG, Liu KD. Fluid balance, diuretic use, and mortality in acute kidney injury. *Clin J Am Soc Nephrol* 2011;6(5):966–973.

42. Bagshaw SM, Darmon M, Ostermann M, et al. Current state of the art for renal replacement therapy in critically ill patients with acute kidney injury. *Intensive Care Med* 2017;43(6):841–854.

43. Pannu N, Gibney RN. Renal replacement therapy in the intensive care unit. *Ther Clin Risk Manag* 2005;1(2):141–150.

44. Vanholder R, Van Biesen W, Hoste E, Lameire N. Pro/con debate: Continuous versus intermittent dialysis for acute kidney injury: A never-ending story yet approaching the finish? *Crit Care* 2011;15(1):204.

45. Khanal N, Marshall MR, Ma TM, Pridmore PJ, Williams AB, Rankin AP. Comparison of outcomes by modality for critically ill patients requiring renal replacement therapy: A single-centre cohort study adjusting for time-varying illness severity and modality exposure. *Anaesth Intensive Care* 2012;40(2):260–268.

46. Wu VC, Ko WJ, Chang HW, et al. Risk factors of early redialysis after weaning from postoperative acute renal replacement therapy. *Intensive Care Med.* 2008;34(1):101–108.

47. Grams ME, Rabb H. The distant organ effects of acute kidney injury. *Kidney Int* 2012;81(10):942–948.

48. Case J, Khan S, Khalid R, Khan A. Epidemiology of acute kidney injury in the intensive care unit. *Crit Care Res Pract* 2013;2013:479730.

49. Tsagalis G. Update of acute kidney injury: Intensive care nephrology. *Hippokratia* 2011;15(Suppl 1):53–68.

50. Bagshaw SM, Laupland KB, Doig CJ, et al. Prognosis for long-term survival and renal recovery in critically ill patients with severe acute renal failure: A population-based study. *Crit Care* 2005;9(6):R700–R709.

51. Lepira F, Amisi EB, Sumaili EK, et al. Acute kidney injury is a powerful independent predictor of mortality in critically ill patients: A multicenter prospective cohort study from kinshasa, the democratic republic of Congo. *BMC Nephrol* 2016;17(1):118.

52. Hoste EA, De Corte W. AKI patients have worse long-term outcomes, especially in the immediate post-ICU period. *Crit Care* 2012;16(4):148.

Section III

Clinical Approach to Infections in
Compromised Hosts in the Critical Care Unit

25 Overwhelming Post-Splenectomy Infections in the Critical Care Unit

Larry I. Lutwick and Jana Preis

CONTENTS

...there is always some little thing that is too big for us.

Don Marquis
Archy and Mehitabel, 1929

CLINICAL PERSPECTIVE

The spleen is the largest lymphoid organ in the body, involved in both blood filtration and host defense against pathogens. It contains stores of immunological cells. Among them are IgM-producing lymphocytes and phagocytes, which remove circulating infected cells and pathogens, particularly polysaccharide-encapsulated bacteria [1].

Although not classically considered a vital organ, an absent or compromised spleen can predispose to severe infection due to loss of normal splenic immunologic function. In particular, mortality is estimated to be as high as 50% in septic post-splenectomy patients, necessitating prompt diagnosis and management [1], usually in the critical care setting. Additionally, preventative measures are used in the asplenic or hyposplenic patient population to avoid this lethal infection, including vaccines and prophylactic antimicrobials.

SPLENIC FUNCTION

Specifically, regarding immunity, both the splenic red pulp and white pulp play important roles to counter-infection. In the red pulp, phagocytosis of IgG- and C3b-tagged infected cells and pathogens occurs, removing opsonized parasite-infected erythrocytes (preventing conditions such as the tickborne infection babesiosis and mosquito borne malaria), as well as other pathogens, in particular polysaccharide-encapsulated bacteria, which evade complimented-mediated lysis and phagocytosis. The white pulp contains both T-cells and B-cells involved with cell-mediated immunity and IgM production, as well as the body's largest reserve of marginal B-cells involved with humoral immunity.

This reserve is not readily replaced by the liver, bone marrow, and lymph nodes after splenectomy and predisposes asplenic patients to infection, especially against encapsulated organisms. Other studies have also demonstrated the spleen's role in bridging adaptive and innate immunity, as well as in modulating the inflammatory cascade [2]. Complete loss of the spleen thus significantly hampers host immune defense, leading to increased risk for infection as well as more rapid and severe infectious disease courses.

The circulation of splenic IgM memory B-cells significantly decreases after splenic removal [3] and is lower in hyposplenic states [4]. Originating in the spleen's marginal zone B (MZB), these cells have a low activation threshold and can rapidly respond to T cell-independent antigens such as those that compose the polysaccharide capsule of many pathogenic bacteria. The response facilitates both the innate and adaptive immune responses. In a mouse model, macrophages in the MZB produce a lectin that protects mice from pneumococcemia [5]. Additionally, splenic neutrophil populations also play a role in the eradication of the pneumococcus [6]. Severe infections can be associated with the overproduction of cytokines, resulting in a "cytokine storm," which can have a detrimental effect.

The spleen can act as an anti-inflammatory agent through nicotinic acetylcholine receptors in the spleen, mediated by the CNS's vagus nerve. The effect is absent in the asplenic mouse [7].

Furthermore, besides a rapid antibacterial response and action to dampen an overactive immune response, the spleen works to clear particulate material in the blood, such as microorganisms. The microvascular system also removes inclusions in red blood cells as they pass through the organ via a remodeling process called pitting. In asplenia and hyposplenic states, nuclear remnants in the RBC called Howell-Jolly bodies can be readily seen by light microscopy and "pocked" RBCs (actually vacuoles denatured hemoglobin) are seen using phase contrast microscopy [8]. The latter are a more sensitive observation than Howell-Jolly bodies for decreased splenic function.

EPIDEMIOLOGY

It is estimated that 25,000 patients undergo surgical splenectomy annually in the United States [1]. Absolute indications for surgical splenectomy include trauma (splenic rupture), splenic cysts and abscesses, and tumor resection, while relative indications include hypersplenism and symptomatic splenomegaly from conditions such as hemolytic anemia, hereditary spherocytosis, and immune thrombocytopenic purpura [9]. In recent decades, partial splenic salvage has the decreased the need for total splenectomy in certain situations such as trauma. However, surgery alone does not account for the estimated 1 million anatomic or functional asplenics in the United States [1], with the addition of congenital asplenia and the many conditions that cause hyposplenism (Table 25.1).

TABLE 25.1
Causes of Functional Asplenia

Autoimmune	Infiltrative	Neoplastic
Lupus erythematosus	Amyloidosis	Sezary syndrome
Sjogren's syndrome	Sarcoidosis	Non-Hodgkin's lymphoma
Rheumatoid arthritis		
Mixed connective tissue disease		Chronic myelogenous leukemia
Hashimoto's thyroiditis		Breast carcinoma
Graves' disease		
Chronic active hepatitis		
Biliary cirrhosis		
Hematologic	**Gastrointestinal**	**Miscellaneous**
Essential thrombocythemia	Celiac disease	Splenic irradiation
Hemophilia	Crohn's disease	Hypopituitarism
Sickle cell hemoglobinopathies	Tropical sprue	Chronic graft vs. host
Fanconi syndrome	Ulcerative colitis	Premature infants
	Whipple's disease	Splenic thrombosis

While asplenic patients may carry some elevated risk of general infection, overwhelming post-splenectomy infection (OPSI), defined as severe sepsis after splenic removal, is a syndrome with high substantial mortality rates [10]. Prior literature reports a wide range of 38%–70% OPSI mortality (with one separate study reporting 10% mortality [11]), with a consensus of a 50% mortality rate [1,2,9,10,12]. Nevertheless, the lifetime risk of asplenic sepsis remains around 5%, with a 0.23%–0.42% annual risk [13].

These figures may not be accurate, as many studies were performed prior to widespread use of pneumococcal conjugate vaccines [1]. The OPSI mortality rates increases in asplenic younger children and infants, in those who are within 2 years of splenectomy, as well as in those with comorbidities such as other causes for immunodeficiency such as corticosteroid use, HIV, diabetes, and alcoholism [1,9,10,13].

A differential risk for OPSI exists, depending on the cause for splenectomy. The highest risk is in autoimmune lymphoproliferative syndrome and thalassemia, intermediate risk is in hereditary spherocytosis and idiopathic thrombocytopenic purpura, and lowest risk is in traumatic or incidental splenectomy [14]. If there is coexisting liver disease, the risk for OPSI is higher, and overall, after one episode of OPSI, the risk of a second is 6-fold higher. Regarding hyposplenics, overall, about 6% of OPSI cases occur in this cohort. Timing wise, about a third of cases occur in the first year following splenectomy, and half occur within 2 years, but cases have also been described 40 years later [14].

CLINICAL PRESENTATION

Unlike most of the syndromes covered in this publication, OPSI in its classic form, a severe sepsis syndrome in a person known to be asplenic or hyposplenic, should be considered to exist as an entity in itself, and the differential diagnosis is more related to the organism rather than the disease state. The various sepsis diagnostic criteria (e.g., systemic inflammatory response syndrome [SIRS], sequential organ failure assessment [SOFA], and acute physiologic assessment and chronic health evaluation [APACHE]) have not been specifically validated in the asplenic population, but clinical suspicion must be high to avoid delay in diagnosis. Thus, fever and significant constitutional symptoms in this cohort should be evaluated and empirically treated immediately.

These patients typically present initially with nonspecific symptoms, including prodromal fever, chills, vomiting, diarrhea, sore throat, muscle aches, fatigue, and headache, similar to that in influenza-like illness [1,9,10]. Often, an asplenic patient will walk into an emergency room with fever, chills, and diarrhea, only to be hypotensive and moribund within hours. It is vitally important for the clinician not to be detoured in his or her thought process into not considering this entity for there are few infectious diseases where a delay in intervention can have such disastrous consequences, which include purpura fulminans with loss of limb, sometimes multiple, and Waterhouse-Friderichsen syndrome (bilateral adrenal hemorrhage) [13].

In order to focus the treating clinician appropriately, the patient without a spleen or with an underlying condition that may produce a functional hyposplenism should have a medical alert necklace or bracelet proclaiming this fact. Additionally, since truth can have a short half-life, the patient and his or her relatives should be aware of relating this fact to the healthcare deliverer at every visit involving an acute febrile illness. Since the splenectomy may be remote in time to the illness, this is even more important. As stated, rarely congenital asplenia may present with severe infections in adulthood, so evidence to support the diagnosis of the absent spleen should be looked for in every presentation of significant febrile illness [14].

Important clues in the diagnosis can be the rapid deterioration in clinical status (often within hours), an appropriate abdominal scar (recall that, in the past, staging laparotomies with splenectomy were performed in Hodgkin's disease and the patient might not know that they were asplenic), and the finding of Howell-Jolly bodies (red blood cell nuclear remnants) on the peripheral blood smear [15]. Historical points of interest will include a vaccination history (remember that the vaccines that people are given in the United States may not be given in other countries), contact with dogs (especially a recent dog bite even how minor it seemed), and living in or recent travel through areas where ticks are common (particularly during the warmer seasons, when the ticks are active). In a traveler, it is important to know if there was travel to a malaria endemic area and what, if any, malaria chemoprophylaxis was used.

DIFFERENTIAL DIAGNOSIS OF RELEVANT PATHOGENS

The hallmarks of organisms that are associated with this clinical entity are a higher risk of infection in the asplenic/hyposplenic cohort of patients and, most importantly, more severe disease in this group of patients. The major players in this arena are bacteria with polysaccharide encapsulation. It is interesting, however, that not all bacteria with such capsules are well-represented in the microbiology of this often-fatal infection. Of note, such common microorganisms such as *Streptococcus pyogenes* (Group A beta-hemolytic streptococcus) and *Klebsiella pneumoniae* are quite rare causes of OPSI.

STREPTOCOCCUS PNEUMONIAE

Streptococcus pneumoniae, the pneumococcus, is a gram-positive lancet-shaped diplococcus and is by far the most significant organism in OPSI. In most large series, it is reported to account for 60%–70% of cases. Literature reviews, however, tend to skew data toward more uncommon microbiology. It is likely that as many as 90% of OPSI cases are caused by *S. pneumoniae*, but in the era of conjugated pneumococcal capsule vaccines, this may decrease.

In general, a predominant capsular type is not found, and the serotype distribution is not different than other forms of invasive pneumococcal infection. Marrie and colleagues in Canada [16] in 2016, however, reported that pneumococcal serotype 22B was found 33-fold more frequently as a cause of invasive pneumococcal disease in asplenics than in individuals with a spleen. This serotype is not present in either of the available vaccines.

Antimicrobial resistance in the pneumococcus has been a growing problem. As reviewed by Kim and colleagues [17], antimicrobial resistance in *S. pneumoniae* is not a new observation, but it was not until 1965 that the first clinical isolate with reduced penicillin susceptibility was reported. By the 1970s and 1980s, fully penicillin-resistant pneumococci as well as those resistance to erythromycin, trimethoprim-sulfamethoxazole, tetracycline, and the fluoroquinolones spread quickly around the world. Certain serotypes were noted to harbor more resistance than others and some with multidrug resistance [18]. Such isolates were associated with more prolonged hospitalization and costs as well as mortality. Ceftriaxone resistance is far less common than penicillin resistance, and vancomycin-resistant strains have not clearly been observed. While 13 valent conjugated pneumococcal vaccines have been effective in controlling more resistant clones like 19A [17], models suggest that there can be future possible deleterious effects of strain-targeted immunization on the frequency of antimicrobial resistance in non-vaccine serotypes [19].

HAEMOPHILUS INFLUENZAE

Although there are a number of different encapsulated (typeable) *H. influenzae* strains, only serotype b (Hib) represents a significant human pathogen. Prior to the introduction of the conjugated type b vaccine, about 10% of OPSI cases were caused by this organism. Like cases of invasive Hib in eusplenic individuals, asplenic infections were primarily in children or in young adults in closed communities such as military recruit camps. In areas of the world where immunization with Hib vaccine is used, the vaccine has dramatically decreased the number of invasive infections with this organism. Other types of *H. influenzae* strains have rarely moved into the void left by Hib [20]. Many strains of *H. influenzae* are beta-lactamase positive, but resistance to ceftriaxone or fluoroquinolones is rare.

NEISSERIA MENINGITIDIS

N. meningitidis, the meningococcus, is usually mentioned in reviews of microbial causes of OPSI. Certainly, invasive meningococcal infection can occur in the asplenic cohort [21]. It is not clear, however, whether this infection is more frequent or more severe in the hyposplenic or asplenic group. Studies on asplenic mice also further support the link to this infection [22]. Ceftriaxone continues to be quite active against these organisms, as do the fluoroquinolones [23].

CAPNOCYTOPHAGA CANIMORSUS AND C. CYNODEGMI

These two organisms, formerly classified as the Centers for Disease Control and Prevention (CDC) group dysgonic fermentor (DF)-2 and DF-2-like, are slender, capnophilic gram-negative bacilli. They are found in the oral cavities of dogs and cats. Classically, the infection is transmitted to man as a zoonosis from a dog bite, and in immunocompetent individuals, the infection tends to be mild. Severe infection rapidly progressing to shock and death can occur in the immunocompromised host, especially the asplenic host [24]. Classically, the illness in asplenics occurs 1–7 days after the bite with gram-negative bacilli, which can be seen on a peripheral blood smear or in a smear of the blood buffy coat in a patient with an eschar at the bite site [25]. Beta-lactamase activity can be found in about 30% of these strains, but sensitivity has been generally demonstrated by ampicillin/sulbactam and the third-generation cephalosporins such as ceftriaxone [26].

BORDETELLA HOLMESII

B. holmesii is a small slow-growing gram-negative coccobacillus that is related to *Bordetella pertussis*, the cause of classical pertussis (whooping cough). *B. holmesii* is an unusual cause of bacteremia. Most individuals with blood cultures positive for this organism are immunocompromised, and asplenia/hyposplenia is the most common risk factor [27]. There are no characteristic clinical or laboratory associations, but most cases appear to occur in individuals less than 20 years old, and the mortality rate is quite low as compared with other causes of post-splenectomy bacteremia. Pittet and colleagues [27] report that there has been no clear consensus for optimal treatment of this organism and that the broad-spectrum cephalosporins may not be the best option. They do cite studies that the fluoroquinolones and the carbapenems have been suggested to be the most effective antimicrobials for *B. holmesii*.

BABESIA SPECIES

Clearly, more severe babesiosis occurs in the immunocompromised host, especially the asplenic [28]. Indeed, the first cases of human babesiosis were reported in asplenic hosts. This tickborne intraerythrocytic parasite is spread by *Ixodes* ticks and can occur in individuals with other *Ixodes*-borne infections at the same time. Although in the United States most of the cases are reported from the northeast and upper Midwest, the geographic range of the tick and its reservoirs seems to be expanding related to climate change and deforestation [29]. Its presentation is usually either asymptomatic in the eusplenic host or as an influenza-like illness with fever and fatigue in the asplenic; however, *Babesia* infection can produce a severe febrile illness with significant hemolysis and end-organ disease, including acute renal injury, acute respiratory distress syndrome, and disseminated intravascular coagulation.

PLASMODIUM SPECIES

Certainly, the spleen plays a significant role in malaria infection [30]. It remains, however, not totally clear whether human *Plasmodium* infection is overtly worse in the asplenic, similar to babesiosis. *Plasmodium falciparum* infection was not altered in an asplenic, partially immune population in a study from Thailand [31], but malaria was both more frequent and severe, as per the report from Malawi [32]. How this relates to malaria occurring in a malaria immunologically naïve asplenic is not clear.

Since pitting of malaria containing RBCs does not occur in the absence of the spleen [28], asplenic and probably hyposplenic individuals will show a higher degree of parasitemia. Delay in the clearance of the parasite from the blood occurs in the asplenic, but this observation may not reflect failure of therapy or resistance to the drug used [33]. Furthermore, *P. falciparum* schizonts and trophozoites can be found in the blood in asplenics, reflecting lack of sequestration [34].

Part of the difference between babesiosis and malaria in the asplenic cohort may reflect the much more recent zoonotic jump of babesiosis into humans, driven by deforestation and climate change. On the other hand, malaria is interwoven with the human immune system for millennia.

LABORATORY EVALUATION

As in any workup of sepsis, laboratory studies, including complete blood count with differential, coagulation studies, renal function tests, liver function tests, and blood gases, should be obtained to assess severity and guide treatment. A peripheral blood smear is useful in seeing Howell-Jolly bodies or Heinz bodies (inclusions containing denatured hemoglobin), which indicate splenic dysfunction, confirming functional asplenia in unclear cases. A Gram stain of the blood buffy coat can be quite useful in rapidly identifying bacteria in the blood. Occasionally, bacteria can be seen in the peripheral smear, a finding that suggests a very high bacterial load and a poor prognosis.

Blood cultures should always be obtained promptly to aid diagnosis and guide antimicrobial choices, although empiric antimicrobials should be initiated prior to finalization of culture results. Rapid diagnostic polymerase chain reaction (PCR) may be used as most commercially available PCR blood culture panel test for the common pathogens of OPSI. In cases of suspected meningitis, lumbar puncture should be performed, although it may be contraindicated in a coagulopathy. As with blood cultures, final CSF fluid results, including culture, should not delay initiation of empiric therapy.

MANAGEMENT

In cases of suspected post-splenectomy infection monitoring should be done in an intensive care unit, as these patients are at risk for fulminant sepsis and multi-organ dysfunction. Fluid resuscitation should be prompt. Empiric antimicrobials should be immediately administered after blood cultures are obtained. These patients are at a high risk for developing septic shock and may require vasopressors and develop ARDS and altered mental status, necessitating mechanical ventilation.

ANTIMICROBIALS

Empiric therapy should be administered immediately after blood cultures are obtained and before blood and other cultures results are available. Of note, there have been no prospective clinical trials defining optimal therapy in the septic asplenic patient [2].

Vancomycin, along with a third-generation cephalosporin, is a generally acceptable regimen and has been shown to reduce mortality to 10%–40% [1,2,10,11]. An alternate empiric regimen includes vancomycin plus a fluoroquinolone [2,13]. These regimens provide coverage against *S. pneumoniae*, *H. influenzae*, and *N. meningitidis*, as well as coverage for *Staphylococcus aureus* and *Enterobacteriaceae* sp. Concern for resistant organisms can justify broadening of empiric therapy; however, cephalosporins are preferred over fluoroquinolones in the case of suspected meningitis. As with any treatment of infection, the therapy should be tailored to accommodate concurrent renal or hepatic dysfunction. Empiric therapy should also be tailored according to local resistance patterns and epidemiological data under the guidance of an infectious diseases physician and antimicrobial stewardship pharmacist.

Ideally, in the outpatient setting, asplenic patients should be instructed to seek medical care if ever febrile. In addition, one dose of amoxicillin, amoxicillin/clavulanate, cefuroxime, or a fluoroquinolone should be previously prescribed to patients take in route to seeking medical care especially if unable to present to a medical facility within 2 hours [1,2] (Table 25.2).

BETA-LACTAM ALLERGY

Antibacterial therapy in patients with a significant beta-lactam allergy can be especially challenging. As mentioned previously, a fluoroquinolone is an acceptable substitute in most cases. Owing to increased prevalence of fluoroquinolone resistance, these regimens should also be tailored to the local resistance patterns and epidemiological data under the guidance of an infectious diseases physician and antimicrobial stewardship pharmacist. Rapid penicillin desensitization can be considered if no other options are available but is generally not feasible in the emergent setting.

TABLE 25.2
Empiric Antibacterial Interventions Against OPSI

Vancomycin plus ceftriaxone

Vancomycin plus cefepime (if there is a suspicion of a ceftriaxone gram-negative-resistant organism)

Vancomycin plus a fluoroquinolone (if significant beta-lactam allergy is present)

IMMUNE ENHANCEMENT METHODOLOGY

INTRAVENOUS GAMMA GLOBULIN

Patients with functional asplenia do not generally have adequate levels of immunoglobulins (in particular, IgM). It has been theorized that intravenous immunoglobulin (IVIG) in the setting of OPSI can improve outcomes. There is strong theoretical evidence and animal data [35,36] supporting the use of IVIG, but clinical evidence is lacking at this time [2]. Nevertheless, some physicians choose to use a short 3-day course of IVIG [13].

GRANULOCYTE-MACROPHAGE COLONY-STIMULATING FACTOR

This modality increases phagocyte bactericidal ability in both asplenic and eusplenic mice. The granulocyte-macrophage colony-stimulating factor treated asplenic mice were observed to have decreased mortality in a model of pneumococcemia [37].

ANTIPROTOZOAN THERAPY BABESIOSIS

While 7–10 days of azithromycin plus atovaquone is generally used for relatively mild babesiosis, a review by Sanchez et al. [38] suggests that clindamycin plus quinine is a better therapy. The treatment of malaria is a more varied affair based on the species of malaria involved and the resistance pattern known for the area and is beyond the scope of this chapter.

MORTALITY

Rapid empiric therapy for OPSI is the best approach in treating OPSI, and a number of studies suggest a lower overall mortality rate. It should be kept in mind that although the risk of OPSI varies depending on the reason for the splenectomy, once the disease develops, there is no such differential risk related to mortality.

PREVENTION

Immunization

Given their immunocompromised state as well as the severe and life-threatening nature of OPSI, asplenic patients are recommended to receive vaccines against *S. pneumoniae*, *N. meningitidis*, *H. influenzae type b*, and influenza virus.

Two vaccines exist for *S. pneumoniae* (a protein-conjugated 13-valent product, PCV13, and a 23-valent non-conjugated polysaccharide one, PPSV23). According to current guidelines, a single dose of PCV13 and a maximum of three doses of PPSV23 should be administered to asplenic adult patients (two before age 65 years and one after). *Neisseria meningitidis* vaccines come in several forms. Either of the quadrivalent meningococcal conjugate vaccines (MenACWY-D or MenACWY-CRM) are recommended for asplenic patients as a two-dose series 2 months apart, followed by boosters every 5 years.

In addition, either of the meningococcal B vaccine series (3-dose MenB-FHbp or 2-dose MenB-4C) are recommended in all adult asplenic patients. The *H. influenzae* type b vaccine is recommended as a routine series during infancy and early childhood, although the series should still be administered to unvaccinated adult asplenic patients or those with unknown vaccination history. Finally, the influenza virus vaccine should be administered yearly, given as an inactivated or recombinant injection, according to the CDC recommendations.

Prior studies investigating prophylactic antibacterial therapy in asplenic patients are limited, performed prior to widespread pneumococcal conjugate vaccine use in infants and children with sickle cell disease [1]. While these studies showed efficacy at that time of reducing the incidence of OPSI in children under 5 years old, it remains unclear whether prophylactic antibacterials are indicated due to the lack of trials investigating the general population and the growing resistance of pneumococcal strains to penicillin today. However, prophylactic antimicrobials are still administered in several situations in the asplenic patient: Asplenic children younger than 5 years old, 1–2 years post-splenectomy, lifelong s/p previous episode of OPSI, or status post dog bites [1].

CLINICAL SUMMARY

- Asplenia is an immunocompromised state predisposing to certain encapsulated bacterial and intraerythrocytic parasitic infections.
- The OPSI carries a high morbidity and mortality.
- *Streptococcus pneumoniae*, the pneumococcus, is by far the most common cause of OPSI.
- Early empiric antimicrobial intervention, usually with vancomycin and ceftriaxone, is key in the management of the febrile asplenic patient.
- Guidance of antimicrobial therapy should be obtained from an infectious diseases physician and antimicrobial stewardship pharmacist.
- Monitoring in a critical care unit is also warranted, as these patients will decompensate quickly.
- Intravenous immunoglobulin has not been well studied but could be used as a supportive adjunct therapy.
- Appropriate vaccination of asplenic patients is a key factor in preventing OPSI.
- Prophylactic antimicrobials have not been well validated in the current asplenic population but continue to be used in certain subpopulations.

REFERENCES

1. Rubin LG, Schaffner W. Care of the asplenic patient. *N Engl J Med* 2014;371:349–356.
2. O'Neal HR, Niven AS, Karam GH. Critical illness in patients with asplenia. *Chest* 2016;150:1394–1402.
3. Kruetzmann S, Rosado MM, Weber H, et al. Human immunoglobulin M memory cells controlled *Streptococcus pneumoniae* infections are generated in the spleen. *J Exp Med* 2003;197:939–945.
4. Di Sabatino A, Rosado MM, Ciccocioppo R, et al. Depletion of immunoglobulin M memory cells is associated splenic hypofunction in inflammatory bowel disease. *Am J Gastroenterol* 2005;100:1788–1795.
5. Lanoue A, Clatworthy MR, Smith P, et al. SIGN-R1 contributes to protection against lethal pneumococcal infections in mice. *J Exp Med* 2004;200:1383–1393.
6. Densiet JF, Surewaard BG, Lee W-Y, Kubes P. Splenic Ly6G^{high} mature and Ly6G^{int} immature neutrophils contribute to eradication of S. pneumoniae. *J Exp Med* 2017;214:1333–1350.
7. Huston JM, Ochani M, Rosas-Ballina M, et al. Splenectomy inactivates the cholinergic anti-inflammatory pathway during lethal endotoxemia and polymicrobial sepsis. *J Exp Med* 2006;203:1623–1628.
8. Willekens FL, Roerdinkholder-Stoelwinder B, Groenen-Dopp YA, et al. Hemoglobin loss from erythrocytes in vivo results from spleen-facilitated vesiculation. *Blood* 2003;101:747–751.
9. Weledji EP. Benefits and risk of splenectomy. *Int J Surg* 2014;12:113–119.
10. DiSabatino A, Carsett R, Corazza GR. Post splenectromy and hyposplenic states. *Lancet* 2011;378:86–97.
11. Sinwer PD. Overwhelming post splenectomy infection syndrome—Review study. *Int J Surg* 2014;12:1314–1316.
12. Hammerquist RJ, Messerschmiddt KA, Pottebaum AA, Hellwig TR. Vaccinations in asplenic adults. *Am J Health Syst Pharm* 2016;73:e220–e228.
13. Davidson RN, Wall RA. Prevention and management of infections in patients without a spleen. *Clin Microbiol Infect* 2001;7:657–660.
14. Lutwick LI. Infections in asplenic patients. In: *Mandell, Bennett and Douglas Principles and Practice of Infectious Diseases* (7th ed.). Churchill Livingstone Elsevier, Philadelphia, PA, 2010; 3865–3872.
15. Hale AJ, LaSalvia M, Kirby JE, Kimball A, Baden R. Fatal purpura fulminans and Waterhouse-Friderichsen syndrome from fulminant *Streptococcus pneumoniae* sepsis in an asplenic young adult. *ID Cases* 2016;6:1–4.
16. Marrie TJ, Tyrrell DJ, Majumdar SR, Eurich DT. Asplenic patients and invasive pneumococcal disease—How bad is it these days? *Int J Infect Dis* 2016;51:27–30.
17. Kim L, McGee L, Tomczyk S, Beall B. Biological and epidemiological features of antibiotic-resistant *Streptococcus pneumoniae* in pre- and post-conjugate vaccine eras: A United States perspective. *Clin Microbiol Rev* 2016;29:525–552.
18. Quach C, Weiss K, Moore D, et al. Clinical aspects and costs of invasive *Streptococcus pneumoniae* infections in children: Resistance vs. susceptible strains. *Int J Antimicrobial Agents*. 2002;20:113–118.
19. Obolski U, Lourenco J, Thompson C, et al. Vaccination can drive an increase in frequencies of antibiotic resistance among nonvaccine serotypes of *Streptococcus pneumoniae*. *Proc Natl Acad Sci USA* 2018;115:3102–3107.
20. Headrick A, Schmit EO, Kimberlin DW. Fulminant *Haemophilus influenza* type a infection in a 4-year-old with previously undiagnosed asplenic heterotaxy. *Pediatr Infect Dis J* 2018;37:e108–e110.
21. Condon RJ, Riley TV, Kelly H. Invasive meningococcal infection after splenectomy. *BMJ* 1994;308:792–793.

22. Loggie BW, Hinchey EJ. Does splenectomy predispose to meningococcal sepsis? An experimental study and clinical review. *J Pediatri Surg* 1986;21:326–330.

23. Gorla MC, Pinhata JMW, Dias UJ, de Moraes C, Lemos AP. Surveillance of antimicrobial resistance in *Neisseria meningitidis* strains isolated from invasive cases in Brazil from 2009 to 2016. *J Med Microbiol* 2018. doi:10.1099/jmm.0.000743.

24. Khawari AA, Myers JW, Ferguson DA, et al. Sepsis and meningitis due to *Capnocytophaga cynodegmi* after splenectomy. *Clin Infect Dis* 2005;40:1709–1710.

25. Kalb R, Kaplan MH, Tenebaum MJ, et al. Cutaneous infection at dog bite wounds associated with fulminant DF-2 septicemia. *Am J Med* 1985;78:687–690.

26. Zajkowska J, Krol M, Falkowski D, Syed N, Kamienska A. *Capnocytophaga canimorsus*—An underestimated danger after dog or cat bite—Review of literature. *Przegl Epidemiol* 2016;70:289–295.

27. Pittet LF, Emonet S, Schrenzel J, Siegrist C-A, Posfay-Barbe KM. Bordetella holmesii: An under-recognized Bordetella species. *Lancet Infect Dis* 2014;14:510–519.

28. Westblade LF, Simon MS, Mathison BA, Kirkman LA. Babesia microti: From mice to ticks to an increasing number of highly susceptible humans. *J Clin Microbiol* 2017;55:2903–2912.

29. Ostfeld RS, Brunner JL: Climate change and ixodes tick-borne diseases of humans. *Philos Trans R Soc Lond B Biol Sci* 2015;370:20140051.

30. del Portillo H, Ferrer M, Brugat T, et al. The role of the spleen in malaria. *Cell Microbiol* 2012;14:343–355.

31. Looareesuwan S, Suntharasamai P, Webster HK, et al. Malaria in splenectomized patients: Report of four cases and review. *Clin Infect Dis* 1993;16:361–366.

32. Bach O, Baier M, Pullwitt A, et al. Falciparum malaria after splenectomy: A prospective controlled study of 33 previously splenectomized Malawian adults. *Trans Roy Soc Trop Med Hyg* 2005;99:861–867.

33. Chativanich K, Udomsangpetch R, McGready R, et al. Central role of the spleen in malaria clearance. *J Infect Di* 2002;185:1538–1541.

34. Ho M, Bannister LH, Looareesuwan S, Suntharasama P. Cytoadherence and ultrastructure of *Plasmodium falciparum*-infected erythrocyte from a splenectomized patient. *Infect Immun* 1992;60:2225–2228.

35. Offenbartl K, Christensen P, Gullstrand P, et al. Treatment of pneumococcal postsplenectomy sepsis in the rat with human gamma-globulins. *J Surg Res* 1986;40:198–201.

36. Camel JE, Kim KS, Tchejeyan GH, et al. Efficacy of passive immunotherapy in experimental postsplenectomy sepsis due to *Haemophilus influenza* type b. *J Pediatr Surg* 1993;28:1441–1445.

37. Hebert JC, O'Reilly M. Granulocyte-macrophage colony-stimulating factor (GM-CSF) enhances pulmonary defenses against pneumococcal infections after splenectomy. *J Trauma* 1996;41:663–666.

38. Sanchez E, Vannier E, Wormser GP, Hu LT. Diagnosis, treatment, and prevention of Lyme disease, human granulocytic anaplasmosis, and babesiosis: A review. *JAMA* 2016;315:1767–1777.

26 Infections in Cirrhosis in the Critical Care Unit

John M. Horne and Laurel C. Preheim

CONTENTS

CLINICAL PERSPECTIVE

Cirrhosis is characterized by fibrosis of the hepatic parenchyma, with regenerative nodules surrounded by scar tissue. It can result from a variety of chronic, progressive liver diseases. The clinical manifestations vary widely, from asymptomatic disease (up to 40% of patients) to fulminant liver failure. Cirrhosis is a major cause of morbidity worldwide. In the United States, cirrhosis has an estimated prevalence of 360 per 100,000 population and accounts for approximately 30,000 deaths annually. The majority of cases in the United States are a result of alcoholic liver disease or chronic infection with hepatitis B or C viruses.

Infection is a common complication of cirrhosis (reviewed in Refs. [1–4]). A Danish death registry study [5] examined long-term survival and cause-specific mortality in 10,154 patients with cirrhosis between 1982 and 1993. The results revealed an increased risk of dying from respiratory infection (fivefold), from tuberculosis (15-fold) and other infectious diseases (22-fold) when compared with the general population. In a study of 501 cirrhotic patients who underwent 781 admissions to a hepatology ward [6], the incidence of proven bacterial infection was 25.6% (60% community-acquired and 40% nosocomial). The most common sites of infection were blood (28%), ascetic fluid (27%), urine (14%), and pleural fluid (4%). Gram-positive isolates exceeded gram-negatives (58% vs. 42%). Prevalence of multi-resistant strains was 23%, and methicillin-resistant *Staphylococcus aureus* (MRSA) and extended-spectrum β-lactamase–producing (ESBL) gram-negative bacteria were isolated most frequently. Survival rates at 3, 6, 12, and 30 months were 83%, 77%, 71%, and 62%, respectively, in uninfected patients vs. 50%, 46%, 41%, and 34%, respectively, in patients diagnosed with infection.

The requirement for intensive care also was associated with decreased survival. Similar findings were reported in a meta-analysis of 13 studies involving 2533 cirrhotic patients treated in critical care units (CCUs) [7]. In-CCU, in-hospital and 6-month mortality was 42.7%, 54.1% and 75%, respectively. Twelve variables related to infection were predictors of in-CCU mortality, including systemic inflammatory response syndrome (SIRS), pneumonia, sepsis-associated refractory oliguria, and fungal infection.

It should be noted that the usual signs and symptoms of infection may be subtle or absent in individuals who have advanced liver disease. Thus, a high index of suspicion is required to ensure that infections are not overlooked in this patient population, especially in those who are hospitalized. Occasionally fever may be due to cirrhosis itself [8], but this must be a diagnosis of exclusion made only when appropriate diagnostic tests, including cultures, have been unrevealing.

ROLE OF THE LIVER IN HOST DEFENSE AGAINST INFECTION

Cirrhosis-associated immune dysfunction (CAID) is a complex phenomenon involving alterations of both innate and acquired immunity, leading to both immunodeficiency and systemic inflammation (reviewed in [9]). Innate immunity is affected by impaired liver synthesis or expression of pattern recognition receptors (PRRs), Toll-like receptors (TLRs), and C-reactive protein (CRP), factors integral to the recognition and elimination of bacterial pathogens. Hepatic Kupffer cells (macrophages) act as scavenger cells to filter blood and, when activated, release cytokines and other inflammatory mediators of innate host defense. Hepatocytes synthesize complement, another important component of innate immune response to infection. Examples of CAID identified by human and experimental animal studies include impairment of chemotaxis, phagocytosis, and intracellular killing by polymorphonuclear leukocytes (PMNL) and monocytes [10–12]; reduction in serum bactericidal activity and opsonic activity [13,14]; depression of serum complement [15–17]; dysregulation of cytokine synthesis and metabolism [18]; and reduced protective efficacy of type-specific antibody [19] and granulocyte colony-stimulating factor [20].

CLASSIFICATION OF LIVER DISEASE SEVERITY

Patients who have cirrhosis are at an increased risk for both community-acquired and nosocomial infections, the majority of which are bacterial. The incidence of infection is highest for patients with the most severe liver disease [21–23]. Accurate assessment for risk of infection is dependent upon proper classification of the extent of liver disease. The Child–Pugh scoring system of liver disease severity [24] is based on five parameters: (i) Serum bilirubin, (ii) serum albumin, (iii) prothrombin time, (iv) ascites, and (v) encephalopathy. A total score is derived from the sum of the points for each of these five parameters. Patients with chronic liver disease are placed in one of three classes (A, B, or C). Despite having some limitations, the modified Child–Pugh scoring system continues to be used by many clinicians to assess the risk of mortality in patients with cirrhosis (Table 26.1).

SPONTANEOUS BACTERIAL PERITONITIS

PATHOGENESIS

Spontaneous bacterial peritonitis (SBP) is the infection of ascitic fluid with no identifiable abdominal source for the infection. SBP is perhaps the most characteristic bacterial infection in cirrhosis, occurring in as many as 20%–30% of cirrhotic patients who are admitted to the hospital with ascites [21,23]. It occurs when normally sterile ascitic fluid is colonized following an episode of transient bacteremia. Historically, aerobic gram-negative bacilli, especially *Escherichia coli*, have caused approximately 75% of SBP infections. Aerobic gram-positive cocci, including *Streptococcus pneumoniae*, *Enterococcus* spp., other streptococci, and *Staphylococcus aureus*, are responsible for most other SBP cases [25,26]. Anaerobes are uncommon causes of SBP, and their presence in ascitic fluid should raise suspicions for bowel perforation. If ascitic fluid cultures yield polymicrobial flora, *Candida albicans* (or other yeast), or *Bacteroides fragilis*, one should suspect a secondary peritonitis caused by an acute abdominal infection.

Because enteric bacteria predominate in SBP, it is thought that the gut is the major source of organisms for this infection. Several mechanisms have been proposed to explain the movement of organisms from the intestinal lumen to the systemic circulation. Cirrhosis-induced depression of the hepatic reticuloendothelial system impairs the liver's filtering function, allowing bacteria to pass from the bowel lumen to the bloodstream via the portal vein. Cirrhosis also is associated with a relative increase in aerobic gram-negative bacilli in the jejunum. A decrease in mucosal blood flow due to acute hypovolemia or drug-induced splanchnic vasoconstriction may compromise the intestinal barrier to enteric flora, thereby increasing the risk of bacteremia. Finally, bacterial translocation may occur with the movement of enteric organisms from the gut lumen through the mucosa to the intestinal lymphatics. From there bacteria can travel through the lymphatic system and enter the bloodstream via the thoracic duct. It is assumed that SBP caused by non-enteric organisms is also due to bacteremia secondary to another site of infection, with subsequent seeding of the peritoneum and ascitic fluid.

Decreased opsonic activity of ascitic fluid also increases the risk of SBP in patients with cirrhosis. Immunoglobulin, complement, and fibronectin are important opsonins in ascitic fluid, and patients with low protein concentrations in their ascitic fluid are especially predisposed to SBP [27,28]. Patients with ascitic fluid protein concentrations below 1 g/dL have a sevenfold increase in the incidence of SBP when compared with patients with higher protein concentrations in ascites [27].

Other risk factors have been associated with SBP, including gastrointestinal bleeding, fulminant hepatic failure, and invasive procedures, such as the placement of peritoneovenous shunts for the treatment of ascites. An elevated bilirubin level also is correlated with a high risk of peritonitis in patients with cirrhosis [28].

DIAGNOSIS

Classic signs and symptoms of peritonitis, including fever, chills, abdominal pain, and increasing ascites may or may not be present in cirrhotic patients who have SBP.

TABLE 26.1
Modified Child–Pugh Classification of Liver Disease Severity

Parameter	Points Assigned		
	1	2	3
Ascites	None	Slight	Moderate/Severe
Encephalopathy	None	Grade 1–2	Grade 3–4
Bilirubin (mg/dL)	<2.0	2.0–3.0	>3.0
Albumin (mg/L)	>3.5	2.8–3.5	<2.8
Prothrombin time (seconds increased)	1–3	4–6	>6.0

Total score	Child–Pugh Class
5–6	A
7–9	B
10–15	C

Abdominal symptoms may be absent in up to one-third of cases. Patients with SBP may present with encephalopathy, gastrointestinal bleeding, or increasing renal insufficiency. Therefore, a high index of suspicion must be maintained in all cases of cirrhotic patients who have ascites and are acutely ill. Non-specific acute-phase proteins such as procalcitonin (PCT) and CRP have been helpful markers of bacterial infection, including SBP, in patients with advanced cirrhosis [29].

A diagnostic paracentesis must be performed on all patients suspected to have SBP. A PMNL count in ascitic fluid of greater than 250 cells/mm³ is highly suggestive of infection. Gram stain of centrifuged ascitic fluid will reveal organisms in approximately 30% of cases. The fluid should be cultured both aerobically and anaerobically. Inoculating some fluid directly into blood culture bottles increases the yield of positive cultures. But this non-quantitative culture technique also increases the risk of false-positives if any skin flora contaminant is introduced into the blood culture bottle at the bedside.

TREATMENT

Historically, SBP has been a severe, frequently fatal infection. In the past decades, mortality rates have dropped from over 90% in the 1970s to the current 20%–40% mortality for patients who have their first diagnosis of SBP. Earlier detection and treatment and the use of non-nephrotoxic antibiotics have contributed to the increased short-term survival. The most common causes of death in patients with SBP are liver failure, gastrointestinal bleeding, and renal failure. One of the greatest threats to long-term survival is the recurrence of SBP, which can occur in 70% of patients [30].

Current clinical practice guidelines published by the European Association for the Study of the Liver [31] and the American Association for the Study of Liver Diseases [32] include recommendations for the diagnosis, treatment, and prevention of SBP. In patients with suspected SBP, empiric therapy should be initiated as soon as possible but not before ascites fluid cultures are obtained. Indications for empiric therapy include the presence of ascites and one or more of the following: temperature greater than 37.8°C (100°F), abdominal pain or tenderness, a change in mental status, and ascitic fluid PMNL count ≥250 cells/mm³.

Clinical trials directly comparing antimicrobial regimens for the treatment of SBP are limited, and no single agent or combination of antibiotics has been proven superior. Most SBP is caused by enteric gram-negatives. However, bacterial SBP also may also be due to other pathogens, including gram-positive streptococci or staphylococci. Thus, initial broad-spectrum therapy using a third-generation cephalosporin is recommended. Cefotaxime, which achieves high serum and ascitic fluid concentrations, has proven efficacy. The recommended dose is 2 g intravenously every 8 hours for 5 days. Ceftriaxone, dosed 1 g every 12 hours, is an alternative. Parenteral fluoroquinolones, such as levofloxacin and ciprofloxacin, may be effective alternatives as well. However, due to the increased likelihood of a fluoroquinolone-resistant pathogen, these agents should be avoided as the empiric therapy in patients who have received a fluoroquinolone for SBP prophylaxis.

Recent studies have documented an increase in the incidence of and mortality due to infections in cirrhotics (including SBP) caused by multidrug-resistant (MDR) bacteria, particularly in patients with nosocomial or healthcare-associated (HCA) infections. The MDR gram-positive pathogens being isolated with increasing frequency include MRSA and vancomycin-resistant *Enterococcus* spp. (VRE). The MDR gram-negative isolates include ESBL-producing strains (*E. coli, Klebsiella pneumoniae, Proteus mirabilis,* and *Pseudomonas aeruginosa*), carbapenemase-producing, colistin-resistant *K. pneumoniae* (KPC, col-R), and metallo-β-lactamase (MBL)-producing *E. coli,* as well as other MDR strains of *P. aeruginosa, Serratia marcescens, Stenotrophomonas maltophilia, Acenitobacter baumannii, Enterobacter* spp. [33–36], and *Burkholderia cepacia* complex [37]. Third-generation cephalosporins remain effective therapy for most infections acquired in the community. However, empiric therapy of nosocomial and HCA infections should take into consideration the local epidemiology and prevalence of MDR pathogens.

Due to the increased incidence of MDR infections, in 2013, the European Association for the Study of the Liver (EASL) recommended substantial changes to empirical antibiotic therapy of infectious in cirrhotic patients [38]. For nosocomial and HCA SBP, empiric therapy should be with intravenous piperacillin/tazobactam or with meropenem (to cover ESBL-producing gram-negatives) ± vancomycin in areas with a high MRSA prevalence. In areas of high VRE prevalence, vancomycin should be replaced by intravenous linezolid or daptomycin.

Excessive and prolonged use of broad-spectrum antibiotics increases the risks of MDR bacterial infections in all patient populations. Use of antimicrobial stewardship principles is mandatory to minimize the risks of inappropriate therapy in cirrhotic patients [39]. These principles include distinguishing between colonization and infection; selecting the safest, most effective agent for the known or suspected infection; consideration of drug-drug interactions and PK/PD parameters in patients with cirrhosis [40,41]; early de-escalation to narrower spectrum therapy when/if allowed by susceptibility testing results; and the use of serial PCT levels as a marker of therapeutic success or failure [29,39].

Deterioration of renal function is the most sensitive predictor of in-hospital mortality in patients with SBP [42]. In a randomized, multicenter comparative study, patients with SBP who received intravenous albumin for plasma volume expansion plus cefotaxime had less renal impairment and significantly lower mortality (22%) than those receiving cefotaxime alone (41%) [43]. The dose of albumin used in this study was 1.5 g/kg of body weight at the time of diagnosis, followed by 1 g/kg on day 3.

PROPHYLAXIS

The use of prophylactic antibiotics decreases the incidence and mortality of bacterial infections, including SBP, in patients who are hospitalized with cirrhosis and ascites [31,32,38]. Cirrhotic patients who recover from SBP also are at the increased risk of subsequent episodes. The 1-year probability of recurrence of SBP in this population has been estimated to approach 70% [44]. Patients with a history of SBP may receive prolonged outpatient prophylaxis with trimethoprim-sulfamethoxazole (TMP-SMX one double strength tablet once daily) or a fluoroquinolone (e.g., ciprofloxacin 500 mg/day or norfloxacin 400 mg/day). Inpatients with ascitic fluid protein concentration <1 g/dL (or 1.5 g/dL per EASL) who are hospitalized for a reason other than SBP or gastrointestinal bleeding should receive either of the above options while hospitalized. Patients with Child–Pugh class B or C cirrhosis and gastrointestinal bleeding can receive ceftriaxone (one g intravenously daily) followed by TMP-SMX (one double-strength tablet daily), ciprofloxacin (500 mg/day) or norfloxacin (400 mg/day) once the patient is able to take medications by mouth [38].

URINARY TRACT INFECTIONS

Urinary tract infections (UTI) account for 25%–40% of infections in hospitalized cirrhotic patients [21,23,45]. The majority have asymptomatic bacteriuria, but approximately one-third have symptomatic infections [23]. Cirrhosis patients have higher rates of asymptomatic bacteriuria and UTI than the general population [46]. The incidence of significant bacteriuria (>10^5 colony-forming units/mL) is higher in women than in men and does not correlate with the severity of the underlying liver disease or with the age of the patient [45]. The presence of an indwelling urinary catheter increases the risk of infection. The most common pathogens are *E. coli* and other aerobic gram-negative coliforms. Cirrhosis is an independent predictor for severe bacteremic UTI caused by MDR *Enterobacteriaceae* [47]. Asymptomatic bacteriuria does not require treatment, particularly in patients with an indwelling urinary catheter. A urine culture should be obtained on any cirrhotic patient suspected to have a UTI. Empiric therapy, when indicated, should be guided by local epidemiologic patterns and prevalence of MDR bacteria [48]. For community-acquired UTI, a third-generation cephalosporin is the appropriate initial therapy. Piperacillin/tazobactam is recommended for nosocomial or HCA UTI, with a carbapenem substituted if infection with an ESBL-producing pathogen is suspected or known. Vancomycin may be added to cover MRSA, although this is an uncommon urinary pathogen. Linezolid should be used if prevalence of VRE is high. Antibiotic adjustments should be based on pathogen identification and microbial susceptibility testing results. Indwelling urinary catheters should be removed as soon as possible to reduce the risk of infection.

BACTEREMIA AND SEPSIS

Cirrhosis predisposes patients to systemic bloodstream infections (BSI) due to intrahepatic blood shunting and impaired bacterial clearance from the portal blood. BSI has been reported to occur in approximately 9% of hospitalized cirrhotic patients [49] and accounts for 20% of the infections diagnosed during their hospital stay [23]. The incidence of BSI increases with the severity of liver disease, and individuals with cirrhosis are more likely to have a diagnosis of sepsis when compared with patients without a diagnosis of cirrhosis [50].

A recent prospective, multicenter study examined the etiology and outcome of BSIs in 312 cirrhotic patients [51]. The BSIs were classified as primary (32%), catheter-related (10%), and secondary (58%). Secondary BSIs included intra-abdominal sources (32%), half of which were SBP, cholangitis (26%), urinary tract (11%), lower respiratory tract (6%), and other (11%). The overall 30-day mortality was 25%, and delayed (>24 hours) or inadequate empirical antibiotic therapies were independently associated with increased rates of mortality. Considering the BSI source, SBP (36%) and pneumonia (31%) were associated with the highest mortality rates, followed by primary BSI (29%). Of the bacterial isolates, 47% were gram-positive and 53% were gram-negative. Among gram-positives, the percentage of staphylococcal isolates did not differ between community-acquired, HCA, and nosocomial BSI. Streptococci were more commonly identified in community-acquired BSIs vs HCA or nosocomial BSIs (p < 0.001). *E. coli* was the most commonly identified gram-negative pathogen but was less likely to cause nosocomial BSI compared with community-acquired or HCA BSIs (p < 0.001). In contrast, the rates of fluoroquinolone-resistant *Enterobacteriaceae*, ESBL-producing *Enterobacteriacea*, and carbapenem-resistant *Enterobacteriacea* were higher in HCA or nosocomial BSIs when compared with community-acquired BSI. Non-fermenting gram-negative bacilli (*P. aeruginosa*, *A. baumannii*, and *S. maltophilia*) and *Candida* spp. were more likely to cause HCA or nosocomial BSIs than community acquired BSIs. Overall, 31% of BSIs were caused by MDR organisms. Prior (<30 days) antimicrobial exposure and prior (<30 days) invasive procedures (e.g., intestinal endoscopic procedures, transjugular intrahepatic portosystemic shunt insertion, and biliary procedures) were associated with increased risk of BSI due to MDR organisms.

Patients with cirrhosis are also at increased risk of sepsis, which can be defined as life-threatening organ dysfunction that occurs because of the dysregulation of the host response to infection. Prompt recognition of sepsis can be challenging since both sepsis and severe cirrhosis can present with similar signs and symptoms. Early goal-directed therapy (EGDT) for sepsis focuses on intensive hemodynamic management to maintain central venous pressure (CVP) of 8–12 mmHg, mean arterial pressure greater than 65 mm Hg, urine output greater than 0.5 mL/kg/h, and central venous oxygen saturation

(Scvo$_2$) of ≥70%. Although the survival benefit of EGDT vs usual care remains controversial, the aims of treatment should focus on correction of hypoperfusion with volume administration and vasopressor support, early administration of appropriate antimicrobial therapy, and source control [52].

The choice of antimicrobial coverage for BSI with or without sepsis must consider the following: (a) Local epidemiology; (b) site of infection onset (community vs. HCA or nosocomial); (c) patient risk factors for MDR infections, including prior antibiotic exposure and colonization status; (d) clinical severity; and and (e) infection source [53]. In general, the recommendations for empiric therapy of BSP apply here as well. Third-generation cephalosporins and fluoroquinolones should be avoided in HCA and nosocomial infections. A β-lactam/β-lactamase inhibitor may be used in settings with low prevalence of ESBL-producing strains. Initiate therapy with a carbapenem in a setting with high prevalence of ESBL-producing strains, de-escalating, if possible, as soon as culture results are available. Provide anti-MRSA coverage in patients with suspected device-related infections and apply therapeutic drug monitoring when indicated (e.g., vancomycin therapy). If time-dependent drugs (e.g., β-lactams) are administered, provide a loading dose and continuous or prolonged infusion [38,53]. The optimal duration of antimicrobial therapy for uncomplicated gram-negative BSIs is unknown. Nelson et al. found cirrhosis to be associated with increased risk of treatment failure in patients receiving ≤10 days of therapy for uncomplicated gram-negative BSI [54]. Their results suggest using >10 days of either intravenous or highly bioavailable oral antimicrobial agents in cirrhotic patients with gram-negative BSI. Finally, it is advisable that BSIs in cirrhotic patients be managed by a multidisciplinary team that includes a hepatologist and an infectious diseases specialist [51].

PNEUMONIA

Respiratory tract infections account for approximately 20% of the infectious diseases that are diagnosed in hospitalized cirrhotic patients [21,23]. In one large retrospective review, pneumonia carried the highest risk of 30- and 90-day mortality (32.0% and 51.0%) among common infections in cirrhotic patients with ascites [55]. Long-term antibiotic prophylaxis may be a risk factor for pneumonia among patients with liver cirrhosis [56]. S. pneumoniae continues to rank first among bacterial pathogens causing community-acquired pneumonia (CAP) in adults [55]. The mortality rate for pneumococcal bacteremia in cirrhotic patients may exceed 50% despite appropriate antibiotic therapy [57]. Other organisms commonly responsible for CAP include Mycoplasma pneumoniae, Chlamydia pneumoniae, Legionella pneumophila, and Haemophilus influenzae. Cirrhosis has been associated with an increased risk of severe CAP caused by A. baumannii [58]. Sputum and blood samples should be obtained for appropriate diagnostic studies, including Gram stain (sputum) and cultures (sputum and blood). Chronic severe liver disease

and/or admission to the intensive care unit are clinical indications for pneumococcal and Legionella urinary antigen testing in patients suspected to have CAP. Appropriate empiric therapy while awaiting the results of cultures and other tests would include an expanded-spectrum cephalosporin plus a macrolide or a β-lactam/β-lactamase inhibitor plus a macrolide or a fluoroquinolone [59].

Hospital-acquired pneumonia (HAP) may be caused by a wide variety of bacteria. It is defined as a pneumonia not incubating at the time of hospital admission, occurring 48 hours or more after admission, and not associated with mechanical ventilation [60]. In this new definition, patients with HAP and ventilator-associated pneumonia (VAP) are in two separate non-overlapping groups, and the term "healthcare-associated pneumonia" has been retired [60]. Common pathogens include aerobic gram-negative bacilli, such as P. aeruginosa, E. coli, K. pneumoniae, S. marcescens, Enterobacter species, Proteus species, and Acinetobacter species. S. aureus and S. pneumoniae predominate among gram-positive pathogens, and the incidence of MRSA nosocomial pneumonia is increasing. A number of risk factors have been identified for MDR bacteria [60] (Table 26.2).

Recommended initial empiric antibiotic therapy for HAP is determined by the patient's risk of mortality and the patient's risk factors, which increase the likelihood of MRSA. Risk factors for mortality include the need for ventilatory support due to pneumonia, and septic shock, while risk factors for MRSA include intravenous antibiotic treatment during the prior 90 days and treatment in a unit where the prevalence of MRSA among S. aureus isolates is not known or is >20% [60].

Initial empiric therapy in patients without risk factors for high mortality should include one of the following: An

---

TABLE 26.2

Risk Factors for Multidrug-Resistant Pathogens

Risk factors for MDR VAP

   Prior intravenous antibiotic use within 90 days

   Septic shock at time of VAP

   ARDS preceding VAP

   Five or more days of hospitalization prior to the occurrence of VAP

   Acute renal replacement therapy prior to VAP onset

Risk factors for MDR HAP

   Prior intravenous antibiotic use within 90 days

Risk factors for MRSA VAP/HAP

   Prior intravenous antibiotic use within 90 days

Risk factors for MDR *Pseudomonas* VAP/HAP

   Prior intravenous antibiotic use within 90 days

Source: Kalil, A.C. et al., *Clin. Infect. Dis.*, 63, e61–e111, 2016.

Abbreviations: ARDS, acute respiratory distress syndrome, HAP, hospital-acquired pneumonia, MDR, multidrug resistant, MRSA, methicillin-resistant *Staphylococcus aureus*, VAP, ventilator-associated pneumonia.

antipseudomonal cephalosporin (e.g., cefepime), antipseudomonal carbapenem (e.g., imipenem or meropenem), piperacillin/tazobactam, an antipseudomonal respiratory fluoroquinolone (levofloxacin) plus vancomycin, or linezolid if MRSA risk factors are present [60]. In patients who have received IV antibiotics during the prior 90 days, with risk factors for high mortality, two antipseudomonal agents from different classes are recommended plus vancomycin or linezolid. Because of increased risks of aminoglycoside-induced nephrotoxicity and ototoxicity, the use of these agents should be avoided in cirrhotic patients, if possible [30].

The recommended empiric treatment for VAP is an antipseudomonal antibiotic such as piperacillin-tazobactam, cefepime, levofloxacin, imipenem, or meropenem. It is suggested to add a second antipseudomonal antibiotic from a separate antibiotic class if there is a risk factor for antimicrobial resistance (Table 26.2), or in units where >10% of gram-negative isolates are resistant to an agent being considered for monotherapy, or in patients in a CCU where local antimicrobial susceptibility rates are not available [60]. Vancomycin or linezolid is added to a VAP regimen for MRSA coverage in patients with any of the following: A risk factor for antimicrobial resistance (Table 26.2), patients being treated in units where >10%–20% of S. aureus isolates are MRSA, or patients in units where the prevalence of MRSA is not known [60].

OTHER INFECTIONS

VIBRIO INFECTIONS

Vibrio bacteria are gram-negative halophilic inhabitants of marine and estuarine environments. Typical infections caused by these organisms include gastroenteritis, wound infections, and septicemia. Infection usually occurs following consumption of contaminated food or water or by cutaneous inoculation through wounds. The most common pathogens include V. cholerae, V. parahaemolyticus, and V. vulnificus. Cirrhosis is a major risk factor for Vibrio infections, likely secondary to dysfunction in portal drainage, hepatocellular damage, and impaired iron metabolism. Liver disease has been associated with a fatal outcome in both wound infections and primary septicemia [61–63]. V. vulnificus, the most virulent of the non-cholera vibrios, can rapidly invade the bloodstream from the gastrointestinal tract. Classic clinical features of V. vulnificus sepsis include the abrupt onset of chills and fever, followed by hypotension, with subsequent development of disseminated skin lesions within 36 hours of onset. The skin lesions progress to hemorrhagic vesicles or bullae and then to necrotic ulcers [62,64]. This syndrome is highly associated with a history of consuming raw oysters. The mortality rate can exceed 50%. Recommended antibiotic therapy for severe infections [65] includes using a third-generation cephalosporin (cefotaxime 2 g intravenously every 8 hours or ceftriaxone 1 g intravenously once daily) plus doxycycline (100 mg orally twice daily) or a fluoroquinolone (e.g., ciprofloxacin). Monotherapy with levofloxacin 750 mg orally or intravenously once daily is another alternative.

INFECTIVE ENDOCARDITIS

Infective endocarditis (IE) is a relatively unusual complication of cirrhosis. In the past, E. coli and S. pneumoniae were commonly implicated in these infections. More recent studies have identified S. aureus as the most common pathogen, along with other gram-positive bacteria such as the Viridans streptococci and Enterococcus species [66,67]. Streptococcus bovis biotypes (recently reclassified as Streptococcus gallolyticus [S. bovis I], Streptococcus lutetiensis [S. bovis II/1], and Streptococcus pasteuriannus [S. bovis II/2]) have emerged as another important cause of bacteremia and IE in patients with chronic liver disease [68,69]. Infective endocarditis caused by S. bovis is commonly associated with bivalvular involvement and a high rate of embolic events.

Features of IE are similar in cirrhotic and non-cirrhotic patients. Predisposing valvular disease and left-sided IE are common (48% aortic valve, 45% mitral valve), and most IE is caused by S. aureus or Streptococcus spp. Cirrhotic patients, however, have higher rates of renal failure, poorer outcomes, and a lower likelihood of valve replacement [70]. The preferred diagnostic tool for IE, the transesophageal echocardiogram, may be contraindicated or dangerous in some cirrhotic patients who are at risk of upper gastrointestinal bleeding.

SPONTANEOUS BACTERIAL EMPYEMA

Spontaneous bacterial empyema is an infection of a pre-existing hydrothorax. The risk of empyema is increased in patients with cirrhosis, especially in those with ascites or gastrointestinal hemorrhage [71]. Spontaneous bacterial peritonitis is present in approximately half of patients who develop empyema. The most common causes of spontaneous bacterial empyema include E. coli, K. pneumoniae, and streptococci, including Enterococcus species and S. gallolyticus. A diagnostic thoracentesis is recommended in patients with cirrhosis who develop pleural effusions and signs and symptoms of infection [72]. Options for empiric therapy include piperacillin/tazobactam or a third-generation cephalosporin or a carbapenem based on local bacterial resistance patterns.

BACTERIAL MENINGITIS

Patients with cirrhosis are at increased risk for bacterial meningitis due to CAID [9] and altered blood-brain barrier permeability related to ammonium metabolism [73]. Severe liver disease is frequently associated with neurologic complications, among which hepatic encephalopathy is the most common. Symptoms of hepatic encephalopathy can include both fever and altered mental status, which can mask the diagnosis of bacterial meningitis. A recent study of 44 cirrhotic patients with acute bacterial meningitis [74] reported the most common symptoms (% of cases) to be headache (93%), fever (80%), and vomiting (41%). Neurologic findings (% of cases) included meningeal signs (52%), altered mental status (57%), and focal abnormalities (14%). S. pneumoniae was the most commonly identified pathogen (50% of cases) based on blood or cerebrospinal fluid (CSF) cultures or CSF pneumococcal antigen detection. Of the 18 cases with positive pneumococcal culture, 10 (56%) were due to penicillin-nonsusceptible strains. *Listeria monocytogenes* was the second leading pathogen (10 cases), followed by *E. coli* (3 cases), *Staphylococcus aureus* (2 cases) and one case each of *S. mitis, S. bovis*, and *Enterococcus faecium*. Seventeen patients (39%) died, and 8 (18%) reported sequelae. Deaths were meningitis-related in 13 cases.

In patients suspected to have bacterial meningitis, it is strongly recommended to determine CSF leukocyte count and protein and glucose concentration and to perform CSF culture and Gram stain. In patients with negative CSF cultures, the causative microorganisms can be identified by polymerase chain reaction or antigen testing. It also is strongly recommended to perform blood cultures before the first dose of antibiotics is administered [75]. Cirrhotic patients with community-acquired meningitis should receive empiric intravenous therapy with a third-generation cephalosporin (ceftriaxone or cefotaxime) *plus* vancomycin *plus* ampicillin [75]. For HCA meningitis or ventriculitis, empiric therapy should include vancomycin *plus* an anti-pseudomonal β-lactam (cefepime, ceftazidime, or meropenem) based on local *in vitro* susceptibility patterns [76].

Clostridium difficile Infections

Clostridium difficile infection (CDI) has been linked to antibiotic therapy, gastric acid suppression, and hospitalization, all of which occur frequently in cirrhosis. Up to 20% of cirrhotic patients are colonized with *C. difficile* [77], which increases their risk for CDI. A case-control study compared 1165 cirrhotic patients who had CDI vs 82,065 cirrhotic patients did not have CDI [78]. Risk factors for CDI included outpatient SBP prophylaxis, inpatient antibiotic exposure, and proton pump inhibitor use. Cirrhotic patients with CDI also had a higher mortality and hospital charges compared with those without CDI.

Antibiotic-associated diarrhea is by far the most common form of CDI, but recurrent bacteremia and liver abscess caused by *C. difficile* has been reported in a patient with cirrhosis [79]. Rifaximin, a rifamycin derivative commonly used as prophylaxis for recurrent hepatic encephalopathy, has been associated with an increased risk of CDI caused by rifaximin-resistant *C. difficile* strains [80].

Cirrhotic patients with unexplained and new-onset ≥3 unformed stools in 24 hours should have a stool toxin test as part of a multistep algorithm (i.e., glutamate dehydrogenase [GDH] plus toxin; GDH plus toxin, arbited by nucleic acid amplification test [NAAT]; and NAAT plus toxin) rather than a NAAT alone for all specimens, received in the clinical laboratory when there are no pre-agreed institutional criteria for patient stool submission [81]. Guidelines now recommend oral vancomycin 125 mg given four times daily for 10 days OR fidaxomicin 200 mg given twice daily for 10 days for the treatment of initial non-severe or severe CDI. For an initial fulminant episode, vancomycin can be administered as 500 mg four times daily by mouth

or nasogastric tube. If ileus is present, vancomycin can be instilled rectally. Intravenously administered metronidazole (500 mg every 8 hours) should be administered, together with oral or rectal vancomycin, particularly if ileus is present [81].

REFERENCES

1. Bunchorntavakul C, Chamroonkul N, Chavalitdhamrong D. Bacterial infections in cirrhosis: A critical review and practical guidance. *World J Hepatol* 2016;8:307–321.
2. Gustot T, Fernández J, Szabo G, et al. Sepsis in alcohol-related liver disease. *J Hepatol* 2017;67:1031–1050.
3. Piotrowski D, Boroń-Kaczmarska A. Bacterial infections and hepatic encephalopathy in liver cirrhosis—Prophylaxis and treatment. *Adv Med Sci* 2017;62:345–356.
4. Piano S, Brocca A, Mareso S, Angeli P. Infections complicating cirrhosis. *Liver Int* 2018;38(Suppl 1):126–133.
5. Sørensen HT, Thulstrup AM, Mellemkjar L, et al. Long-term survival and cause-specific mortality in patients with cirrhosis of the liver: A nationwide cohort study in Denmark. *J Clin Epidem* 2003;56:88–93.
6. Dionigi E, Garcovich M, Borzio M, et al. Bacterial infections change natural history of cirrhosis irrespective of liver disease severity. *Am J Gastroenterol* 2017;112:588–596.
7. Weil D, Levesque E, McPhail M, et al. Prognosis of cirrhotic patients admitted to intensive care: A meta-analysis. *Ann Intensive Care* 2017;7:33–46.
8. Singh N, Yu VL, Wagener MM, et al. Cirrhotic fever in the 1990s: A prospective study with clinical implications. *Clin Infect Dis* 1997;24:1135–1138.
9. Noor MT, Manoria P. Immune dysfunction in cirrhosis. *J Clin Transl Hepatol* 2017;5:50–58.
10. Rajkovic IA, Williams R. Abnormalities of neutrophil phagocytosis, intracellular killing, and metabolic activity in alcoholic cirrhosis and heptatitis. *Hepatology* 1986;6:252–262.
11. Gentry MJ, Snitily MU, Preheim LC. Phagocytosis of *Streptococcus pneumoniae* measured in vitro and in vivo in a rat model of carbon tetrachloride-induced liver cirrhosis. *J Infect Dis* 1995;171:350–355.
12. Gentry MJ, Snitily MU, Preheim LC. Decreased uptake and killing of *Streptococcus pneumoniae* within the lungs of cirrhotic rats. *Immunol Infect Dis* 1996;6:43–47.
13. Fierer J, Finley F. Serum bactericidal activity against *Escherichia coli* in patients with cirrhosis of the liver. *J Clin Invest* 1979;63:912–921.
14. Lister PD, Mellencamp MA, Preheim LC. Serum-sensitive *Escherichia coli* multiply in cirrhotic serum. *J Lab Clin Med* 1992;120:633–638.
15. Mellencamp MA, Preheim LC. Pneumococcol pneumonia in a rat model of cirrhosis: Effects of cirrhosis on pulmonary defense mechanisms against *Streptococcus pneumoniae*. *J Infect Dis* 1991;163:102–108.
16. Homann C, Varming K, Hogasen K, et al. Acquired C3 deficiency in patients with alcoholic cirrhosis predisposes to infection and increased mortality. *Gut* 1997;40:544–549.
17. Alcantara RB, Preheim LC, Gentry MJ. The role of pneumolysin's complement-activating activity during pneumococcal bacteremia in cirrhotic rats. *Infect Immun* 1999;67:2862–2866.
18. Baudouin B, Roucloux I, Crusiaux A, et al. Tumor necrosis factor a and interleukin 6 plasma levels in infected cirrhotic patients. *Gastroenterol* 1993;104:1492–1497.

19. Preheim LC, Mellencamp MA, Snitily MU, et al. Effect of cirrhosis on the production and efficacy of pneumococcal capsular antibody in a rat model. *Am Rev Respir Dis* 1992;146:1054–1058.

20. Preheim LC, Snitily MU, Gentry MJ. Effects of granulocyte colony-stimulating factor in cirrhotic rats with pneumococcal pneumonia. *J Infect Dis* 1996;174:225–228.

21. Caly WR, Strauss E. A prospective study of bacterial infections in patients with cirrhosis. *J Hepatol* 1993;18:353–358.

22. Yoshida H, Hamada T, Inuzuka S, et al. Bacterial infections in cirrhosis, with and without hepatocellular carcinoma. *Am J Gastroenterol* 1993;88:2067–2071.

23. Borzio M, Salerno F, Piantoni L, et al. Bacterial infection in patients with advanced cirrhosis: A multicentre prospective study. *Digest Liver Dis* 2001;33:41–48.

24. Pugh RN, Murray-Lyon IM, Dawson JL, et al. Transection of the oesophagus for bleeding oesophageal varices. *Br J Surg* 1973;60:646–649.

25. Rimola A, Navasa M, Arroyo V. Experience with cefotaxime in the treatment of spontaneous bacterial peritonitis in cirrhosis. *Diagn Microbiol Infect Dis* 1995;22:141–145.

26. Runyon BA, McHutchison JG, Antillon MR, et al. Short-course versus long-course antibiotic treatment of spontaneous bacterial peritonitis. *Gastroenterol* 1991;100:1737–1742.

27. Runyon BA. Low-protein-concentration ascitic fluid is predisposed to spontaneous bacterial peritonitis. *Gastroenterol* 1986;91:1343–1346.

28. Andreu M, Sola R, Sitges-Serra A, et al. Risk factors for spontaneous bacterial peritonitis in cirrhotic patients with ascites. *Gastroenterol* 1993;104:1133–1138.

29. Papp M, Vitalis Z, Altorjay I, et al. Acute phase proteins in the diagnosis and prediction of cirrhosis-associated bacterial infections. *Liver Int* 2012;32:603–611.

30. Rimola A, Garcia-Tsao G, Navasa M, et al. Diagnosis, treatment and prophylaxis of spontaneous bacterial peritonitis: A consensus document. *J Hepatol* 2000;32:142–153.

31. European Association for the Study of the Liver. EASL clinical practice guidelines on the management of ascites, spontaneous bacterial peritonitis, and hepatorenal syndrome in cirrhosis. *J Hepatol* 2010;53:397–417.

32. Runyan BA, ASSLD. Introduction to the revised American association for the study of liver diseases practice guideline management of adult patients with ascites due to cirrhosis 2012. *Hepatology* 2013;57;1651–1653.

33. Tandon P, Delisle A, Topal JE, Garcia-Tsao G. High prevalence of antibiotic-resistant bacterial resistant infections among patients with cirrhosis at a US liver center. *Clin Gastroenterol Hepatol* 2012;10:1291–1298.

34. Alexopoulou A, Vasilieva L, Agiasotelli D, et al. Extensively drug-resistant bacteria are an independent predictive factor of mortality in 130 patients with spontaneous bacterial peritonitis or spontaneous bacteremia. *World J Gastroenterol* 2016;22:4049–4056.

35. Salerno F, Borzio M, Pedicino C, et al. The impact of infection by multidrug-resistant agents in patients with cirrhosis. A multicenter prospective study. *Liver Int* 2017;37:71–79.

36. Lutz P, Nischalke HD, Krämer B, et al. Antibiotic resistance in healthcare-related and nosocomial spontaneous bacterial peritonitis. *Eur J Clin Invest* 2017;47:44–52.

37. Taneja S, Kumar P, Gautam V, et al. Spontaneous bacterial peritonitis by *Burkholderia cepacian* Complex: A rare, difficult to treat infection in decompensated cirrhotic patients. *J Clin Exp Hepatol* 2017;7:102–106.

38. Jalan R, Fernandez J, Wiest R, et al. Bacterial infections in cirrhosis: A position statement based on the EASL special conference 2013. *J Hepatol* 2014;60:1310–1324.

39. Zuccaro V, Columpsi P, Sacchi P, et al. Antibiotic stewardship and empirical antibiotic treatment: How can they get along? *Dig Liver Dis* 2017;49:579–584.

40. Lewis JH, Stine JG. Review article: Prescribing medications in patients with cirrhosis—A practical guide. *Aliment Pharmacol Ther* 2013;37:1132–1156.

41. Halilovic J, Heintz BH. Antibiotic dosing in cirrhosis. *Am J Health-Sys Pharm* 2014;71:1621–1634.

42. Follo A, Llovet JM, Navasa M, et al. Renal impairment after spontaneous bacterial peritonitis in cirrhosis: Incidence, clinical course, predictive factors, and prognosis. *Hepatology* 1994;20:1495–1501.

43. Sort P, Navasa M, Arroyo V, et al. Effect of intravenous albumin on renal impairment and mortality in patients with cirrhosis and spontaneous bacterial peritonitis. *N Engl J Med* 1999;341:403–409.

44. Titó L, Rimola A, Ginés P, et al. Recurrence of spontaneous bacterial peritonitis in cirrhosis: Frequency and predictive factors. *Hepatology* 1988;8:27–31.

45. Rabinovitz M, Prieto M, Gavaler JS, et al. Bacteriuria in patients with cirrhosis. *J Hepatol* 1992;16:73–76.

46. Ye C, Kumar D, Carbonneau M, et al. Asymptomatic bacteriuria is an independent predictor of urinary tract infections in an ambulatory cirrhotic population: A prospective evaluation. *Liver Int* 2014;34:e39–e44.

47. Lee YC, Hsiao CY, Hung MC, et al. Bacteremic urinary tract infection caused by multidrug-resistant *Enterobacteriaceae* are associated with severe sepsis at admission. *Medicine* 2016;95:1–7.

48. Acevedo J. Multiresistant bacterial infections in liver cirrhosis: Clinical impact and new empirical antibiotic treatment policies. *World J Hepatol* 2015;7:916–921.

49. Kuo CH, Changchien CS, Yang CY, et al. Bacteremia in patients with cirrhosis of the liver. *Liver* 1991;11:334–339.

50. Foreman MG, Mannino DM, Moss M. Cirrhosis as a risk factor for sepsis and death. Analysis of the national hospital discharge summary. *Chest* 2003;124:1016–1020.

51. Bartoletti M, Giannella M, Lewis R, et al. A prospective multicentre study of the epidemiology and outcomes of bloodstream infection in cirrhotic patients. *Clin Microbiol Infect* 2018;24:546e1–546e8.

52. McLaughlin D, Shellenback L. Sepsis in patients with cirrhosis. *AACN Adv Crit Care* 2016;27:408–419.

53. Bartoletti M, Giannella M, Lewis RE, Viale P. Bloodstream infections in patients with liver cirrhosis. *Virulence* 2016;7:309–319.

54. Nelson AN, Justo JA, Bookstaver PB, et al. Optimal duration of antimicrobial therapy for uncomplicated gram-negative blood stream infections. *Infection* 2017;45:613–620.

55. Hung TH, Tseng CW, Hsieh YH, et al. High mortality of pneumonia in cirrhotic patients with ascites. *BMC Gastroenterol* 2013;13:25.

56. Cuomo G, Brancaccio G, Stornaiuolo G, et al. Bacterial pneumonia in patients with liver cirrhosis, with or without HIV co-infection: A possible definition of antibiotic prophylaxis associated pneumonia (APAP). *Infect Dis* 2017;50:2,125–132.

57. Gransden WR, Eykyn SJ, Phillips I. Pneumococcal bacteremia: 325 episodes diagnosed at St. Thomas's Hospital. *Br Med J* 1985;290:505–508.

58. Chen M, Hsueh P, Lee L, et al. Severe community-acquired pneumonia due to *Acinetobacter baumannii*. *Chest* 2001; 120:1072–1077.

59. Mandell LA, Wunderink RG, Anzueto A, et al. Infectious diseases society of America/American thoracic society consensus guidelines on the management of community-acquired pneumonia in adults. *Clin Infect Dis* 2007;44:S27–S72.

60. Kalil AC, Metersky ML, Klompas M, et al. Management of adults with hospital-acquired and ventilator-associated pneumonia: 2016 clinical practice guidelines by the Infectious diseases society of America and the American thoracic society. *Clin Infect Dis* 2016;63(5):e61–e111.

61. Hlady WG, Klontz KC. The epidemiology of *Vibrio* infections in Florida, 1981–1993. *J Infect Dis* 1996;173:1176–1183.

62. Matsumoto K, Ohshige K, Fujita N, et al. Clinical features of *Vibrio vulnificus* infections in the coastal areas of the Ariake Sea, Japan. *J Infect Chemother* 2010;16:272–279.

63. Syue L-S, Chen P-L, Wu C-J, et al. Monomicrobial *Aeromonas* and *Vibrio* bacteremia in cirrhotic adults in southern Taiwan: Similarities and differences. *J Micribiol Immunol Infect* 2016;49:509–515.

64. Oliver JD. Wound infections caused by *Vibrio vulnificus* and other marine bacteria. *Epidemiol Infect* 2005;133:383–391.

65. Chiang S, Chuang Y. *Vibrio vulnificus* infection: Clinical manifestations, pathogenesis, and antimicrobial therapy. *J Microbiol Immunol Infect* 2003;36:81–88.

66. McCashland TM, Sorrell MF, Zetterman RK. Bacterial endocarditis in patients with chronic liver disease. *Am J Gastroenterol* 1994;89:924–927.

67. Hsu RB, Chen RJ, Chu SH. Infective endocarditis in patients with liver cirrhosis. *J Formos Med Assoc* 2004;103:355–358.

68. Gonzalez-Quintela A, Martinez-Rey C, Castroagudin JF, et al. Prevalence of liver disease in patients with *Streptococcus bovis* bacteremia. *J Infect* 2001;42:116–119.

69. Tripodi MF, Adinolfi LE, Ragone E, et al. *Streptococcus bovis* endocarditis and its association with chronic liver disease: An underestimated risk factor. *Clin Infect Dis* 2004;38:1394–1400.

70. Fernández Guerrero ML, González López J, Górgolas M. Infective endocarditis in patients with cirrhosis of the liver: A model of infection in the frail patient. *Eur J Clin Microbiol Infect Dis* 2010;29:1271–1275.

71. Shen TC, Chen CH, Lai HC, et al. Risk of empyema in patients with chronic liver disease and cirrhosis: A nationwide, population-based cohort study. *Liver Int* 2017;37:862–870.

72. Xiol X, Castellví JM, Guardiola J, et al. Spontaneous bacterial empyema in cirrhotic patients: A prospective study. *Hepatology* 1996;23:719–723.

73. Cabellos C, Viladrich PF, Ariza J, et al. Community-acquired bacterial meningitis in cirrhotic patients. *Clin Microbiol Infect* 2008;14:35–40.

74. Pagliano P, Boccia G, De Caro F, Esposito S. Bacterial meningitis complicating the course of liver cirrhosis. *Infection* 2017;45:795–800.

75. van de Beek D, Cabellos C, Dzupova O, et al. ESCMID guideline: Diagnosis and treatment of acute bacterial meningitis. *Clin Microbiol Infect* 2016;22:S37–S62.

76. Tunkel AR, Hasbun R, Bhimraj A, et al. 2017 infectious diseases society of America's clinical practice guidelines for healthcare-associated ventriculitis and meningitis. *CID* 2017;64:e34–e65.

77. Yan D, Chen Y, Tao L, Huang Y, et al. *Clostridium difficile* colonization and infection in patients with hepatic cirrhosis. *J Med Microbiol* 2017;66:1483–1488.

78. Bajaj JS, Ananthakrishnan AN, Hafeezullah M, et al. *Clostridium difficile* is associated with poor outcomes in patients with cirrhosis: A national and tertiary center perspective. *Am J Gastroenterol* 2010;105:106–113.

79. Morioka H, Mitsutaka I, Kuzuya T, et al. Recurrent bacteremia and liver abscess caused by *Clostridium difficile*. A case report. *Medicine* 2017;96:35(e7969).

80. Reigadas E, Alcalá L, Gómez J, et al. Breakthrough *Clostridium difficile* infection in cirrhotic patients receiving rifaximin. *CID* 2018;66:1086–1091.

81. McDonald LC, Gerding DN, Johnson S, et al. Clinical practice guidelines for *Clostridium difficile* infection in adults and children: 2017 update by the Infectious diseases society of America (IDSA) and society for healthcare epidemiology of America (SHEA). *CID* 2018;66:987–994.

27 Febrile Neutropenia in the Critical Care Unit

Perrine Parize, Anne Pouvaret, Paul-Louis Woerther, Frédéric Pène, and Olivier Lortholary

CONTENTS

CLINICAL PERSPECTIVE

Patients with neutropenia have an increased susceptibility to infection. Among these patients, those with long duration of neutropenia (>7 days) and very low count of neutrophils (<100 cells/mm^3) are at high risk for fungal and bacterial infections and subsequent sepsis or septic shock. The survival of critically ill neutropenic cancer patients has improved over time, and these patients are increasingly admitted to the critical care unit (CCU) [1,2]. Empirical bactericidal antibiotic therapy targeting most threatening microorganisms should be initiated promptly to all neutropenic patients at the onset of fever. In critically ill patients, empirical therapeutic decisions are more complex and have a tremendous impact on the outcome. In the era of growing antimicrobial resistance, these decisions are challenging and must lay on a collaborative approach involving intensivists, hematologists/oncologists, infectious disease specialists, and microbiologists. Recent international guidelines for empirical antibacterial therapy for febrile neutropenic patients are not dedicated to seriously ill patients; however, specific management strategies are proposed for this population [3–6]. This review aims to summarize existing guidelines and current strategies for the management of neutropenic patients in the CCU.

NEUTROPENIC PATIENTS' SPECIFIC FEATURES

PROGNOSIS OF CRITICALLY ILL NEUTROPENIC PATIENTS IN CCU

Prognosis of critically ill cancer patients was very poor two decades ago, so that their admission to CCU was limited by triage policies only because of cancer status. However, improvement of survival of these patients has been confirmed in a large cohort study of neutropenic patients hospitalized for severe sepsis or septic shock during the 2000s, with a hospital mortality rate reaching 43%, which tended to that observed in non-cancer patients' mortality rate [1,7]. Improved outcomes can be explained by several factors. First, therapeutic advances in oncohematology have been obtained over recent years. Second, prevention, better understanding, and management of organ dysfunction in CCU have also contributed to a higher survival rate. Third, iatrogenic toxicity, including that of antineoplastic chemotherapy, is managed better.

Nevertheless, some factors have been independently associated with unfavorable outcome in febrile neutropenic severe patients: The presence of at least one non-infectious acute condition (hemophagocytic lymphohistiocytosis, tumor lysis syndrome, toxicity of chemotherapy, bleeding, and venous thromboembolism), neurologic, respiratory, or hepatic failure. On the other hand, some factors have been identified as associated with a better survival, e.g., initial combination antibiotherapy, including an aminoglycoside and early catheter removal [1]. Neutropenia and its expected duration, though, should not be used as a criterion to limit admission in CCU [5]. Indeed, several studies failed to prove the impact of neutropenia or its duration on the prognosis of critically ill cancer patients [8,9]. Admission to CCU should not be delayed, since any delay is independently associated with an increased mortality [2]. The underlying disease and its status are no longer considered as a prognostic factor for critically ill cancer patients in CCU [8].

Necessity of life-prolonging interventions such as mechanical ventilation or renal replacement therapy has been reported as poor prognostic factor for 30-day mortality but not the length of these interventions [9]. These data encourage intensivists and oncohematologists to maintain close and forthright collaboration, with high-quality communication, in order to anticipate admission in CCU and prevent organ failure with less invasive procedures [10].

A special case that deserves to be mentioned is that of the allogeneic hematopoietic stem cell transplantation (allo-HSCT) patients. Indeed, that population used to have an extremely grim prognosis in the 1990s, especially when mechanical ventilation was required. Hospital mortality has improved thanks to reduced intensity conditioning, early CCU admission, and advances in hematology and in CCU management, but allo-HSCT remains an independent variable associated with mortality among neutropenic patients admitted to the CCU, with mechanical ventilation as a main determinant of short-term survival [10]. However, the use of non-invasive procedures as high-flow oxygen therapy combined with non-invasive ventilation may decrease mechanical ventilation requirement, even if such strategies have not been specifically investigated in that population. Among the prognostic factors of critically ill allo-HSCT, presence of graft versus host disease and the number of organ failure at admission are relevant [11] while neutropenia is not. Admission of allo-HSCT patient in CCU for sepsis relies on a policy of triage hard to define, with a case-by-case decision [12].

Given the potential severe outcome of febrile neutropenia, identification of sepsis in cancer patients is of particular importance. The Multinational Association for Supportive Care in Cancer (MASCC) score has been developed and validated for the management of febrile neutropenia [13]. It provides to physicians in emergency departments a decisional tool for outpatient care decision [6]. It has no application for high-risk patients and cannot be used as a prognostic indicator for complications, although it has been reported that a low MASCC risk index score of <21 was associated with an increased risk for septic shock in febrile neutropenic patients [14]. Other methods, such as the Clinical Index of Stable Febrile Neutropenia, are currently tested to detect patients that might be apparently stable but have an occult high risk of complications [15]. Thus, this new index includes performance status >2, the stress-induce hyperglycemia, chronic obstructive pulmonary disease, chronic cardiovascular disease, mucositis National Cancer Institute (NCI) grade >2, and monocytes<200/μL [16]. The procedure has been validated in patients with different types of solid cancers but not with hematological malignancies.

New sepsis definitions have been recently been set, with a new risk stratification to facilitate earlier recognition and more timely management of patients with sepsis: Absence of organ dysfunction, sepsis, and septic shock [17]. Those definitions are based on the evaluation by the Sequential Organ Failure Assessment (SOFA) score and quick-SOFA (qSOFA), while the previous sepsis definitions were set with the Systemic Inflammatory Response Syndrome (SIRS) score [18]. Only two studies with discordant results have evaluated and compared the accuracy of these scores for mortality in cancer patients admitted to CCU with infections or febrile neutropenia. One of them reported a better discriminative power than SIRS for predicting hospital and CCU mortality [19]. The second one concludes that even if qSOFA score was an independent

factor predicting sepsis and CCU admission in patients with febrile neutropenia, its performance remained inferior to that of the MASCC score, with a poor sensitivity of 14% for predicting sepsis but a high specificity of 98% [20]. Thus, predictive models may be helpful for some groups of febrile neutropenia but cannot be applied to the overall population. Severity of illness scores, such as Simplified Acute Physiology Score (SAPS II) in febrile neutropenic patients in hematology wards, appear to be inaccurate for predicting mortality [21].

INTESTINAL MICROBIOTA OF NEUTROPENIC PATIENTS

Intestinal microbiota, composed of 10^{11} bacteria per gram of feces, the majority of which are strict anaerobes (>99%), plays the role of barrier regarding the acquisition of exogenous bacteria. This function, also called colonization resistance, can be defined as the process resulting in the removal of bacteria administered by mouth. Under physiologic conditions, colonization resistance allows the clearance of potentially pathogenic bacteria (dominated by aerotolerant gram-negative bacilli, such as enterobacteria, or non-fermenter gram-negative bacilli, such as *Pseudomonas* spp.), which remain transient or minority. In patients treated for cancer, selective pressure related to exposure to both cytotoxic drugs and antimicrobial agents has a major impact on the intestinal microbiota [22]. As a result, these treatments induce a reduction of the colonization resistance and, in this way, ease the acquisition of exogenous and potentially multidrug resistant (MDR) bacteria [23]. In the same time, they also select indigenous resistant bacteria, while the more susceptible ones are cleared. Finally, intestinal microbiota is found enriched with more and more resistant and potentially pathogenic bacteria and appears as a major reservoir of pathogens, especially for neutropenic patients. Infectious risk is even more significant when these patients are hospitalized in CCU, where they can be exposed to nosocomial infections linked to invasive procedures such as ventilator-associated pneumonias.

In patients receiving high-dose chemotherapy, the mucosal toxicity together with neutropenia favors the risk of digestive translocation, i.e., the crossing of intestinal wall by bacteria originating from the intestinal microbiota. For that reason, intestinal microbiota is of paramount importance in the understanding and management of infection in patients with profound and sustained neutropenia, especially when bacterial translocation is suspected. Since bacterial carriage is the mandatory prerequisite for infection, knowledge about MDR bacteria carriage (when available) should always be considered in the choice of the antimicrobial molecule, and resort to broad-spectrum antibiotics may be recommended, particularly in the absence of any microbiological and clinical documentation. It has been shown a long time ago that among all the species inhabiting the gut, the predominant aerotolerant bacterial species may be the most at risk to translocate in neutropenic patients [24]. Moreover, this observation has been confirmed with NGS tools during neutropenia in allo-HSCT [25]. The correlation between the risk of translocation with an ESBL-EB and the level of the fecal carriage of this bacteria has also been observed in a cohort of neutropenic patients with bacteremia [26], supporting the value of the assessment of MDR bacteria carriage in the choice of empirical antibiotic treatment.

To counter the risk of intestinal translocation, strategies based on antimicrobial prophylaxis have been proposed in patients with profound and sustained neutropenia, with an enteral antibiotic containing most often fluoroquinolones but also tobramycin and/or colistin. Despite the fact that fluroquinolones-based antimicrobial prophylaxis has been found to significantly decrease the frequency of neutropenic fevers and infection-related mortality in some neutropenic patients [27], their use remains a matter of debate because of the risk of acquisition and selection of MDR bacteria, as recently shown in allo-HSCT recipients [28]. This link between fluoroquinolones' exposure and MDR incite to abandon this strategy and prefers empiric antibiotic protocols based on local monitoring of resistance [29]. Although still under study, the fecal microbiota transplantation has been proposed to decolonize carriers of extensively antimicrobial-resistant opportunistic pathogens and prevent difficult-to-treat infections. This strategy has provided adequate results at least in the short term [30] and may be used in the future.

PHARMACODYNAMICS AND PHARMACOKINETICS OF ANTIBACTERIAL DRUGS IN THE MANAGEMENT OF FEBRILE NEUTROPENIA

The pharmacokinetics and pharmacodynamics of antibacterial agents could be altered in patients with neutropenia with potentially reduced serum, tissue, and body fluid concentrations, leading to decreased bacterial activities of these agents [31]. Pharmacokinetic changes are multifactorial in these patients and probably not only related to the low count of neutrophils. Antipseudomonal beta-lactams are the cornerstone of empirical therapy in febrile neutropenia and are frequently initiated as monotherapy at the onset of fever. High-dosage regimen and loading dose immediately followed by continuous infusion (ceftazidime) [32] or long infusions (piperacilline-tazobactam) have been associated with improved pharmacokinetic parameters in patients with neutropenia. Moreover, patients with neutropenia have an increased clearance of glycopeptides and an increased volume of distribution, suggesting the use of higher initial doses and monitoring of the trough serum concentrations in this population [33–35]. Optimal dosages for teicoplanin and amikacin have been specifically evaluated during febrile neutropenia [35,36]. Lastly, some data suggest that the pharmacokinetics of fluoroquinolones is not significantly modified during neutropenia [37]. In addition to modifications related to neutropenia, there are a variety of factors that influence the dosing of any individual antibiotic in CCU, including increased volume of distribution and organ failures. These numerous factors lead to hardly predictable anti-infectious dosing in critically ill neutropenic patients. Therefore, in these patients, if the loading dose appears of critical importance, then therapy should be reviewed daily and adjusted in the light of changes in patient organ function and results of monitoring of trough serum concentrations [31,38].

SPECIFIC CCU ENTITIES

Neutropenic Enterocolitis (Typhlitis)

Typhlitis complicates cytotoxic chemotherapy such as high-dose cytarabine [39]. Clinical manifestations include fever, abdominal cramping, abdominal distention, occlusion, pain and/or tenderness, diarrhea, and intestinal bleeding. A systematic abdominal CT scan with contrast enhancement may help in the diagnosis, as typhlitis diagnostic criteria include the presence of profound neutropenia, bowel wall thickening greater than 4 mm of any segment of the bowel at least 30 mm length in CT, and the exclusion of other diagnosis. Most of the time, colonoscopy or recto-sigmoidoscopy is not warranted first-line but may be required in a second phase; however, these exams are associated with a high risk of perforation.

The management of typhlitis is conservative when possible, including broad-spectrum antibiotic, symptomatic measures, and parenteral nutrition in severe cases [39]. A surgical management is justified by uncontrolled bleeding despite transfusion, suspicion of gastrointestinal perforation, and clinical deterioration despite adequate conservative management [40]. When indicated, surgery should not be delayed in critically ill neutropenic patients suspected, as the lack of surgical management is associated with unfavorable prognostic.

Perianal Cellulitis

Perianal cellulitis should be systematically sought in neutropenic patients, as it could be associated with sepsis or septic shock in this population [41]. The management of perianal cellulitis could be conservative in the absence of septic shock or fluctuation/collection evidenced during diagnostic workup and includes a broad-spectrum antibiotic therapy active on anaerobes, *Enterococcus*, *Enterobacteriaceae*, and *Pseudomonas aeruginosa* and antifungal therapy targeting *Candida*. In case of conservative management, the patients should be monitored cautiously by surgeons. Surgery is always required in cellulitis-induced septic shock or in case of fluctuation/collection [40].

Fungemia

In a cohort of 3417 patients with candidemia in Paris (3666 isolates), 1164 (34.1%) had a solid tumor (45.7% digestive tract) and 586 (17.1%) had a hematological malignancy (41.8% lymphoma and 33.5% acute leukemia) [42]. The hematology patients were significantly younger, more often pre-exposed to antifungals, more often infected by *C. tropicalis*, *C. krusei*, or *C. kefyr*, and more often treated in the first instance with an echinocandin. Compared with inpatients who were not in CCU at the time of fungemia, those in CCU were less frequently infected by *C. parapsilosis*, had more recent surgery, and died more frequently before day 8 and day 30. An increase in crude mortality over time in CCU was observed only in oncology patients [42]. In the same cohort, 338 episodes of fungemia due to uncommon yeasts were also analyzed. Thirty-five different species were identified (27 ascomycetes and 8 basidiomycetes), of which 11 had caspofungin MIC 50 >0.25 mg/L and 15 had fluconazole minimal inhibitory concentration (MIC) 50 >4 mg/L. Hematological malignancies and prior exposure to antifungal drugs were independent predisposing factors for uncommon species. Infections due to *C. kefyr*-related species and *Trichosporon* spp. remained associated with hematological malignancies, those due to the *Geotrichum* group were associated with acute leukemia. Infections due to *Trichosporon* spp. or fungus of the *Geotrichum* group were associated with prior exposure to caspofungin but not to fluconazole [43].

Invasive Aspergillosis

Invasive pulmonary aspergillosis (IPA) is documented in up to 15% of hematology patients requiring intensive care for acute respiratory failure [44]. Clinical signs and symptoms of IPA are non-specific, and the diagnosis is based on clinical and imaging findings, cultures, indirect tests (galactomannan antigen in bronchoalveolar lavage > serum and specific PCR), and more rarely histology. Patients at high risk of IPA are mainly neutropenic patients with a history of hematological malignancies or allogeneic HSCT; however, new risk factors have been identified, including chronic obstructive pulmonary disease, liver failure, cirrhosis, and post-influenza infections. In neutropenic patients, diagnosis of IPA can be made in the days before admission to CCU or after admission in patients initially admitted for non-documented acute respiratory failure [44]. The mortality of these patients is high; however, the use of voriconazole has been associated with lower mortality rates.

INITIAL MANAGEMENT OF NEUTROPENIC PATIENTS IN CCU

Diagnostic Workup

Infections in neutropenic patients often progress rapidly, leading to hemodynamic instability and other life-threatening complications requiring admission to the CCU. The spectrum of potential pathogens is broad, and early diagnosis is necessary for adequate treatment. That's why, at admission, a careful assessment should be performed to help localize the site of infection and adapt the initial treatment: Relevant targeted medical history, including previous infections, previous administered antibiotics, and prophylaxis, combined with a detailed physical examination. Symptoms and signs of infections are often unapparent or attenuated, as a result of the impaired inflammatory response [45]. For example, swelling, erythema, pus formation, and exudates are absent. Fever may be the only sign suggesting an infection. The rate of clinically documented infections in neutropenic patients with sepsis or septic shock is around 30% [1]. Lungs, gastrointestinal tract, and skin or soft tissue are the three main sites of infections, accounting for more than 90% of clinically documented infections. Physical examination should be repeated daily. Special attention should be devoted to the perianal area, site of fissures complicated with cellulitis, central catheter sites where slight erythema or tenderness may be the only evidence of tunnel infection, the peritoneal signs and/or abdominal tenderness, and intestinal bleeding, which may be compatible with neutropenic enterocolitis [46]. Oral cavity should be examined for signs of mucositis. This examination requires that the patient is undressed, so that the skin can be fully inspected. Indeed, skin lesions can be the only manifestation of a systemic infection or even its portal of entry, as illustrated by fusariosis [47] or aspergillosis [48].

Biomarkers have been developed to help physicians distinguish between infectious and non-infectious fever and also between bacteriological and viral infections. Even though C-reactive protein (CRP) has some inconsistencies and limitations, its serial measurement can be used for further therapeutic response assessment [49]. The CRP level should be serially assessed. In septic neutropenic cancer patients, CRP level is significantly higher in comparison with non-neutropenic cancer patients, with a similar course [50]. It is widely agreed that high concentrations of CRP are associated with bacterial infections and low concentrations with viral, even if not absolute. Thus, CRP provides a valuable tool as a therapeutic decision support for infections in neutropenic critically ill cancer patients [49]. Although preliminary studies looked promising [51], current data in literature do not support the use of procalcitonin measurement for routine analysis in febrile neutropenia, since as a marker of infection, its sensitivity ranges from 42% to 72% and its specificity from 64% to 89%. It may be useful in the outcome prediction but seems to be not superior to CRP [52].

Microbiological documentation is an issue of great importance in order to adapt antibiotherapy and limit resistance emergence. In total, 10%–55% of patients have microbiologically documented infections, with bacteremia only documented in 10%–20% [1,53]. At least two sets of blood cultures should be drawn, with collection from each lumen of the central venous catheter and from a peripheral vein site. In patients without central venous catheter, two sets of blood cultures should be sent from two separate peripheral puncture sites. Colonization by antibiotic resistant bacteria has to be sought, especially for patients with hematological malignancies who received prior broad-spectrum antibacterial therapy. Other specimens should be driven by clinical signs, such as detection of *Clostridium difficile* toxins in case of diarrheas and urine sample for bacterial culture.

Febrile patients with prolonged neutropenia need a special attention, as they are prone to develop invasive fungal infections, viral reactivation such as cytomegalovirus, adenovirus, and human herpes virus 6 infections.

When invasive fungal infections are suspected for patients with deep prolonged neutropenia and persistent or recurrent fever despite broad-spectrum antibiotics, fungal biomarkers may provide valuable assistance, at least in those not receiving mold active prophylaxis [54]. They constitute an indirect mycological test used as a criterion by the European Organization for Research and Treatment of Cancer/Invasive Fungal Infections Cooperative Group and the National Institute of Allergy and Infectious Diseases Mycoses Study Group to diagnose probable invasive fungal infections [55]. Therefore, galactomannan (GM) antigen can be detected for the diagnosis of aspergillosis in plasma, serum, bronchoalveolar lavage fluid, and cerebrospinal fluid, keeping in mind the reasons of false-positive reactions. β-D-glucan antigen can be detected in serum and help for the diagnosis of invasive fungal disease other than mucormycosis. Combining GM antigen test and real-time MycAssay *Aspergillus* polymerase chain reaction (PCR) could be beneficial for early diagnosis and treatment of invasive aspergillosis in febrile neutropenia but require more studies [56,57].

In case of cutaneous lesions, skin biopsy should be performed promptly for direct examination of the specimen and bacterial and fungal cultures. Furthermore, herpes simplex virus, and varicella-zoster virus PCR should be performed if vesicles are present, in addition to histopathology analysis.

Diagnostic imaging examinations are based on clinical examination. Even if chest X-ray is commonly recommended as a first evaluation for neutropenic fever, considering intermediate or high-resolution chest computed tomography (CT) is important, owing to its better sensitivity for detecting earlier abnormalities in neutropenic patients, even if outcome is not improved [58]. As the main admission reason in CCU for febrile neutropenia is acute respiratory failure [1], CT scan is of great value to orientate bronchial endoscopy for bronchoalveolar lavage. Pulmonary biopsies should be proposed case-by-case with a multidisciplinary approach [5].

Abdominal CT should be performed for patients showing signs evocative of neutropenic enterocolitis, in particular patients following cytotoxic chemotherapy with mucositis. The CT scan can show complications such as perforation [46].

Finally, physicians should be aware that a wide range of non-infectious diagnosis can cause temperature elevation: Drugs, thromboembolisms, neoplastic fever, cytokines release, and transfusion-related events. Thus, initial evaluation reevaluation must be performed. Indeed, treating non-infectious causes with antimicrobial therapy may lead to adverse health effects, by delaying adequate treatment and increasing toxicity and risk for antimicrobial resistance acquisition.

ANTI-INFECTIOUS STRATEGY

Prophylaxis and Protective Isolation

The benefit of protective isolation in prevention of invasive fungal infection seems to be correlated with neutropenia severity. As a consequence, protective isolation might be of interest in patients with deep (neutrophil count less than 500 cells/mm^3) and prolonged neutropenia (more than 7 days), including high-efficiency air filtration, if available, geographic isolation, and technical isolation (face mask and cap) [59]. However, protective isolation should not delay CCU admission or limit patient's clinical monitoring or decrease the quality of care [5]. Anti-*Aspergillus* prophylaxis and specific antiviral and *Pneumocystis* prophylaxis may be continued in CCU if indicated in the management of the underlying malignancy [60,61].

Empirical Antibacterial Therapy in CCU

In patients with neutropenia, fever should always lead to consider the possibility of an ongoing infection that requires the immediate introduction of an appropriate empirical antimicrobial treatment (Figure 27.1). Indeed, any delay in the initiation of the treatment has been significantly and independently associated with poorer outcome in these patients [62–65]. The aim of empiric therapy in neutropenic patients admitted in CCU is thus to cover the most likely and most virulent pathogens. An escalation approach could be chosen [3], with an initial empirical therapy secondarily broadened if the patient remains hemodynamically unstable to cover drug-resistant gram-negative and gram-positive organisms, as well as anaerobes. However, a de-escalation strategy is frequently preferred for seriously ill patients (sepsis or septic shock), initiating a broad initial empirical regimen and then de-escalating to a narrower-spectrum therapy in function of microbiology laboratory findings and outcome [4].

Combination antibiotic therapy, including an antipseudomonal β-lactam and an aminoglycoside, is recommended by most experts in neutropenic patients with sepsis and septic shock, as this combination has been associated with lower mortality [1,66]. A recent study showed that a short course of gentamicin was not associated with faster reversal of shock or improved survival in patients with sepsis or septic shock [67]. However, this study was conducted in a setting with low prevalence of antimicrobial resistance and was contradictory with previous studies [1,68]. Therefore, depending on the local prevalence of resistance, a short course of aminoglycoside in combination with antipseudomonal β-lactam may be considered as an empirical therapy in critically ill neutropenic patients, in order to broaden the bacterial spectrum. The β-lactam should be carefully chosen at the admission in CCU, taking into account the therapeutic history of the patient, his MDR bacteria carriage, his organic failures, and the local bacterial epidemiology and prevalence resistance patterns [4]. An anti-pseudomonal β-lactam (cefepime, ceftazidime, or piperacillin-tazobactam) in combination with

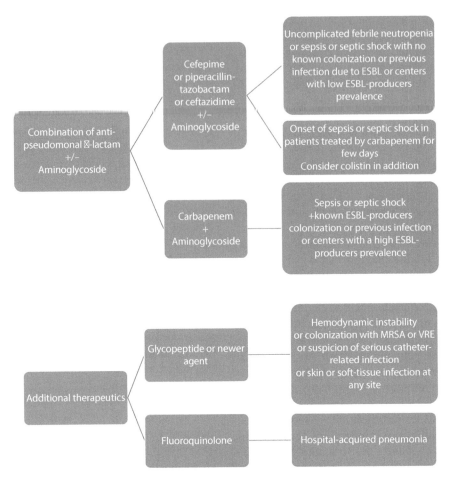

FIGURE 27.1   Initial empirical antibacterial treatment in neutropenic patient in the CCU.

an aminoglycoside could be initiated for patients with no history of carriage or previous infection with resistant bacteria. However, in centers where resistant pathogens are regularly seen at the onset of febrile neutropenia or when the patient has known carriage or previous infection with a resistant bacterium, a combination of carbapenem and aminoglycoside could be recommended [3,4]. Finally, if the patient had been treated with carbapenem for a few days before the onset of sepsis or septic shock, an infection due to a carbapenem-resistant bacteria is suspected (carbapenemase-producing gram-negative bacteria or more frequently bacteria with carbapenem-induced membrane impermeability), and a treatment associating a non-carbapenem anti-pseudomonal beta-lactam, an aminoglycoside, could be preferred with the addition of colistin, depending on the local bacterial epidemiology [4,69].

Other Therapeutics Depends on Diagnostic Orientation

The addition of a glycopeptide is recommended for hemodynamically unstable patients or in case of suspected central venous catheter-related infection, skin or soft tissue infection, or severe mucositis. Coverage of resistant gram-positive microorganisms with a glycopeptide or newer agents could also be indicated in settings of high methicillin-resistant staphylococcus aureus (MRSA) or *vancomycin-resistant enterococcus (VRE)*.

The management of typhlitis or perianal cellulitis requires a broad-spectrum antibiotic therapy active on anaerobes, *Enterococcus*, *Enterobacteriaceae*, and *Pseudomonas aeruginosa*. An empiric treatment against *Candida* spp. should also be added in absence of clinical improvement. The main differential diagnosis of typhlitis is *Clostridium difficile* colitis, and a search for *C. difficile* toxin in stool should be systematic [39].

For neutropenic patients with hospital-acquired pneumonia, a double anti-pseudomonal/gram-negative coverage could be appropriate, and the initiation of a fluoroquinolone should be discussed [70]. A fluoroquinolone would also cover *Legionella*, particularly in case of profound monocytopenia, such as in patients with hairy cell leukemia.

Antifungal Therapy in CCU

In CCU, antifungal therapy should be considered in patients who are clinically unstable and in patients with findings suggestive of invasive fungal infection. The choice of an empiric agent depends on fungus potentially responsible for the clinical presentation, previous antifungal prophylaxis, and toxicity profiles [3]. An echinocandin is preferred if *Candida* spp.-invasive infection is suspected due to the high incidence of fluconazole resistant *Candida* in CCU, the benefit of this therapeutic class in case of septic shock and the favorable profile of tolerance [71–73]. In patients with pulmonary or sinus findings suggesting an invasive mold infection, anti-fungal treatment relies on voriconazole or lipid formulation of amphotericin B [74]. A lipid formulation of amphotericin B is preferred when a Mucorales infection is suspected [75], if the suspected invasive infection occurred while the patient was treated by azole as prophylaxis or if a voriconazole-resistant *Aspergillus* spp. is suspected (patient from the Netherlands) [76]. Hepatic and renal dysfunctions should be taken into consideration when choosing an antifungal drug. Moreover, when an azole agent is preferred, drug-drug inter-action should be anticipated, and trough serum concentrations monitored.

NON-ANTIMICROBIAL MANAGEMENT

Catheter Removal

Immediate indwelling catheter removal is recommended in neutropenic patients with septic shock or sepsis, as the removal has been associated with increased survival in these populations [1].

Granulocyte Colony-Stimulating Factor

Only limited data are available on the benefit of granulocyte colony-stimulating factor (G-CSF) in CCU [5]. The use of G-CSF seems associated with a reduction of the time to neu-trophil recovery but does not influence the overall mortality. Moreover, in patients with pulmonary infiltrates during neu-tropenia, G-CSF may induce a worsening of respiratory status with a risk of acute respiratory distress syndrome (ARDS). Thus, G-CSF is generally not recommended for the manage-ment of febrile neutropenic patients. This treatment should be used only on a case-by-case basis after consulting an oncologist or a hematologist and stopped before neutropenia recovery in patients at risk of worsening of respiratory status (pre-existing respiratory failure or pulmonary infection) [77,78].

Granulocyte Transfusion

To date, no well-designed study supports or refutes the benefit of granulocyte transfusion in neutropenic patients with severe infection. Little data on this topic are available, and existing studies are often underpowered [79]. A recent study demon-strated a good feasibility of granulocyte transfusion, with evi-dence of efficacy, but on the other hand, this treatment could be associated with severe complications (allo-immunization and transfusion-related acute lung injury) [80]. Therefore, granulocyte transfusions cannot be recommended in routine use in neutropenic patients in CCU and should be considered in specific situations such as severe cellulitis or uncontrolled invasive fungal infections after a collaborative discussion.

Routine Management of Severe Sepsis and Septic Shock

Routine management of sepsis and septic shock was recently modified by the emergence of therapeutic strategies that dem-onstrated an improvement in survival in septic shock patients. Most of measures retained in the latest Surviving Sepsis Campaign Guidelines have not been specifically assessed in neutropenic patients [81]. However, most of these treatments,

including fluid therapy, vasoactive medications, transfusion, mechanical ventilation, glucose control, and renal replace-ment therapy, are applicable to patients with malignancies.

ADAPTATION OF MANAGEMENT

ADJUSTMENT OF THE INITIAL ANTIMICROBIAL REGIMEN

Bacterial identification following initial microbiological workup may help in de-escalating antibiotic therapy [4]:

- In case of documented infection, the patient should be treated according to the organism identified. A switch to an appropriate narrower-spectrum β-lactam is recommended, using *in vitro* susceptibility tests. Antibiotics given in combination should be discon-tinued (aminoglycosides, quinolones, and colistin) if the patient is stable or improving. If used empirically, glycopeptide antibiotics should probably be discon-tinued after 72 hours if no resistant gram-positive cocci have been identified or if the infection is due to a bacterium susceptible to the β-lactam prescribed.
- In case of non-documented infection, the initial β-lactam should be maintained. Antibiotics given in combination should be discontinued (aminogly-cosides, quinolones, and colistin) if the patient is stable or improving. If used empirically, glycopep-tide antibiotics should probably be discontinued after 72 hours if no resistant gram-positive cocci have been identified or if the infection is due to a bacte-rium susceptible to the β-lactam.
- In case of clinical deterioration, the diagnostic workup should be pursued, an escalation of bacte-rial and fungal empirical therapy should be consid-ered, and the source of infection should be controlled (drainage, surgery, catheter removal, etc.) [3–5].

DURATION OF ANTIBIOTIC THERAPY IN FEBRILE NEUTROPENIA

Most studies evaluating the optimal duration of empirical antibiotic therapy in neutropenic patients exclude severely ill patients [4]; therefore, the continuation of antibiotics until neu-trophil recovery is a standard approach for high-risk patients with neutropenia persisting more than 7 days [3]. However, for febrile patients admitted in CCU for reasons other than sepsis (tumor lysis syndrome, hemorrhagic syndrome, non-infectious acute respiratory failure, etc.), empirical antibiotics should probably be discontinued after 72 hours or more of apy-rexia if they were hemodynamically stable since presentation, irrespective of their neutrophil count or expected duration of neutropenia, as recommended by the european conference on infections in leukemia (ECIL)-4 guidelines [4,82]. These patients should be kept hospitalized for a few days under close observation if still neutropenic, and an antibiotic therapy should be re-started urgently in case of fever recurrence.

Even when the neutrophil recovery occurs in CCU, the total course duration of the antimicrobial treatment is usually of at least 7 days for sepsis of unknown origin, with discontinuation after a minimum of 2 afebrile days in patients hemodynamically stable, while for clinically and/or microbiologically documented infections, the duration of antibiotic therapy is guided by the diagnostic and evolution.

REFERENCES

1. Legrand M, Max A, Peigne V, et al. Survival in neutropenic patients with severe sepsis or septic shock. *Crit Care Med* 2012;40:43–49.
2. Azoulay E, Mokart D, Pène F, et al. Outcomes of critically ill patients with hematologic malignancies: Prospective multicenter data from France and Belgium—A groupe de recherché respiratoire en réanimation onco-hématologique study. *J Clin Oncol* 2013;31:2810–2818.
3. Freifeld AG, Bow EJ, Sepkowitz KA, et al. Clinical practice guideline for the use of antimicrobial agents in neutropenic patients with cancer: 2010 update by the infectious diseases society of America. *Clin Infect Dis* 2011;52:427–431.
4. Averbuch D, Orasch C, Cordonnier C, et al. European guidelines for empirical antibacterial therapy for febrile neutropenic patients in the era of growing resistance: Summary of the 2011 4th European conference on infections in leukemia. *Haematologica* 2013;98:1826–1835.
5. Schnell D, Azoulay E, Benoit D, et al. Management of neutropenic patients in the intensive care unit (NEWBORNS EXCLUDED) recommendations from an expert panel from the French Intensive Care Society (SRLF) with the French Group for Pediatric Intensive Care Emergencies (GFRUP), the French Society of Anesthesia and Intensive Care (SFAR), the French Society of Hematology (SFH), the French Society for Hospital Hygiene (SF2H), and the French Infectious Diseases Society (SPILF). *Ann Intensive Care* 2016;6:90.
6. Klastersky J, de Naurois J, Rolston K, et al. Management of febrile neutropaenia: ESMO clinical practice guidelines. *Ann Oncol Off J Eur Soc Med Oncol* 2016;27:v111–v118.
7. Regazzoni CJ, Irrazabal C, Luna CM, Poderoso JJ. Cancer patients with septic shock: Mortality predictors and neutropenia. *Support Care Cancer Off J Multinatl Assoc Support Care Cancer* 2004;12:833–839.
8. Darmon M, Azoulay E, Alberti C, et al. Impact of neutropenia duration on short-term mortality in neutropenic critically ill cancer patients. *Intensive Care Med* 2002;28:1775–1780.
9. Mokart D, Darmon M, Resche-Rigon M, et al. Prognosis of neutropenic patients admitted to the intensive care unit. *Intensive Care Med* 2015;41:296–303.
10. Azoulay E, Pène F, Darmon M, et al. Managing critically Ill hematology patients: Time to think differently. *Blood Rev* 2015;29:359–367.
11. Lengliné E, Chevret S, Moreau AS, et al. Changes in intensive care for allogeneic hematopoietic stem cell transplant recipients. *Bone Marrow Transplant* 2015;50:840–845.
12. Saillard C, Blaise D, Mokart D. Critically ill allogeneic hematopoietic stem cell transplantation patients in the intensive care unit: Reappraisal of actual prognosis. *Bone Marrow Transplant* 2016;51:1050–1061.
13. Klastersky J, Paesmans M, Rubenstein EB, et al. The multinational association for supportive care in cancer risk index: A multinational scoring system for identifying low-risk febrile neutropenic cancer patients. *J Clin Oncol Off J Am Soc Clin Oncol* 2000;18:3038–3051.
14. Ahn S, Lee YS, Lim KS, Lee JL. Adding procalcitonin to the MASCC risk-index score could improve risk stratification of patients with febrile neutropenia. *Support Care Cancer Off J Multinatl Assoc Support Care Cancer* 2013;21:2303–2308.
15. Carmona-Bayonas A, Jiménez-Fonseca P, Viriuzela Echaburu J, et al. The time has come for new models in febrile neutropenia: A practical demonstration of the inadequacy of the MASCC score. *Clin Transl Oncol Off Publ Fed Span Oncol Soc Natl Cancer Inst Mex* 2017;19:1084–1090.
16. Carmona-Bayonas A, Gómez J, González-Billalabeitia E, et al. Prognostic evaluation of febrile neutropenia in apparently stable adult cancer patients. *Br J Cancer* 2011;105:612–617.
17. Singer M, Deutschman CS, Seymour CW, et al. The third international consensus definitions for sepsis and septic shock (Sepsis-3). *JAMA* 2016;315:801–810.
18. Levy MM, Fink MP, Marshall JC, et al. 2001 SCCM/ESICM/ACCP/ATS/SIS international sepsis definitions conference. *Intensive Care Med* 2003;29:530–538.
19. Costa TR, Nassar Jr A, Caruso P. Accuracy of SOFA, qSOFA and SIRS scores for mortality in cancer patients admitted to an intensive care unit with suspected infection. *J Crit Care* 2018;45:52–57.
20. Kim M, Ahn S, Kim WY, et al. Predictive performance of the quick sequential organ failure assessment score as a screening tool for sepsis, mortality, and intensive care unit admission in patients with febrile neutropenia. *Support Care Cancer Off J Multinatl Assoc Support Care Cancer* 2017;25:1557–1562.
21. Blot F, Cordonnier C, Buzyn A, et al. Severity of illness scores: Are they useful in febrile neutropenic adult patients in hematology wards? A prospective multicenter study. *Crit Care Med* 2001;29:2125–2131.
22. Zhernakova A, Kurilshikov A, Bonder MJ, et al. Population-based metagenomics analysis reveals markers for gut microbiome composition and diversity. *Science* 2016;352:565–569.
23. Borgmann S, Pfeifer Y, Becker L, et al. Findings from an outbreak of carbapenem-resistant *Klebsiella pneumoniae* emphasize the role of antibiotic treatment for cross transmission. *Infection* 2018;46:103–112.
24. Tancrède CH, Andremont AO. Bacterial translocation and gram-negative bacteremia in patients with hematological malignancies. *J Infect Dis* 1985;152:99–103.
25. Taur Y, Xavier JB, Lipuma L, et al. Intestinal domination and the risk of bacteremia in patients undergoing allogeneic hematopoietic stem cell transplantation. *Clin Infect Dis* 2012;55:905–914.
26. Woerther PL, Micol JB, Angebault C, et al. Monitoring antibiotic-resistant enterobacteria faecal levels is helpful in predicting antibiotic susceptibility of bacteraemia isolates in patients with haematological malignancies. *J Med Microbiol* 2015;64:676–681.
27. Gafter-Gvili A, Fraser A, Paul M, Leibovici L. Meta-analysis: Antibiotic prophylaxis reduces mortality in neutropenic patients. *Ann Intern Med* 2005;142(12 Pt 1):979–995.
28. Averbuch D, Tridello G, Hoek J, et al. Antimicrobial resistance in gram-negative rods causing bacteremia in hematopoietic stem cell transplant recipients: Intercontinental prospective study of the infectious diseases working party of the European bone marrow transplantation group. *Clin Infect Dis* 2017;65:1819–1828.
29. Averbuch D, Cordonnier C, Livermore DM, et al. Targeted therapy against multi-resistant bacteria in leukemic and hematopoietic stem cell transplant recipients: Guidelines of the 4th European conference on infections in leukemia (ECIL-4, 2011). *Haematologica* 2013;98:1836–1847.

30. Bar-Yoseph H, Hussein K, Braun E, Paul M. Natural history and decolonization strategies for ESBL/carbapenem-resistant Enterobacteriaceae carriage: Systematic review and meta-analysis. *J Antimicrob Chemother* 2016;71:2729–2739.

31. Lortholary O, Lefort A, Tod M, et al. Pharmacodynamics and pharmacokinetics of antibacterial drugs in the management of febrile neutropenia. *Lancet Infect Dis* 2008;8:612–620.

32. Dalle JH, Gnansounou M, Husson MO, et al. Continuous infusion of ceftazidime in the empiric treatment of febrile neutropenic children with cancer. *J Pediatr Hematol Oncol* 2002;24:714–716.

33. Zimmermann AE, Katona BG, Plaisance KI. Association of vancomycin serum concentrations with outcomes in patients with gram-positive bacteremia. *Pharmacotherapy* 1995;15:85–91.

34. Le Normand Y, Milpied N, Kergueris MF, Harousseau JL. Pharmacokinetic parameters of vancomycin for therapeutic regimens in neutropenic adult patients. *Int J Biomed Comput* 1994;36:121–125.

35. Lortholary O, Tod M, Rizzo N, et al. Population pharmacokinetic study of teicoplanin in severely neutropenic patients. *Antimicrob Agents Chemother* 1996;40:1242–1247.

36. Tod M, Lortholary O, Seytre D, et al. Population pharmacokinetic study of amikacin administered once or twice daily to febrile, severely neutropenic adults. *Antimicrob Agents Chemother* 1998;42:849–856.

37. Smith GM, Leyland MJ, Farrell ID, Geddes AM. Preliminary evaluation of ciprofloxacin, a new 4-quinolone antibiotic, in the treatment of febrile neutropenic patients. *J Antimicrob Chemother* 1986;18(Suppl D):165–174.

38. McKenzie C. Antibiotic dosing in critical illness. *J Antimicrob Chemother* 2011;66(Suppl 2):ii25–ii31.

39. Nesher L, Rolston KV. Neutropenic enterocolitis, a growing concern in the era of widespread use of aggressive chemotherapy. *Clin Infect Dis* 2013;56:711–717.

40. Badgwell BD, Cormier JN, Wray CJ, et al. Challenges in surgical management of abdominal pain in the neutropenic cancer patient. *Ann Surg* 2008;248:104–109.

41. Morcos B, Amarin R, Abu Sba' A, et al. Contemporary management of perianal conditions in febrile neutropenic patients. *Eur J Surg Oncol* 2013;39:404–407.

42. Lortholary O, Renaudat C, Sitbon K, et al. The risk and clinical outcome of candidemia depending on underlying malignancy. *Intensive Care Med* 2017;43:652–662.

43. Bretagne S, Renaudat C, Desnos-Ollivier M, et al. Predisposing factors and outcome of uncommon yeast species-related fungaemia based on an exhaustive surveillance programme (2002–2014). *J Antimicrob Chemother* 2017;72:1784–1793.

44. Burghi G, Lemiale V, Seguin A, et al. Outcomes of mechanically ventilated hematology patients with invasive pulmonary aspergillosis. *Intensive Care Med* 2011;37:1605–1612.

45. Urabe A. Clinical features of the neutropenic host: Definitions and initial evaluation. *Clin Infect Dis* 2004;39:S53–S55.

46. Rodrigues FG, Dasilva G, Wexner SD. Neutropenic enterocolitis. *World J Gastroenterol* 2017;23:42–47.

47. Nucci M, Varon AG, Garnica M, et al. Increased incidence of invasive fusariosis with cutaneous portal of entry, Brazil. *Emerg Infect Dis* 2013;19:1567–1572.

48. Bernardeschi C, Foulet F, Ingen-Housz-Oro S, et al. Cutaneous invasive aspergillosis: Retrospective multicenter study of the French invasive-aspergillosis registry and literature review. *Medicine* 2015;94:e1018.

49. Ketema EB. Value of CRP as a marker of infection in cancer patients with febrile neutropenia: Review. *IJPSR* 2016;7:278–283.

50. Póvoa P, Souza-Dantas VC, Soares M, Salluh JI. C-reactive protein in critically ill cancer patients with sepsis: Influence of neutropenia. *Crit Care* 2011;15:R129.

51. Bernard L, Ferrière F, Casassus P, et al. Procalcitonin as an early marker of bacterial infection in severely neutropenic febrile adults. *Clin Infect Dis* 1998;27:914-915.

52. Sakr Y, Sponholz C, Tuche F, et al. The role of procalcitonin in febrile neutropenic patients: Review of the literature. *Infection* 2008;36:396.

53. Legrand M, Max A, Schlemmer B, et al. The strategy of antibiotic use in critically ill neutropenic patients. *Ann Intensive Care* 2011;1:22.

54. Duarte RF, Sánchez-Ortega I, Cuesta I, et al. Serum galactomannan-based early detection of invasive aspergillosis in hematology patients receiving effective antimold prophylaxis. *Clin Infect Dis* 2014;59:1696–1702.

55. De Pauw B, Walsh TJ, Donnelly JP, et al. Revised definitions of invasive fungal disease from the European Organization for Research and Treatment of Cancer/Invasive Fungal Infections Cooperative Group and the National Institute of Allergy and Infectious Diseases Mycoses Study Group (EORTC/MSG) Consensus Group. *Clin Infect Dis Off Publ Infect Dis Soc Am* 2008;46:1813–1821.

56. Aslan M, Oz Y, Aksit F, Akay OM. Potential of polymerase chain reaction and galactomannan for the diagnosis of invasive aspergillosis in patients with febrile neutropenia. *Mycoses* 2015;58:343–349.

57. Suarez F, Lortholary O, Buland S, et al. Detection of circulating *Aspergillus* fumigatus DNA by real-time PCR assay of large serum volumes improves early diagnosis of invasive aspergillosis in high-risk adult patients under hematologic surveillance. *J Clin Microbiol* 2008;46:3772–3777.

58. Heussel CP, Kauczor HU, Heussel GE, et al. Pneumonia in febrile neutropenic patients and in bone marrow and blood stem-cell transplant recipients: Use of high-resolution computed tomography. *J Clin Oncol Off J Am Soc Clin Oncol* 1999;17:796–805.

59. Levine AS, Siegel SE, Schreiber AD, et al. Protected environments and prophylactic antibiotics. A prospective controlled study of their utility in the therapy of acute leukemia. *N Engl J Med* 1973;288:477–483.

60. Alberti C, Bouakline A, Ribaud P, et al. Relationship between environmental fungal contamination and the incidence of invasive aspergillosis in haematology patients. *J Hosp Infect* 2001;48:198–206.

61. Mellinghoff SC, Panse J, Alakel N, et al. Primary prophylaxis of invasive fungal infections in patients with haematological malignancies: 2017 update of the recommendations of the infectious diseases working party (AGIHO) of the German Society for Haematology and Medical Oncology (DGHO). *Ann Hematol* 2018;97:197–207.

62. Tumbarello M, Sali M, Trecarichi EM, et al. Bloodstream infections caused by extended-spectrum-beta-lactamase-producing *Escherichia coli*: Risk factors for inadequate initial antimicrobial therapy. *Antimicrob Agents Chemother* 2008;52:3244–3252.

63. Cornejo-Juárez P, Pérez-Jiménez C, Silva-Sánchez J, et al. Molecular analysis and risk factors for *Escherichia coli* producing extended-spectrum β-lactamase bloodstream infection in hematological malignances. *PLOS ONE* 2012;7:e35780.

64. Gudiol C, Bodro M, Simonetti A, et al. Changing aetiology, clinical features, antimicrobial resistance, and outcomes of bloodstream infection in neutropenic cancer patients. *Clin Microbiol Infect* 2013;19:474–479.

65. Ortega M, Marco F, Soriano A, et al. Analysis of 4758 *Escherichia coli* bacteraemia episodes: Predictive factors for isolation of an antibiotic-resistant strain and their impact on the outcome. *J Antimicrob Chemother* 2009;63:568–574.

66. Leibovici L, Paul M, Poznanski O, et al. Monotherapy versus beta-lactam-aminoglycoside combination treatment for gram-negative bacteremia: A prospective, observational study. *Antimicrob Agents Chemother* 1997;41:1127–1133.

67. Ong DSY, Frencken JF, Klein Klouwenberg PMC, et al. Short-course adjunctive gentamicin as empirical therapy in patients with severe sepsis and septic shock: A prospective observational cohort study. *Clin Infect Dis* 2017;64:1731–1736.

68. Kumar A, Zarychanski R, Light B, et al. Early combination antibiotic therapy yields improved survival compared with monotherapy in septic shock: A propensity-matched analysis. *Crit Care Med* 2010;38:1773–1785.

69. Jacobs DM, Safir MC, Huang D, et al. Triple combination antibiotic therapy for carbapenemase-producing *Klebsiella pneumoniae*: A systematic review. *Ann Clin Microbiol Antimicrob* 2017;16:76.

70. Kalil AC, Metersky ML, Klompas M, et al. Management of adults with hospital-acquired and ventilator-associated pneumonia: 2016 clinical practice guidelines by the infectious diseases society of America and the American thoracic society. *Clin Infect Dis* 2016;63:e61–e111.

71. Pappas PG, Kauffman CA, Andes DR, et al. Clinical practice guideline for the management of candidiasis: 2016 update by the infectious diseases society of America. *Clin Infect Dis* 2016;62:e1–e50.

72. Ullmann AJ, Akova M, Herbrecht R, et al. ESCMID* guideline for the diagnosis and management of candida diseases 2012: Adults with haematological malignancies and after haematopoietic stem cell transplantation (HCT). *Clin Microbiol Infect* 2012;18(Suppl 7):53–67.

73. Bailly S, Leroy O, Azoulay E, et al. Impact of echinocandin on prognosis of proven invasive candidiasis in ICU: A post-hoc causal inference model using the AmarCAND2 study. *J Infect* 2017;74:408–417.

74. Patterson TF, Thompson GR 3rd, Denning DW, et al. Practice guidelines for the diagnosis and management of aspergillosis: 2016 update by the infectious diseases society of America. *Clin Infect Dis* 2016;63:e1–e60.

75. Cornely OA, Arikan-Akdagli S, Dannaoui E, et al. ESCMID and ECMM joint clinical guidelines for the diagnosis and management of mucormycosis 2013. *Clin Microbiol Infect* 2014;20(Suppl 3):5–26.

76. Lestrade PP, van der Velden WJFM, Bouwman F, et al. Epidemiology of invasive aspergillosis and triazole-resistant *Aspergillus* fumigatus in patients with haematological malignancies: A single-centre retrospective cohort study. *J Antimicrob Chemother* 2018;73:1389–1394.

77. Azoulay E, Darmon M, Delclaux C, et al. Deterioration of previous acute lung injury during neutropenia recovery. *Crit Care Med* 2002;30:781–786.

78. Rhee CK, Kang JY, Kim YH, et al. Risk factors for acute respiratory distress syndrome during neutropenia recovery in patients with hematologic malignancies. *Crit Care* 2009;13:R173.

79. Estcourt LJ, Stanworth SJ, Hopewell S, et al. Granulocyte transfusions for treating infections in people with neutropenia or neutrophil dysfunction. *Cochrane Database Syst Rev* 2016;4:CD005339.

80. Price TH, Boeckh M, Harrison RW, et al. Efficacy of transfusion with granulocytes from G-CSF/dexamethasone-treated donors in neutropenic patients with infection. *Blood* 2015;126:2153–2161.

81. Rhodes A, Evans LE, Alhazzani W, et al. Surviving sepsis campaign: International guidelines for management of sepsis and septic shock: 2016. *Intensive Care Med* 2017;43:304–377.

82. Aguilar-Guisado M, Espigado I, Martín-Peña A, et al. Optimisation of empirical antimicrobial therapy in patients with haematological malignancies and febrile neutropenia (How Long study): An open-label, randomised, controlled phase 4 trial. *Lancet Haematol* 2017;4:e573–e583.

28 Infections Related to Steroids and Immunosuppressive Agents in the Critical Care Unit

Gülden Yilmaz and Müge Ayhan

CONTENTS

CLINICAL PERSPECTIVE

This chapter focuses on the management of patients with infectious complications—especially serious infectious complications defined as fatal, life-threatening, or causing prolonged hospitalization—taking exogenous glucocorticoids (GC) and/or biologic agents for chronic autoimmune or inflammatory diseases in critical care unit.

GLUCOCORTICOIDS

Since their discovery in the 1940s, corticosteroids remained the central component of anti-inflammatory and immuno-suppressive therapy. They can be used for replacement in adrenal insufficiency at physiologic doses and for rheumatologic, pulmonary, neurological, hematologic, dermatologic, and gastrointestinal diseases at higher doses. They are very efficient for the indications stated previously but also have various adverse effects, including osteoporosis, adrenal suppression, hyperglycemia, psychiatric disorders, dyslipidemia, cardiovascular diseases, and hematologic and immunologic changes. In this chapter, considerations and management of infectious complications in a patient who can be followed up in critical care are discussed. This section will focus on the mechanisms of action, effects on immune system, and common opportunistic infections observed in patients using glucocorticoids.

Available exogenously used corticosteroids are analogues of hormones that are excreted from adrenal gland. All human cells have glucocorticoid receptors (GRs) on the cell membrane and in the cytoplasm. They have several effects on the immune system.

Most of anti-inflammatory and immunosuppressive actions of glucocorticoids are related with transcription effects of GR agonism, which regulates transcription of various genes in leukocytes up and down. Some anti-inflammatory effects of GCs start within minutes, and these fast effects are independent of the transcriptional effects of GR. The GCs repress many proinflammatory cytokines and chemokines, cell adhesion molecules, and some enzymes that have a role in host inflammatory response by inhibiting the transcription of many genes. Glucocorticoids inhibit vasodilatation and increase vascular permeability. They cause demargination of leukocytes from vascular endothelium, and this is seen as an increase in white blood cell count. Demargination causes a decrease in leukocyte entry and activity on the inflammation and infection sites. The GCs also inhibit macrophage and neutrophil phagocytosis, which plays a role in microbial killing and presentation of antigens.

The most well-documented adverse effects of GCs are infectious complications. Owing to immunosuppressive and anti-inflammatory effects of GCs, patients receiving exogenous GCs have a potential risk of infection. This risk is dose- and cumulative dose-dependent. Daily prednisone of 10 mg or higher doses (or its equivalent of other GCs) or a greater cumulative dose of 700 mg increases the infection risk as compared with the control group. In addition to dose, some other factors, including underlying disease, patient's age, and concomitant usage of other immunosuppressive therapy, affect the risk of infection.

Infectious complications include bacterial infections; reactivation of tuberculosis (TB) or toxoplasmosis; viral infections, including herpes virus and varicella zoster virus; and reactivation of viral hepatitis and fungal infections.

TYPES OF INFECTIONS

PNEUMOCYSTIS JIROVECII PNEUMONIA

Pneumocystis jirovecii pneumonia (PJP) is a life-threatening infection that mostly occurs in immunosuppressed patients. These infections are commonly seen in HIV/AIDS but can also be observed in patients taking high-dose prolonged GC therapy and other iatrogenic immunosuppression therapies. Transplant patients and HIV/AIDS patients take prophylaxis to prevent PJP.

Mortality of PJP in non-HIV infected patients is higher than that in HIV patients and is approximately 40%. Routine PJP prophylaxis in all patients taking GCs is not recommended, but it should be taken into account case by case. There is a poor understanding of what is the minimum dose and duration of corticosteroids that may constitute a significant risk of a patient acquiring PJP, as this has not been definitively determined in the literature and actually varies greatly among sources. Some studies showed that in patients taking ≥20 mg prednisone or its equivalent for ≥4 weeks, if another risk factor, or another immunosuppressive agent is present, prophylaxis for PJP should be considered. Some other studies that are well supported in the literature noted that a median daily dose of 30 mg of prednisone or the equivalent for 12 weeks is a significant risk factor.

First choice for prophylaxis is trimethoprim-sulfamethoxazole 160/800 mg (double strength) dosed either daily or three times weekly. Alternative regimens include atovaquone and dapsone.

TUBERCULOSIS

Chronic administration of glucocorticoids has been shown to render patients susceptible to mycobacterial infection and cause reactivation of latent bacilli.

There are many mechanisms by which glucocorticoids can increase the risk of TB. Systemic glucocorticoids have effects on the cellular immune response, which is important for TB control. Several previous reports have demonstrated that glucocorticoids inhibited proliferation of antigen-specific T-cells. Also, GCs increased apoptosis and decreased interferon (IFN)-γ secretion. These were observed in cultured T-cells after glucocorticoid administration.

The lower limit of prednisone dosing that increases the risk is unclear. The Centers for Disease Control and Prevention and the American Thoracic Society identified prednisone 15 mg daily for 1 month as the threshold for increased risk, based on dosing identified in previous studies, as the one that suppresses the tuberculin skin test. In one case-control study, the adjusted odds ratio of TB was 2.8 (95% confidence interval, 1.0–7.9) for <15 mg daily prednisone vs. 7.7 (95% confidence interval, 2.8–21.4) for >15 mg daily prednisone (or equivalent). Risk of infection remains high in patients who are considered recent users (i.e., glucocorticoid use in 120–180 days before TB). In this study, it was defined that patients diagnosed with TB are more likely to be smokers, underweight, diabetic and have lung disease.

The testing for determining high risk for TB progression and appropriate treatment can prevent active TB. Patients who have clinical history of TB risk factors, such as known contact with a person infected with TB, living or moving from a TB endemic area, and substance abuse should be tested before initiation of immunosuppressive therapy.

HERPES ZOSTER

Herpes zoster (HZ) is a significant global problem that results from reactivation of the latent varicella zoster virus within the sensory ganglia. Older age, female gender, ethnicity, and depression are the potential risk factors. In addition, cellular immune dysfunction in certain conditions (e.g., HIV infection or lymphomas) is another risk factor triggering the HZ infection. In half of HZ-infected patients, some complications such as postherpetic neuralgia (PHN), ophthalmic zona, meningoencephalitis, and secondary bacterial infections occur.

Immunosuppressive medications cause an increased risk of HZ. Use of glucocorticoids shows a dose-dependent association with HZ.

BIOLOGIC AGENTS

Since biologic agents targeting proinflammatory cytokines (tumor necrosis factor [TNF], interleukin [IL]-1, IL-6, IL-12, IL-17, and IL-27), B-cell molecules (B-cell activating factor and CD-20), and T-cell costimulatory molecules (CD-80 and alfa-4-integrin) have substantially advanced the treatment of immunological disorders, the management of chronic inflammatory and autoimmune diseases has substantially changed. Especially, anti-TNF agents are a major therapeutic breakthrough in the treatment of the diseases mentioned previously. Two types of anti-TNFs are currently available: Monoclonal antibodies (infliximab, adalimumab, certolizumab, and golimumab) and soluble receptors (etanercept). However, because of immunological properties, clinical trials and postmarketing data of these agents highlighted some adverse events, including infections. The excessive infection risk seems particularly in the first 6 months and higher for patients receiving anti-TNF monoclonal antibodies than for those receiving soluble TNF-α receptor. In these studies, serious infection was defined as the infection requiring admission to the hospital or prolongation of hospitalization or leading to death.

The patients receiving biologic agents are at a high risk of infection because of both the disease itself and the immunosuppressive therapies before and after biologic agents. The Food and Drug Administration (FDA) warns about serious infections, including TB, bacterial sepsis, and invasive fungal and other opportunistic infections, in patients receiving anti-TNFs and suggests to discontinue the biologic agent if a patient develops a serious infection or sepsis.

The FDA recommends about performing test for latent TB—if positive, starting treatment for TB prior to therapy; if negative, monitoring all patients for active TB during treatment.

TUBERCULOSIS

Biologic agents targeting TNF or inhibiting other proinflammatory cytokines are associated with an increased risk of infection with intracellular or extracellular pathogens. Mycobacterium and other granulomatous agents are sequestered within granulomas, and TNF-α is the main mediator for maintaining granuloma structure. The use of TNF-α antagonists is accompanied by the risk of reactivation of latent TB infection, often in extrapulmonary sites, with disseminated forms, and sometimes, it can be fatal, especially in the first 6 months of the treatment. Reactivation of TB may be associated with substantial mortality (7%). In addition, biologic agents other than TNF-antagonists also have a risk of the reactivation of TB. Among TNF antagonists, the risk is higher with infliximab and adalimumab than with etanercept. Abatacept, etanercept, and tocilizumab have an intermediate risk, and anakinra and rituximab have a lower risk of reactivating TB.

It seems that there is a need for appropriate screening (careful history, tuberculin skin test, chest radiograph, and gamma interferon-based assays) and subsequent prophylaxis in patients taking these agents. Recommended treatment regimens for latent TB vary from isoniazid alone for 6–9 months to rifampicin alone for 4 months to both drugs combined for 3 months. It is reported that after the initiation of TB screening recommendations before anti-TNF initiation among rheumatoid arthritis (RA) patients, TB reactivation decreased from an incidence rate ratio of 19 to 1.8 compared with general population. Although uncommon, since TB reactivation in patients with a history of treatment of latent TB before anti-TNF therapy has been described, clinicians should be aware of the risk along the therapy.

OPPORTUNISTIC INFECTIONS

Tumor necrosis factor is a major proinflammatory cytokine that plays a role in intracellular killing mechanisms and formation of granulomas by activating macrophage effector functions, adhesion processes, and chemoattraction. Therefore, in patients receiving TNF antagonists, serious infections, especially caused by intracellular microorganisms, including *Listeria monocytogenes*, *Salmonella* spp., *Nocardia, Candida, Aspergillus*, and other fungus may occur. The French study estimated that the risk of legionellosis in patients on anti-TNF therapy is more than 13 times that of the general population, even higher with infliximab or adalimumab. Nocardiosis and actinomycosis have also been reported on biologic agent treatment.

The increasing risk of fungal infections was reported with anti-TNF agents and biologic agents targeting IL-17 (e.g., secukinumab). The study analyzing BIOBADASER data from Spain reported *Candida albicans* as the most common

fungus among anti-TNF users in RA patients, with the other fungi being *Aspergillus fumigatus, Malassezia furfur*, and *Pityrosporum ovale*. Invasive aspergillosis with pulmonary presentations or dissemination must be kept in mind in this population. Histoplasmosis, a life-threatening granulomatous infection, has mainly been reported in endemic areas (Northern America, Central and South America, Africa, Asia, and Australia). Most of the cases have lung involvement and are sometimes associated with fever, skin or mucous disorders, hepatosplenomegaly, and adenomegaly. Cryptococcosis, coccidioidomycosis, mucormycosis, and blastomycosis are other occasionally reported fungal infections.

PNEUMOCYSTIS JIROVECII PNEUMONIA

Pneumocystis jirovecii pneumonia is one of the most prevalent opportunistic infections that can lead to lethal respiratory dysfunction. It can be observed in patients both with autoimmune diseases and undergoing immunosuppressive treatment. From a postmarketing surveillance in Japan, it was reported that 0.44% of patients receiving infliximab and 0.18% of those receiving etanercept developed PCP. The study recently reported, including not only TNF-α inhibitors (infliximab, etanercept, and adalimumab) but also the IL-6 inhibitor (tocilizumab), revealed the PCP rate as 1.28%, with the identified significant risk factors as age at least 65 years, coexisting pulmonary disease, and use of glucocorticoids. They also mentioned that RA patients with two or three risk factors for PCP who are receiving biologic therapy can benefit from prophylaxis, which was defined as trimethoprim-sulfamethoxazole (80/400 mg) given every day or two tablets given three times weekly. The other risk factors for PCP highlighted by other studies are leukopenia <500/mm^3, hypoalbuminemia, and lymphopenia.

OTHER SERIOUS INFECTIONS

In a study analyzing the infectious complications associated with anti-TNFs in rheumatic patients, the infection incidence was 53.09/1000 patient-years, similar to previous reports. Attributable mortality was 3%, and they emphasized that when a relevant infection occurs, it has an impact on mortality. Besides, it was mentioned that the individual risk of severe infections also depends on the presence of comorbidities and on any prior use of other immunosuppressive therapies, especially glucocorticoids. Strangfeld et al. emphasized the high risk of infections in patients above 60 years, presenting with a chronic renal or lung disease, with a history of severe infection, or concomitant corticosteroid treatment (>7.5 mg/day).

Infectious complications with significant mortality included pneumonia, sepsis, TB, abdominal infection, and endocarditis. The highest mortality rates were reported with mycobacteria and gram-negative bacteria (6.6% and 4.9%, respectively). The common microorganisms identified as cause of pneumonia, with 9% relevant mortality, were *Staphylococcus aureus*, *Legionella* spp., *Streptococcus pneumoniae*, *Pseudomonas aeruginosa*, *Cytomegalovirus*, and *Aspergillus fumigatus*. In a study from France, lower respiratory tract infections were the most frequently reported severe infection, followed by soft tissue infections and pneumococcal, and annual influenza vaccination is therefore justified in these patients.

Patients taking biologic agents should be considered at individual infectious risk in light of comorbidities; concomitant treatments; and history of vaccinations, travels, and prophylaxis (Table 28.1).

TABLE 28.1
Biologic Immunosuppressive/Immunomodulator Agents

TNF inhibitors	Mechanisms of Action
• Etanercept	Reduction of circulating TNF via soluble receptor; partial blockade
• Infliximab	Antibody inactivates TNF-α; biologic activity documented at 2 months
• Adalimumab	TNF reduction via antibody to TNF-α; prevents its binding to TNF-v receptor
• Certolizumab	A pegylated mAb under investigation, conferring a longer half-life
• Golimumab	A mAb with activity targeting circulating and membrane-bound TNF, pending approval
IL-1 inhibition	
• Anakinra	IL-1 receptor antagonist
• Canakinumab	A specific human mAb targeted against IL-1β
• Rilonacept	It binds IL-1β and IL-1α with high affinity and potently inhibits IL-1 activity
IL-6 inhibition	
• Tocilizumab	Antibody to IL-6 receptor
• Sarilumab	Human monoclonal antibody that inhibits IL-6 receptor signaling targets and binds with high affinity to soluble and membrane-bound IL-6 receptors
IL-17 inhibition	
• Secukinumab	A mAb against IL-17
• Ixekizumab	A mAb against IL-17
IL-12/23 blockage	
• Ustekinumab	Inhibits activity of IL-12 and IL-23
Costimulation blockage	
• Abatacept	Protein mimics natural CTLA-4; binds CD80 and CD86 on APC, blocking CD28 on T cell and thus costimulation and activation
B-cell depletion and inhibition	
• Rituximab	B-cell lysis via chimeric antibody to CD20
• Belimumab	mAb directed against soluble B lymphocyte stimulator (BLyS)

REFERENCES

1. Stuck AE, Minder CE, Frey FJ. Risk of infectious complications in patients taking glucocorticosteroids. *Rev Infect Dis* 1989;11(6):954–963.
2. Yale SH, Limper AH. *Pneumocystis carinii pneumonia* in patients without acquired immunodeficiency syndrome: Associated illness and prior corticosteroid therapy. *Mayo Clin Proc* 1996;71:5.
3. Green H, Paul M, Vidal L, Leibovici L. Prophylaxis of *Pneumocystis pneumonia* in immunocompromised non-HIV-infected patients: Systematic review and meta-analysis of randomized controlled trials. *Mayo Clin Proc* 2007;82(9):1052–1059.
4. Caplan A, Fett N, Rosenbach M, Werth VP, Micheletti RG. Prevention and management of glucocorticoid-induced side effects: A comprehensive review infectious complications and vaccination recommendations. *J Am Acad Dermatol* 2017;76:191–198.
5. Jick SS, Lieberman ES, Rahman MU, Choi HK. Glucocorticoid use, other associated factors, and the risk of tuberculosis. *Arthritis Rheum* 2006;55:19–26.
6. Liebling M, Rubio E, Le S. Prophylaxis for *Pneumocystis jiroveci pneumonia*: Is it a necessity in pulmonary patients on high-dose, chronic corticosteroid therapy without AIDS? *Expert Rev Respir Med* 2015;9(2):171–181.
7. Klein NC, Go CH-U, Cunha BA. Infections associated with steroid use. *Infect Dis Clin* 2001;15(2):423–432.
8. Youssef J, Novosad SA, Winthrop KL. Infection risk and safety of corticosteroid use. *Rheum Dis Clin North Am* 2016;42(1):157–176.
9. Boyman O, Comte D, Spertini F. Adverse reactions to biologic agents and their medical management. *Nat Rev Rheumatol* 2014;10(10):612–627.
10. Kourbeti IS, Ziakas PD, Mylonakis E. Biologic therapies in rheumatoid arthritis and the risk of opportunistic infections: A meta-analysis. *Clin Infect Dis* 2014;58(12):1649–1657.
11. Liao TL, Chen YM, Liu HJ, et al. Risk and severity of herpes zoster in patients with rheumatoid arthritis receiving different immunosuppressive medications: A case–control study in Asia. *BMJ Open* 2017;7:e014032.
12. Kopylov U, Aif W. Risk of Infections with biological agents. *Gastroenterol Clin* 2014;43(3):509–524.
13. Koç E. Ustekinumab. *Arch Turk Dermatol Venerol* 2016;50(Suppl 1):43–45.
14. Fala L. Cosentyx (Secukinumab): First IL-17A antagonist receives FDA approval for moderate-to-severe plaque psoriasis. *Am Health Drug Benefits* 2016;9(Spec Feature):60–63.
15. Dubois EA, Rissmann R, Cohen AF. Rilonacept and canakinumab. *Br J Clin Pharmacol*. 2011;71(5):639–641.
16. Blanchard E, Truchetet ME, Machelart I, et al. Respiratory infections associated with anti_TNFalpha agents. *Med Mal Infect* 2017;47:3865–3872.
17. The Food and Drug Administration. Available at: http://www.fda.gov. Accessed on February 2018.
18. Hou JK, Kramer JR, Richardson P, et al. Tuberculosis screening and reactivation among a national cohort of patients with inflammatory bowel disease treated with tumor necrosis falpha antagonists. *Inflamm Bowel Dis* 2017;23(2):254–260.

19. Theis VS, Rhodes JM. Review article: Minimizing tuberculosis during anti-tumour necrosis factor alpha treatment of inflammatory bowel disease. *Aliment Pharmacol Ther* 2008;27:19–30.

20. Katsuyama T, saito K, Kubo S, et al. Prophylaxis for *Pneumocystis pneumonia* in patients with rheumatoid arthritis treated with biologics, based on risk factors found in a retrospective study. *Res Ther* 2014;16:43–51.

21. Koike T, Harigai M, Inokuma S, et al. Postmarketing surveillance of safety and effectiveness of etanercept in Japanese patients with rheumatoid arthritis. *Mod Rheumatol* 2011;21:343–351.

22. Perez-Sola MJ, Torre-Cisneros J, Perez-Zafrilla B, et al. BIOBADASER study group. Infections in patients treated with tumor necrosis factor antagonists: Incidence, etiology and mortality in the BIOBADASER registry. *Med Clin (Barc)* 2011;137(12):533–540.

23. Strangfeld A, eveslage M, Schneider M, et al. Treatment benefit or survival of hte fittests: What drives the time dependent decrease in serious infection rates under TNF inhibition and what does this imply for the individual patient? *Ann Rheum Dis* 2011;70(11):1914–1920.

29 Infections in Solid Organ Transplant Recipients Admitted to the Critical Care Unit

Almudena Burillo, Patricia Muñoz, and Emilio Bouza

CONTENTS

This chapter compiles the information regarding the most frequently encountered infections in solid organ transplant (SOT) patients admitted to critical care units (CCUs). Where no reliable data are available, perspectives based on our own experience and opinion are presented. Given the broad scope of this topic, the chapter is divided into 10 sections covering the burden and etiology of infection, its diagnosis, treatment, and challenges that remain, such as effective prevention measures.

THE BURDEN OF THE PROBLEM

Solid organ transplant recipients may require CCU admission for different reasons, and infection is one of the most important. Between 5% and 50% of candidates for organ transplantation await the transplant procedure in a CCU, and, once over, most of them spend a mean of 4–7 days there for life support [1–6]. If CCU stay is prolonged due to postsurgical complications, the probability of acquiring an in-hospital infection increases significantly.

Most days spent in the CCU after receiving a SOT will be under intense immunosuppression [7]. However, transplant recipients may require CCU re-admission at any time, owing to both infectious and non-infectious complications such as severe rejection, bleeding, organ dysfunction, etc.

Infections are the most common indication for admission of a SOT recipient to an emergency department (35%). Severe sepsis (11.7%) is the most common reason for CCU entry [8]. The incidence of sepsis is 20%–60% of all SOT recipients, with an in-hospital mortality of 5%–40% [9,10].

Figures regarding infection and CCU admission indicate that one-half of all febrile days in liver transplant recipients occurs in the CCU, and in 87% of these, the cause is infection [11].

PRINCIPLES OF CARE FOR SOT CANDIDATES AND RECIPIENTS IN THE CCU

Critical care for SOT candidates and recipients is often guided by medical and surgical intensive care unit protocols. A SOT patient usually carries a higher risk of infection than the standard non-immunocompromised patient. The key factors that a responsible physician needs to know regarding patient history are summarized in the acronym PHISIO:

- **P**atient:
  - Type of transplant and how long ago it occurred. Surgical procedure: Technical details, anastomosis, etc. Genetic factors in the recipient (Human Leukocyte Antigen [HLA], pattern recognition receptors, and toll-like receptors). Level of immunosuppression.

- Medical **Hi**story [12]:
  - Infection status of the donor. Mismatch in transplant serology. Travel in the previous 3 months. Antibiotics in the previous 3 months. History of rejection. Administration of T-cell depleting therapy for induction or treatment of rejection. Recent sick contact, new sexual contact, or exposure to animals. Administration of antimicrobial prophylaxis at present. Dialysis at present.
- Diagnostic **S**yndrome [12]:
  - Bloodstream infection. Central-line infection. Sepsis. Pneumonia. Intra-abdominal infection. Urinary tract infection (UTI). Other.
- Diagnostic **I**nformation:
  - Tests ordered and information collected to establish etiology.
- **O**ther.
  - Management. Prevention.

ANAMNESIS AND PHYSICAL EXAMINATION TO ESTABLISH A CLINICAL SYNDROME

Risk factors for infection should be carefully identified in all SOT patients admitted to the CCU, as these may suggest an etiology and clinical syndrome.

Pre-transplantation history, e.g., serological status regarding microorganisms such as cytomegalovirus (CMV), hepatitis virus, and *Toxoplasma* spp., etc. may yield valuable information.

Information should be compiled, including previous infection or colonization, exposure to tuberculosis (TBC), contact with animals, raw food ingestion, gardening, prior antimicrobial therapy or prophylaxis, vaccines or immunosuppressors, and contact with a contaminated environment or persons [13,14]. History of residence or travel to endemic areas of regional mycosis [15] or *S. stercoralis* may be essential to detect these diseases [16]. Exposure to ticks may be crucial to diagnose entities such as human monocytic ehrlichiosis, which is potentially lethal in immunosuppressed patients [17].

Certain factors may increase the risk of bacterial and fungal infection in the early post-transplant period, such as a long duration of surgery (over 8 hours), blood transfusion in excess of six units, allograft dysfunction, pulmonary or neurological problems, diaphragm dysfunction, renal failure, hyperglycemia, poor nutritional state, or thrombocytopenia [18–24].

Fever in CCU SOT patients should be considered an emergency. In our opinion, a basic tenet of the management of a SOT recipient with fever is that anamnesis and physical examination data should be directly obtained by the infectious disease (ID) consultant, who should not rely on second-hand information. This may be more useful than many expensive and time-consuming tests.

An *aggressive diagnostic approach* is necessary when dealing with febrile compromised CCU hosts, since it has been reported that many infectious complications remain undiagnosed [25].

Approximately 25% of febrile episodes do not present with an apparent focus and do not allow for a straight syndromic approach [26]. Thus, the patient's medical history, type of transplantation, and time after surgery are essential data.

MOST COMMON CLINICAL SYNDROMES

PNEUMONIA

Pneumonia accounts for 30%–80% of infections suffered by SOT recipients and for the vast majority of fever episodes in the CCU (41% of all febrile infections during the first 7 days of CCU stay and 14% of those thereafter) [11]. Pneumonia is among the leading causes of infectious mortality in this population [27]. Its crude mortality exceeds 40% in most series [28–31]. In the most recent series, harmful pathogens and worse outcome were less common than previously reported [32].

Pneumonia in SOT patients can be divided into three categories. Postoperative pneumonia occurs in the CCU and, usually, as a consequence of prolonged mechanical ventilation. The second group is related to the patient's immunosuppression and occurs mainly with months 2–6 of transplantation but also beyond this time in patients that remain profoundly immunosuppressed. Up to 95% of post-transplant cases of pneumonia occur within the first 6 months [32,33]. Finally, there is a category of pneumonia occurring late after transplantation in patients under only maintenance immunosuppression. These infections are typically caused by common pathogens and are usually not related to immunosuppression state.

The incidence of pneumonia is highest in heart-lung transplant (H-LT) (22%) and orthotopic liver transplant (OLT) recipients (17%), intermediate in heart transplant (HT) recipients (5%), and lowest in kidney transplant (KT) patients (1%–2%) [30,34,35].

In an HT series in Spain, the etiology of pneumonia could be established in 61% of the cases [51]. Bacteria caused 91% of cases, fungi 9%, and viruses 6%. Pneumonia caused by gram-negative bacilli appeared a median of 9 days after transplant, and episodes caused by gram-positive cocci, fungi, *M. tuberculosis/Nocardia* spp., and viruses after medians of 11, 80, 145, and 230 days, respectively. *Legionella* spp. should always be included in the differential diagnosis [36–40].

Pneumonia is less common after KT (8%–16%), although it remains a significant cause of morbidity [30,34,35]. Most frequent etiologies are *Staphylococcus aureus*, *P. aeruginosa*, *Acinetobacter* spp., and *Haemophilus influenzae* [41] (Table 29.1).

An etiologic diagnosis should be attempted through different techniques, meaning careful tailoring to every single patient. Blood and respiratory samples for the detection of bacteria, mycobacteria, fungi, and viruses and urine for *Legionella pneumophila* and *S. pneumoniae* antigen detection must be sent to the laboratory. Nucleic acid amplification test (NAAT) techniques may help improve diagnostic sensitivity [42]. If pleural fluid is present, it should also be

TABLE 29.1

Likely Etiologies of Pneumonia According to Infiltrate and Radiologic Patterns

	Likely Etiology	
Radiologic Pattern	Acute[a]	Subacute
Consolidation	Bacteria (*S. pneumoniae*, gram-negative rods, *Legionella* spp., *S. aureus*) (1–2 weeks) Embolism, atelectasis Hemorrhage Acute graft rejection in lung transplant recipients CMV (2–3 months or later if prophylaxis)	*Aspergillus* (30 days), *Nocardia* spp., tuberculosis (9–23 months), drug-related, *P. jirovecii*, *Legionella* spp., HSV, VZV, *Toxoplasma* spp., Bronchiolitis obliterans
Interstitial	Edema Transfusions (Bacteria)	Virus (CMV, influenza, parainfluenza, RSV, EBV), *P. jirovecii*, bacteria (fungi, *Nocardia*, tuberculosis), drugs
Nodular	(Bacteria, edema)	Fungi, *Nocardia* spp., *R. equi*, tuberculosis (*P. jirovecii*, CMV)

Abbreviations: CMV, cytomegalovirus; HSV, herpes simplex virus; VZV, varicella-zoster virus; RSV, respiratory syncytial virus; EBV, Epstein–Barr virus.

[a] Acute: requiring attention within 24 hours. Less common possibilities indicated between brackets.

analyzed. Pneumonia is the infection with the higher related mortality rate, and this holds true for SOT recipients. Thus, after obtaining adequate samples, prompt empirical therapy is highly recommended.

SURGICAL SITE INFECTION

Following transplant, complications in the proximity of the surgical site must always be investigated. Surgical problems leading to devitalized tissue, anastomosis disruption, or fluid collections markedly predispose the patient to potentially lethal infections.

In the early post-transplantation period, KT and pancreas transplant recipients (PT) recipients are prone to surgical site infection (SSI), perigraft hematoma, lymphocele, and urinary fistula [43]. In 55 of 1400 consecutive KTs in Spain, incisional SSI was detected within a median of 20 days of transplantation. The most frequently isolated pathogens were *Escherichia coli* (31.7%), *P. aeruginosa* (13.3%), *Enterococcus faecalis* (11.6%), *Enterobacter* spp. (10%), and coagulase-negative staphylococci (8.3%). Risk factors were diabetes mellitus and use of sirolimus [44]. In another study, risk factors for SSI in KT recipients included chronic glomerulonephritis, delayed graft function, reoperation, acute

graft rejection, diabetes mellitus, and a high body mass index [45].

The OLT recipients are at risk of portal vein thrombosis, hepatic vein occlusion, hepatic artery thrombosis, and biliary stricture formation and leaks.

The HT recipients are at risk of mediastinitis and infection at the aortic suture line resulting in mycotic aneurysm. Patients who had an LT carry the risk of disruption of the bronchial anastomosis.

Surgical site infection is frequent in intestinal transplant recipients, and so, the use of a mesh for abdominal wall closure should be avoided [46,47].

Surgical site infection requires rapid debridement and effective antimicrobial therapy and should prompt the exclusion of adjacent cavities or organ involvement.

INTRA-ABDOMINAL INFECTION

In OLT recipients, intra-abdominal infections may be responsible for 50% of bacterial complications along with significant morbidity [48], including intra-abdominal abscess, biliary tree infection, and peritonitis [49,50]. Risk factors are prolonged duration of surgery, transfusion of large volumes of blood products, choledochojejunostomy (Roux-en-Y) instead of a choledochostomy (duct-to-duct) for biliary anastomosis, repeat abdominal surgery, biliary-tract dehiscence or obstruction, intra-abdominal hematoma, vascular problems in the allograft (e.g., thrombosis of the hepatic artery or ischemia of the biliary tract may condition cholangitis episodes and liver abscesses), previous antibiotic therapy, and CMV infection [51]. Occasionally, complications will appear after a procedure such as a liver biopsy or a cholangiography. These infections may be bacteremic, and OLT recipients show the highest rate of secondary bloodstream infections (BSI) [52]. Most common microorganisms include *Enterobacteriaceae*, enterococci, anaerobes and *Candida* spp.

In a series published by Singh et al., the biliary tree was the origin of 9% of infections associated with fever in SOT patients in the CCU [11]. Biliary anastomosis leaks may give rise to peritonitis or perihepatic collections, cholangitis, or liver abscesses [53–55]. Orthotopic liver transplants are especially predisposed to cholangitis. Recent data suggest that duct-to-duct biliary anastomosis stented with a T tube tends to be associated with more postoperative complications [56]. A percutaneous aspirate with culture of the fluid is required to confirm infection. T-tube culture is unreliable since it may only reflect colonization.

Hepatic abscesses are frequently associated with hepatic artery thrombosis, which occurs in up to 7% of patients [57]. Occasionally, the only manifestations are unexplained fever and relapsing subacute bacteremia; 40%–45% of liver abscesses are associated with bacteremia. Prolonged antibiotic therapy, drainage, and even retransplantation may be required to improve the outcome in these patients. Catheter drainage was successful in 70% of cases. The mortality rate was 42% [58].

MEDIASTINITIS

In HT and LT recipients, the possibility of mediastinitis (2%–9%) should be considered. Heart transplant recipients have a higher risk of postsurgical mediastinitis and sternal osteomyelitis than other heart surgery patients [59]. Mediastinitis may initially appear just as fever or bacteremia of unknown origin. Inflammatory signs in the sternal wound, sternal dehiscence, and purulent drainage may appear later. The most commonly involved microorganisms are staphylococci, but gram-negative rods represented at least a third of our cases. *Mycoplasma* spp., mycobacteria, and other less common pathogens should be suspected in "culture-negative" SSI [60,61]. Bacteremia of unknown origin during the first month after HT should always suggest the possibility of mediastinitis [62]. Risk factors are prolonged hospitalization before surgery, early chest re-exploration, and low-output syndrome in adults. Aspiration of fluid collections in the mediastinum is critical to guide therapy [63,64]. Treatment consists of surgical debridement and repair, and antimicrobial treatment for 3–6 weeks.

URINARY TRACT INFECTION

Urinary tract infections (UTIs) are the most frequent form of bacterial complication affecting KT recipients [65–68]. Their incidence in recent series of patients not receiving prophylaxis has been reported to vary from 5% to 36% [69,70]. The pretransplant history of UTI increases the risk of infection after transplantation [71]. Some authors have described a cumulative incidence of acute pyelonephritis (APN) after KT of 18.7%. The risk of developing APN was found higher in female (64%) than in male recipients and correlated with the frequency of recurrent UTI and rejection episodes. Multivariate analysis identified APN as an independent risk factor for a decline in renal function (p = 0.034) [72].

Notwithstanding, UTI is not a common cause of CCU admission. These infections usually present with a lack of systemic symptoms, with or without accompanying localized urinary symptoms; ureteral obstruction due to anastomosis site stenosis; hydronephrosis, or, less frequently, APN, and sepsis [73]. The most common pathogens include *Enterobacteriaceae*, enterococci, staphylococci, and *Pseudomonas* spp. [74]. Other less frequent microorganisms, such as *Salmonella* spp., *Candida* spp., and *Corynebacterium urealyticum* pose specific management problems in this population [75]. It is also important to remember the possibility of infection caused by unusual pathogens such as *Mycoplasma hominis*, *M. tuberculosis*, or BK polyomavirus (BK) and JC polyomavirus (JC). Unless another source of fever is readily apparent, any febrile KT patient with an abrupt deterioration in renal function should be treated with empiric antibacterial therapy aimed at gram-negative bacteria, including *P. aeruginosa*, after first obtaining blood and urine cultures, especially in the first 3 months of transplantation [76,77]. Examination of the iliac fossa is particularly important after KT. Tenderness, erythema, fluctuance, or an increased allograft size may indicate the presence of an infection caused by a microorganism resistant to antimicrobial resistance to drugs commonly used to prevent UTI in these patients such as cotrimoxazole or quinolones; thus, these drugs should not be selected for empirical therapy of severe UTI [78,79].

GASTROINTESTINAL INFECTION

Abdominal pain and diarrhea are detected in up to 20% of SOT recipients [80]. Possible manifestations of gastrointestinal (GI) infections also include bleeding, jaundice, nausea or vomiting, odynophagia, dysphagia, or just weight loss [81]. Gastrointestinal symptoms were present in up to 51% of HT patients in recent series, although in only 15% of cases were these significant enough to warrant endoscopic, radiologic, or surgical procedures [81].

Diarrhea is a significant problem in SOT recipients admitted to the CCU, with a myriad of potential causes: Allograft rejection; enteral nutrition; intestinal ischemia resulting from medication (e.g., antibiotics, immunosuppressants); post-transplantation lymphoproliferative disorders; and infections due to *C. difficile*, CMV, adenovirus, norovirus, rotavirus, *Cryptosporidium* spp., and microsporidia [82–86]. A gastric lymphoma called mucosa-associated lymphoid tissue (MALT) lymphoma, which usually responds to the eradication of *Helicobacter pylori* [87], may develop in KT patients.

Cytomegalovirus and *C. difficile* are the most common causes of infectious diarrhea in SOT patients [88–91]. Cytomegalovirus may involve the whole GI tract, although the duodenum and stomach are the most frequent sites involved [92]. Frequent clinical presentations are nausea, vomiting, abdominal pain, increased stool output, fever, and even GI bleeding. The differential diagnosis should include diverticulitis, intestinal ischemia, cancer, and Epstein–Barr virus (EBV)-associated lymphoproliferative disorders. Practically, all patients with GI CMV will return a positive NAAT in blood or GI tract mucosa [93]. The natural history of CMV disease associated with SOT has been modified as a result of the widespread use of potent immunosuppressants and antiviral prophylaxis, and severe late forms are now detected [94]. Hypogammaglobulinemia may also justify severe or relapsing forms of CMV after SOT [95].

Clostridium difficile is more common in SOT patients who frequently receive antimicrobial agents, and up to 20%–25% of patients may experience relapse [96–98]. The incidence of *C. difficile* infection is increasing. The SOT recipients have many risk factors for developing *C. difficile*-associated diarrhea (CDAD): Surgery, frequent hospital admissions, the use of proton pump inhibitors, antimicrobial exposure, and immunosuppression. The most common clinical presentation is diarrhea, which may be unusually severe [99,100]. In a recent series, 5.7% of KT or PT patients developed fulminant CDAD presenting with toxic megacolon, and these patients underwent colectomy [88]. The absence of diarrhea is a poor prognostic factor. Significant leukocytosis may be a useful clue. Occasionally, patients present with an acute abdomen [101] or an inflammatory pseudotumor [102]. Fresh stool samples should be analyzed for the presence of toxin producing *C. difficile*. The reference method for diagnosis is NAAT alone or a multistep testing algorithm (e.g., glutamate dehydrogenase (GDH)-plus toxin and NAAT-plus toxin) [103]. *C. difficile*-associated diarrhea may occur in coincidence with CMV GI infection [96,104].

Whenever possible, the first step in managing diarrhea and colitis caused by *C. difficile* is discontinuation of the antibiotic therapy that precipitated the disease. About 15%–25% of patients respond within a few days. Patients with severe disease should be treated with oral vancomycin or fidaxomicin 200 mg, twice daily, for 10 days. Recent reports of severe clinical forms suggest that vancomycin tapering and fidaxomicin may be preferable for especially virulent strains. The reader is referred to the Infectious Diseases Society of America (IDSA) guidelines on this subject [103]. The prescription of probiotics such as *Saccharomyces boulardii* or *Lactobacillus* spp. for the prophylaxis of CDAD remains controversial, and we do not recommend this practice in CCU patients, as severe invasive disease by *S. boulardii* has been described [105].

A substantial proportion of patients (10%–25%) suffer relapse usually 3–10 days after treatment has been discontinued, even with no further antibiotic therapy. Nearly all patients respond to another course of antibiotics if given early. The frequency of relapse is lower with fidaxomicin [106]. Multiple relapses may be challenging to manage. Several measures have been used: gradual tapering of the dosage of vancomycin over 1–2 months, "pulse-dose" vancomycin, anion-exchange resins to absorb *C. difficile* toxin A, vancomycin plus rifampin, or a specific anti-*C. difficile* toxin B immunoglobulin (bezlotoxumab). Fecal transplant is a safe and effective option in SOT recipients [50].

Infectious enteritis is especially frequent in intestinal transplant recipients (39%). Viral agents are the cause in two-thirds of cases. In a recent series, there were 14 cases of viral enteritis (one of CMV, eight of rotavirus, four of adenovirus, and one of EBV), three bacterial (*C. difficile*), and three protozoan infections (one *Giardia lamblia*, two *Cryptosporidium* spp.). The bacterial infections tended to present earlier than the viral infections; the most frequent presenting symptom was diarrhea [107].

Immunosuppressive drugs, such as mycophenolate mofetil (MMF), cyclosporine A (CSA), tacrolimus, and sirolimus, are all associated with diarrhea. Reports exist of an incidence of diarrhea of 13%–38% for regimens containing CSA and MMF and 29%–64% for regimens, including tacrolimus and MMF [108]. Rarely, graft-versus-host disease (GVHD), lymphoproliferative disorder, de novo inflammatory bowel disease (IBD), or colon cancer may present as diarrhea. A flare-up of pre-existing IBD is also not uncommon after OLT.

Accordingly, the first step in the management of a patient with fever and diarrhea or abdominal pain should be to try to exclude CMV and *C. difficile*. If clinical manifestations persist thereafter, a broader differential diagnosis and more sophisticated diagnostic techniques should be considered, as there are reports of SOT recipients with infections caused by Norwalk virus [109], rotavirus [110], adenovirus [111], EBV [112], *Cryptosporidium parvum* [113], and *Isospora belli* [114,115], among others. Notwithstanding, the cause of acute diarrhea remains unidentified in one out of three patients [89].

CENTRAL NERVOUS SYSTEM INFECTION

The detection of CNS symptoms in SOT should immediately raise the suspicion of infection [116]. Fever, headache, altered mental status, seizures, focal neurological deficit, or a combination of these signs should prompt a neuroimaging study [80]. Non-infectious causes include immunosuppression-associated leukoencephalopathy [117], toxic and metabolic etiologies, stroke, and malignancy [118]. Therapy with OKT3 monoclonal antibodies has been related to the emergence of acute aseptic meningitis (CSF pleocytosis with negative cultures, fever, and transient cognitive dysfunction) [119]. Infectious progressive dementia has been related to JC virus, herpes simplex, CMV, and EBV [118].

The most common causes of meningoencephalitis in SOT patients are herpes viruses, followed by *L. monocytogenes*, *C. neoformans*, and *Toxoplasma gondii*. The ubiquitous neurotropic virus human herpes virus (HHV)-6 is known to cause febrile syndromes and exanthema subitum in children. Less commonly, and particularly in SOT patients, it may cause hepatitis, bone marrow suppression, interstitial pneumonitis, and meningoencephalitis [120–126]. A growing body of evidence suggests that the most significant effects of HHV-6 and HHV-7 reactivation on OLT outcomes may be mediated indirectly by their interactions with CMV [123]. An independent predictor of invasive fungal infection is HHV-6 viremia [127].

Central nervous system CMV infection is fairly uncommon in SOT recipients. It may affect the brain (diffuse encephalitis, ventriculoencephalitis, and cerebral mass lesions) or the spinal cord (transverse myelitis and polyradiculomyelitis). Diagnosis should be based on clinical presentation, results of imaging and virological markers. Encephalitis caused by herpes simplex virus (HSV) has also been described [128,129].

Among other causes of encephalitis, West Nile virus (WNV) has emerged as an important cause of several outbreaks of febrile illness and encephalitis in North America. In recent reports, 11 SOT patients with naturally acquired WNV encephalitis were identified (four KT, two stem cell, two OLT, one LT, and two KT/PT recipients) [130–132]. Donor-derived WNV has also been described [133].

The most common occurrence of *Listeria monocytogenes* infection is 2–6 months post-transplant [134]. Its incidence has significantly been reduced by cotrimoxazole prophylaxis [135]. *Listeria* spp. infections may present as isolated bacteremia or with associated meningitis [136–138]. Cerebritis/abscess due to *L. monocytogenes*, without meningeal involvement, is less common [139].

Nocardiosis is usually observed between 1 and 6 months post-transplantation. Risk factors are high calcineurin inhibitor trough levels in the month before diagnosis (OR, 6.11), use of tacrolimus (OR, 2.65) and corticosteroid dose (OR, 1.12) at the time of diagnosis, patient age (OR, 1.04), and length of CCU stay after SOT (OR, 1.04) [140]. The clinical presentation of nocardiosis includes pneumonia, focal CNS lesions, and skin involvement [116,141–145]. Brain abscesses due to *Nocardia* spp. are multiple in 40% of cases and may show ring enhancement.

The incidence of cryptococcosis after SOT is 2.6%–5%. The CNS is involved in 25%–72% of patients [146–149]. *Cryptococcus* spp. is mostly a cause of meningitis, pneumonia, and skin lesions [150–153]. In a recent series, survival at 6 months tended to be lower in patients whose CSF cultures at 2 weeks were positive compared with those whose CSF cultures were negative (50% vs. 91%, p = 0.06) [154]. No correlation was found between CSF or serum cryptococcal antigen titer and outcome or CSF sterilization at 2 weeks [155].

Focal brain infection (seizures or focal neurologic abnormalities) may be caused by *Listeria* spp., *Toxoplasma gondii*, fungi (*Aspergillus* spp., Mucorales, phaeohyphomycetes, or dematiaceous fungi), post-transplantation lymphoproliferative disease, or *Nocardia* spp. Brain abscesses are relatively uncommon (0.6%) in SOT patients, and *Aspergillus* spp. cause most of them (78%) [156], followed by *T. gondii* and *N. asteroides*. Fever was uncommon and was documented in only 45% of OLT recipients with brain abscesses [157].

Scedosporium, zygomycetes, and other uncommon fungi are being increasingly detected as significant CNS pathogens in SOT recipients [158–164].

Toxoplasmosis was more prevalent when prophylaxis with cotrimoxazole was not provided [165,166]. Its incidence is higher in HT recipients. The disease usually occurred within 3 months of transplantation, and fever, neurological disturbances, and pneumonia were primary clinical features [167]. The donor was the likely source of transmission in most recipients [168]. The mortality rate was high (around 60%). Disseminated toxoplasmosis should be considered in the differential diagnosis of immunocompromised patients with culture-negative sepsis syndrome, particularly if combined with neurologic, respiratory, or unexplained skin lesions [169,170].

Other parasite infections such as Chagas disease, neurocysticercosis, schistosomiasis, and strongyloidiasis are exceedingly less common [171].

BLOODSTREAM INFECTION, CATHETER-RELATED INFECTION, INFECTIVE ENDOCARDITIS

As other patients requiring critical care, catheter-related bloodstream infections (CR-BSI) are a potential threat for severe infection after SOT. In a study performed by our group in HT recipients, CR-BSI accounted for 16% of BSI [172]. In HT recipients, the incidence of BSI was 15.8%. BSI episodes were detected a median of 51 days after transplantation. Independent risk factors for BSI after HT were hemodialysis (OR 6.5; 95% CI 3.2–13), prolonged CCU stay (OR 3.6; 95% CI 1.6–8.1), and viral infection (OR 2.1; 95% CI 1.1–4).

Bloodstream infection was a risk factor for mortality (OR 1.8; 95% CI 1.2–2.8) [172]. Main BSI origins were the lower respiratory tract (LRT) (23%), urinary tract (20%), and CR-BSI (16%). Directly attributable mortality of BSI was 12.2%.

Infective endocarditis is a rare event in the SOT population (1.7%–6%), yet it may be an underappreciated sequela of hospital-acquired infection [173]. In this last study, the spectrum of organisms causing infective endocarditis was distinctly different in SOT patients than in the general population; 50% of infections were due to *Aspergillus fumigatus* or *S. aureus*, but only 4% were due to viridans streptococci. Fungal infections predominated early on (accounting for 6 of 10 cases of endocarditis within 30 days of transplantation), while bacterial infections caused most cases after this time point (80%). In 80% [37] of the 46 SOT recipients, there was no underlying valve disease. Seventy-four percent [34] of these 46 cases were associated with previous hospital-acquired infection, notably CR-BSI and SSI. The overall mortality rate was 57%, and over 50% of fatal cases were not suspected while the patient was alive [173].

In this population, CMV, *Toxoplasma* spp. and parvovirus B19 may cause myocarditis. Therapy for established infections is similar to that used in other immunosuppressed patients.

FEVER OF UNKNOWN ORIGIN

Undoubtedly, the most common alarm sign suggesting infection is fever. Fever in the recipient of a SOT has been defined as an oral temperature of 37.8°C detected on at least two occasions during a 24-hour period [11]. Antimetabolite immunosuppressive drugs, MMF and azathioprine, are associated with significantly lower maximum temperatures and leukocyte counts [174]. However, it is important to remember that fever and infections do not always come together. The absence of fever does not exclude infection. In a recent series, 40% of OLT recipients with documented infection (mainly fungal) were afebrile [175]. What is more, the absence of a febrile response has been found to be a predictor of poor outcome in OLT patients with bacteremia [176].

NON-INFECTIOUS CAUSES OF FEVER

In a recent study, 87% of febrile episodes detected in OLT patients in the CCU were due to infections and 13% were of a non-infectious nature [11]. Rejection, malignancy, adrenal insufficiency, and drug-induced fever were the most common non-infectious causes.

Fever is common in the first 48 hours of surgery and after specific procedures.

Malignancy, mainly lymphoproliferative disease, is relatively common after SOT and may initially present as a febrile episode (80%) [177–179]. This usually occurs longer after transplantation [180]. Acute adrenal insufficiency should be excluded in SOT patients admitted to a CCU because of sepsis or surgery, mainly when corticosteroids have been withdrawn and drugs that accelerate the degradation of cortisol (phenytoin, rifampin) are administered [181]. However, although analytical adrenal insufficiency is frequent in SOT patients, prospective studies suggest that supplemental steroids are not needed in most cases even under stress [182–184]. Another setting of potential adrenal insufficiency is KT recipients returning to dialysis [185,186]. Occasionally, lymphoproliferative disease may present with adrenal insufficiency after OLT [187].

Drugs such as OKT3, antithymocyte globulin, everolimus, antimicrobials, interferon, and anticonvulsants may also cause fever in this population [188,189]. The temporal relationship with the drug is usually a diagnostic clue. New induction therapies such as basiliximab have been related to fewer side effects and fewer CMV infections [190].

Other causes of non-infectious fever include thromboembolic disease, hematoma reabsorption, pericardial effusions, tissue infarction, hemolytic uremic syndrome, and transfusion reaction. Non-cardiogenic pulmonary edema (pulmonary reimplantation response) is a common finding after LT (50%–60%) and may occasionally lead to a differential diagnosis with pneumonia. This condition prolongs mechanical ventilation and CCU stay but does not affect survival [191].

ETIOLOGIC AGENTS

After an anamnesis, medical history, and physical examination, syndromic diagnosis is possible. This is when a "checklist" of the main causal agents of infection in transplanted patients should be drawn up, systematically oriented to the particular syndrome. However obvious the etiological diagnosis, no possibility should be ruled out. We must not forget that we are dealing with patients in whom a second and third cause of infection is not rare.

The most common agents are summarized in Table 29.2.

Thus, the post-transplant interval is divided into early (first month), intermediate (from month 2 to 6), and late (from then onwards) periods after transplantation (Table 29.3). In the *first month*, the two major causes of infection are pre-existing infections in the donor or recipient and infectious complications related to surgery. The *intermediate* period is characterized by intense immunosuppression, and therefore, opportunistic microorganism infections predominate. *Late* infections occur in a patient with a stable, yet reduced level of immunosuppression

TABLE 29.3

Chronology of Most Common Infections and Causative Microorganisms in Severely Ill SOT Recipients

Chronology of Infection	Most Common Syndromes
Early infection (1 month post-transplant)	Bacterial infection
	Pneumonia
	Surgical wound infection
	Deep infections near the surgical site
	Intra-abdominal abscesses
	Urinary tract infection
	Catheter-related infection
	Bloodstream infection
	Antibiotic-associated diarrhea
	Viral infection
	Herpes simplex stomatitis
	HHV-6 infection
	Primary CMV disease
	Infections transmitted with the allograft
	Invasive aspergillosis or candidiasis
Intermediate infection (2–6 months post-transplant)	Opportunistic infections: Bacterial, tuberculosis, nocardiosis, invasive aspergillosis, other fungal infections, viral diseases, toxoplasmosis
Late infection (beyond 6 months post-transplant)	Common community-acquired infections
	Respiratory tract infections
	Urinary tract infections
	Varicella-zoster infections
	CMV, adenovirus
	Other opportunistic microorganisms: Listeriosis, *Cryptococcus* spp., *P. jiroveciii*

Abbreviations: HHV, human herpes virus; CMV, cytomegalovirus.

and present as community-acquired infections in normal hosts (except for patients showing chronic rejection and GVHD). The risk of nosocomial and opportunistic infection in SOT recipients peaks during the first 6 months, but more recently, it has been shown that related mortality after 6 months is only slightly lower, and this source of infection is still a significant burden [192].

TABLE 29.2
Incidence of Infections (%) in SOT Recipients

Type of Infection	Type of Transplant				
	Liver	Kidney	Heart	Lung, Heart-Lung	Pancreas, Kidney-Pancreas
Bacterial	33–68	47	21–30	54	35
Cytomegalovirus	22–29	8–32	9–35	39–41	50
Herpes-simplex virus	3–44	53	1–42	10–18	6
Varicella-zoster virus	5–10	4–12	–12	8–15	9
Candida spp.	1–26	2	1–5	10–16	32
Filamentous fungi	2–4	1–2	3–6	3–19	3

TOOLS FOR AN ETIOLOGIC SEARCH

Initial investigations and tests for all patients with suspected infection include blood cell count and differential test, liver function tests, microscopic examination of urine, and the following:

- Blood cultures and differential blood cultures if a central venous catheter (CVC) is in place.
- Blood CMV PCR.
- Syndrome/symptom-specific investigations.
  - Respiratory tract infection: Chest X-ray; if abnormal, consider chest CT; nasopharyngeal swab/aspirate for NAAT of respiratory virus; *L. pneumophila* serogroup 1 and *S. pneumoniae* urinary antigens. If pneumonia is suspected, samples should also be submitted for bacteria, mycobacteria, and fungi detection.
  - Intra-abdominal infection: Abdominal ultrasound or CT; *C. difficile* toxin and NAAT, as appropriate.
  - Urinary tract infection: Urine culture.

Viral screening tests for CMV should be ordered if the patient is still in the high-risk early post-transplantation period or has recently been treated for rejection or if clinical findings are strongly suggestive of CMV disease. Late-onset CMV disease is not uncommon in a CMV-seronegative patient receiving an organ from a CMV-seropositive donor in whom an extended course of antiviral prophylaxis was discontinued 4–8 weeks earlier. A lumbar puncture with a cranial CT scan (including the paranasal sinus) need not be a routine part of the initial workup of febrile transplant recipients. However, a CSF sample should be obtained from patients with headache or other neurologic complaints or signs.

A NAAT is available for adenovirus, HSV, influenza A and B, RSV and other respiratory viruses, rotavirus, norovirus, sapovirus, and other GI pathogens. Most common herpesviruses can also be easily detected. Most laboratories also offer specific NAAT for *Bordetella pertussis*.

Direct testing of specimens by NAAT is also used for CSF samples (e.g., *Neisseria meningitidis*, *S. pneumoniae*, *H. influenzae*, herpes simplex virus, VZV, CMV, EBV, enterovirus, JC, and BK).

In a patient with a clear infection site, assessment should focus on quickly obtaining adequate samples for culture and smears from that site. Gram staining requires expertise but may provide valuable rapid information (5 minutes) on the quality of the specimen and whether gram-negative or -positive rods or cocci are present. It may reveal yeast and occasionally molds, parasites, *Nocardia* spp., and even mycobacteria. The amount of material and the number of organisms limit detection sensitivity.

Also available is the group A *streptococcus* antigen detection test directly performed on the skin and soft tissue samples [193].

As already mentioned, in case of diarrhea, *C. difficile* should be investigated.

Acid-fast stain and fluorochrome stains for mycobacteria or *Nocardia* spp. require a lengthier laboratory procedure (30–60 minutes). New techniques, such as polymerase chain reaction (PCR) and interferon-gamma quantification, achieve more rapid and accurate diagnoses. *M. tuberculosis* complex PCR is very useful in smear-positive specimens. In smear-negative samples, its sensitivity is ~70% [42]. Cultures and PCR for detection of *M. tuberculosis* should be ordered for all SOT patients in whom infection is suspected.

Fungal infections should be aggressively pursued in colonized patients and in those with risk factors. Isolation of *Candida* spp. or *Aspergillus* spp. from superficial sites may indicate infection. Early stages of fungal infection may be challenging to detect [194,195]. Fungal elements may be rapidly detected in wet mounts with potassium hydroxide or immunofluorescent calcofluor white stain. In approximately 50% of patients, an Indian ink preparation allows the identification of encapsulated *C. neoformans*, particularly in CSF. The latex agglutination test or enzyme immunoassay cryptococcal antigen shows a higher sensitivity. The fluorescent antibody stains, toluidine blue O and NAAT, permit the detection of *P. jirovecii*. The detection of *H. capsulatum* antigen is quite sensitive and the detection of *Aspergillus* spp. antigen is useful, although its efficiency is lower than in hematological patients [196–198]. When a fungal infection is suspected, a fundus examination, blood and respiratory cultures, *Aspergillus* spp. and *Cryptococcus* spp. antigen detection tests, and NAAT are mandatory.

Parasite infections are uncommon, but toxoplasmosis and leishmaniasis should be considered if the diagnosis remains elusive. Serology, bone marrow culture, or NAAT usually provides a diagnosis. The possibility of a *Toxoplasma* spp. primary infection should be considered when a seronegative recipient receives a graft from a seropositive donor. The risk of primary toxoplasmosis (R-D+) is over 50% in HT, 20% in OLT, and <1% in KT recipients.

Leishmaniasis is another parasite that should be excluded, though it is exceedingly uncommon after SOT. It may present as fever, pancytopenia, and splenomegaly. The relapse rate in SOT recipients is approximately 25%. The benefits of PCR monitoring of blood for secondary prophylaxis or preemptive therapy have not been confirmed [199].

It is essential to check the diagnostic procedures offered by the microbiology department for the various infectious syndromes: Type of sample, volume, instructions on how to obtain it, container, guidelines for transport, turnaround time until a result is issued, available results, and their interpretation. If the hospital's microbiology department does not offer a particular test, samples are sent to the corresponding reference laboratory. Microbiological samples from SOT patients should always be managed in microbiology laboratories equipped for a "fast track" diagnostic approach for the rapid search of pathogens and susceptibility testing, including fast, expert-guided reporting of results via a microbiology hotline [200].

Diagnostic imaging by (18)F-fluoro-2-deoxy-D-glucose (FDG) positron emission tomography/computed tomography

(PET/CT) for infection diagnosis in SOT recipients shows a sensitivity, specificity, positive predictive value (PPV), and negative predictive value (NPV) of 78%, 90%, 78% and 90%, respectively, and a global accuracy of 86% [201]. This procedure was used to modify the therapeutic strategy in 40% of cases. The authors of this study concluded that FDG PET/CT should be considered in patients with a severe unexplained inflammatory syndrome or fever of unknown origin (FUO) and inconclusive conventional imaging or to discriminate active from silent lesions previously detected by standard imaging, particularly when malignancy is suspected [201].

Multimodality imaging with the use of combined indium-labeled WBC scintigraphy and CT served to detect infection within a retained left ventricular assist device tubing in an HT recipient with a diagnosis of fever of unknown origin [202].

The HIV infection, *Brucella* spp., and syphilis are infections that can be rapidly diagnosed serologically.

MANAGEMENT

Fever is not harmful in itself, and accordingly, it should not be systematically reduced. Studies have shown that fever enhances several host defense mechanisms (chemotaxis, phagocytosis, and opsonization) [80]. Besides, antibiotics may be more active at higher body temperatures. If needed to avoid recurrent shivering and an associated increase in metabolic demands, antipyretic drugs should be given at regular intervals.

After obtaining the previously mentioned samples, empiric antimicrobials should be promptly started in all SOT patients with suspicion of bacterial infection and in a toxic or unstable clinical situation. They are also recommended if a focus of infection is apparent, in the early post-transplant setting in which nosocomial infection is prevalent, or when there has been a recent increase in immunosuppression. In a stable patient without an apparent source of infection, further diagnostic tests should be carried out, withholding antibiotics and considering non-infectious causes.

We have recently observed that only 58.5% of patients with BSI at our center received appropriate empirical antimicrobial therapy. Inadequate treatment was related to an extended hospital stay and a higher risk of CDAD, overall mortality rate, and infection-related mortality [203]. In patients with suspicion of sepsis, once blood cultures are obtained, empirical broad-spectrum antimicrobials guided by the clinical condition of the patient and the presumed origin of infection should be promptly started. When results of blood cultures are available, antibiotics should be adjusted according to the susceptibility patterns of the isolates. This antibacterial de-escalation strategy attempts to balance the need to provide appropriate, initial antibacterial treatment while limiting the emergence of antibacterial resistance [204].

The selection of the antimicrobial should be based on the likely origin of infection, prevalent bacterial microbiota, the rate of antimicrobial resistance, and previous use of antimicrobials by the patient. In our series of HT patients with bacteremia, gram-negative microorganisms predominated

(55.3%), followed by gram-positive organisms (44.6%). Gram-negatives accounted for 54% of infections in the first month, 50% in months 2–6, and 72% thereafter (p = 0.3) [172].

The possibility of antimicrobial drug interactions, mainly with CSA and tacrolimus, is genuine and significantly impacts the choice of antimicrobial. There are three categories of antimicrobial interactions with CSA and tacrolimus. First, the antimicrobial agents such as rifampin, isoniazid, and nafcillin upregulate the metabolism of immunosuppressive drugs, resulting in decreased blood levels and an increased possibility of graft rejection. Second, the antimicrobial agents such as the macrolides erythromycin, clarithromycin, and to lesser extent azithromycin and the azoles ketoconazole, itraconazole, and to a lesser extent fluconazole and the newer azoles downregulate immunosuppressive drug metabolism with the opposite effect of increased blood levels and an increased risk of nephrotoxicity and overimmunosuppression. Finally, there may be synergistic nephrotoxicity when therapeutic levels of immunosuppressive agents are combined with therapeutic concentrations of aminoglycosides, amphotericin B, and vancomycin, and high therapeutic doses of cotrimoxazole and fluoroquinolones.

OUTCOMES OF INFECTIONS IN SOT PATIENTS

Among all-cause in-hospital mortality in SOT patients, approximately 10% of deaths are related to infection [192,205]. Bloodstream infection still represents a significant cause of mortality and graft loss after SOT. In a recent study, the 30-day case-fatality rate from the onset of BSI was 11.4% [50]. Mortality may reach 50% when bacteremia is accompanied by septic shock [206,207].

Infection is a leading cause of death in HT (30% of early deaths, 45% of deaths from 1–3 months, and 9.7% thereafter) [208]. Infectious complications, including pneumonia, bacteremia, and sepsis, emerged as significant predictors of overall mortality in extended criteria HT recipients [209].

In febrile LT patients, mortality on day 14 (24% vs. 0%, p = 0.001) and day 30 (34% vs. 5%, p = 0.001) was significantly higher in those in the CCU, as compared with non-CCU patients [11]. Risk factors for mortality in SOT patients in CCUs include pneumonia and mechanical ventilation, a creatinine level >1.5 mg/dL, and a worse acute physiology and chronic health evaluation (APACHE) score [7,175,210].

In another series, mortality among KT recipients admitted to the CCU was 11%, and infection was the cause of six out of seven deaths [211].

PREVENTION

Solid organ transplant patients admitted to the CCU should receive all measures available to prevent hospital-acquired infection. The first of such measures, when feasible, could be to avoid CCU admission.

Prevention is essential to fight against infection. As for any other patient admitted to the CCU, main efforts in SOT patients should be directed toward avoiding nosocomial infections during their stay in the unit [212]. We should highlight the prevention of surgical wound infection during transplant surgery, the prevention of acquired pneumonia during mechanical ventilation, and the measures necessary to minimize the risk of CR-BSI. Preventive measures applicable to intensely immunocompromised patients are also particularly relevant and will undoubtedly contribute to avoiding unnecessary admissions to CCU (https://www.cdc.gov/infectioncontrol/guidelines/index.html). Appropriate vaccines for adult SOT recipients are especially important and frequently overlooked. Emphasis should be placed on vaccination against influenza, pneumococcus, and herpes zoster virus, among others.

CONCLUSIONS

To improve the success of solid organ transplantation, infections in transplant patients need to be effectively diagnosed and treated. This still remains a challenge today. Diagnostic tests for infection are frequently initiated when clinical symptoms arise, which in immunocompromised patients are often late in the disease course. Thus, clinicians must be extra vigilant of the possibility of severe infection through a comprehensive diagnostic approach, including the assessment of infection mimics.

The data that need to be collected because of their paramount importance include immunosuppressants, surgery, patient ID epidemiology (e.g., previous infections, colonization state, prior antibiotics, and community-acquired and endemic infections), and hospital microbiologic epidemiology.

An accurate microbiologic diagnosis is needed to avoid unnecessary toxicities and interactions associated with therapy often requiring invasive diagnostic procedures. The cornerstone of patient management is the early administration of antimicrobials, removal of infectious fluid collections or devitalized tissues, and when feasible, the reduction of immunosuppressive treatment.

REFERENCES

1. Miller LW, Naftel DC, Bourge RC, et al. Infection after heart transplantation: A multiinstitutional study. Cardiac transplant research database group. *J Heart Lung Transplant* 1994;13:381–392.
2. Plöchl W, Pezawas L, Artemiou O, Grimm M, Klepetko W, Hiesmayr M. Nutritional status, ICU duration and ICU mortality in lung transplant recipients. *Intensive Care Med* 1996;22:1179–1185.
3. Hsu J, Griffith BP, Dowling RD, et al. Infections in mortally ill cardiac transplant recipients. *J Thorac Cardiovasc Surg* 1989;98:506–509.
4. Cisneros AC, Montero CA, Moreno GE, García GI, Guillén RF, García FC. Complications of liver transplant in intensive care. Experience in 130 cases. *Rev Clin Esp* 1991;189:264–267.
5. Plevak DJ, Southorn PA, Narr BJ. Intensive-care unit experience in the Mayo liver transplantation program: The first 100 cases. *Mayo Clin Proc* 1989;64:433–445.
6. Bindi ML, Biancofiore G, Pasquini C, et al. Pancreas transplantation: Problems and prospects in intensive care units. *Minerva Anestesiol* 2005;71:207–221.
7. Singh N, Gayowski T, Wagener MM. Intensive care unit management in liver transplant recipients: Beneficial effect on survival and preservation of quality of life. *Clin Transplant* 1997;11:113–120.
8. Trzeciak S, Sharer R, Piper D, et al. Infections and severe sepsis in solid-organ transplant patients admitted from a university-based ED. *Am J Emerg Med* 2004;22:530–533.
9. Linares L, Garcia-Goez JF, Cervera C, et al. Early bacteremia after solid organ transplantation. *Transplant Proc* 2009;41:2262–2264.
10. Hsu RB, Chang CI, Fang CT, Chang SC, Wang SS, Chu SH. Bloodstream infection in heart transplant recipients: 12-year experience at a university hospital in Taiwan. *Eur J Cardiothorac Surg* 2011;40:1362–1367.
11. Singh N, Chang FY, Gayowski T, Wagener M, Marino IR. Fever in liver transplant recipients in the intensive care unit. *Clin Transplant* 1999;13:504–511.
12. Program TSHS-UHNAS. Empiric management of common infections in solid organ transplant patients 2017. Available at: https://docs.wixstatic.com/ugd/550306_a68800e702bd4c-7c9e8c25c622b3f891.pdf. Accessed on January 22, 2019.
13. Papanicolaou GA, Meyers BR, Meyers J, et al. Nosocomial infections with vancomycin-resistant *Enterococcus faecium* in liver transplant recipients: Risk factors for acquisition and mortality. *Clin Infect Dis* 1996;23:760–766.
14. Duchini A, Goss JA, Karpen S, Pockros PJ. Vaccinations for adult solid-organ transplant recipients: Current recommendations and protocols. *Clin Microbiol Rev* 2003;16:357–364.
15. Braddy CM, Heilman RL, Blair JE. Coccidioidomycosis after renal transplantation in an endemic area. *Am J Transplant* 2006;6:340–345.
16. Martín-Rabadán P, Muñoz P, Palomo J, Bouza E. Strongyloidiasis: The Harada-Mori test revisited. *Clin Microbiol Infect* 1999;5:374–376.
17. Tan HP, Stephen Dumler J, Maley WR, et al. Human monocytic ehrlichiosis: An emerging pathogen in transplantation. *Transplantation* 2001;71:1678–1680.
18. Detre KM, Belle SH, Carr MA, et al. A report from the NIDDK liver transplantation database. In: Terasaki P. ed., *Clinical Transplants*. Los Angeles, UCLA Tissue Typing Laboratory, 1989;129–141.
19. Lafayette RA, Paré G, Schmid CH, et al. Pretransplant renal dysfunction predicts poorer outcome in liver transplantation. *Clin Nephrol* 1997;48:159–164.
20. Deschênes M, Belle SH, Krom RA, et al. Early allograft dysfunction after liver transplantation: A definition and predictors of outcome. National Institute of Diabetes and Digestive and Kidney Diseases Liver Transplantation Database. *Transplantation* 1998;66:302–310.
21. Reilly J, Mehta R, Teperman L, et al. Nutritional support after liver transplantation: A randomized prospective study (see comments). *JPEN J Parenter Enteral Nutr* 1990;14:386–391.
22. Gurakar A, Hassanein T, Van Thiel DH. Right diaphragmatic paralysis following orthotopic liver transplantation. *J Okla State Med Assoc* 1995;88:149–153.
23. Hoppe L, Bressane R, Lago LS, et al. Risk factors associated with cytomegalovirus-positive antigenemia in orthotopic liver transplant patients. *Transplant Proc* 2004;36:961–963.
24. Gavalda J, Len O, San Juan R, et al. Risk factors for invasive aspergillosis in solid-organ transplant recipients: A case-control study. *Clin Infect Dis* 2005;41:52–59.
25. Petty LA, Te HS, Pursell K. A case of Q fever after liver transplantation. *Transpl Infect Dis* 2017;19:e12737.

26. Chang FY, Singh N, Gayowski T, et al. *Staphylococcus aureus* nasal colonization and association with infections in liver transplant recipients. *Transplantation* 1998;65:1169–1172.

27. Dizdar OS, Ersoy A, Akalin H. Pneumonia after kidney transplant: Incidence, risk factors, and mortality. *Exp Clin Transplant* 2014;12:205–211.

28. Mermel LA, Maki DG. Bacterial pneumonia in solid organ transplantation. *Semin Respir Infect* 1990;5:10–29.

29. Jimenez-Jambrina M, Hernandez A, et al. Pneumonia after heart transplantation in the XXI century: A multicenter prospective study. *45th Interscience Conference on Antimicrobial Agents and Chemotherapy* 2005.

30. Chang GC, Wu CL, Pan SH, et al. The diagnosis of pneumonia in renal transplant recipients using invasive and noninvasive procedures. *Chest* 2004;125:541–547.

31. Torres A, Ewig S, Insausti J, et al. Etiology and microbial patterns of pulmonary infiltrates in patients with orthotopic liver transplantation. *Chest* 2000;117:494–502.

32. Giannella M, Munoz P, Alarcon JM, et al. Pneumonia in solid organ transplant recipients: A prospective multicenter study. *Transpl Infect Dis* 2014;16:232–241.

33. Cisneros JM, Muñoz P, Torre-Cisneros J, et al. Pneumonia after heart transplantation: A multiinstitutional study. *Clin Infect Dis* 1998;27:324–331.

34. Gupta RK, Jain M, Garg R. *Pneumocystis carinii* pneumonia after renal transplantation. *Indian J Pathol Microbiol* 2004;47:474–476.

35. Renoult E, Georges E, Biava MF, et al. Toxoplasmosis in kidney transplant recipients: Report of six cases and review. *Clin Infect Dis* 1997;24:625–634.

36. Fraser TG, Zembower TR, Lynch P, et al. Cavitary *Legionella* pneumonia in a liver transplant recipient. *Transpl Infect Dis* 2004;6:77–80.

37. Singh N, Gayowski T, Wagener M, et al. Pulmonary infections in liver transplant recipients receiving tacrolimus. Changing pattern of microbial etiologies. *Transplantation* 1996;61:396–401.

38. Nichols L, Strollo DC, Kusne S. Legionellosis in a lung transplant recipient obscured by cytomegalovirus infection and *Clostridium difficile* colitis. *Transpl Infect Dis* 2002;4:41–45.

39. Horbach I, Fehrenbach FJ. Legionellosis in heart transplant recipients. *Infection* 1990;18:361–363.

40. Sivagnanam S, Podczervinski S, Butler-Wu SM, et al. Legionnaires' disease in transplant recipients: A 15-year retrospective study in a tertiary referral center. *Transpl Infect Dis* 2017;19:e12745.

41. Kara S, Sen N, Kursun E, et al. Pneumonia in renal transplant recipients: A single-center study. *Exp Clin Transplant* 2018;16(Suppl 1):122–125.

42. Muñoz P, Rodriguez C, Bouza E. *Mycobacterium tuberculosis* infection in recipients of solid organ transplants. *Clin Infect Dis* 2005;40:581–587.

43. Singh RP, Farney AC, Rogers J, et al. Analysis of bacteremia after pancreatic transplantation with enteric drainage. *Transplant Proc* 2008;40:506–509.

44. Ramos A, Asensio A, Munez E, et al. Incisional surgical site infection in kidney transplantation. *Urology* 2008;72:119–123.

45. Menezes FG, Wey SB, Peres CA, et al. Risk factors for surgical site infection in kidney transplant recipients. *Infect Control Hosp Epidemiol* 2008;29:771–773.

46. Zanfi C, Cescon M, Lauro A, et al. Incidence and management of abdominal closure-related complications in adult intestinal transplantation. *Transplantation* 2008;85:1607–1609.

47. Perdiz LB, Furtado GH, Linhares MM, et al. Incidence and risk factors for surgical site infection after simultaneous pancreas-kidney transplantation. *J Hosp Infect* 2009;72:326–331.

48. Ho MC, Wu YM, Hu RH, et al. Surgical complications and outcome of living related liver transplantation. *Transplant Proc* 2004;36:2249–2251.

49. Asensio A, Ramos A, Cuervas-Mons V, et al. Effect of antibiotic prophylaxis on the risk of surgical site infection in orthotopic liver transplant. *Liver Transpl* 2008;14:799–805.

50. Kritikos A, Manuel O. Bloodstream infections after solid-organ transplantation. *Virulence* 2016;7:329–340.

51. Garcia Prado ME, Matia EC, Ciuro FP, et al. Surgical site infection in liver transplant recipients: Impact of the type of perioperative prophylaxis. *Transplantation* 2008;85:1849–1854.

52. Bellier C, Bert F, Durand F, et al. Risk factors for Enterobacteriaceae bacteremia after liver transplantation. *Transpl Int* 2008;21:755–763.

53. Rerknimitr R, Sherman S, Fogel EL, et al. Biliary tract complications after orthotopic liver transplantation with choledochocholedochostomy anastomosis: Endoscopic findings and results of therapy. *Gastrointest Endosc* 2002;55:224–231.

54. Piecuch J, Witkowski K. Biliary tract complications following 52 consecutive orthotopic liver transplants. *Ann Transplant* 2001;6:36–38.

55. Testa G, Malago M, Broelseh CE. Complications of biliary tract in liver transplantation. *World J Surg* 2001;25:1296–1299.

56. Elola-Olaso AM, Diaz JC, Gonzalez EM, et al. Preliminary study of choledochocholedochostomy without T tube in liver transplantation: A comparative study. *Transplant Proc* 2005;37:3922–3923.

57. Stange BJ, Glanemann M, Nuessler NC, et al. Neuhaus P. Hepatic artery thrombosis after adult liver transplantation. *Liver Transpl* 2003;9:612–620.

58. Tachopoulou OA, Vogt DP, Henderson JM, et al. Hepatic abscess after liver transplantation: 1990–2000. *Transplantation* 2003;75:79–83.

59. Munoz P, Menasalvas A, Bernaldo de Quiros JC, et al. Postsurgical mediastinitis: A case-control study. *Clin Infect Dis* 1997;25:1060–1064.

60. Thaler F, Gotainer B, Teodori G, et al. Mediastinitis due to *Nocardia asteroides* after cardiac transplantation. *Intensive Care Med* 1992;18:127–128.

61. Levin T, Suh B, Beltramo D, Samuel R. *Aspergillus* mediastinitis following orthotopic heart transplantation: Case report and review of the literature. *Transpl Infect Dis* 2004;6:129–131.

62. Smart FW, Naftel DC, Costanzo MR, et al. Risk factors for early, cumulative, and fatal infections after heart transplantation: A multiinstitutional study. *J Heart Lung Transplant* 1996;15:329–341.

63. Bernabeu-Wittel M, Cisneros JM, Rodriguez-Hernandez MJ, et al. Suppurative mediastinitis after heart transplantation: Early diagnosis with CT-guided needle aspiration. *J Heart Lung Transplant* 2000;19:512–514.

64. Benlolo S, Mateo J, Raskine L, et al. Sternal puncture allows an early diagnosis of poststernotomy mediastinitis. *J Thorac Cardiovasc Surg* 2003;125:611–617.

65. Veroux M, Giuffrida G, Corona D, et al. Infective complications in renal allograft recipients: Epidemiology and outcome. *Transplant Proc* 2008;40:1873–1876.

66. Muñoz P. Management of urinary tract infections and lymphocele in renal transplant recipients. *Clin Infect Dis* 2001;33:S53–S57.

67. Tolkoff Rubin NE, Rubin RH. Urinary tract infection in the immunocompromised host. Lessons from kidney transplantation and the AIDS epidemic. *Infect Dis Clin North Am* 1997;11:707–717.
68. Chacon-Mora N, Pachon Diaz J, Cordero Matia E. Urinary tract infection in kidney transplant recipients. *Enferm Infecc Microbiol Clin* 2017;35:255–259.
69. Kahan BD, Flechner SM, Lorber MI, et al. Complications of cyclosporine-prednisone immunosuppression in 402 renal allograft recipients exclusively followed at a single center for from one to five years. *Transplantation* 1987;43:197–204.
70. Ghasemian SM, Guleria AS, Khawand NY, Light JA. Diagnosis and management of the urologic complications of renal transplantation. *Clin Transplant* 1996;10:218–223.
71. Rizvi SJ, Chauhan R, Gupta R, Modi P. Significance of pretransplant urinary tract infection in short-term renal allograft function and survival. *Transplant Proc* 2008;40:1117–1118.
72. Pelle G, Vimont S, Levy PP, et al. Acute pyelonephritis represents a risk factor impairing long-term kidney graft function. *Am J Transplant* 2007;7:899–907.
73. Kalil AC, Sandkovsky U, Florescu DF. Severe infections in critically ill solid organ transplant recipients. *Clin Microbiol Infect* 2018;24:1257–1263.
74. Sharma M, Rani S, Johnson LB. Effect of time after transplantation on microbiology of urinary tract infections among renal transplant recipients. *Transpl Infect Dis* 2008;10:145–148.
75. Lopez-Medrano F, Garcia-Bravo M, Morales JM, et al. Urinary tract infection due to *Corynebacterium urealyticum* in kidney transplant recipients: An underdiagnosed etiology for obstructive uropathy and graft dysfunction-results of a prospective cohort study. *Clin Infect Dis* 2008;46:825–830.
76. Peterson PK, Anderson RC. Infection in renal transplant recipients. Current approaches to diagnosis, therapy, and prevention. *Am J Med* 1986;81:2–10.
77. Vidal E, Cervera C, Cordero E, et al. Management of urinary tract infection in solid organ transplant recipients: Consensus statement of the Group for the Study of Infection in Transplant Recipients (GESITRA) of the Spanish Society of Infectious Diseases and Clinical Microbiology (SEIMC) and the Spanish Network for Research in Infectious Diseases (REIPI). *Enferm Infecc Microbiol Clin* 2015;33:679.e1–79.e21.
78. Senger SS, Arslan H, Azap OK, et al. Urinary tract infections in renal transplant recipients. *Transplant Proc* 2007;39:1016–1017.
79. Di Cocco P, Orlando G, Mazzotta C, et al. Incidence of urinary tract infections caused by germs resistant to antibiotics commonly used after renal transplantation. *Transplant Proc* 2008;40:1881–1884.
80. Singh N. Posttransplant fever in critically ill transplant recipients. In: Singh N, Aguado JM eds. *Infectious Complications in Transplant Patients.* Kluwer Academic Publishers, 2000. ISBN 0-7923-7972-1:113-32.
81. Laskin B, Goebel J. Clinically "silent" weight loss associated with mycophenolate mofetil in pediatric renal transplant recipients. *Pediatr Transplant* 2008;12:113–116.
82. Godt C, Regnery A, Schwarze B, et al. A rare cause of ulcerative colitis—Diarrhoea and perianal bleeding due to posttransplant lymphoproliferative disorder (PTLD). *Z Gastroenterol* 2009;47:283–287.
83. Ramos A, Ortiz J, Asensio A, et al. Risk factors for *Clostridium difficile* diarrhea in patients with solid organ transplantation. *Prog Transplant* 2016;26:231–237.
84. Lee LY, Ison MG. Diarrhea caused by viruses in transplant recipients. *Transpl Infect Dis* 2014;16:347–358.
85. Lanternier F, Amazzough K, Favennec L, et al. *Cryptosporidium* spp. infection in solid organ transplantation: The nationwide "TRANSCRYPTO" study. *Transplantation* 2017;101:826–830.
86. Lanternier F, Boutboul D, Menotti J, et al. Microsporidiosis in solid organ transplant recipients: Two *Enterocytozoon bieneusi* cases and review. *Transpl Infect Dis* 2009;11:83–88.
87. Ponticelli C, Passerini P. Gastrointestinal complications in renal transplant recipients. *Transpl Int* 2005;18:643–650.
88. Keven K, Basu A, Re L, et al. *Clostridium difficile* colitis in patients after kidney and pancreas-kidney transplantation. *Transpl Infect Dis* 2004;6:10–14.
89. Ginsburg PM, Thuluvath PJ. Diarrhea in liver transplant recipients: Etiology and management. *Liver Transpl* 2005;11:881–890.
90. Altiparmak MR, Trablus S, Pamuk ON, et al. Diarrhoea following renal transplantation. *Clin Transplant* 2002;16:212–216.
91. Kottaridis PD, Peggs K, Devereux S, Goldstone AH, Mackinnon S. Simultaneous occurrence of *Clostridium difficile* and Cytomegalovirus colitis in a recipient of autologous stem cell transplantation. *Haematologica* 2000;85:1116–1117.
92. Kaplan B, Meier-Kriesche HU, Jacobs MG, et al. Prevalence of cytomegalovirus in the gastrointestinal tract of renal transplant recipients with persistent abdominal pain. *Am J Kidney Dis* 1999;34:65–68.
93. Peter A, Telkes G, Varga M, et al. Endoscopic diagnosis of cytomegalovirus infection of upper gastrointestinal tract in solid organ transplant recipients: Hungarian single-center experience. *Clin Transplant* 2004;18:580–584.
94. Boobes Y, Al Hakim M, Dastoor H, et al. Late cytomegalovirus disease with atypical presentation in renal transplant patients: Case reports. *Transplant Proc* 2004;36:1841–1843.
95. Sarmiento E, Fernandez-Yanez J, Munoz P, et al. Hypogammaglobulinemia after heart transplantation: Use of intravenous immunoglobulin replacement therapy in relapsing CMV disease. *Int Immunopharmacol* 2005;5:97–101.
96. Munoz P, Palomo J, Yanez J, Bouza E. Clinical microbiological case: A heart transplant recipient with diarrhea and abdominal pain. Recurring *C. difficile* infection. *Clin Microbiol Infect* 2001;7:451–452, 58–59.
97. West M, Pirenne J, Chavers B, et al. *Clostridium difficile* colitis after kidney and kidney-pancreas transplantation. *Clin Transplant* 1999;13:318–23.
98. Apaydin S, Altiparmak MR, Saribas S, Ozturk R. Prevalence of *Clostridium difficile* toxin in kidney transplant recipients. *Scand J Infect Dis* 1998;30:542.
99. Nadir A, Wright HI, Naz-Nadir F,et al. Atypical *Clostridium difficile* colitis in a heart transplant recipient. *J Heart Lung Transplant* 1995;14:606–607.
100. Mistry B, Longo W, Solomon H, Garvin P. *Clostridium difficile* colitis requiring subtotal colectomy in a renal transplant recipient: A case report and review of literature. *Transplant Proc* 1998;30:3914.
101. Schenk P, Madl C, Kramer L, et al. Pneumatosis intestinalis with *Clostridium difficile* colitis as a cause of acute abdomen after lung transplantation. *Dig Dis Sci* 1998;43:2455–2458.
102. Lykavieris P, Fabre M, Pariente D, et al. *Clostridium difficile* colitis associated with inflammatory pseudotumor in a liver transplant recipient. *Pediatr Transplant* 2003;7:76–79.
103. McDonald LC, Gerding DN, Johnson S, et al. Clinical practice guidelines for *Clostridium difficile* infection in adults and children: 2017 update by the Infectious Diseases Society of America (IDSA) and Society for Healthcare Epidemiology of America (SHEA). *Clin Infect Dis* 2018;66:987–994.

104. Veroux M, Puzzo L, Corona D, et al. Cytomegalovirus and *Clostridium difficile* ischemic colitis in a renal transplant recipient: A lethal complication of anti-rejection therapy? *Urol Int* 2007;79:177–179.

105. Munoz P, Bouza E, Cuenca-Estrella M, et al. *Saccharomyces cerevisiae* fungemia: An emerging infectious disease. *Clin Infect Dis* 2005;40:1625–1634.

106. Cornely OA, Miller MA, Louie TJ, et al. Treatment of first recurrence of *Clostridium difficile* infection: Fidaxomicin versus vancomycin. *Clin Infect Dis* 2012;55(Suppl 2):S154–S161.

107. Ziring D, Tran R, Edelstein S, et al. Infectious enteritis after intestinal transplantation: Incidence, timing, and outcome. *Transplantation* 2005;79:702–709.

108. Bunnapradist S, Neri L, Wong W, et al. Incidence and risk factors for diarrhea following kidney transplantation and association with graft loss and mortality. *Am J Kidney Dis* 2008;51:478–486.

109. Florescu DF, Hill LA, McCartan MA, Grant W. Two cases of norwalk virus enteritis following small bowel transplantation treated with oral human serum immunoglobulin. *Pediatr Transplant* 2008;12:372–375.

110. Stelzmueller I, Wiesmayr S, Swenson BR, et al. Rotavirus enteritis in solid organ transplant recipients: An underestimated problem? *Transpl Infect Dis* 2007;9:281–285.

111. Lee BE, Pang XL, Robinson JL, et al. Chronic norovirus and adenovirus infection in a solid organ transplant recipient. *Pediatr Infect Dis J* 2008;27:360–362.

112. Hranjec T, Bonatti H, Roman AL, et al. Benign transient hyperphosphatasemia associated with Epstein–Barr virus enteritis in a pediatric liver transplant patient: A case report. *Transplant Proc* 2008;40:1780–1782.

113. Denkinger CM, Harigopal P, Ruiz P, Dowdy LM. *Cryptosporidium parvum*-associated sclerosing cholangitis in a liver transplant patient. *Transpl Infect Dis* 2008;10:133–136.

114. Koru O, Araz RE, Yilmaz YA, et al. Case report: Isospora belli infection in a renal transplant recipent. *Turkiye Parazitol Derg* 2007;31:98–100.

115. Atambay M, Bayraktar MR, et al. A rare diarrheic parasite in a liver transplant patient: Isospora belli. *Transplant Proc* 2007;39:1693–1695.

116. Singh N, Husain S. Infections of the central nervous system in transplant recipients. *Transpl Infect Dis* 2000;2:101–111.

117. Singh N, Bonham A, Fukui M. Immunosuppressive-associated leukoencephalopathy in organ transplant recipients. *Transplantation* 2000;69:467–472.

118. Ponticelli C, Campise MR. Neurological complications in kidney transplant recipients. *J Nephrol* 2005;18:521–528.

119. Min DI, Monaco AP. Complications associated with immunosuppressive therapy and their management. *Pharmacotherapy* 1991;11:119S–125S.

120. Lehto JT, Halme M, Tukiainen P, et al. Human herpesvirus-6 and -7 after lung and heart-lung transplantation. *J Heart Lung Transplant* 2007;26:41–47.

121. Montejo M, Ramon Fernandez J, Testillano M, et al. Encephalitis caused by human herpesvirus-6 in a liver transplant recipient. *Eur Neurol* 2002;48:234–235.

122. Singh N, Paterson DL. Encephalitis caused by human herpesvirus-6 in transplant recipients: Relevance of a novel neurotropic virus. *Transplantation* 2000;69:2474–2479.

123. Razonable RR, Paya CV. The impact of human herpesvirus-6 and -7 infection on the outcome of liver transplantation. *Liver Transpl* 2002;8:651–658.

124. Benito N, Ricart MJ, Pumarola T, et al. Infection with human herpesvirus 6 after kidney-pancreas transplant. *Am J Transplant* 2004;4:1197–1199.

125. Nash PJ, Avery RK, Tang WH, et al. Encephalitis owing to human herpesvirus-6 after cardiac transplant. *Am J Transplant* 2004;4:1200–1203.

126. Ljungman P, Singh N. Human herpesvirus-6 infection in solid organ and stem cell transplant recipients. *J Clin Virol* 2006;37(Suppl 1):S87–S91.

127. Rogers J, Rohal S, Carrigan DR, et al. Human herpesvirus-6 in liver transplant recipients: Role in pathogenesis of fungal infections, neurologic complications, and outcome. *Transplantation* 2000;69:2566–2573.

128. Gomez E, Melon S, Aguado S, et al. Herpes simplex virus encephalitis in a renal transplant patient: Diagnosis by polymerase chain reaction detection of HSV DNA. *Am J Kidney Dis* 1997;30:423–427.

129. Bamborschke S, Wullen T, Huber M, et al. Early diagnosis and successful treatment of acute cytomegalovirus encephalitis in a renal transplant recipient. *J Neurol* 1992;239:205–208.

130. Wadei H, Alangaden GJ, Sillix DH, et al. West nile virus encephalitis: An emerging disease in renal transplant recipients. *Clin Transplant* 2004;18:753–758.

131. Kleinschmidt-DeMasters BK, Marder BA, Levi ME, et al. Naturally acquired West Nile virus encephalomyelitis in transplant recipients: Clinical, laboratory, diagnostic, and neuropathological features. *Arch Neurol* 2004;61:1210–1220.

132. DeSalvo D, Roy-Chaudhury P, Peddi R, et al. West Nile virus encephalitis in organ transplant recipients: Another high-risk group for meningoencephalitis and death. *Transplantation* 2004;77:466–469.

133. Winston DJ, Vikram HR, Rabe IB, et al. Donor-derived West Nile virus infection in solid organ transplant recipients: Report of four additional cases and review of clinical, diagnostic, and therapeutic features. *Transplantation* 2014;97:881–889.

134. Ascher NL, Simmons RL, Marker S, Najarian JS. Listeria infection in transplant patients. Five cases and a review of the literature. *Arch Surg* 1978;113:90–94.

135. Munoz P, Munoz RM, Palomo J, et al. *Pneumocystis carinii* infection in heart transplant recipients. Efficacy of a weekend prophylaxis schedule. *Medicine* 1997;76:415–422.

136. Wiesmayr S, Tabarelli W, Stelzmueller I, et al. *Listeria* meningitis in transplant recipients. *Wien Klin Wochenschr* 2005;117:229–233.

137. Limaye AP, Perkins JD, Kowdley KV. *Listeria* infection after liver transplantation: Report of a case and review of the literature. *Am J Gastroenterol* 1998;93:1942–1944.

138. van Veen KE, Brouwer MC, van der Ende A, van de Beek D. Bacterial meningitis in solid organ transplant recipients: A population-based prospective study. *Transpl Infect Dis* 2016;18:674–680.

139. Mylonakis E, Hohmann EL, Calderwood SB. Central nervous system infection with *Listeria monocytogenes*. 33 years' experience at a general hospital and review of 776 episodes from the literature. *Medicine* 1998;77:313–336.

140. Coussement J, Lebeaux D, van Delden C, et al. *Nocardia* infection in solid organ transplant recipients: A multicenter European case-control study. *Clin Infect Dis* 2016;63:338–345.

141. Shin JH, Lee HK. Nocardial brain abscess in a renal transplant recipient. *Clin Imaging* 2003;27:321–324.

142. Palomares M, Martinez T, Pastor J, et al. Cerebral abscess caused by *Nocardia asteroides* in renal transplant recipient. *Nephrol Dial Transplant* 1999;14:2950–2952.

143. Arduino RC, Johnson PC, Miranda AG. Nocardiosis in renal transplant recipients undergoing immunosuppression with cyclosporine. *Clin Infect Dis* 1993;16:505–512.

144. Husain S, McCurry K, Dauber J, et al. *Nocardia* infection in lung transplant recipients. *J Heart Lung Transplant* 2002;21:354–359.

145. Coussement J, Lebeaux D, Rouzaud C, Lortholary O. *Nocardia* infections in solid organ and hematopoietic stem cell transplant recipients. *Curr Opin Infect Dis* 2017;30:545–551.

146. Marik PE. Fungal infections in solid organ transplantation. *Expert Opin Pharmacother* 2006;7:297–305.

147. Husain S, Wagener MM, Singh N. *Cryptococcus neoformans* infection in organ transplant recipients: variables influencing clinical characteristics and outcome. *Emerg Infect Dis* 2001;7:375–381.

148. Singh N, Gayowski T, Wagener MM, Marino IR. Clinical spectrum of invasive cryptococcosis in liver transplant recipients receiving tacrolimus. *Clin Transplant* 1997;11:66–70.

149. Singh N, Rihs JD, Gayowski T, Yu VL. Cutaneous cryptococcosis mimicking bacterial cellulitis in a liver transplant recipient: Case report and review in solid organ transplant recipients. *Clin Transplant* 1994;8:365–368.

150. Rakvit A, Meyerrose G, Vidal AM, et al. Cellulitis caused by *Cryptococcus neoformans* in a lung transplant recipient. *J Heart Lung Transplant* 2005;24:642.

151. Gupta RK, Khan ZU, Nampoory MR, Mikhail MM, Johny KV. Cutaneous cryptococcosis in a diabetic renal transplant recipient. *J Med Microbiol* 2004;53:445–449.

152. Baumgarten KL, Valentine VG, Garcia-Diaz JB. Primary cutaneous cryptococcosis in a lung transplant recipient. *South Med J* 2004;97:692–695.

153. Basaran O, Emiroglu R, Arikan U, et al. Cryptococcal necrotizing fasciitis with multiple sites of involvement in the lower extremities. *Dermatol Surg* 2003;29:1158–1160.

154. Singh N, Lortholary O, Alexander BD, et al. Antifungal management practices and evolution of infection in organ transplant recipients with cryptococcus neoformans infection. *Transplantation* 2005;80:1033–1039.

155. Singh N, Alexander BD, Lortholary O, et al. Pulmonary cryptococcosis in solid organ transplant recipients: Clinical relevance of serum cryptococcal antigen. *Clin Infect Dis* 2008;46:e12–e18.

156. Simon DM, Levin S. Infectious complications of solid organ transplantations. *Infect Dis Clin North Am* 2001;15:521–549.

157. Bonham CA, Dominguez EA, Fukui MB, et al. Central nervous system lesions in liver transplant recipients: Prospective assessment of indications for biopsy and implications for management. *Transplantation* 1998;66:1596–1604.

158. Shoham S, Pic-Aluas L, Taylor J, et al. Transplant-associated *Ochroconis gallopava* infections. *Transpl Infect Dis* 2008;10:442–428.

159. Satirapoj B, Ruangkanchanasetr P, Treewatchareekorn S, et al. *Pseudallescheria boydii* brain abscess in a renal transplant recipient: first case report in Southeast Asia. *Transplant Proc* 2008;40:2425–2427.

160. Husain S, Munoz P, Forrest G, et al. Infections due to *Scedosporium apiospermum* and *Scedosporium prolificans* in transplant recipients: Clinical characteristics and impact of antifungal agent therapy on outcome. *Clin Infect Dis* 2005;40:89–99.

161. Nucci M. Emerging moulds: *Fusarium*, *Scedosporium* and zygomycetes in transplant recipients. *Curr Opin Infect Dis* 2003;16:607–612.

162. Islam MN, Cohen DM, Celestina LJ, Ojha J, Claudio R, Bhattacharyya IB. Rhinocerebral zygomycosis: An increasingly frequent challenge: Update and favorable outcomes in two cases. *Oral Surg Oral Med Oral Pathol Oral Radiol Endod* 2007;104:e28–e34.

163. Aslani J, Eizadi M, Kardavani B, et al. Mucormycosis after kidney transplantations: Report of seven cases. *Scand J Infect Dis* 2007;39:703–706.

164. Singh N, Gayowski T, Singh J, Yu VL. Invasive gastrointestinal zygomycosis in a liver transplant recipient: Case report and review of zygomycosis in solid-organ transplant recipients. *Clin Infect Dis* 1995;20:617–620.

165. Munoz P, Arencibia J, Rodriguez C, et al. Trimethoprim-sulfamethoxazole as toxoplasmosis prophylaxis for heart transplant recipients. *Clin Infect Dis* 2003;36:932–933.

166. Baden LR, Katz JT, Franck L, et al. Successful toxoplasmosis prophylaxis after orthotopic cardiac transplantation with trimethoprim-sulfamethoxazole. *Transplantation* 2003;75:339–343.

167. Fernandez-Sabe N, Cervera C, Farinas MC, et al. Risk factors, clinical features, and outcomes of toxoplasmosis in solid-organ transplant recipients: A matched case-control study. *Clin Infect Dis* 2012;54:355–361.

168. Botterel F, Ichai P, Feray C, et al. Disseminated toxoplasmosis, resulting from infection of allograft, after orthotopic liver transplantation: Usefulness of quantitative PCR. *J Clin Microbiol* 2002;40:1648–1650.

169. Arnold SJ, Kinney MC, McCormick MS, et al. Disseminated toxoplasmosis. Unusual presentations in the immunocompromised host. *Arch Pathol Lab Med* 1997;121:869–873.

170. Robert-Gangneux F, Meroni V, Dupont D, et al. Toxoplasmosis in transplant recipients, Europe, 2010–2014. *Emerg Infect Dis* 2018;24:1497–1504.

171. Walker M, Zunt JR. Parasitic central nervous system infections in immunocompromised hosts. *Clin Infect Dis* 2005;40:1005–1015.

172. Rodriguez C, Munoz P, Rodriguez-Creixems M, et al. Bloodstream infections among heart transplant recipients. *Transplantation* 2006;81:384–391.

173. Paterson DL, Dominguez EA, Chang FY, et al. Infective endocarditis in solid organ transplant recipients. *Clin Infect Dis* 1998;26:689–694.

174. Sawyer RG, Crabtree TD, Gleason TG, et al. Impact of solid organ transplantation and immunosuppression on fever, leukocytosis, and physiologic response during bacterial and fungal infections. *Clin Transplant* 1999;13:260–265.

175. Singh N, Gayowski T, Wagener MM, Marino IR. Pulmonary infiltrates in liver transplant recipients in the intensive care unit. *Transplantation* 1999;67:1138–1144.

176. Singh N, Paterson DL, Gayowski T, et al. Predicting bacteremia and bacteremic mortality in liver transplant recipients. *Liver Transpl* 2000;6:54–61.

177. Crespo-Leiro MG, Alonso-Pulpon L, Vazquez de Prada JA, et al. Malignancy after heart transplantation: Incidence, prognosis and risk factors. *Am J Transplant* 2008;8:1031–1039.

178. Kasiske BL, Snyder JJ, Gilbertson DT, Wang C. Cancer after kidney transplantation in the United States. *Am J Transplant* 2004;4:905–913.

179. Heo JS, Park JW, Lee KW, et al. Posttransplantation lymphoproliferative disorder in pediatric liver transplantation. *Transplant Proc* 2004;36:2307–2308.

180. Chang FY, Singh N, Gayowski T, et al. Fever in liver transplant recipients: Changing spectrum of etiologic agents. *Clin Infect Dis* 1998;26:59–65.

181. Singh N, Gayowski T, Marino IR, Schlichtig R. Acute adrenal insufficiency in critically ill liver transplant recipients. Implications for diagnosis. *Transplantation* 1995;59:1744–1745.

182. Hummel M, Warnecke H, Schüler S, et al. Risk of adrenal cortex insufficiency following heart transplantation. *Klin Wochenschr* 1991;69:269–273.

183. Bromberg JS, Alfrey EJ, Barker CF, et al. Adrenal suppression and steroid supplementation in renal transplant recipients. *Transplantation* 1991;51:385–390.

184. Bromberg JS, Baliga P, Cofer JB, et al. Stress steroids are not required for patients receiving a renal allograft and undergoing operation. *J Am Coll Surg* 1995;180:532–536.

185. Rodger RS, Watson MJ, Sellars L, et al. Hypothalamic-pituitary-adrenocortical suppression and recovery in renal transplant patients returning to maintenance dialysis. *Q J Med* 1986;61:1039–1046.

186. Sever MS, Türkmen A, Yildiz A, et al. Fever in dialysis patients with recently rejected renal allografts. *Int J Artif Organs* 1998;21:403–407.

187. Khan A, Ortiz J, Jacobson L, et al. Posttransplant lymphoproliferative disease presenting as adrenal insufficiency: Case report. *Exp Clin Transplant* 2005;3:341–344.

188. Dorschner L, Speich R, Ruschitzka F, et al. Everolimus-induced drug fever after heart transplantation. *Transplantation* 2004;78:303–304.

189. Shin S, Kim YH, Kim SH, et al. Incidence and differential characteristics of culture-negative fever following pancreas transplantation with anti-thymocyte globulin induction. *Transpl Infect Dis* 2016;18:681–689.

190. Mourad G, Rostaing L, Legendre C, et al. Sequential protocols using basiliximab versus antithymocyte globulins in renal-transplant patients receiving mycophenolate mofetil and steroids. *Transplantation* 2004;78:584–590.

191. Khan SU, Salloum J, O'Donovan PB, et al. Acute pulmonary edema after lung transplantation: The pulmonary reimplantation response. *Chest* 1999;116:187–194.

192. San Juan R, Aguado JM, Lumbreras C, et al. Incidence, clinical characteristics and risk factors of late infection in solid organ transplant recipients: Data from the RESITRA study group. *Am J Transplant* 2007;7:964–971.

193. Petts DN, Lane A, Kennedy P, et al. Direct detection of groups A, C and G streptococci in clinical specimens by a trivalent colour test. *Eur J Clin Microbiol Infect Dis* 1988;7:34–39.

194. Muñoz P, de la Torre J, Bouza E, et al. Invasive aspergillosis in transplant recipients. A large multicentric study. *36th Interscience Conference of Antimicrobial Agents and Chemotherapy.* 1996.

195. Paterson DL, Singh N. Invasive aspergillosis in transplant recipients. *Medicine* 1999;78:123–138.

196. Husain S, Kwak EJ, Obman A, et al. Prospective assessment of Platelia *Aspergillus* galactomannan antigen for the diagnosis of invasive aspergillosis in lung transplant recipients. *Am J Transplant* 2004;4:796–802.

197. Kwak EJ, Husain S, Obman A, et al. Efficacy of galactomannan antigen in the Platelia *Aspergillus* enzyme immunoassay for diagnosis of invasive aspergillosis in liver transplant recipients. *J Clin Microbiol* 2004;42:435–438.

198. Fortun J, Martin-Davila P, Alvarez ME, et al. *Aspergillus* antigenemia sandwich-enzyme immunoassay test as a serodiagnostic method for invasive aspergillosis in liver transplant recipients. *Transplantation* 2001;71:145–149.

199. Gajurel K, Dhakal R, Deresinski S. Leishmaniasis in solid organ and hematopoietic stem cell transplant recipients. *Clin Transplant* 2017;31:e12867.

200. Bouza E, Munoz P, Burillo A. Role of the clinical microbiology laboratory in antimicrobial stewardship. *Med Clin North Am* 2018;102:883–898.

201. Muller N, Kessler R, Caillard S, et al. (18)F-FDG PET/CT for the diagnosis of malignant and infectious complications after solid organ transplantation. *Transpl Infect Dis* 2017;51:58–68.

202. Roman CD, Habibian MR, Martin WH. Identification of an infected left ventricular assist device after cardiac transplant by indium-111 WBC scintigraphy. *Clin Nucl Med* 2005;30:16–17.

203. Bouza E, Sousa D, Munoz P, et al. Bloodstream infections: A trial of the impact of different methods of reporting positive blood culture results. *Clin Infect Dis* 2004;39:1161–1169.

204. Hand J. Strategies for antimicrobial stewardship in solid organ transplant recipients. *Infect Dis Clin North Am* 2018;32:535–550.

205. Donnelly JP, Locke JE, MacLennan PA, et al. Inpatient mortality among solid organ transplant recipients hospitalized for sepsis and severe sepsis. *Clin Infect Dis* 2016;63:186–194.

206. Candel FJ, Grima E, Matesanz M, et al. Bacteremia and septic shock after solid-organ transplantation. *Transplant Proc* 2005;37:4097–4099.

207. Moreno A, Cervera C, Gavalda J, et al. Bloodstream infections among transplant recipients: Results of a nationwide surveillance in Spain. *Am J Transplant* 2007;7:2579–2586.

208. Hosenpud JD, Bennett LE, Keck BM, et al. The registry of the international society for heart and lung transplantation: Fifteenth official report-1998. *J Heart Lung Transpl* 1998;17:656–668.

209. Rajagopal K, Lima B, Petersen RP, et al. Infectious complications in extended criteria heart transplantation. *J Heart Lung Transpl* 2008;27:1217–1221.

210. Pelletier SJ, Schaubel DE, Punch JD, et al. Hepatitis C is a risk factor for death after liver retransplantation. *Liver Transpl* 2005;11:434–440.

211. Sadaghdar H, Chelluri L, Bowles SA, Shapiro R. Outcome of renal transplant recipients in the ICU. *Chest* 1995;107:1402–1405.

212. Johnson JR. Hospital-onset infections: A patient safety issue. *Ann Intern Med* 2003;139:233–234.

30 Care of Critically Ill Patients with HIV

Joseph Metmowlee Garland, Andrew Levinson, and Edward Wing

CONTENTS

Care of HIV-infected patients in the critical care unit (CCU) has changed dramatically since the infection was first recognized in the United States in 1981. The purpose of this chapter is to review the important aspects of care of HIV-infected patients in the CCU, with a primary focus on the United States and developed countries. The epidemiology, initial approach to diagnosis and treatment of HIV (including the newest antiretroviral guidelines), common syndromes and their management in the CCU, and typical co-morbidities and opportunistic infections (OIs) of HIV patients will be discussed.

The HIV epidemic was first recognized in 1981 in Los Angeles and New York and primarily affected men who have sex with men (MSM) and injection drug users. Transmission occurred through sex (anal receptive or vaginal) or blood (e.g., blood products or sharing needles). The epidemiology of HIV changed dramatically with the introduction of antiretroviral drugs, usually three drugs in combination, in 1996. Until that year, the number of cases and deaths in the United States steadily increased. After that date both cases and deaths fell dramatically although both continued at disturbingly high rates, particularly in high risk populations. In 2018, it is estimated that there are 1.1 million individuals living with HIV in the United States, 15% of whom are unaware of the diagnosis. There were 37,600 new cases in 2017, and 70% were gay or bisexual men [1].

THE CHANGING EPIDEMIOLOGY OF HIV CARE IN THE CCU

THE PRE-ANTIRETROVIRAL THERAPY ERA

In the pre-antiretroviral therapy (ART) era, CCU diagnoses in HIV-infected patients were dominated by respiratory failure, frequently due to *Pneumocystis jirovecii* and bacterial pneumonia, including nosocomial pneumonia [2]. Other AIDS-associated OIs also occurred frequently [3–5]. Mortality was highest in the early years of the epidemic. In a series from the San Francisco General Hospital from 1981–1985, the in-hospital mortality from *Pneumocystis* pneumonia (PCP), the most frequent diagnosis, was 86%. It fell to 60% in 1986–1988 and to 29% in 1996–1999 (post-ART) [3,6]. The initial improvement may have been due in part to the addition of corticosteroids for treatment of PCP [6]. Similar decreases in mortality were noted in other series during the same time period. An even more dramatic improvement occurred with the initial introduction of ART [7–9]. In this era, the diagnosis of PCP, mechanical ventilation, HIV-related illness, pneumothorax, and shock predicted mortality. CD4 count was not associated with mortality [8,10–13].

THE ART ERA

In the era of ART, respiratory failure, sepsis, and neurological disease have become the most common reasons for CCU admission [14–22]. Compared to the pre-ART era, rates of PCP, *Toxoplasma* encephalitis, and tuberculosis have decreased; rates of bacterial pneumonia have not changed; and rates of cancer, cardiovascular, pulmonary, hepatic, and renal disease, and non-pulmonary sepsis have each increased [9]. In general, in those with lower respiratory tract infections, bacterial pneumonia accounts for 60%, PCP for 10%–20%, mycobacterial disease for 15%, and viruses and fungi for small percentages [23]. In the CCU, HIV-infected patients may have higher rates of gram-positive sepsis and bacterial pneumonia, whereas HIV-negative patients have more gram-negative sepsis, though this is variable across populations [17].

Although OIs have decreased dramatically since the introduction of ART, they continue to account for an important proportion of either CCU admitting diagnoses or concurrent diagnoses, particularly in newly diagnosed HIV-infected patients. Concomitantly, the prevalence of chronic diseases, including cancer, cardiac, pulmonary, hepatic, and renal disease have increased. These increases are associated with a significant increase of the average age of HIV-infected patients, from 39 years old to 47 years old.

Intensive care unit or hospital mortality rates in the ART era have ranged from approximately 9% to 50% [8,12,15–19,23,24]. Risk factors for higher mortality include severe sepsis, high APACHE score, age, hepatitis C infection, acute kidney injury, hepatic cirrhosis, low albumin, mechanical ventilation, and PCP-associated pneumothorax. The relationship between CD4 count, ART use in the CCU, and mortality has not been consistently shown. Mortality for HIV-infected patients in the CCU in developing countries is higher than in developed countries [25].

When HIV-infected patients admitted to the CCU were compared with HIV-uninfected patients in the CCU, HIV-infected patients tended to be younger, have a greater rate of mechanical ventilation, but lesser rates of underlying cardiovascular disease, diabetes mellitus, and chronic renal dialysis [12,17,19,26]. In most but not all series, no differences in mortality were noted between HIV-infected and -uninfected patients [9,10,17,19,24,27].

DIAGNOSIS AND INTERPRETING RESULTS OF HIV DIAGNOSIS

Since 2013, the US Preventive Services Task Force has recommended routine HIV testing in all individuals ages 15–65 years [28]. Despite this recommendation for universal testing, almost a quarter of new HIV diagnoses still occur when the patient already has an AIDS diagnosis (CD4 count <200 or AIDS-defining condition). Because of the regularity of late diagnosis, it is important to include HIV in the differential for many patients presenting to the CCU and to offer routine testing.

Diagnosing HIV in the CCU is important, as HIV infection often alters the differential diagnosis and may dictate additional diagnostic workup. Standard testing is through use of a fourth-generation enzyme-linked immunosorbent assay test, with confirmation by HIV-1 and HIV-2 antibodies, and nucleic acid if these are both negative. The window from acquisition to positivity with fourth-generation testing is 18–45 days. If HIV is diagnosed, it is important to pursue further testing to characterize the stage of disease, including checking a CD4 count and HIV viral load. However, clinicians should remember that CD4 counts obtained in the CCU setting can be deceptive, as critical illness alone will lead to a decrease in circulating CD4-positive cells, as cells are redistributed from the circulation to activated tissue. A clue to the presence of this phenomenon is a CD4 count/CD4 percentage discrepancy. In steady state, a CD4 count

of 200 is roughly equivalent to a CD4 percentage of 14%. Clinicians should suspect a "falsely" low CD4 count in patients with a low CD4 count but higher-than-expected percentage.

When patients with a known or new HIV diagnosis are admitted to the CCU, it is important to remember issues of patient confidentiality with any visitors or family members. Most US states have laws specifically governing disclosure of HIV diagnosis, and clinicians should respect the patient's wishes, as well as local laws, when speaking with family members and visitors.

ANTIRETROVIRAL THERAPY IN THE CCU

The field of HIV management has changed rapidly, and for many clinicians, treatment priorities and antiretroviral medications have changed since they last studied HIV. Many standard-of-care agents today were not the drugs of choice, or even in existence, just a few years ago. While it is beyond the scope of this chapter, and also of the average critical care clinician, to offer an expert opinion on current antiretroviral management, a basic understanding of current treatment approaches and medications is important.

GENERAL GUIDELINES ON INITIATION OF TREATMENT

Studies have established that initiation of ART early in HIV disease is generally associated with improved outcomes. Since 2012, the US Department of Health and Human Services (DHHS) has recommended ART treatment for all HIV-infected individuals, regardless of CD4 count. This recommendation is based on data from the TEMPRANO and START trials, both of which showed a significant mortality benefit of early ART initiation [29,30]. Additionally, the HPTN052 and PARTNER trials demonstrated a benefit of early treatment initiation as a means of preventing HIV transmission to others, that is, "treatment as prevention" [31,32]. These studies have led to universal treatment recommendations, and now, the vast majority of HIV-infected patients in the developed world are taking ART. Even in the setting of active OIs, in which the clinician must balance benefit with the risk of immune reconstitution inflammatory syndrome (IRIS), evidence has shifted toward early treatment. Studies have now shown that early treatment initiation clearly demonstrates a mortality benefit, with just a few notable exceptions [33]. Management of OIs and timing of ART will be addressed later in this chapter in more detail.

MANAGING ANTIRETROVIRAL TREATMENT DECISIONS IN THE CCU

It is important to consider the potential benefits and risks of starting ART in the CCU setting. There are two distinct clinical scenarios to consider: Patients who are stably on ART and patients who are not on therapy due to a new diagnosis, a decision not to start therapy, or poor adherence. As these are different clinical scenarios, we will address them separately.

Patients Stably on ART

Perhaps the most common scenario in modern CCUs is that of HIV-infected patients who are already stably on ART. There are a number of issues raised by an CCU admission that can involve complex decision making around continuing antiretrovirals, including the following:

1. *Drug-drug interactions* between some antiretrovirals and commonly used CCU drugs, particularly regimens containing the CYP3A4 antagonists ritonavir and cobicistat
2. *Concerns about absorption*, due to modification of gastric pH (which can be of concern with integrase inhibitors, rilpivirine, and atazanavir), or impaired gut motility due to ileus
3. *Administration concerns* in the setting of lack of enteral access, gastric tubes, or ileus
4. *Concern for precipitating IRIS*
5. *Renal insufficiency* and the possibility of drug-induced renal insufficiency, as well as the need for dose-adjustment in the setting of changes in renal function
6. *Hepatic insufficiency* and the fact that a number of antiretrovirals are contraindicated with advanced liver disease

There is no consensus statement on maintenance of ART in the CCU setting, because there remains a lack of data specific to the CCU. However, data generally support continuation of a patient's antiretroviral regimen, if feasible, as higher mortality has been seen in patients with treatment interruption [30]. The benefits of continuing ART, including maintaining virologic control, avoidance of precipitating viral rebound, and avoidance of the development of antiretroviral resistance, are substantial. Therefore, in the absence of a compelling reason for stopping ART, antiretroviral medications should be continued in HIV-infected patients admitted to the CCU [34].

However, situations can occur in an CCU setting that necessitate stopping or holding ART for patients, such as drug toxicity; intercurrent illnesses that preclude oral intake, such as gastroenteritis or pancreatitis; surgical procedures; and interrupted access to drugs [35]. In these situations, stopping ART for a short time would be indicated. Considerations when making this decision would include duration of the expected treatment interruption, administration requirements of the antiretroviral medications (e.g., with or without food), and the half-life of the individual drug components of the patient's regimen. The *Guidelines for the Use of Antiretroviral Agents in Adults and Adolescents Living with HIV* from the US Department of Health and Human Services (DHHS) are generally considered standard of care for treatment guidance in the United States. These

guidelines state that "discontinuation of ART may result in viral rebound, immune decompensation, and clinical progression. Thus, planned interruptions of ART are not generally recommended. However, unplanned interruption of ART may occur under certain circumstances." Very brief interruptions (i.e., less than 1–2 days) because of a medical/surgical procedure can usually be accomplished by holding all drugs in the regimen. Short-term interruptions (i.e., less than 2 weeks), may be needed if severe or life-threatening drug toxicity or unexpected inability to take oral medications occurs; in these situations, all components of the drug regimen should be stopped simultaneously, regardless of drug half-life [35].

If ART discontinuation is needed but can be planned, consideration of the half-life of each individual component of the regimen is helpful, as component drugs with long half-lives may raise the risk of development of resistance. If all components have similar half-lives, all regimen components should be stopped, and later restarted, simultaneously. However, if drugs have substantially different half-lives, functional monotherapy with one agent may occur and result in an increased risk of development of resistance to that drug. In those situations, staggered switching, or replacing the concerning component before stopping, can be considered. The optimal time sequence for staggered discontinuation of regimen components, or replacement of the component, has not been determined, so this should be undertaken with expert consultation. Planned long-term discontinuation (greater than 2 weeks) is not recommended [35].

Patients Who Are Not on ART

It is also common to encounter patients in the CCU setting who are not currently receiving ART. This includes individuals who present with a new diagnosis of HIV and individuals with known HIV infection who are not taking medications, perhaps after being lost to care, due to struggling with medication adherence, or through a decision by the patient and/or their providers. In these settings, clinical context is important to determining whether to initiate ART. As noted previously, concerns about drug toxicity, drug-drug interactions, absorption, administration, risk for immune reconstitution inflammatory syndrome, and any acute renal or hepatic insufficiency should be considered. Additionally, for patients who are not expected to continue ART after leaving the hospital due to a history of poor adherence, restarting ART only to have it stopped a short while later raises the risk of the development of resistant virus. Clinicians must weigh the aforementioned concerns against the potential benefit of improved immunologic response, overall immunologic recovery, and prevention of OIs.

A number of non-randomized trials have attempted to address whether ART should be initiated in the CCU; however, all studies to date have the limitation of being retrospective. Additionally, the heterogeneity of clinical presentation in the patient populations likely biases results, as the sickest patients may not have the option of starting antiretrovirals due to ileus, lack of enteral access, or acute renal or hepatic failure. This would result in poorer outcomes being observed in this group but would actually reflect a sicker cohort rather than indicate a true benefit to ART initiation. With those caveats, the data that exist do suggest a benefit to starting ART in the critical care setting. A 2017 systematic review and meta-analysis looked both at the continuation and at the initiation of ART during the CCU stay and reviewed data from 1584 patients in 12 studies, all retrospective. A reduction in short-term mortality with the use of antiretroviral treatment during the CCU stay was found, as was a trend for lower long-term mortality [36]. Therefore, clinician should carefully consider starting ART even in an CCU setting.

ART IN THE SETTING OF AN OPPORTUNISTIC INFECTION

Recent studies have helped illuminate the benefits and risks of initiating ART in the setting of an active opportunistic infection. While the benefits of virologic control are obvious, including improvement in overall immune function and decreased risk of concurrent OI, early initiation of ART in the setting of an active OI is also known to be associated with a higher risk of IRIS, which carries with it serious morbidity and mortality. Due to fear of IRIS, clinicians often delayed ART initiation until the OI had been successfully treated. However, the benefit of this approach was unproven. In 2009, the AIDS Clinical Trials Group published the results of ACTG A5164, which compared strategies of "early ART," given within 14 days of starting acute OI treatment, and "deferred ART," given after acute OI treatment was completed. The results clearly showed that the early ART arm had fewer events of AIDS progression and death and a longer time to AIDS progression or death. The early ART arm also had a shorter time to achieving a CD4 count above 50 cells/mL and no increase in adverse events [33]. These results were largely driven by patients with *Pneumocystis jirovecii* pneumonia (present in 63% of patients), though the study included many different OIs. Further studies in developing world settings have generally supported this same conclusion about the benefits of early ART initiation in the presence of an active OI, with the CaMELIA, SAPIT, and STRIDE (A5221) trials showing a mortality benefit in patients with tuberculosis and CD4 cell counts below 50 cells/mL who received early treatment within 2 weeks after initiating tuberculosis therapy [37–39]. This has resulted in a reversal of clinical practice, with early ART favored for most OIs.

An important distinction must be made for a few CNS infections, specifically for cryptococcal meningitis and tuberculous meningitis. For these two entities, data actually suggest *poorer* outcomes with early ART initiation, likely due to a more life-threatening presentation of IRIS in the brain, leading to risk of herniation and death. A 2010 trial in patients with cryptococcal meningitis in Zimbabwe first showed worsened outcomes with early ART initiation [40]. This trial was criticized because of its use of

oral fluconazole rather than intravenous amphotericin B. However, the COAT trial, published in 2014, confirmed this finding in patients who received amphotericin B and fluconazole for the induction phase of their OI treatment. The 26-week mortality was significantly higher in the early ART arm, with the excess deaths occurring early, within 2–5 weeks after diagnosis. The effect was even more notable in patients with few white blood cells in their CSF (<5/mm^3). Based on these findings, the authors suggested deferring ART initiation in patients with cryptococcal meningitis until at least 5 weeks after diagnosis of the cryptococcal infection [41]. In a similar vein, a 2011 trial in early treatment initiation in tuberculous meningitis showed no difference in 9-month mortality (which was very high in both groups) or time to new AIDS events or death but significantly more grade 4 adverse events in the immediate-treatment arm than in the deferred ART group. These results led the authors to conclude that early ART does not improve outcomes in patients with HIV-associated tuberculous meningitis and that an increased risk of grade 4 adverse events supports delaying initiation of ART in HV-associated tuberculous meningitis [42].

In summary, data have shown that in the setting of most OIs, early ART initiation is beneficial and recommended. However, in the case of cryptococcal meningitis and tuberculous meningitis, deferring ART for at least 5 weeks after diagnosis of the OI is likely warranted.

THE ANTIRETROVIRALS

While a complete review of all antiretrovirals would be beyond the scope of this chapter, it is important for clinicians to familiarize themselves with the most commonly prescribed antiretrovirals in the United States. Currently available antiretrovirals fall into five classes:

1. *Nucleotide/nucleoside reverse transcriptase inhibitors (NRTIs)*: Nucleotide or nucleoside analogs that lack a 3'-hydroxyl group on the deoxyribose moiety, causing chain termination and thus inhibition of viral reverse transcriptase
2. *Non-nucleotide reverse transcription inhibitors (NNRTIs)*: Inhibitors of the reverse transcriptase enzyme that are not nucleotide analogs
3. *Protease inhibitors (PIs)*: Inhibitors of the viral protease, an enzyme necessary for proteolytic cleavage of protein precursors necessary for the production of an infectious viral particle. These agents end with the suffix "-navir."
4. *Entry inhibitors*: Including fusion inhibitors and CCR5 antagonists; these are not first-line and only used in salvage regimens
5. *Integrase inhibitors or integrase strand transfer inhibitors (InSTIs)*: Drugs that block the viral integrase, which is responsible for integrating the reverse-transcribed viral DNA into the host genome. These agents end with the suffix "-tegravir."

Treatment of HIV since 1996 has utilized the concept of "combination antiretroviral therapy" (ART, also called "HAART"), which involves treating HIV-infected patients with multiple agents targeting multiple steps in the viral replication cycle. This overcomes the virus's ability to mutate and evolve resistance to a single agent. A complete regimen is generally composed of three active agents (three drugs to which the virus is not believed to harbor resistance), though there are clinical situations in which fewer or more agents are used. The US DHHS maintains HIV treatment guidelines that are considered standard-of-care for HIV providers in the United States. They are available online at https://aidsinfo.nih.gov/guidelines, and are updated frequently. The last decade has seen a major shift in recommended treatment guidelines such that two NRTI's plus an InSTI are now recommended as the components of all first-line therapies for patients initiating HIV treatment. Here, we will briefly review the first-line agents. Please also see Table 30.1 for further details on these agents.

Nucleotide/Nucleoside Reverse Transcriptase Inhibitors

The NRTI class includes several agents, including zidovudine (AZT), the first antiretroviral available for treatment of HIV. Nearly all recommended regimens today involve use of two NRTI's. These are generally a combination of lamivudine or emtricitabine (a fluorinated version of lamivudine with a longer half-life—8–10 hours vs. 5–7—and otherwise similar properties) with either tenofovir disoproxil fumarate (TDF), tenofovir alafenamide (TAF), or abacavir sulfate. **Lamivudine and emtricitabine** are cytosine analogs with good oral bioavailability. They are excreted renally and require dose-adjustment in the setting of renal failure. They have an excellent side effect profile and a high therapeutic index [43,44]. Tenofovir is a component of nearly all DHHS recommended regimens and was first marketed as **tenofovir disoproxil fumarate (TDF)**. TDF is an ester prodrug of tenofovir diphosphate. It is approximately 25% bioavailable, with a half-life of 14 hours. It is primarily excreted in the urine and requires dose-adjustment for a creatinine clearance less than 50. Its most concerning side effects include both development of progressive renal failure and development of a Fanconi-like syndrome, though these are both rare, occurring in less than 2% of patients; long-term bone density loss and diarrhea in ~10% of patients are other known side effects [45]. In terms of drug-drug interactions, cumulative drug toxicities are important to consider when administered with other potentially nephrotoxic agents. **Tenofovir alafenamide (TAF)**, introduced in 2015, is also a prodrug of tenofovir diphosphate, similar to TDF. Unlike its predecessor TDF, however, it is not converted in the plasma and remains unchanged until it is intracellular within lymphoid cells. This allows for administration of much lower oral doses. At comparable intracellular levels, TAF has 90% lower circulating levels, thus the oral equivalent of 300 mg of TDF is 25 mg of TAF. TAF is associated with far less, if any, nephrotoxicity, and much less bone loss, and it does not require any dose adjustment

above a creatinine clearance of 30 mL/min. Difference in serum transporters leads to slightly different drug-drug interactions than seen with TDF, so TAF should not be co-administered with carbamazepine, oxcarbazepine, phenobarbital, phenytoin, and rifamycins (rifabutin, rifampin, rifapentine) [46]. **Abacavir sulfate** is the last commonly used NRTI. It is rapidly absorbed, 83% bioavailable and widely distributed. It has a brief half-life but intracellular concentration allows for once-daily dosing. It is hepatically metabolized and therefore does not require dose adjustment in renal disease, but is not recommended in advanced liver disease (Child–Pugh scores over six). Abacavir has been associated with a hypersensitivity reaction that is linked to a specific major histocompatibility complex class I allele HLA-B*5701, and genetic testing for the presence of this allele must be performed before its usage as the presence of the allele is considered a contraindication to usage of the drug [47]. Abacavir has been also associated with an increased risk of cardiovascular disease in several large cohorts, though the association has not been seen in pooled datasets from randomized trials, and therefore this association remains controversial [47–50]. Abacavir is a component of one first-line treatment regimen.

Integrase Inhibitors

Integrase inhibitors (InSTIs) entered clinical care with the approval of raltegravir by the US FDA in 2007. They have quickly become the backbone of initial treatment regimens due to their excellent tolerability, relatively few drug-drug interactions, and low incidence of pre-existing resistance. All three currently available agents are part of first-line regimens. **Raltegravir** is well-absorbed and has a half-life of 9 hours. It is hepatically metabolized by glucuronidation and is not affected by even severe renal dysfunction, or moderate hepatic dysfunction. It has a good side effect profile, though drug-induced hypersensitivity syndrome (DIHS) and a creatine kinase elevation that can range from mild to frank rhabdomyolysis, have been observed. Headache, diarrhea, and nausea have also been observed with this drug. There are very few drug-drug interactions of clinical consequence besides rifampin and divalent cations, which inhibit oral absorption of all integrase inhibitors [51]. **Elvitegravir** is almost always prescribed as part of a combination pill of elvitegravir, cobicistat, emtricitabine, and TDF (Stribild, by Gilead), or elvitegravir, cobicistat, emtricitabine, and TAF (Genvoya, by Gilead). It has a half-life of 8.7 hours when administered with a CYP 3A4 inhibitor (such as cobicistat). It is hepatically metabolized and requires no adjustment for renal impairment. Because it must be co-administered with a CYP 3A4 inhibitor, there are a large number of drug-drug interactions to consider (see "cobicistat" section). Divalent cations, as discussed above, inhibit intestinal absorption of elvitegravir [52]. **Dolutegravir** has a half-life of 13–15 hours, allowing for once-daily dosing without boosting. It is metabolized through UGT1A1, with a minor contribution for CYP3A4. It does not require dose adjustment

TABLE 30.1

Potential Toxicities, Major Drug-Drug Interactions, and Other Clinically Useful Characteristics of Commonly Used Antiretroviral Drugs

Antiretroviral Drug	Formulation	Potential Toxicities	Major Drug-Drug Interactions with Commonly Prescribed CCU Medications	Recommended Minimum Creatinine Clearance	Need for Hepatic Adjustment	Can it be Crushed, Dispersed, or Given in Liquid Formulation[a,b]?
Single Tablets						
Stribild	TDF, emtricitabine, elvitegravir, cobicistat	TDF: Renal toxicity, Fanconi syndrome, decreased bone density, diarrhea, lactic acidosis Elvitegravir: Nausea, rash, headache Cobicistat: Diarrhea, GI upset	Amiodarone, quinidine, carbamazepine, phenytoin, phenobarbital, rifampin, inhaled salmeterol, bosentan, rivaroxaban, sildenafil *Use with caution:* Statins, midazolam, triazolam, voriconazole, fentanyl, warfarin	70 mL/min	None	Case reports and PK data in healthy volunteers suggest successful viral suppression and bioequivalence with crushed pills in food or enteral feeds though cobicistat and elvitegravir are not soluble in water.
Genvoya	TAF, emtricitabine, elvitegravir, cobicistat	TAF: Diarrhea, lactic acidosis Elvitegravir: Nausea, rash, headache Cobicistat: Diarrhea, GI upset	Amiodarone, quinidine, carbamazepine, oxcarbazepine, phenytoin, phenobarbital, rifampin, inhaled salmeterol, bosentan, rivaroxaban, sildenafil *Use with caution:* Statins, midazolam, triazolam, voriconazole, fentanyl, warfarin	30 mL/min	None	Crushing or splitting tablets has not been studied and is not recommended. TAF is soluble in water but it has a bitter and burnt flavor.
Triumeq	Abacavir, lamivudine, dolutegravir	Abacavir: N/v, headache. Possible increased CV risk Lactic acidosis Hypersensitivity in HLA-B5701-positive patients Dolutegravir: Headache, insomnia, GI upset	Dofetilide, carbamazepine, oxcarbazepine, phenytoin, phenobarbital, ganciclovir, divalent cations, rifampin	50 mL/min	Do not use if Childs B, Contraindicated for Childs C	Package insert states that though there are no studies, PK is expected to be equivalent. PK data in healthy volunteers are clinically comparable.
Atripla	TDF, emtricitabine, efavirenz	TDF: Renal toxicity, Fanconi syndrome, decreased bone density, diarrhea, lactic acidosis Efavirenz: Depression, vivid dreams, somnolence	IV midazolam, rifampin, rifabutin, voriconazole, carbamazepine, dabigatran, phenytoin, tacrolimus, methadone, warfarin	50 mL/min	Contraindicated for Childs C	In case reports, bioequivalence of crushed tablets was not met, though clinical implications are unknown. Efavirenz is not water-soluble, so crushing is not recommended.

(Continued)

TABLE 30.1 *(Continued)*
Potential Toxicities, Major Drug-Drug Interactions, and Other Clinically Useful Characteristics of Commonly Used Antiretroviral Drugs

Antiretroviral Drug	Formulation	Potential Toxicities	Major Drug-Drug Interactions with Commonly Prescribed CCU Medications	Recommended Minimum Creatinine Clearance	Need for Hepatic Adjustment	Can it be Crushed, Dispersed, or Given in Liquid Formulation a,b?
Complera	TDF, emtricitabine, rilpivirine	TDF: Renal toxicity, Fanconi syndrome, decreased bone density, diarrhea, lactic acidosis Rilpivirine: Depression, rash, GI upset	Carbamazepine, dexamethasone, PPIs, H2 blockers, antacids, phenytoin, phenobarbital, oxcarbazepine, rifampin, dabigatran	50 mL/min	None	Splitting or crushing has not been studied and is not recommended. Rilpivirine is insoluble in water across a wide pH range.
Odefsey	TAF, emtricitabine, rilpivirine	TAF: Diarrhea, lactic acidosis Rilpivirine: Depression, rash, GI upset	Carbamazepine, dexamethasone, PPIs, H2 blockers, antacids, phenytoin, phenobarbital, oxcarbazepine, rifampin, dabigatran	30 mL/min	None	Splitting or crushing has not been studied and is not recommended. Rilpivirine is insoluble in water across a wide pH range.
Others						
Truvada	TDF, emtricitabine	Renal toxicity, Fanconi syndrome, decreased bone density, diarrhea, lactic acidosis	Dabigatran, other nephrotoxic agents	50 mL/min	None	Multiple case reports support bioequivalence of crushed vs oral tablets.
Descovy	TAF, emtricitabine	Diarrhea, lactic acidosis	Carbamazepine, oxcarbazepine, phenobarbital, phenytoin, rifamycins	30 mL/min	None	Crushing or splitting tablets has not been studied and is not recommended. TAF is soluble in water but it has a bitter and burnt flavor.
Epzicom	Abacavir, lamivudine	N/v, headache. Possible increased CV risk. Lactic acidosis.	Ganciclovir, valganciclovir, methadone	50 mL/min	Do not use if Childs B, contraindicated for Childs C	No studies, but film-coated immediate release tablet, predicted to have good absorption. Abacavir and lamivudine also both have liquid formulations.
Prezista, Norvir *or* Prezcobix	Darunavir + ritonavir *or* Darunavir/cobicistat	Diarrhea, n/v, rash	Amiodarone, quinidine, carbamazepine, oxcarbazepine, phenytoin, phenobarbital, rifampin, inhaled salmeterol, bosentan, rivaroxaban, sildenafil *Use with caution:* Statins, midazolam, triazolam, voriconazole, fentanyl, warfarin	None	Not recommended for Childs C	Case reports and PK data in healthy volunteers suggest successful viral suppression and bioequivalence with crushed pills in food or enteral feeds. Darunavir is also available in liquid formulation

(Continued)

TABLE 30.1 (Continued)
Potential Toxicities, Major Drug-Drug Interactions, and Other Clinically Useful Characteristics of Commonly Used Antiretroviral Drugs

Antiretroviral Drug	Formulation	Potential Toxicities	Major Drug-Drug Interactions with Commonly Prescribed CCU Medications	Recommended Minimum Creatinine Clearance	Need for Hepatic Adjustment	Can it be Crushed, Dispersed, or Given in Liquid Formulation[a,b]?
Reyataz, Norvir or Evotaz	Atazanavir, ritonavir or Atazanavir/cobicistat	Jaundice, unconjugated hyperbilirubinemia, diarrhea, n/v	PPIs and H2 blockers, Amiodarone, quinidine, carbamazepine, oxcarbazepine, phenytoin, phenobarbital, rifampin, inhaled salmeterol, bosentan, rivaroxaban, sildenafil *Use with caution:* Statins, midazolam, triazolam, voriconazole, fentanyl, warfarin	None	Do not use if Childs B, Contraindicated for Childs C	Atazanavir capsules may be opened and mixed with food. Atazanavir and ritonavir are both also available as liquid formulations. Manufacturer recommends that Evotaz can be swallowed whole and advises against crushing.
Isentress	Raltegravir	Elevated CK, rhabdomyolysis, rash, including DIHS	Rifampin, divalent cations	None	Not studied in Childs C (no data)	Crushing pills is not recommended. Granules absorb faster and affect levels. Both chewable tablets and oral suspensions are available. Note that they are not bioequivalent (400 mg oral tablet = 300-mg oral chewable = 100-mg oral suspension)
Tivicay	Dolutegravir	Headache, insomnia, GI upset	Dofetilide, carbamazepine, oxcarbazepine, phenytoin, phenobarbital, ganciclovir, divalent cations, rifampin	None	Not recommended in Childs C	Case reports and PK data in healthy volunteers suggest successful viral suppression and bioequivalence with crushed pills in food or enteral feed.

[a] Foisy M and Tseng A. "Liquid Drug formulations." Toronto General Hospital Immunodeficiency Clinic web resource: http://hivclinic.ca/main/drugs_extra_files/LIQUID%20DRUG%20FORMULATIONS.pdf.

[b] Foisy M, Hughes C, Lamb S, Tseng A. "Oral antiretroviral administration: Information on crushing and liquid drug formulations." Toronto General Hospital Immunodeficiency Clinic web resource: http://www.hivclinic.ca/main/drugs_extra_files/Crushing%20and%20Liquid%20ARV%20Formulations.pdf.

for renal disease. It does have some drug-drug interactions with other antivirals, including the uncommonly used protease inhibitors fosamprenavir and tipranavir, and the NNRTIs efavirenz and etravirine. Co-administration with rifampin requires dolutegravir dosing be increased to twice-daily. Antacids and other divalent cations should not be administered within 6 hours prior or 2 hours after dolutegravir. Side effects are rare but include insomnia, headache, and rare GI side effects. Dolutegravir has a high genetic barrier to resistance and is often used in patients with underlying resistance mutations [53]. **Bictegravir**, the newest integrase inhibitor, received FDA approval in 2018 and is marketed in a combination tablet with TAF and emtricitabine (Biktarvy, by Gilead). Similar to dolutegravir, it has a half-life of 18 hours, allowing for once-daily dosing. It is metabolized equally by both CYP3A4 and glucuronidation UGT 1A1. There is no dose-adjustment required for even advanced renal disease. Drug-drug interactions are expected to be relatively few because of its multiple pathways to metabolism, but data are not yet published confirming this. It has a high barrier to resistance. Side effects in early trials appear comparable to dolutegravir [54].

CYP3A4 INHIBITORS (THE "BOOSTERS")

Ritonavir and **cobicistat** are both administered as part of some HIV treatment regimens but are not active agents in terms of suppressing viral activity (ritonavir does have antiviral properties, but when administered at significantly higher doses). They are structurally similar molecules, with similar effects on inhibition of cytochrome P450, predominantly, but not exclusively, 3A4. Both are renal multidrug and toxin extrusion protein 1 (MATE1) inhibitors in the kidney, causing increases in serum creatinine of 10%–15%. Both can be associated with a number of side effects, particularly diarrhea and dyslipidemia. These agents are of particular importance to note in the critical care setting because of their numerous drug-drug interactions through their CYP3A4 inhibition. Several agents are contraindicated for co-administration, including alfuzosin, amiodarone, carbamazepine, phenytoin, phenobarbital, bosentan, inhaled salmeterol, rivaroxaban, ergotamines, high-dose sildenafil, oral midazolam, and triazolam. Close monitoring is recommended for clarithromycin, clonazepam, metoprolol, azole antifungals, atorvastatin, and rosuvastatin, among others [55]. Please see Table 30.1 for more details.

RECOMMENDED REGIMENS

The DHHS guidelines classify seven regimens as "Recommended Initial Regimens for Most People with HIV." They are recommended with equal weight. All these regimens incorporate NRTIs and InSTIs as their constituent components. First-line regimens as of 5/2020 are as follows:

- Bictegravir/TAF/emtricitabine (Biktarvy, Gilead)
- Dolutegravir/abacavir/lamivudine (Triumeq, Viiv)—only for patients who are HLA-B*5701-negative and without hepatitis B co-infection

- Dolutegravir (Tivicay, Viiv) plus (emtricitabine or lamivudine) plus (TAF or TDF)
- Dolutegravir/lamivudine (Dovato, Viiv)—except for individuals with HIV RNA >500,000, HBV co-infection, or patients without prior genotype testing
- Raltegravir (Isentress, Merck) plus (emtricitabine or lamivudine) plus (TAF or TDF)

OTHER AGENTS

The DHHS Guidelines do not recommend switching patients who are virally suppressed and tolerating their regimens to newer agents; therefore, some patients who present to the hospital will be on older, alternative, or salvage regimens containing agents other than those listed above. These patients generally should not have their regimen changed in the CCU setting unless a clear compelling reason (e.g., toxicity) is identified. We will not review all of the agents, but will briefly touch on three still commonly in use. **Efavirenz** is a component of the combination tablet TDF/emtricitabine/efavirenz (Atripla) and is still commonly prescribed. Efavirenz has a very long half-life of 40–55 hours once steady state is achieved. It is an inducer of CYP3A4 and an inhibitor of CYP2C9 and CYP2C19, and has drug-drug interactions with rifamycins, voriconazole, many anticonvulsants, and methadone. It has a number of side effects, which has led to its removal from the first-line recommended agents list, most notably depression with a twofold increased risk of suicidality, vivid dreams, and somnolence [56]. **Darunavir** is the most commonly prescribed protease inhibitor still used today. It is generally well-tolerated and has a high genetic barrier to resistance. It should always be boosted by ritonavir or cobicistat. Ritonavir-boosted darunavir has a half-life of 15 hours. It is hepatically metabolized and does not require dose-adjustment for renal failure. Because of its co-administration with a CYP3A4 inhibitor, there are a number of drug-drug interactions. Alfazosin, cisapride, ergot derivatives, triazolam, oral midazolam, simvastatin, rifampin, and high-dose sildenafil are contraindicated. Side effects include diarrhea (>10%), rash, dyslipidemia, and, rarely, hepatitis [57]. **Atazanavir** is also a protease inhibitor. It is the only protease inhibitor that may be given without ritonavir or cobicistat boosting, though CYP3A4 boosting of atazanavir is still preferred. The recommended unboosted dose is 400-mg daily. If co-administered with ritonavir or cobicistat, it is given as a 300-mg daily dose. Its half-life is 7 hours unboosted and 12 hours with CYP3A4 boosting. It is hepatically metabolized and does not require dose-adjustment for renal failure. Because of its co-administration with a CYP3A4 inhibitor, there are a number of drug-drug interactions, similar to darunavir above (see Table 30.1). Additionally, atazanavir is highly dependent on gastric pH for absorption, and therefore its absorption will be inhibited using H2-blockers, proton-pump inhibitors, and other gastric-pH-lowering agents. It must be taken with food. Side effects include nausea, diarrhea, rash, abdominal pain, dyspepsia, headache, and fatigue. A benign unconjugated hyperbilirubinemia and mild jaundice are common with atazanavir, due to atazanavir's inhibition of UGT1A1, which is responsible for bilirubin conjugation. Atazanavir is also a rare cause of nephrolithiasis [58].

CONCLUSIONS REGARDING ANTIRETROVIRALS

In summary, ART is recommended in the CCU setting for all patients who are already on therapy at admission, and should strongly be considered in those who are not, but who are presenting with advanced disease, an opportunistic infection, or a clinical presentation suggestive of HIV-related disease. In the absence of enteral access or in settings in which short-term discontinuation of ARVs is necessary, all antivirals should all be discontinued and then restarted simultaneously unless there is a significant difference in half-life of the drugs (e.g., efavirenz). There are no constructible regimens of IV/IM formulations currently, and attempts to switch a patient's oral regimen to an IV/IM proxy are not recommended. Many of the current regimens are crushable and amenable to tube feeding once enteral access is regained (see Table 30.1). In the setting of OIs, ARV initiation is generally recommended, and understanding that there may be an increased risk of IRIS that will require further management. Exceptions to this recommendation include CNS disease with *Cryptococcus* spp. and tuberculosis.

Treatment guidelines have shifted rapidly, and now, all first-line regimens contain two NRTI drugs combined with an InSTI. When strategizing on a regimen, the state of the patient's renal and hepatic function should be taken into consideration, as should the potential for drug-drug interactions. When available, expert consultation with an infectious disease or HIV specialist is strongly recommended.

MANAGEMENT OF COMMON DIAGNOSES

SEPSIS/SEPTIC SHOCK

Severe sepsis and septic shock are leading causes of CCU admission and have high predicted morbidity and mortality in HIV-infected patients. In general, the management of septic shock in HIV-infected patients should be the same as for non-infected patients and should follow recommended guidelines [59].

Initial emphasis should be on the rapid detection and triage to critical care of patients presenting with severe sepsis and septic shock. Ideally, appropriate microbiologic cultures, including blood, should be quickly obtained before antibiotic initiation, in order to increase the likelihood of making an accurate diagnosis and in order to appropriately de-escalate antimicrobial therapy later [59,60].

It is absolutely essential that appropriate antibiotics be initiated in patients with severe sepsis and septic shock, preferably within one hour of identification, as such an approach has been shown to decrease both mortality and subsequent multi-organ dysfunction [61–63]. Broad

spectrum therapy, including antimicrobial therapies and, if clinically suspected, anti-fungal and/or anti-viral therapies, should be initiated against all likely pathogens based on the patient's clinical presentation and most recent CD4 count, if known. Known community resistance patterns and suspected anatomic location of the infection should be taken into account when choosing initial anti-microbial therapies. Of note, in one prospective cohort study of HIV-infected patients in CCUs, compared to non-infected critically ill patients, HIV-infected patients were not found to have increased rates of colonization of drug-resistant organisms; therefore, different antibiotic choices should generally not be made for HIV-infected patients than HIV-negative patients regarding resistant organisms [64]. Initial broad-spectrum antimicrobial therapy should be narrowed once the patient is clinically improving and/or resistance patterns and drug sensitivities are available [59]. As in the non-HIV-infected patient, immediate source control is essential and any potential sources of ongoing infection, such as intra-vascular catheters or abscesses, should be immediately addressed.

Perhaps equally as important as antibiotic administration is the simultaneous provision of appropriate fluid resuscitation. Initial fluid resuscitation of HIV-infected patients with severe sepsis and septic shock should be based on best practices developed in HIV-negative patient populations. It is recommended that patients should receive an initial fluid resuscitation of 30 mL crystalloid/kg in the first three hours after presentation. Further fluid resuscitation should be based on hemodynamic monitoring, dynamic assessment of a patient's volume status, and the clearance of lactate [59]. Vasopressors should be initiated if a patient in septic shock is not responsive to initial fluid resuscitation and should be titrated to a goal MAP of 65 mmHg [59]. The administration of IV hydrocortisone should be considered in patients who are not responding initially to fluids and vasopressors, although this remains controversial [65,66].

In addition, all septic patients should have a target glucose level of ≤180 [67]. Tighter glucose control may result in increased mortality. All patients should have appropriate venous thromboembolism prophylaxis and, if at risk of bleeding, stress-ulcer prophylaxis [59]. Clinicians should remember that there are some drug-drug interactions with acid-suppressing medications and antiretrovirals (integrase inhibitors, rilpivirine, and atazanavir in particular).

RESPIRATORY FAILURE

As previously discussed, acute hypoxic respiratory failure remains one the most common reasons for CCU admission for patients with HIV. While the percentage of CCU deaths from acute respiratory failure has significantly declined over the last three decades, patients with HIV/AIDS still have a significantly increased risk of dying from acute respiratory failure when admitted to the CCU [68].

Infectious reasons for acute respiratory failure include PCP, bacterial pneumonia, fungal pneumonia, and viral pneumonia.

As in the general population, the most common pathogens for bacterial pneumonia in the United States and other developed countries in patients with HIV/AIDS are *Streptococcus pneumoniae*, *Haemophilus influenza*, *Staphylococcus aureus*, and *Pseudomonas aeruginosa*. Less common but still clinically important causes of pneumonia are *Mycobacterium tuberculosis*, *Pneumocystis jirovecii*, *Cryptococcus neoformans*, *Histoplasma capsulatum*, *Coccidioides immitis*, *Aspergillus* spp., CMV, and influenza virus [22,69–71].

Diagnosis and treatment of pneumonia should follow generally accepted guidelines [72,73]. The cardinal clinical findings of cough, fever, dyspnea, and sputum production may not always be helpful in diagnosing pneumonia in immunocompromised patients. In addition, not all patients may present with fever, tachycardia, or tachypnea. Similarly, leukocytosis, while helpful, may not be present, and particular attention should be paid to diagnosing patients who have leukopenia. Every effort should be made to obtain two sets of blood cultures and an adequate sputum culture at time of clinical diagnosis, ideally before the initiation of antimicrobial therapy, in order to help guide subsequent treatment de-escalation [73].

Current guidelines do not recommend the use of biomarkers such as C-reactive protein and procalcitonin (PCT) to diagnose pneumonia, but PCT may be helpful in non-HIV-infected patients in de-escalating antibiotics once initiated [73]. It should be noted, however, that almost all studies of using PCT to guide antibiotic therapy have excluded HIV-infected patients [74,75].

Appropriate triage to the CCU of patients with pneumonia can be challenging and dependent on the resources of the specific health care system and community [76]. In general, patients who show signs of confusion, renal failure or other organ failure, and hypoxemia not yet receiving mechanical ventilation, should be considered for CCU admission. Scoring systems and predictive models such as the pneumonia severity index (PSI) [77] confusion, urea, respiratory rate, blood pressure plus age ≥ 65 years (CURB-65) [78], and predisposition, insult, response, and organ dysfunction (PIRO) [79] can be helpful in assisting and identifying patients at high risk of clinical decompensation. One of the most recent pneumonia predictive models, PIRO, may be particularly helpful in predicting outcomes in patients with HIV as it takes immunocompromised status into account in its risk score calculation [79]. In treating patients with severe CAP, underlying cardiac and pulmonary disease, in addition to HIV, can delay recognition and significantly increase morbidity and mortality. Many HIV-infected patients have chronic lung disease and cardiac disease at baseline, which significantly increases the risk of clinical decompensation from pneumonia [80].

While recent studies have suggested there may be a benefit to using steroids as an adjunct therapy to treating patients hospitalized for community-acquired pneumonia (CAP) [81], this remains controversial; additionally, HIV-infected patients were excluded from the study, so the results may not be applicable [82]. In contrast, for HIV-infected patients diagnosed with PCP with even just mildly impaired oxygenation and gas exchange at time of diagnosis, adjunctive therapy with corticosteroids can significantly increase survival and slow disease progression [83–85].

In terms of treatment for severe CAP requiring CCU admission, most patients with severe CAP can be treated with a fluoroquinolone or a beta-lactam and a macrolide. However, those with multi-drug resistant risk factors, most notably recent antibiotic use, or risk of community acquired MRSA, should be given additional appropriate antibiotic coverage [72]. Of note, one recent prospective cohort surveillance study found an increased rate of colonization of community associated MRSA in HIV-infected patients [74].

With regards to ventilator associated pneumonia and hospital acquired pneumonia, recently revised guidelines emphasize selecting initial empiric treatment based on known local susceptibility patterns. Initial therapy should usually include an antibiotic with gram-positive, including MRSA, activity, and an antibiotic with gram-negative, including anti-pseudomonal, activity. Coverage for *Staphylococcus* including MRSA, *Pseudomonas*, and other gram-negative organisms should be considered [73].

In suspected ventilator-associated pneumonia, the evidence for obtaining a quantitative broncheoalveolar lavage (BAL) versus obtaining a non-quantitative tracheal aspirate remains controversial; of note, many of these studies excluded immunocompromised patients with HIV [86,87]. Current guidelines recommend noninvasive semi-quantitative culture via endotracheal aspirate over quantitative BAL culture [72]. In HIV-infected patients where the tracheal aspirate is non-diagnostic, where the patient is severely immunocompromised, or where *Pneumocystis* is in the differential, bronchoscopy with BAL still should strongly be considered. In all cases the initial empiric treatment should be de-escalated based on the culture data obtained whenever possible.

There may be a benefit to using high flow nasal cannula oxygen devices and non-invasive positive pressure ventilation in patients with acute hypoxemic respiratory failure with the hope of preventing intubation [88]. The early administration of these devices is performed to improve both oxygenation and ventilation without endotracheal intubation and to decrease work of breathing for patients in respiratory distress. Two potential advantages of using such a strategy before clinical deterioration are that the immunocompromised patient can avoid intubation and mechanical ventilation, and associated ventilator acquired infections [22]. However, one recent randomized trial that administered high flow oxygen via a nasal cannula device to immunocompromised patients with hypoxemic respiratory failure found no benefit when compared to similar patients offered standard oxygen therapy without a high flow device [89].

For patients that are mechanically ventilated for pneumonia, it is important that best practices be followed to avoid increased mortality from mechanical ventilation. In mechanically ventilated patients with pneumonia who meet current definitions for ARDS [90], a ventilation strategy using low tidal volumes of 6–8 cc/kg ideal body weight should be followed [91,92]. One large retrospective study found that lower tidal volume ventilation is independently associated with reduced mortality in HIV-infected patients with acute lung injury and respiratory failure [91]. In addition, positive end-expiratory pressure (PEEP) should be used to lower the fraction of inspired oxygen administered (FIO_2) to safe levels to avoid potential oxygen toxicity [93]. If peak pressures on the ventilator remain high, or if there is difficulty with lowering the FIO_2 or ventilating at targeted low tidal volumes utilizing a lung-protective strategy, alternative therapies such as extracorporeal membrane oxygenation (ECMO) should be considered. There may be a benefit to the early use of neuromuscular blockade and proning in patients who develop severe ARDS [94,95].

Extracorporeal membrane oxygenation is an alternative to standard positive mechanical ventilation in patients with hypoxic respiratory failure that uses cardio-pulmonary bypass technology to temporarily provide gas exchange via large vascular cannulae and an external device. Patients on ECMO must be systemically anticoagulated. Extracorporeal membrane oxygenation can be considered in patients who are unable to be supported by standard positive pressure mechanical ventilation or those that are unable to be oxygenated or ventilated adequately using a lung protective strategy [96].

In the last decade, there has been increasing use of ECMO in critical care at tertiary referral centers; however, there is yet to be high quality randomized controlled trials to support its use and significant cost. The largest ECMO trial, the CESAR trial, randomized ARDS patients to care at a tertiary center where ECMO was available [97]. However, a significant percentage of the patients randomized to the tertiary center ultimately did not end up receiving ECMO. A criticism of the study has been that the significantly decreased mortality found in the treatment group was not due just to ECMO but also perhaps because patients received other best practices for ARDS management. Specifically, regarding patients with HIV, the current evidence for the use of ECMO with respiratory failure is limited to case reports. Most of the case reports involve patients with severe PCP who were unable to be oxygenated with conventional positive pressure mechanical ventilation [98–101].

For HIV-infected patients who are mechanically ventilated, it is important that protocolized approaches for removing the patient from the ventilator are implemented [102,103]. Meticulous attention should be given to providing appropriate sedation and analgesia if the patient is mechanically ventilated and all patients should have a daily wakening trial paired with their weaning trial [104]. A combined approach can result in decreased time on the ventilator, decreased length of CCU and hospital stay, and decreased mortality.

OPPORTUNISTIC INFECTIONS

In the ART era, respiratory failure secondary to bacterial pneumonia and sepsis are the most common reasons for admission to the CCU for HIV-infected patients. The OIs

TABLE 30.2
Opportunistic Infections in HIV+ Patients

Pathogen/Disease	Typical Manifestations[a]	Diagnosis	Treatment
Pneumocystis jirovecii	Dyspnea, central ground-glass infiltrates	BAL; DFA stain	Trimethoprim-sulfamethoxazole (TMP/SMX) +/−CS
Candida esophagitis	Pain on swallowing with oral thrush	+/− endoscopy	Fluconazole
Tuberculosis	Pulmonary or extra-pulmonary (adenopathy, hepatic)	AFB stain, culture X-gen sputum, tissue	INH/Pyr/Etha/Rif
Mycobacterium-avium complex (MAC)	Adenopathy, weight loss, abdominal pain, cough	AFB stain and culture blood, sputum, tissue	Clarithromycin, ethambutol +/− rifabutin
Cerebral toxoplasmosis	Focal neurological signs; multiple ring-enhancing lesions	CT/MRI; +IgG toxo Ab	Pyrimethamine/sulfadizine or TMP/SMX
Cryptococcal meningitis	Headache, malaise, confusion	+CSF India Ink or Crypto antigen	Amphotericin/flucytosine followed by fluconazole

Note: Other OIs and tumors occur in HIV+ patients with CD4 counts less than 200 at lower rates. These include disseminated herpes viruses such as herpes simplex, herpes zoster, and CMV, histoplasmosis, progressive multifocal leukoencephalopathy (JC virus), cryptosporidiosis, Kaposi's sarcoma, and non-Hodgkin's B cell lymphoma.

[a] Fever is typical for most infections with OIs.

due to immunodeficiency remain an important consideration in patients with CD4 counts less than 200/microliter (Table 30.2).

PNEUMOCYSTIS JIROVECII PNEUMONIA

Pneumocystis jirovecii pneumonia (PCP) remains the most important opportunistic infection in HIV-infected CCU patients in the developed world [105]. Of note, approximately 25% of PCP cases occur in patients unaware of their HIV diagnosis. Mortality has fallen from over 75% in the early pre-ART era [11] to 5%–15% currently. HIV-infected patients usually present with weeks of dyspnea, cough, and fever. The chest X-ray typically has a diffuse, perihilar pattern of ground glass opacities. More diffuse disease with consolidation may occur in untreated patients [106]. Importantly, PCP can present with a range of unusual features including a completely clear chest X-ray; cysts, which are usually multiple and bilateral; nodules; mediastinal and hilar lymphadenopathy; and pneumothorax [107]. Diagnosis either by induced sputum (sensitivity 50%–90%) or bronchoalveolar lavage (sensitivity approaches 100%) is made using direct fluorescent antibody stain [6,108,109]. The preferred treatment is trimethoprim/sulfamethoxazole either intravenously or orally [110]. Up to 50%–80% of patients will develop drug reactions to trimethoprim/sulfamethoxazole including rash, hepatitis, nephritis, neutropenia, and thrombocytopenia [110]. Alternative treatments include pentamidine, which is more toxic; trimethoprim plus dapsone; atovaquone; or primaquine plus clindamycin, which are less effective. Patients with moderate to severe PCP ($PaO_2 < 70$ mmHg) should be started on prednisone.

ESOPHAGEAL CANDIDIASIS

Esophageal candidiasis is characterized by pain on swallowing and is usually accompanied by oral-pharyngeal white plaques. *Candida albicans* is the usual cause and treatment is indicated with systemic fluconazole for esophageal disease.

TUBERCULOSIS

Patients with HIV are at high risk for *Mycobacterium tuberculosis* disease, particularly if the CD4 count is less than 200 cells/microliter. While the incidence of tuberculosis has declined markedly in developed countries [14], cases do occur and it is important to determine risk factors including exposure and country of origin. The rates in developing countries remain high and are a significant cause of CCU admission [24]. Manifestations in critically ill patients are pulmonary in 50% and disseminated, often with adenitis, in 45%. Mortality rates range from 52%–68% and are much higher in those with multi-drug resistant TB [25,111]. Concurrent HIV treatment is indicated by recently published guidelines [112]. Drug interactions may occur between ART and rifamycins as part of anti-tuberculous regimens.

MYCOBACTERIUM AVIUM COMPLEX DISEASE

Mycobacterium avium complex disease (MAC) occurs in patients with CD4 count < 50 cells/microliter and HIV viral loads generally >10,000. Manifestations are nonspecific and include fever, weight loss, cough, and abdominal pain. Lymphadenopathy, either detected on physical exam or by imaging, is an important clue. Diagnosis is definitively made by culture of the organism either from blood or lymph node. Treatment is with clarithromycin plus ethambutol +/− rifampin or rifabutin. IRIS is common in HIV-infected, treatment-naive patients with MAC who are started on ART.

CEREBRAL TOXOPLASMOSIS

Neurological disease remains a significant cause for admission to the CCU in patients with HIV. In those with CD4 counts <100 cells/microliter, toxoplasma encephalitis is an important consideration. Patients usually present with some combination of headache, confusion, and focal neurological deficits. Seizures may occur. Imaging with CT or MRI typically shows multiple ring-enhancing lesions. Positive IgG antibodies for *Toxoplasma gondii* support the diagnosis. The preferred treatment is sulfadiazine and pyrimethamine, with leucovorin. If there is sulfa intolerance, then clindamycin can be combined with pyrimethamine plus leucovorin. Trimethoprim/sulfamethoxazole has also been used successfully.

CRYPTOCOCCUS NEOFORMANS MENINGITIS

The incidence of cryptococcal meningitis has decreased in the ART era but continues to occur in those with a CD4 count of <100 cells/microliter. Patients typically present with headache, malaise, and fever that develop over several weeks. Some patients may have a stiff neck. A positive CSF cryptococcal antigen or India ink preparation is diagnostic. Imaging before the lumbar puncture is important to rule out mass lesions or hydrocephalus. Treatment is with amphotericin and flucytosine for a two-week induction phase, followed by oral fluconazole for an eight-week consolidation phase. Maintenance fluconazole is then continued for a minimum of one year, and until the CD4 count is >100 cells/microliter. ART should not be started for the first 5 weeks of treatment because of concern for IRIS.

OTHER NEUROLOGICAL CONDITIONS

Other causes of CNS mass lesions that produce focal neurological signs in patients with low CD4 counts include CNS lymphoma (often presenting as one lesion that may be ring enhancing) and progressive multifocal leukoencephalopathy caused by JC virus (usually non-ring enhancing lesions in the white matter). The HIV virus itself may cause encephalopathy, and herpes viruses including herpes simplex 1 and 2, varicella zoster, and cytomegalovirus, can cause encephalitis with characteristic MRI findings. CMV retinitis characterized by pathognomonic retinal hemorrhages and exudates may occur in patients with CD4 counts less than 200 cells/microliter.

Other OIs and tumors are listed in Table 30.1.

IMMUNE RECONSTITUTION INFLAMMATORY SYNDROME

The Immune Reconstitution Inflammatory Syndrome (IRIS) is a complication of initiation of ART in a severely immunocompromised patient. IRIS can be defined as either a paradoxical worsening of treated OIs ("paradoxical IRIS"), or the unmasking of previously subclinical, untreated infections ("unmasking IRIS"). IRIS is described as occurring any time between 4 weeks and one year after initiating ART, though rare otherwise clinically compatible cases may present earlier or later than this. There is significant morbidity to IRIS, as up to 50% of IRIS cases require hospitalization, and often require extensive testing and both diagnostic and therapeutic procedures [113].

Studies demonstrate a wide range in frequency of presentation of IRIS, which can be identified in anywhere between

10%–50% of patients initiating ART [114–119]. In general, risk is associated with lower CD4 counts at treatment initiation. Additionally, some opportunistic infections and diseases have a higher risk of the development of IRIS. MAC, CMV retinitis, cryptococcal meningitis, PML, and tuberculosis are all higher risk, while IRIS is uncommonly seen with Kaposi sarcoma or herpes zoster [120]. The immunopathological process that causes clinical IRIS is not fully understood, but data from clinicopathological and immunological studies suggest that IRIS results from exaggerated and dysregulated cellular immune responses to the associated pathogen [120].

Diagnosis of IRIS depends on the presentation. Unmasking IRIS is diagnosed based on a clinical presentation of an OI in the setting of initiation of ART. The diagnostic workup is driven by the clinical presentation and usually involves blood cultures, mycobacterial isolators on serum, sputum for bacterial and AFB staining and culture if respiratory symptoms or radiographic findings are suggestive, imaging such as CT abdomen and pelvis or brain imaging if symptoms are suggestive, a retinal exam if any eye symptoms are present, a lymph node biopsy if any lymphadenopathy is present (particularly asymmetric), and further additional workup as dictated by symptoms. Paradoxical IRIS is diagnosed based on a clinical scenario of a known opportunistic infection initially improving and then deteriorating, with clinical features suggestive of the same opportunistic infection. Concurrent reduction in HIV viral load and often a rise in the CD4 count in response to ART initiation make this a compatible clinical syndrome. Alternative causes, such as a concurrent infection, drug reaction, or resistant OI should be excluded.

There are limited treatment options for IRIS. In all but life-threatening cases, ART should be continued, as there is a clear mortality benefit associated with ART even in the setting of IRIS [33,37–39]. Examples of clinical situations in which stopping ART might be considered would be life-threatening tuberculous meningitis or PML. NSAID use may be helpful in milder disease, but there are no clinical trial data on efficacy, and this recommendation is based on data from case series and expert opinion [121,122]. There are a few case reports of success with other agents, including pentoxifylline, montelukast, thalidomide, and hydroxychloroquine [122].

The only treatment for IRIS for which there are randomized clinical trial data is corticosteroids. In a clinical trial of patients with tuberculosis IRIS, patients were randomized to prednisone 1.5 mg/kg per day for two weeks then decreased to 0.75 mg/kg per day for an additional two weeks, versus placebo. The steroid treatment arm had a significant reduction in hospitalization and outpatient therapeutic procedures, more rapid improvement of symptoms, improvement in quality of life, and an improvement in chest X-ray findings. Of note, 10 of the 55 patients had a clinical relapse after the four-week course of steroids ended, suggesting that it is too short for some; in the patients switched to open label corticosteroid use (35), duration was based on clinical response and the median was 84 days. No difference in mortality was seen,

but immediately life-threatening cases were excluded from analysis [123]. Steroids have also independently been shown to improve mortality in cases of TB meningitis, regardless of HIV status [124]. The use of steroids is described with OIs other than tuberculosis as well, though this usage has not been studied with as much rigor. Several case series of disseminated *Mycobacterium avium* complex with MAC-IRIS have demonstrated a clinical response to steroid administration [125,126]. In cryptococcal meningitis, several case reports and retrospective studies have noted clinical benefit in the use of corticosteroids for severe paradoxical IRIS with *Cryptococcus*, though there are no clinical trial data [127,128]. Many clinicians will still advocate the use of corticosteroids in cryptococcal IRIS [113]. Use of corticosteroids in PML, however, is controversial. Some series have shown a clinical benefit, including a systematic review that showed good neurologic recovery in 7/12 patients who received corticosteroids for PML-IRIS [129]. However, inflammation on imaging and CSF sampling (e.g., a CSF pleocytosis) is often associated with improved clinical outcomes and therefore corticosteroids have also been posited to risk blunting the protective response in some patients [130]. As there are no clinical trial data, corticosteroids should be used with caution in PML. It is important to note that unlike in other forms of IRIS, steroids are not recommended in Kaposi sarcoma due to a worsening of disease [113,131–133].

MORBIDITIES IN THE AGING HIV POPULATION

The age of the HIV population in the US and other economically developed countries has been increasing since the introduction of effective ART. Approximately 50% of the HIV-infected population of the United States is currently over the age of 50 and by the year 2030, 70% will be over the age of 50. As the age of the HIV-infected population has increased, the prevalence of co-morbidities associated with aging, such as cardiovascular disease, osteoporosis, renal impairment, and metabolic disorders, has also increased [134]. Patients with HIV also have increased rates of multi-morbidity, defined as two or more chronic conditions, which is associated with increased morbidity and mortality [135].

Because the incidence of co-morbidities, as well as other markers of aging, is increased in HIV-infected patients compared to age matched HIV-uninfected people, aging is believed to be accelerated in HIV-infected patients. Other hallmarks of aging including biomarkers of low level inflammation, epigenetic and chromosomal abnormalities, and metabolic changes are all consistent with accelerated aging. Thus, HIV-infected patients admitted to the CCU have an increased rate of co-morbidities and multi-morbidity that have either been diagnosed or are unrecognized and may have increased markers of biological age. A brief discussion of the important co-morbidities is given below.

Cardiovascular disease: Data from the Veteran Aging Cohort, a large cross sectional study, indicated that HIV-infected patients have a 50% increased risk for acute myocardial infarction [136]. These findings have been confirmed in other studies and have been extended to cerebrovascular disease as well [137–139]. A recent modeling study indicates that the lifetime CVD risk is increased for HIV-infected men compared to those uninfected [140]. In addition, the type of cardiovascular disease may differ. For example, an analysis of HIV-infected patients with acute myocardial infarction indicated that 50% had a type 2 MI (T2MI) caused by a mismatch between oxygen supply and demand, rather than coronary occlusion, which occurs in 80% of HIV-uninfected patients [141]. Thus, physicians caring for patients in the CCU should have a high level of suspicion for cardiovascular disease as a complicating factor in the care of HIV-infected patients.

Metabolic disorders: HIV-infected patients are at greater risk than the general population for the metabolic syndrome and diabetes mellitus if they are obese [142]. HIV-infected patients now have obesity rates greater than 30%, and consequently the rates of metabolic syndrome, insulin resistance, and diabetes mellitus are now increasing [143].

Chronic kidney disease: Chronic kidney disease is increased in HIV-infected patients at all ages compared to the general population and is particularly a risk for those who are aged, black, have diabetes mellitus, have low CD4 counts, or have high viral loads [134,144–146]. In addition, certain antiretrovirals, particularly tenofovir disoproxil fumarate, can be nephrotoxic. In the CCU, acute renal failure, which is increased in those with chronic kidney disease, increases the risk for mortality [147].

Liver disease: Patients with HIV are at increased risk for chronic liver disease secondary to hepatitis B and C, alcoholism, and obesity. Patients with these conditions may have increased inflammation and fibrosis leading to cirrhosis. Pharmacological considerations, liver toxicity, and liver failure are all important factors in the CCU.

Others: In addition to these co-morbidities, patients with HIV are at increased risk for osteoporosis and fractures; neurocognitive disorders; and malignancies, particularly skin and lung cancer, as well as virally related tumors including cervical and anal cancer, B cell lymphomas, and Kaposi's sarcoma [134,148].

CONCLUSION

In summary, it is important to consider routine HIV testing for patients in the CCU to avoid a missed diagnosis that might change management. For patients with a known HIV diagnosis, the care of HIV-infected patients in the CCU is largely the same as the care of HIV-uninfected populations. It is crucial, however, to understand current ART regimens, drug-drug interactions and toxicities, the risk and management of OIs, and HIV-associated comorbidities.

ACKNOWLEDGMENTS

The authors would like to thank Amy Brotherton, PharmD, for her assistance with the development of Table 30.1.

REFERENCES

1. https://www.cdc.gov/hiv/statistics/overview/index.html. 2017.
2. Franzetti F, Grassini A, Piazza M, et al. Nosocomial bacterial pneumonia in HIV-infected patients: Risk factors for adverse outcome and implications for rational empiric antibiotic therapy. *Infection* 2006;34:9–16.
3. Wachter RM, Russi MB, Bloch DA, Hopewell PC, Luce JM. *Pneumocystis carinii* pneumonia and respiratory failure in AIDS. Improved outcomes and increased use of intensive care units. *Am Rev Respir Dis* 1991;143:251–256.
4. Wachter RM, Luce JM, Turner J, Volberding P, Hopewell PC. Intensive care of patients with the acquired immunodeficiency syndrome. Outcome and changing patterns of utilization. *Am Rev Respir Dis* 1986;134:891–896.
5. Rosen MJ, Clayton K, Schneider RF, et al. Intensive care of patients with HIV infection: Utilization, critical illnesses, and outcomes. Pulmonary Complications of HIV Infection Study Group. *Am J Respir Crit Care Med* 1997;155:67–71.
6. Morris A, Creasman J, Turner J, Luce JM, Wachter RM, Huang L. Intensive care of human immunodeficiency virus-infected patients during the era of highly active antiretroviral therapy. *Am J Respir Crit Care Med* 2002;166:262–267.
7. Casalino E, Wolff M, Ravaud P, Choquet C, Bruneel F, Regnier B. Impact of HAART advent on admission patterns and survival in HIV-infected patients admitted to an intensive care unit. *AIDS* 2004;18:1429–1433.
8. Narasimhan M, Posner AJ, DePalo VA, Mayo PH, Rosen MJ. Intensive care in patients with HIV infection in the era of highly active antiretroviral therapy. *Chest* 2004;125:1800–1804.
9. van Lelyveld SF, Wind CM, Mudrikova T, van Leeuwen HJ, de Lange DW, Hoepelman AI. Short- and long-term outcome of HIV-infected patients admitted to the intensive care unit. *Eur J Clin Microbiol Infect Dis* 2011;30:1085–1093.
10. Vincent B, Timsit JF, Auburtin M, et al. Characteristics and outcomes of HIV-infected patients in the ICU: Impact of the highly active antiretroviral treatment era. *Intensive Care Med* 2004;30:859–866.
11. Khouli H, Afrasiabi A, Shibli M, Hajal R, Barrett CR, Homel P. Outcome of critically ill human immunodeficiency virus-infected patients in the era of highly active antiretroviral therapy. *J Intensive Care Med* 2005;20:327–333.
12. Akgun KM, Tate JP, Pisani M, et al. Medical ICU admission diagnoses and outcomes in human immunodeficiency virus-infected and virus-uninfected veterans in the combination antiretroviral era. *Crit Care Med* 2013;41:1458–1467.
13. Vargas-Infante YA, Guerrero ML, Ruiz-Palacios GM, et al. Improving outcome of human immunodeficiency virus-infected patients in a Mexican intensive care unit. *Arch Med Res* 2007;38:827–833.
14. Barbier F, Roux A, Canet E, et al. Temporal trends in critical events complicating HIV infection: 1999–2010 multicentre cohort study in France. *Intensive Care Med* 2014;40:1906–1915.
15. Chiang HH, Hung CC, Lee CM, et al. Admissions to intensive care unit of HIV-infected patients in the era of highly active antiretroviral therapy: Etiology and prognostic factors. *Crit Care* 2011;15:R202.

16. Powell K, Davis JL, Morris AM, Chi A, Bensley MR, Huang L. Survival for patients With HIV admitted to the ICU continues to improve in the current era of combination antiretroviral therapy. *Chest* 2009;135:11–17.

17. Wiewel MA, Huson MA, van Vught LA, et al. Impact of HIV infection on the presentation, outcome and host response in patients admitted to the intensive care unit with sepsis; a case control study. *Crit Care* 2016;20:322.

18. Coquet I, Pavie J, Palmer P, et al. Survival trends in critically ill HIV-infected patients in the highly active antiretroviral therapy era. *Crit Care* 2010;14:R107.

19. Cribbs SK, Tse C, Andrews J, Shenvi N, Martin GS. Characteristics and outcomes of HIV-infected patients with severe sepsis: Continued risk in the post-highly active antiretroviral therapy era. *Crit Care Med* 2015;43:1638–1645.

20. Nickas G, Wachter RM. Outcomes of intensive care for patients with human immunodeficiency virus infection. *Arch Intern Med* 2000;160:541–547.

21. Sarkar P, Rasheed HF. Clinical review: Respiratory failure in HIV-infected patients—a changing picture. *Crit Care* 2013;17:228.

22. Akgun KM, Miller RF. Critical care in human immunodeficiency virus-infected patients. *Semin Respir Crit Care Med* 2016;37:303–317.

23. Turtle L, Vyakernam R, Menon-Johansson A, Nelson MR, Soni N. Intensive care usage by HIV-positive patients in the HAART era. *Interdiscip Perspect Infect Dis* 2011;2011:Article ID 847835.

24. Adlakha A, Pavlou M, Walker DA, et al. Survival of HIV-infected patients admitted to the intensive care unit in the era of highly active antiretroviral therapy. *Int J STD AIDS* 2011;22:498–504.

25. Amancio FF, Lambertucci JR, Cota GF, Antunes CM. Predictors of the short- and long-term survival of HIV-infected patients admitted to a Brazilian intensive care unit. *Int J STD AIDS* 2012;23:692–697.

26. Medrano J, Alvaro-Meca A, Boyer A, Jimenez-Sousa MA, Resino S. Mortality of patients infected with HIV in the intensive care unit (2005 through 2010): Significant role of chronic hepatitis C and severe sepsis. *Crit Care* 2014;18:475.

27. Dickson SJ, Batson S, Copas AJ, Edwards SG, Singer M, Miller RF. Survival of HIV-infected patients in the intensive care unit in the era of highly active antiretroviral therapy. *Thorax* 2007;62:964–968.

28. Force UPST. Final Update Summary: Human Immunodeficiency Virus (HIV) infection: Screening. 2016.

29. Group TAS, Danel C, Moh R, et al. A trial of early antiretrovirals and isoniazid preventive therapy in Africa. *N Engl J Med* 2015;373:808–822.

30. Group ISS, Lundgren JD, Babiker AG, et al. Initiation of antiretroviral therapy in early asymptomatic HIV infection. *N Engl J Med* 2015;373:795–807.

31. Cohen MS, Chen YQ, McCauley M, et al. Prevention of HIV-1 infection with early antiretroviral therapy. *N Engl J Med* 2011;365:493–505.

32. Rodger AJ, Cambiano V, Bruun T, et al. Sexual activity without condoms and risk of HIV transmission in serodifferent couples when the HIV-positive partner is using suppressive antiretroviral therapy. *JAMA* 2016;316:171–181.

33. Zolopa A, Andersen J, Powderly W, et al. Early antiretroviral therapy reduces AIDS progression/death in individuals with acute opportunistic infections: A multicenter randomized strategy trial. *PLOS ONE* 2009;4:e5575.

34. Lanoix JP, Andrejak C, Schmit JL. Antiretroviral therapy in intensive care. *Med Mal Infect* 2011;41:353–358.

35. Panel on Antiretroviral Guidelines for Adults and Adolescents. Guidelines for the Use of Antiretroviral Agents in Adults and Adolescents Living with HIV. Department of Health and Human Services. NIH, 2017.

36. Andrade HB, Shinotsuka CR, da Silva IRF, et al. Highly active antiretroviral therapy for critically ill HIV patients: A systematic review and meta-analysis. *PLOS ONE* 2017;12:e0186968.

37. Blanc FX, Sok T, Laureillard D, et al. Earlier versus later start of antiretroviral therapy in HIV-infected adults with tuberculosis. *N Engl J Med* 2011;365:1471–1481.

38. Abdool Karim SS, Naidoo K, Grobler A, et al. Integration of antiretroviral therapy with tuberculosis treatment. *N Engl J Med* 2011;365:1492–1501.

39. Havlir DV, Kendall MA, Ive P, et al. Timing of antiretroviral therapy for HIV-1 infection and tuberculosis. *N Engl J Med* 2011;365:1482–1491.

40. Makadzange AT, Ndhlovu CE, Takarinda K, et al. Early versus delayed initiation of antiretroviral therapy for concurrent HIV infection and cryptococcal meningitis in sub-Saharan Africa. *Clin Infect Dis* 2010;50:1532–1538.

41. Boulware DR, Meya DB, Muzoora C, et al. Timing of antiretroviral therapy after diagnosis of cryptococcal meningitis. *N Engl J Med* 2014;370:2487–2498.

42. Torok ME, Yen NT, Chau TT, et al. Timing of initiation of antiretroviral therapy in human immunodeficiency virus (HIV)-associated tuberculous meningitis. *Clin Infect Dis* 2011;52:1374–1383.

43. Saag MS. Emtricitabine, a new antiretroviral agent with activity against HIV and hepatitis B virus. *Clin Infect Dis* 2006;42:126–131.

44. Perry CM, Faulds D. Lamivudine. A review of its antiviral activity, pharmacokinetic properties and therapeutic efficacy in the management of HIV infection. *Drugs* 1997;53:657–680.

45. Pozniak A. Tenofovir: What have over 1 million years of patient experience taught us? *Int J Clin Pract* 2008;62:1285–1293.

46. Gibson AK, Shah BM, Nambiar PH, Schafer JJ. Tenofovir alafenamide. *Ann Pharmacother* 2016;50:942–952.

47. Rizzardini G, Zucchi P. Abacavir and lamivudine for the treatment of human immunodeficiency virus. *Expert Opin Pharmacother* 2011;12:2129–2138.

48. Strategies for Management of Anti-Retroviral Therapy I, Groups DADS. Use of nucleoside reverse transcriptase inhibitors and risk of myocardial infarction in HIV-infected patients. *AIDS* 2008;22:F17–F24.

49. Brothers CH, Hernandez JE, Cutrell AG, et al. Risk of myocardial infarction and abacavir therapy: No increased risk across 52 GlaxoSmithKline-sponsored clinical trials in adult subjects. *J Acquir Immune Defic Syndr* 2009;51:20–28.

50. Ding X, Andraca-Carrera E, Cooper C, et al. No association of abacavir use with myocardial infarction: Findings of an FDA meta-analysis. *J Acquir Immune Defic Syndr* 2012;61:441–447.

51. Sharma M, Walmsley SL. Raltegravir as antiretroviral therapy in HIV/AIDS. *Expert Opin Pharmacother* 2014;15:395–405.

52. Perry CM. Elvitegravir/cobicistat/emtricitabine/tenofovir disoproxil fumarate single-tablet regimen (Stribild(R)): A review of its use in the management of HIV-1 infection in adults. *Drugs* 2014;74:75–97.

53. Shah BM, Schafer JJ, Desimone JA, Jr. Dolutegravir: A new integrase strand transfer inhibitor for the treatment of HIV. *Pharmacotherapy* 2014;34:506–520.

54. Clinical Pharmacology of the HIV Integrase Strand Transfer Inhibitor Bictegravir. Oral presentation at CROI 2017, Seattle, WA, 2017.

55. Capetti A, Rizzardini G. Cobicistat: A new opportunity in the treatment of HIV disease? *Expert Opin Pharmacother* 2014;15:1289–1298.

56. Vrouenraets SM, Wit FW, van Tongeren J, Lange JM. Efavirenz: A review. *Expert Opin Pharmacother* 2007;8:851–871.

57. Deeks ED. Darunavir: A review of its use in the management of HIV-1 infection. *Drugs* 2014;74:99–125.

58. Croom KF, Dhillon S, Keam SJ. Atazanavir: A review of its use in the management of HIV-1 infection. *Drugs* 2009;69:1107–1140.

59. Rhodes A, Evans LE, Alhazzani W, et al. Surviving sepsis campaign: International guidelines for management of sepsis and septic shock: 2016. *Intensive Care Med* 2017;43:304–377.

60. Pollack LA, van Santen KL, Weiner LM, Dudeck MA, Edwards JR, Srinivasan A. Antibiotic stewardship programs in U.S. acute care hospitals: Findings From the 2014 National Healthcare Safety Network Annual Hospital Survey. *Clin Infect Dis* 2016;63:443–449.

61. Kumar A, Roberts D, Wood KE, et al. Duration of hypotension before initiation of effective antimicrobial therapy is the critical determinant of survival in human septic shock. *Crit Care Med* 2006;34:1589–1596.

62. Ferrer R, Martin-Loeches I, Phillips G, et al. Empiric antibiotic treatment reduces mortality in severe sepsis and septic shock from the first hour: Results from a guideline-based performance improvement program. *Crit Care Med* 2014;42:1749–1755.

63. Dorobat CM, Dorobat G, Bejan C, et al. Antibiotic therapy in severe sepsis in HIV-positive patients. *Rev Med Chir Soc Med Nat Iasi* 2012;116:714–717.

64. Cobos-Trigueros N, Rinaudo M, Sole M, et al. Acquisition of resistant microorganisms and infections in HIV-infected patients admitted to the ICU. *Eur J Clin Microbiol Infect Dis* 2014;33:611–620.

65. Annane D, Sebille V, Charpentier C, et al. Effect of treatment with low doses of hydrocortisone and fludrocortisone on mortality in patients with septic shock. *JAMA* 2002;288:862–871.

66. Sprung CL, Annane D, Keh D, et al. Hydrocortisone therapy for patients with septic shock. *N Engl J Med* 2008;358:111–124.

67. Investigators N-SS, Finfer S, Chittock DR, et al. Intensive versus conventional glucose control in critically ill patients. *N Engl J Med* 2009;360:1283–1297.

68. Soeiro Ade M, Ruppert AD, Canzian M, Parra ER, Farhat C, Capelozzi VL. Demographic, etiological, and histological pulmonary analysis of patients with acute respiratory failure: A study of 19 years of autopsies. *Clinics (Sao Paulo)* 2011;66:1193–1197.

69. Lopez-Aldeguer J, Iribarren JA, Valencia E, et al. Outcomes in HIV-infected patients admitted due to pandemic influenza. *Enferm Infecc Microbiol Clin* 2012;30:608–612.

70. Gilroy SA, Bennett NJ. Pneumocystis pneumonia. *Semin Respir Crit Care Med* 2011;32:775–782.

71. Martinez E, Marcos MA, Hoyo-Ulloa I, et al. Influenza A H1N1 in HIV-infected adults. *HIV Med* 2011; 12:236–245.

72. Mandell LA, Wunderink RG, Anzueto A, et al. Infectious Diseases Society of America/American Thoracic Society consensus guidelines on the management of community-acquired pneumonia in adults. *Clin Infect Dis* 2007;44 Suppl 2:S27–S72.

73. Kalil AC, Metersky ML, Klompas M, et al. Management of adults with hospital-acquired and ventilator-associated pneumonia: 2016 Clinical practice guidelines by the Infectious Diseases Society of America and the American Thoracic Society. *Clin Infect Dis* 2016;63:e61–e111.

74. Popovich KJ, Hota B, Aroutcheva A, et al. Community-associated methicillin-resistant *Staphylococcus aureus* colonization burden in HIV-infected patients. *Clin Infect Dis* 2013;56:1067–1074.

75. Bele N, Darmon M, Coquet I, et al. Diagnostic accuracy of procalcitonin in critically ill immunocompromised patients. *BMC Infect Dis* 2011;11:224.

76. Balkema CA, Irusen EM, Taljaard JJ, Zeier MD, Koegelenberg CF. A prospective study on the outcome of human immunodeficiency virus-infected patients requiring mechanical ventilation in a high-burden setting. *QJM* 2016;109:35–40.

77. Fine MJ, Auble TE, Yealy DM, et al. A prediction rule to identify low-risk patients with community-acquired pneumonia. *N Engl J Med* 1997;336:243–250.

78. Lim WS, van der Eerden MM, Laing R, et al. Defining community acquired pneumonia severity on presentation to hospital: An international derivation and validation study. *Thorax* 2003;58:377–382.

79. Lisboa T, Diaz E, Sa-Borges M, et al. The ventilator-associated pneumonia PIRO score: A tool for predicting ICU mortality and health-care resources use in ventilator-associated pneumonia. *Chest* 2008;134:1208–1216.

80. Smit M, Hallett T. Respiratory co-morbidities in people with HIV. *Lancet Infect Dis* 2016;16:152.

81. Siemieniuk RA, Meade MO, Alonso-Coello P, et al. Corticosteroid therapy for patients hospitalized with community-acquired pneumonia: A systematic review and meta-analysis. *Ann Intern Med* 2015;163:519–528.

82. Blum CA, Nigro N, Briel M, et al. Adjunct prednisone therapy for patients with community-acquired pneumonia: A multi-centre, double-blind, randomised, placebo-controlled trial. *Lancet* 2015;385:1511–1518.

83. Moon SM, Kim T, Sung H, et al. Outcomes of moderate-to-severe Pneumocystis pneumonia treated with adjunctive steroid in non-HIV-infected patients. *Antimicrob Agents Chemother* 2011;55:4613–4618.

84. Montaner JS, Lawson LM, Levitt N, Belzberg A, Schechter MT, Ruedy J. Corticosteroids prevent early deterioration in patients with moderately severe *Pneumocystis carinii* pneumonia and the acquired immunodeficiency syndrome (AIDS). *Ann Intern Med* 1990;113:14–20.

85. Gagnon S, Boota AM, Fischl MA, Baier H, Kirksey OW, La Voie L. Corticosteroids as adjunctive therapy for severe *Pneumocystis carinii* pneumonia in the acquired immunodeficiency syndrome. A double-blind, placebo-controlled trial. *N Engl J Med* 1990;323:1444–1450.

86. Canadian Critical Care Trials G. A randomized trial of diagnostic techniques for ventilator-associated pneumonia. *N Engl J Med* 2006;355:2619–2630.

87. Fagon JY. Diagnosis and treatment of ventilator-associated pneumonia: Fiberoptic bronchoscopy with bronchoalveolar lavage is essential. *Semin Respir Crit Care Med* 2006;27:34–44.

88. Frat JP, Thille AW, Mercat A, et al. High-flow oxygen through nasal cannula in acute hypoxemic respiratory failure. *N Engl J Med* 2015;372:2185–2196.

89. Lemiale V, Mokart D, Mayaux J, et al. The effects of a 2-h trial of high-flow oxygen by nasal cannula versus Venturi mask in immunocompromised patients with hypoxemic acute respiratory failure: A multicenter randomized trial. *Crit Care* 2015;19:380.

90. Force ADT, Ranieri VM, Rubenfeld GD, et al. Acute respiratory distress syndrome: The Berlin definition. *JAMA* 2012;307:2526–2533.

91. Meade MO, Cook DJ, Guyatt GH, et al. Ventilation strategy using low tidal volumes, recruitment maneuvers, and high positive end-expiratory pressure for acute lung injury and acute respiratory distress syndrome: A randomized controlled trial. *JAMA* 2008;299:637–645.

92. Acute Respiratory Distress Syndrome N, Brower RG, Matthay MA, et al. Ventilation with lower tidal volumes as compared with traditional tidal volumes for acute lung injury and the acute respiratory distress syndrome. *N Engl J Med* 2000;342:1301–1308.

93. Brower RG, Lanken PN, MacIntyre N, et al. Higher versus lower positive end-expiratory pressures in patients with the acute respiratory distress syndrome. *N Engl J Med* 2004;351:327–336.

94. Guerin C, Reignier J, Richard JC, et al. Prone positioning in severe acute respiratory distress syndrome. *N Engl J Med* 2013;368:2159–2168.

95. Papazian L, Forel JM, Gacouin A, et al. Neuromuscular blockers in early acute respiratory distress syndrome. *N Engl J Med* 2010;363:1107–1116.

96. Brodie D, Bacchetta M. Extracorporeal membrane oxygenation for ARDS in adults. *N Engl J Med* 2011;365:1905–1914.

97. Peek GJ, Mugford M, Tiruvoipati R, et al. Efficacy and economic assessment of conventional ventilatory support versus extracorporeal membrane oxygenation for severe adult respiratory failure (CESAR): A multicentre randomised controlled trial. *Lancet* 2009;374:1351–1363.

98. Morley D, Lynam A, Carton E, et al. Extracorporeal membrane oxygenation in an HIV-positive man with severe acute respiratory distress syndrome secondary to pneumocystis and cytomegalovirus pneumonia. *Int J STD AIDS* 2017;29(2):198–202.

99. Ali HS, Hassan IF, George S. Extra corporeal membrane oxygenation to facilitate lung protective ventilation and prevent ventilator-induced lung injury in severe Pneumocystis pneumonia with pneumomediastinum: A case report and short literature review. *BMC Pulm Med* 2016;16:52.

100. Cawcutt K, Gallo De Moraes A, Lee SJ, Park JG, Schears GJ, Nemergut ME. The use of ECMO in HIV/AIDS with *Pneumocystis jirovecii* pneumonia: A case report and review of the literature. *ASAIO J* 2014;60:606–608.

101. De Rosa FG, Fanelli V, Corcione S, et al. Extra Corporeal Membrane Oxygenation (ECMO) in three HIV-positive patients with acute respiratory distress syndrome. *BMC Anesthesiol* 2014;14:37.

102. Ely EW, Baker AM, Dunagan DP, et al. Effect on the duration of mechanical ventilation of identifying patients capable of breathing spontaneously. *N Engl J Med* 1996;335:1864–1869.

103. Esteban A, Frutos F, Tobin MJ, et al. A comparison of four methods of weaning patients from mechanical ventilation. Spanish Lung Failure Collaborative Group. *N Engl J Med* 1995;332:345–350.

104. Girard TD, Kress JP, Fuchs BD, et al. Efficacy and safety of a paired sedation and ventilator weaning protocol for mechanically ventilated patients in intensive care (Awakening and Breathing Controlled trial): A randomised controlled trial. *Lancet* 2008;371:126–134.

105. Siegel M, Masur H, Kovacs J. *Pneumocystis jirovecii* pneumonia in human immunodeficiency virus infection. *Semin Respir Crit Care Med* 2016;37:243–256.

106. Crans CA, Jr, Boiselle PM. Imaging features of *Pneumocystis carinii* pneumonia. *Crit Rev Diagn Imaging* 1999;40:251–284.

107. Richards PJ, Riddell L, Reznek RH, Armstrong P, Pinching AJ, Parkin JM. High resolution computed tomography in HIV patients with suspected *Pneumocystis carinii* pneumonia and a normal chest radiograph. *Clin Radiol* 1996;51:689–693.

108. Thomas CF, Jr., Limper AH. Pneumocystis pneumonia. *N Engl J Med* 2004;350:2487–2498.

109. Turner D, Schwarz Y, Yust I. Induced sputum for diagnosing *Pneumocystis carinii* pneumonia in HIV patients: New data, new issues. *Eur Respir J* 2003;21:204–208.

110. Siegel MO, Ghafouri S, Ajmera R, Simon GL. Immune reconstitution inflammatory syndrome, human herpesvirus 8 viremia, and HIV-associated multicentric Castleman disease. *Int J Infect Dis* 2016;48:49–51.

111. Bonarek M, Morlat P, Chene G, et al. Prognostic score of short-term survival in HIV-infected patients admitted to medical intensive care units. *Int J STD AIDS* 2001;12:239–244.

112. Nahid P, Dorman SE, Alipanah N, et al. Official American thoracic society/centers for disease control and prevention/ infectious diseases society of America clinical practice guidelines: Treatment of drug-susceptible tuberculosis. *Clin Infect Dis* 2016;63:e147–e195.

113. Meintjes G, Scriven J, Marais S. Management of the immune reconstitution inflammatory syndrome. *Curr HIV/AIDS Rep* 2012;9:238–250.

114. Lawn SD, Bekker LG, Myer L, Orrell C, Wood R. Cryptococcocal immune reconstitution disease: A major cause of early mortality in a South African antiretroviral programme. *AIDS* 2005;19:2050–205.

115. Kumarasamy N, Chaguturu S, Mayer KH, et al. Incidence of immune reconstitution syndrome in HIV/tuberculosis-coinfected patients after initiation of generic antiretroviral therapy in India. *J Acquir Immune Defic Syndr* 2004;37:1574–1576.

116. Narita M, Ashkin D, Hollender ES, Pitchenik AE. Paradoxical worsening of tuberculosis following antiretroviral therapy in patients with AIDS. *Am J Respir Crit Care Med* 1998;158:157–161.

117. French MA, Lenzo N, John M, et al. Immune restoration disease after the treatment of immunodeficient HIV-infected patients with highly active antiretroviral therapy. *HIV Med* 2000;1:107–115.

118. Jevtovic DJ, Salemovic D, Ranin J, Pesic I, Zerjav S, Djurkovic-Djakovic O. The prevalence and risk of immune restoration disease in HIV-infected patients treated with highly active antiretroviral therapy. *HIV Med* 2005;6:140–143.

119. Boulware DR, Meya DB, Bergemann TL, et al. Clinical features and serum biomarkers in HIV immune reconstitution inflammatory syndrome after cryptococcal meningitis: A prospective cohort study. *PLoS Med* 2010;7:e1000384.

120. Muller M, Wandel S, Colebunders R, et al. Immune reconstitution inflammatory syndrome in patients starting antiretroviral therapy for HIV infection: A systematic review and meta-analysis. *Lancet Infect Dis* 2010;10:251–261.

121. Achenbach CJ, Harrington RD, Dhanireddy S, Crane HM, Casper C, Kitahata MM. Paradoxical immune reconstitution inflammatory syndrome in HIV-infected patients treated with combination antiretroviral therapy after AIDS-defining opportunistic infection. *Clin Infect Dis* 2012;54:424–433.

122. Marais S, Wilkinson RJ, Pepper DJ, Meintjes G. Management of patients with the immune reconstitution inflammatory syndrome. *Curr HIV/AIDS Rep* 2009;6:162–171.

123. Meintjes G, Wilkinson RJ, Morroni C, et al. Randomized placebo-controlled trial of prednisone for paradoxical tuberculosis-associated immune reconstitution inflammatory syndrome. *AIDS* 2010;24:2381–2390.

124. Thwaites GE, Nguyen DB, Nguyen HD, et al. Dexamethasone for the treatment of tuberculous meningitis in adolescents and adults. *N Engl J Med* 2004;351:1741–1751.

125. Riddell J, Kaul DR, Karakousis PC, Gallant JE, Mitty J, Kazanjian PH. Mycobacterium avium complex immune reconstitution inflammatory syndrome: Long term outcomes. *J Transl Med* 2007;5:50.

126. Phillips P, Bonner S, Gataric N, et al. Nontuberculous mycobacterial immune reconstitution syndrome in HIV-infected patients: Spectrum of disease and long-term follow-up. *Clin Infect Dis* 2005;41:1483–1497.

127. Lortholary O, Fontanet A, Memain N, et al. Incidence and risk factors of immune reconstitution inflammatory syndrome complicating HIV-associated cryptococcosis in France. *AIDS* 2005;19:1043–1049.

128. Venkataramana A, Pardo CA, McArthur JC, et al. Immune reconstitution inflammatory syndrome in the CNS of HIV-infected patients. *Neurology* 2006;67:383–388.

129. Tan K, Roda R, Ostrow L, McArthur J, Nath A. PML-IRIS in patients with HIV infection: Clinical manifestations and treatment with steroids. *Neurology* 2009;72:1458–1464.

130. Berger JR. Steroids for PML-IRIS: A double-edged sword? *Neurology* 2009;72:1454–1455.

131. Crane HM, Deubner H, Huang JC, Swanson PE, Harrington RD. Fatal Kaposi's sarcoma-associated immune reconstitution following HAART initiation. *Int J STD AIDS* 2005;16:80–83.

132. Volkow PF, Cornejo P, Zinser JW, Ormsby CE, Reyes-Teran G. Life-threatening exacerbation of Kaposi's sarcoma after prednisone treatment for immune reconstitution inflammatory syndrome. *AIDS* 2008;22:663–665.

133. Gill PS, Loureiro C, Bernstein-Singer M, Rarick MU, Sattler F, Levine AM. Clinical effect of glucocorticoids on Kaposi sarcoma related to the acquired immunodeficiency syndrome (AIDS). *Ann Intern Med* 1989;110:937–940.

134. Rasmussen LD, May MT, Kronborg G, et al. Time trends for risk of severe age-related diseases in individuals with and without HIV infection in Denmark: A nationwide population-based cohort study. *Lancet HIV* 2015;2:e288–e298.

135. Guaraldi G, Orlando G, Zona S, et al. Premature age-related comorbidities among HIV-infected persons compared with the general population. *Clin Infect Dis* 2011;53:1120–1126.

136. Freiberg MS, Chang CC, Kuller LH, et al. HIV infection and the risk of acute myocardial infarction. *JAMA Intern Med* 2013;173:614–622.

137. Sico JJ, Chang CC, So-Armah K, et al. HIV status and the risk of ischemic stroke among men. *Neurology* 2015;84:1933–1940.

138. Obel N, Thomsen HF, Kronborg G, et al. Ischemic heart disease in HIV-infected and HIV-uninfected individuals: A population-based cohort study. *Clin Infect Dis* 2007;44:1625–1631.

139. Klein DB, Leyden WA, Xu L, et al. Declining relative risk for myocardial infarction among HIV-positive compared with HIV-negative individuals with access to care. *Clin Infect Dis* 2015;60:1278–1280.

140. Losina E, Hyle EP, Borre ED, et al. Projecting 10-year, 20-year, and lifetime risks of cardiovascular disease in persons living with human immunodeficiency virus in the United States. *Clin Infect Dis* 2017;65:1266–1271.

141. Crane HM, Paramsothy P, Drozd DR, et al. Types of myocardial infarction among human immunodeficiency virus-infected individuals in the United States. *JAMA Cardiol* 2017;2:260–267.

142. Brown TT, Cole SR, Li X, et al. Antiretroviral therapy and the prevalence and incidence of diabetes mellitus in the multicenter AIDS cohort study. *Arch Intern Med* 2005;165:1179–1184.

143. Willig AL, Overton ET. Metabolic complications and glucose metabolism in HIV infection: A review of the evidence. *Curr HIV/AIDS Rep* 2016;13:289–296.

144. Ando M, Tsuchiya K, Nitta K. How to manage HIV-infected patients with chronic kidney disease in the HAART era. *Clin Exp Nephrol* 2012;16:363–372.

145. Abraham AG, Althoff KN, Jing Y, et al. End-stage renal disease among HIV-infected adults in North America. *Clin Infect Dis* 2015;60:941–949.

146. Cohen SD, Kopp JB, Kimmel PL. Kidney diseases associated with human immunodeficiency virus infection. *N Engl J Med* 2017;377:2363–2374.

147. Randall DW, Brima N, Walker D, et al. Acute kidney injury among HIV-infected patients admitted to the intensive care unit. *Int J STD AIDS* 2015;26:915–921.

148. Wing EJ. HIV and aging. *Int J Infect Dis* 2016;53:61–68.

149. Foisy M, Tseng A. Liquid drug formulations. Toronto General Hospital Immunodeficiency Clinic. Available at: http://hivclinic.ca/main/drugs_extra_files/LIQUID%20DRUG%20FORMULATIONS.pdf. Accessed on January 15, 2018.

150. Foisy M, Hughes C, Lamb S, Tseng A. Oral antiretroviral administration: Information on crushing and liquid drug formulations. Toronto General Hospital Immunodeficiency Clinic. Available at: http://www.hivclinic.ca/main/drugs_extra_files/Crushing%20and%20Liquid%20ARV%20Formulations.pdf. Accessed on January 15, 2018.

Section IV

Antimicrobial Therapy and Antibiotic Stewardship in the Critical Care Unit

31 Principles of Antibiotic Stewardship in the Critical Care Unit

Cheston B. Cunha

CONTENTS

CLINICAL PERSPECTIVE

Infectious disease (ID) clinicians, particularly those with expertise in antibiotic therapy, have traditionally been the stewards of antimicrobial therapy. The principles of optimal antibiotic use are now included in antibiotic stewardship programs (ASPs). Effective ASPs are dependent on hospital-wide efforts involving the coordination of activities and interventions under the leadership of the ID clinician ASP team leader. The ID ASP team leader and support group of ID trained clinical pharmacists (PharmDs) provide expert consultation and guidance in optimizing antibiotic therapy. The ASP includes coordination with the medical microbiology laboratory and infection control (IC) and hospital epidemiology. The success of the program is dependent on the ID clinicians ASP teams' financial support of hospital administration and medical education of the staff (Table 31.1).

The primary ASP task is to optimize antibiotic therapy while containing antibiotic resistance and adverse effects, e.g., drug side effects, *C. difficile*, in a cost-effective manner. The effectiveness of various ASP interventions is best assessed using prospective audits. Prospective audits are the best way to assess the effectiveness of ASP initiatives in each hospital. With ASPs, one size does not fit all; what works in one hospital doesn't apply or work in another. Certainly, the devil is in the details.

The ASP initiatives in the critical care unit (CCU) are an important subset of hospital-wide ASP efforts, but some ASP concerns take on added importance in the CCU setting, e.g., appropriate antibiotic spectrum, optimal dosing based on pharmacokinetic/pharmacodynamic (PK/PD) considerations, and antibiotic resistance (Table 31.2).

This chapter is an overview of CCU-focused ASP principles obtained in the following chapters elsewhere in the book: fever in the CCU, severe CAP in the CCU, NA/CAP treatment/containment of multiresistant organisms (MDROs), approach to *C. difficile* diarrhea (CDD)/ *C. difficile* colitis (CDC), and clinical approach to antibiotic failure. This chapter is a synopsis of the most critical ASP aspects in the CCU [1].

TABLE 31.1

Antimicrobial Stewardship

Colonization vs. Infection

- Treat infection, not colonization.
- Provide empiric coverage primarily directed against the most probable pathogens causing the infection at the body site.
- Avoid "covering" or "chasing" multiple organisms cultured that are not (pathogens and non-pathogens) at the body site cultured.
- Colonization of respiratory secretions, wounds, or urine with "water" (*S. maltophilia*, *B. cepacia*, and *P. aeruginosa*) or skin organisms (MSSA, MRSA, CoNS, VSE, and VRE) is the rule.

Narrow- vs. Broad-Spectrum Therapy

- Narrow- vs. broad-spectrum therapy does not prevent resistance; e.g., in treating *E. coli* urosepsis, switching from a carbapenem (broad spectrum) to ampicillin (narrow spectrum) may actually increase resistance potential.
- Narrow- vs. broad-spectrum therapy may not be clinically superior to well-chosen broad-spectrum therapy, e.g., switching from ceftriaxone (broad spectrum) to penicillin in treating *S. pneumoniae* has no clinical rationale or clinical advantage and has no effect on controlling resistance.
- Antibiotic resistance is not related to spectrum narrowness or broadness, e.g., levofloxacin (broad spectrum but "low resistance potential") vs. ampicillin (narrow spectrum but "high resistance potential").

(Continued)

TABLE 31.1 (*Continued*)

Antimicrobial Stewardship

Antibiotic Resistance

- The best way to control resistance is a selectively restricted formulary and restricting "high resistance potential" antibiotics, e.g., imipenem (not meropenem or ertapenem), ceftazidime (not other third of fourth GC), and gentamicin/tobramycin (not amikacin).
- Some antibiotics may be restricted for other reasons, e.g., excessive vancomycin (IV not PO) use predisposes to VRE emergence, and vancomycin may cause cell wall thickening in *S. aureus*, resulting in permeability-related resistance (to vancomycin and other antibiotics, e.g., daptomycin).
- Excessive restriction of antibiotics may impair timely effective therapy and does not, per se, decrease resistance.
- Preferentially select antibiotics (all other things being equal) with a "low resistance potential." Avoid, if possible, "high resistance potential" antibiotics, e.g., macrolides (for respiratory infections) and TMP-SMX (for UTIs).
- Since resistance is, in part, concentration dependent, subtherapeutic or low antibiotic tissue concentrations (all other things being equal) predispose to resistance.
- Suboptimal dosing or usual dosing with inadequate tissue penetration, e.g., into the body fluids or undrained abscesses (source control is key), predisposes to resistance.

Monotherapy vs. Combination Therapy

- Preferably use monotherapy, whenever possible, to cover the most likely pathogen or cultured pathogen clinically relevant to the site of infection.
- Combination therapy should be avoided if possible. Always try to preferentially use monotherapy.
- Monotherapy is usually less expensive than combination therapy and has less potential for adverse effects and drug-drug interactions.
- Combination therapy is often used for potential synergy (rarely occurs and if used must be based on microbiology laboratory synergy studies), to increase spectrum (preferable to use monotherapy with same spectrum), or to prevent resistance (except for TB).

PO and IV-to-PO Switch Antibiotic Therapy

- Wherever possible, treat with entirely oral antibiotic therapy instead of IV therapy.
- Switch from IV-to-PO antibiotic therapy after clinical defervescence (usually <72 hours).
- Early IV-to-PO switch therapy eliminates phlebitis and IV line-associated infections.

Antibiotic De-escalation

- De-escalation is problematic if based on microbiology data alone, without site-pathogen correlation.
- De-escalation is appropriate in the setting of broad-spectrum coverage of "presumed urosepsis," which can be narrowed after the uropathogen is identified in blood/urine.
- In intubated/ventilate patients, microbiology data from respiratory secretion cultures are usually misleading and not representative of NP or VAP lung pathogens.
- In patients with NP or VAP, it is more prudent to treat the most likely pathogen, e.g., *P. aeruginosa* (even if not cultured from respiratory secretions), than to be misguided into treating multiple colonizing organisms in respiratory secretions.
- De-escalation can be harmful if microbiology data is misleading, e.g., represents colonization rather than being reflective of the pathogen (underlying bone pathogen, not ulcer organisms), e.g., diabetic foot ulcers/chronic osteomyelitis or sacral ulcers/chronic osteomyelitis.

C. difficile Diarrhea/Colitis

- Preferentially select antibiotics (all other things being equal) with low *C. difficile* potential.
- Predisposing factors to *C. difficile* include relatively few antibiotics, e.g., clindamycin, β-lactams, ciprofloxacin.
- Many antibiotics have little *C. difficile* potential, e.g., aminoglycosides, aztreonam, macrolides, TMP-SMX, colistin, polymyxin B, daptomycin, Q/D, doxycycline, minocycline, tigecycline, vancomycin, and linezolid.
- Some antibiotics are protective against *C. difficile*, e.g., doxycycline and tigecycline.
- Always consider non-antibiotic factors that may predispose to *C. difficile*, e.g., cancer chemotherapy, anti-depressants, statins, and PPIs.
- Also consider person-to-person spread or acquisition for the environment.

Abbreviations: MSSA, methicillin-susceptible Staphylococcus aureus; MRSA, methicillin-resistant Staphylococcus aureus; CoNS, coagulase negative staphylococci; VSE, vancomycin-susceptible enterococci; VRE, vancomycin-resistant enterococci.

ASP CONSIDERATION IS APPROPRIATE SPECTRUM AND AVOIDANCE OF EXCESSIVE OR UNNECESSARY COVERAGE

BLOOD CULTURE POSITIVITY VS. BACTEREMIA

Empiric antimicrobial therapy should be directed against the most likely pathogens at the site of infection. Unless clinically relevant to the infection site, isolates from blood or various body sites should not be "covered," i.e., *Staphylococcus aureus* cultured from urine (*S. aureus* is not a uropathogen).

The CCU clinicians must carefully differentiate positive blood cultures from true bacteremia. With few exceptions,

aerobic gram-negative bacilli (GNB) are rarely skin contaminants during venipuncture and usually point to a GI or GU track source, and accordingly, the empiric antibiotic selected should be active against the most common GNBs for the GI/GU tract until subsequent diagnoses or isolate identification localize the organ infected (with its most likely pathogens).

In contrast, the situation is more complicated with blood cultures (BCs) positive for gram-positive cocci (GPC). There are three determinants of blood culture significance with GPC in BCs. First is the BC positive (1/4–2/4), i.e., 1/4 BC with GPC, in clusters, likely represents a skin containment and does not represent bacteremia. The degree of BC positive with GPC in

TABLE 31.2

Pharmacokinetic/Pharmacodynamic Considerations

Antibiotics	Optimal Dosing Strategies
Concentration-Dependent Antibiotics (Cmax:MIC)	
• Quinolones • Doxycycline • Aminoglycosides • Tigecycline • Vancomycin (if MIC >1 µg/mL, use 2 g (IV) q12h) • Polymyxin B • Colistin	Use highest effective dose without toxicity
Time Dependent Antibiotics (T > MIC)	
• PCN: Maintain concentrations > MIC for >60% of the dosing interval • β-lactams: Maintain concentrations > MIC for >75% of the dosing interval • Carbapenems: Maintain concentrations > MIC for >40% of the dosing interval • Vancomycin (if MIC <1 µg/mL, use 1 g (IV) q12h)	Use high doses (which increase serum concentrations and which also increases T > MIC for more of the dosing interval)

Source: Cunha, C.B., and Cunha, B.A. (Eds.), *Antibiotic Essentials* (16th ed.), Jay Pee Medical Publishers, New Delhi, India, 2018.
Abbreviation: MIC, minimum inhibitory concentration.

clusters predicts likely bacteremia and should prompt a search for a source, e.g., skin abscesses, bone/joint infections, central venous catheter (CVC) associated bacteremia, and acute bacterial endocarditis (ABE). Sources that are not generations of high-grade GPC bacteremias (3/4–4/4 BC) are the lungs, abdomen (if no recent intra-abdominal surgery), and urinary tract infection (no percutaneous procedures). The second consideration is time to positive cultures (TTPC). *S. aureus* and *S. epididymitis*, i.e., coagulase-negative staphylococci (CoNS), have short replication times, and *bona fide* infection should become positive in <2 days TTPC. If the TTPC with GPC in clusters is >2 days, its clinical significance should be questioned.

The third diagnostic consideration is the arrangement of GPC in the BC isolate, i.e., diplococci (*S. pneumoniae*), pairs/chains (streptococci), or clusters (*S. aureus* or CoNS). Nearly always, GPC in pairs/chains represent *bona fide* pathogens, and even 1/4 BC has clinical relevance. The arrangement of GPC in BC should direct the diagnostic workup to determine the source of the bacteremia, i.e., diplococci (*S. pneumoniae*) indicates upper/lower respiratory source. If GPC are in chains, then the differential diagnosis (DDx) is between Group A streptococci (GAS)/Group B streptococci (GBS) and Group D enterococci, i.e., vancomycin-sensitive enterococci (VSE) and vancomycin-resistant enterococci (VRE). The organism isolated provides the clue to site/origin of the bacteria; e.g., VSE or VRE indicates a hepatobiliary or GU source, and GAS/GBS indicates a skin source.

The interpretation of enterococci in BCs should also take into account possible BC contamination during venipuncture, e.g., 1/4 BC positive for VSE or VRE should be considered a skin contaminant until proven otherwise. In contrast, if the clinical presentation is that of a GI/GU source, then 1/4 BC positive for VSE/VRE should be researched as clinically significant.

Another common clinical problem with interpreting the clinical relevance of GCs positive for GPC is that of the viridans streptococci (VS). In BCs, the VS appear in pairs/chains. Their clinical significance depends on degree of BC positivity and potential organ source. First, 1/4–2/4 nearly always represents

skin contamination during venipuncture. In contrast, 3/4 or 4/4 BCs positive for VS likely represent an intra-abdominal source (abscess depending on species, i.e., *Streptococcus intermedius*) versus subacute bacterial endocarditis (SBE). If the patient has SBE, BC positivity will be high grade (3/4–4/4+ BCs) and will continuously be accompanied by the clinical features of SBE. If the 4/4 BC isolate VS was *S. intermedius*, then an intra-abdominal source (hepatic/abdominal abscess) should be suspected, since this species doesn't cause SBE. The converse is also helpful clinically, i.e., even in the presence of a cardiac murmur, 1/4–2/4 BC+ for NS effectively rules over SBE from further diagnostic consideration [2].

Avoidance of Excessive and Unnecessary Coverage

The most common ASP examples of excessive/unnecessary spectrum is that of the ampiric treatment of potential ventilator-associated pneumonia (pVAP). In many cases in the CCU, the criteria for pVAP is non-specific and not diagnostic. In the CCU, there are many patients without pVAP who have fever, leukocytosis, and new pulmonary infiltrates due to non-pulmonary causes, e.g., chronic heart failure (CHF), pulmonary hemorrhage, pulmonary drug reactions, and pulmonary emboli.

If pVAP is likely, coverage should be directed against the usual aerobic GNB VAP pathogens, i.e., *P. aeruginosa* (the most virulent, but not the most common) and other GNB, but not *B. cepacia*, *S. maltophilia*, *Acinetobacter* sp., *Enterobacter* sp. Serratia marcesens, and *K. pneumoniae* are relatively rare causes of VAP [2].

Gram-positive cocci, particularly *S. aureus* (methicillin-sensitive *S. aureus* [MSSA]/methicillin-resistant *S. aureus* [MRSA]), are common colonizers of respiratory secretions in ventilated patients, but MSSA/MRSA are not the causes of NP/VAP. As many of a third of ventilated CCU patients will have respiratory secretion cultures positive for MSSA/MRSA. Colonization of respiratory secretion results from other colonizer selective pressure. If an antibiotic is selected from empiric NP/VAP coverage and has limited antibiotic

S. aureus activity, MSSA/MRSA will emerge as the aerobic GNB are suppressed/eliminated; e.g., ceftazidime has a limited anti-*S. aureus* activity [1].

The most common ASP error in the CCU is unnecessary coverage for MSSA/MRSA cultures from respiratory secretions in ventilated patients. While *bona fide* MSSA/MRSA CAP does occur in patients with influenza, it's clinical presentation is remarkable and should allow selective us of anti-Staph therapy in these patients. Clinical features have been well described for decades. Influenza with MSSA/MRSA CAP presents with abrupt onset of high fevers, bloody sputum, organisms/elastin fibers in respiratory secretions, and rapid cavitation with thick walled cavities. In purported cases of MSSA/MRSA NP/VAP, these features are not present. If actually MSSA/MRSA NP/VAP exists, the high mortality rate, as seen in MSSA/MRSA CAP with influenza, would have been obvious to clinicians and a frequent autopsy finding. In four decades of searching for *bona fide* cases of MSSA/MRSA BP/VAP, there are few, if any convincing cases. Even if a sporadic case is reported, that does not make MSSA/MRSA one of the usual pathogens of NP/VAP that should be "covered."

Over the years, epidemiologic data has triumphed. Clinical findings and empiric MSSA/MRSA coverage with vancomycin have been used extensively. Unless accompanied by the imaging and clinical findings characteristic of MSSA/MRSA CAP, the NP/VAP patient should not be "covered" with vancomycin. Certainly, in patients not colonized (negative MRSA nasal swabs), vancomycin should not be used. Furthermore, it has been shown that in colonized pVAP patients, vancomycin does not improve outcomes, since MRSA is a non-pathogen in NP/VAP [2].

The other common clinical ASP concern is that of unnecessary "double coverage" for pVAP due to aerobic GNBs. "Double coverage" was a necessity few decades ago, when there were few antibiotics with excellent anti-*P. aeruginosa* activity, e.g., gentamicin, and with/without possible synergy, two drugs were considered better than one, e.g., an anti-pseudomonas penicillin or cephalosporin plus an aminoglycoside. "Double coverage" may have a limited place in the rare scenario of *bona fide P. aeruginosa* NP/VAP. Like MSSA/MRSA pneumonia, *P. aeruginosa* causes a necrotizing pneumonia, with rapid cavitation in <72 hours. Again, this is not diagnosed based on respiratory secretion cultures of ventilated patients.

Experience over the years has indicated that well-selected empiric monotherapy, e.g., meropenem, is as effective as "double drug" for anti-*P. aeruginosa* coverage. Unless the particular stain (causing infection tracheobronchitis or NP) does not colonize, then "relatively resistant strains" could be tested for synergy. Synergy should not be assumed, since two drugs used together may be indifferent or antagonistic. Synergy is the exception rather than the rule and rarely useful for non-ID physicians in practice [1,2].

CONTROLLING ANTIBIOTIC RESISTANCE IN THE CCU

The most difficult ASP goals are the prevention of resistance and limitation of its spread in the CCU and hospital. There are two components that need to work in concert for optimal effect. Controlling resistance depends on not promoting resistance by careful antibiotic selection, as well as limiting the spread of MDROs by effective infection control (IC) containment methods and isolation protocols.

The main CCU resistance problems are centered on IC to prevent MDRO spread and limit the spread of clonal resistance. For this reason, it is essential to ASPs that there is close coordination with the microbiology laboratory and IC. Since IC is separate from clinical ID services, only non-IC intervention are discussed here.

Clearly, it is preferable to prevent than to contain antibiotic resistance problems. Most physicians do not consider the "resistance potential" of antibiotics. It is a common misconception that antibiotic resistance is dependent on the volume/duration of use (years after available) and is inevitable. Furthermore, resistance potential is not related to antibiotic class. Antibiotic resistance from the practitioner's perspective is best approached by considering the antibiotic "resistance potential" of antibiotics. Practically, antibiotics may be considered as "high or low resistance potential" antibiotics. "Low resistance potential" antibiotics are those whose use has been associated with few, if any, resistance problems. Regardless of the volume/duration of use, "low resistance potential" antibiotics have maintained their effectiveness over time, e.g., doxycycline. In contrast, "high resistance potential" antibiotics may cause resistance with limited use and, of course, even more resistance with more use, e.g., ceftazidime. With each antibiotic, resistance is limited to one or two organisms but not across the antibiotic's spectrum. For example, ciprofloxacin, a "high resistance potential" antibiotic, remains effective against most pathogens in its spectrum, and resistance is largely limited to *S. aureus* and *S. pneumoniae* (Table 31.3).

Resistance is unrelated to antibiotic class in that each class contains both "high and low resistance" potential antibiotics. Among carbapenems, all are "low resistance potential" antibiotics, except imipenem, a "high resistance potential" antibiotic. Similarly, third-generation cephalosporins are "low resistance potential" antibiotics, except ceftazidime, a "high resistance potential" antibiotic.

Clinically, applying these principles in the CCU, if the antibiotic choice (proper spectrum, activity, side effects, etc.) is between a "high and low resistance potential" antibiotic, preferentially select the "low resistance potential" antibiotic, i.e., for UTI due to GNB, from a resistance perspective, levofloxacin alone would be preferable to ciprofloxacin. Similarly, among carbapenems, meropenem would be preferable to imipenem. Among the aminoglycosides, amikacin would be preferable to gentamicin or tobramycin.

Antibiotic resistance potential aside, unnecessary or prolonged antibiotic therapy may have untoned effects, i.e., selecting out MDRO strains (in body fluids, i.e., wounds, respiratory secretions, and urine).

Clinically, most MDROs are colonizers of body fluids. While these organisms cause infection, more often, they are only colonizers not requiring treatment. Importantly, colonization should not be treated regardless of the organism [2,3].

TABLE 31.3

Antibiotic Resistance Potential

"High Resistance Potential" Antibiotics (*Antibiotics to Avoid*)	
IV Antibiotics	**PO Antibiotics**
Ciprofloxacin	Gentamicin or tobramycin
Organism often resistant: *E. coli*	Organism often resistant: *P. aeruginosa*
TMP-SMX	Ceftazidime
Organism often resistant: *E. coli*	Organism often resistant: *P. aeruginosa*
Imipenem	Ciprofloxacin
Organism often resistant: *P. aeruginosa*	Organism often resistant: *E. coli*
	TMP-SMX
	Organism often resistant: *E. coli*

"Low Resistance Potential" Antibiotics (*Preferred Antibiotics*)			
IV Antibiotics		**PO Antibiotics**	
Meropenem	Levofloxacin	Doxycycline	Nitrofurantoin[a]
Amikacin	Aztreonam	Minocycline	Methenamine salts[a]
Ceftriaxone	Cefepime	Levofloxacin	Fosfomycin[a]
Doxycycline	Colistin		
Tigecycline	Polymyxin B		

Source: Cunha, B.A., *Med Clin North Am*, 84, 1407–1429, 2000; Cunha, B.A., *Lancet*, 357, 1307–1308, 2001; Cunha, C.B., and Cunha, B.A. (Eds.), *Antibiotic Essentials*, 17th ed., Jaypee Medical Publishers, New Delhi, India, 2020.

Abbreviation: TMP-SMX, trimethoprim/sulfamethoxazole.

[a] For uncomplicated lower UTIs.

The reasons not to treat or "cover" colonized body fluids are several. First, colonization rarely proceeds to infection, e.g., prolonged MSSA/MRSA colonization of respiratory secretions with MRSA does not precede, predispose to, or eventually result in MRSA NP/VAP [4,5].

Colonization is more difficult to eliminate than infection is to cure. Most antibiotics do not have the PK/PD characteristics to penetrate well into body fluids. As a result, not only the subinhibitory concentration in body fluids cannot eliminate the colonizing organisms, but prolonged exposure to low-level antibiotic concentration predisposes to antibiotic resistance.

The ASP implications are clear. There is no rational for treating colonies, organisms in respiratory secretions, or urine. First, do no harm is the operation principle here. "Covering" colonizers with antibiotics is futile but may worsen resistance and/or predispose to superinfection with other pathogens, i.e., MDROs or yeasts. Besides covering only the usual pathogens using "low resistance potential" antibiotics, other useful resistance-preventative principles include using monotherapy vs. unnecessary multiple antibiotics and treat infection (not colonization) only for the shortest duration of therapy needed to effect cure [7–9] (Tables 31.4 and 31.5).

C. DIFFICILE DIARRHEA AND COLITIS

There are special ASP considerations re: *C. difficile* in the CCU. The first consideration always is correct diagnosis. In the CCU setting, there are factors that may confuse the unwary.

First, all loose stools are not due to *C. difficile*. In the CCU, the use of enteral feeds is common. Enteral feeds are frequently accompanied by loose stools, and stools are frequently tested for *C. difficile*. It is important to appreciate that enteral feeds are protective against *C. difficile*. Aside from *C. difficile* testing often unnecessary, a simple diagnostic test is to decrease the euteal feed by 75% or hold for 1 day. If the number of loose stools greatly diminishes in the next 12–24 hours, the loose stools were due to the enteral feed, not *C. difficile*. Be careful, however, since if the patient is a *C. difficile* carrier, stools will test positive for *C. difficile*, but the patient does not have *C. difficile*.

All loose stools need not be tested for *C. difficile*, particularly those on laxatives or stool softeners. With laxatives/stool softeners, indeed, diarrhea has fewer episodes per day (usually <6 soft/semi-formed stools) rather than the many watery stools (20–30 liquid stools per day with CDD). As with the enteral feeds in patients, the patient on laxatives/stool softeners may test *C. difficile* positive if they were asymptomatic *C. difficile* carriers.

TABLE 31.4
Resistance Potential of Selected Antibiotics

"High Resistance Potential" Antibiotics To Avoid	Usual Organism(s) Resistance to Each Antibiotic	Preferred "Low Resistance Potential" Antibiotic Alternatives in Same Class	Preferred "Low Resistance Potential" Antibiotic Alternatives in Different Classes
Aminoglycosides			
Gentamicin or Tobramycin	*P. aeruginosa*	Amikacin	Levofloxacin, colistin, cefepime
Cephalosporins			
Ceftazidime	*P. aeruginosa*	Cefepime	Levofloxacin, colistin, polymyxin B
Tetracyclines			
Tetracycline	*S. pneumoniae*	Doxycycline, minocycline	Levofloxacin, moxifloxacin
Quinolones			
Ciprofloxacin	*S. pneumoniae*	Levofloxacin, moxifloxacin	Doxycycline
Ciprofloxacin	*P. aeruginosa*	Levofloxacin	Amikacin, colistin, cefepime
Glycopeptides			
Vancomycin	MSSA	None	Linezolid, daptomycin, minocycline, tigecycline
	MRSA		
Carbapenems			
Imipenem	*P. aeruginosa*	Meropenem, doripenem	Amikacin, cefepime, colistin, polymyxin B
Macrolides			
Azithromycin	*S. pneumoniae*	None	Doxycycline, levofloxacin, moxifloxacin
Dihydrofolate Reductase Inhibitors			
TMP-SMX	*S. pneumonia*	None	Doxycycline, levofloxacin, moxifloxacin

Abbreviation: TMP-SMX, trimethoprim/sulfamethoxazole.

TABLE 31.5
Empiric Antibiotic Therapy of Selected MDR Pathogens

Potential MDR Pathogens	Preferred Therapy	Alternate Therapy
MRSA	Tigecycline	Clindamycin (CA-MRSA)
	Minocycline	Doxycycline (CA-MRSA)
	Ceftaroline	TMP-SMX (CA-MRSA)
	Quinupristin/dalfopristin	
	Linezolid	
	Daptomycin	
	Vancomycin	
VRE	Tigecycline	Chloramphenicol
	Minocycline	
	Quinupristin/dalfopristin	
	Daptomycin[a]	
	Linezolid	
	Nitrofurantoin[b]	
	Fosfomycin[b]	
Klebsiella	Meropenem[c]	Levofloxacin
	Cefepime[c]	Moxifloxacin
	Amikacin[c]	Colistin
	Aztreonam	Doxycycline
	Tigecycline[c]	
	Polymyxin B	
	Nitrofurantoin[b]	
	Fosfomycin[b]	

(Continued)

TABLE 31.5 (*Continued*)
Empiric Antibiotic Therapy of Selected MDR Pathogens

Potential MDR Pathogens	Preferred Therapy	Alternate Therapy
Enterobacter	Ceftriaxone	Second-generation
	TMP-SMX	cephalosporins
	Cefepime[c]	Ticarcillin/clavulanate
	Meropenem[c]	Piperacillin/tazobactam
	Amikacin	Levofloxacin
	Aztreonam	Moxifloxacin
	Polymyxin B	Colistin
	Tigecycline[c]	
	Ceftazidime/avibactam	
	Ceftolozane/tazobactam	
	Nitrofurantoin[b]	
	Fosfomycin[b]	
Serratia	Ceftriaxone	Second-generation
	Cefepime[c]	cephalosporin
	TMP-SMX	Piperacillin/tazobactam
	Meropenem[c]	Levofloxacin[c]
	Amikacin[c]	Moxifloxacin
	Aztreonam	Colistin
	Polymyxin B	
	Tigecycline[c]	
	Ceftazidime/avibactam	
	Ceftolozane/tazobactam	
	Fosfomycin[b]	
P. aeruginosa	Meropenem[c]	Gentamicin
(Meropenem susceptible)	Aztreonam	Tobramycin
	Amikacin[c]	Piperacillin/tazobactam
	Ciprofloxacin	Cefoperazone
	Levofloxacin[c]	Doripenem
	Polymyxin B	Colistin
	Doxycycline[b]	
	Fosfomycin[b]	
P. aeruginosa	Doripenem	Colistin
(Meropenem resistant)	Polymyxin B	
	Amikacin[c]	
	Ceftazidime/avibactam	
	Ceftolozane/tazobactam	
	Meropenem/verobactam	
CRE[b]	Tigecycline[c]	Colistin
	Ceftazidime/avibactam	Aztreonam
	Meropenem/verobactam	
	Polymyxin B	
	Nitrofurantoin[b]	
	Fosfomycin[b]	
Acinetobacter[b]	TMP-SMX	Aztreonam
	Amikacin[c]	Gentamicin
	Minocycline	Tobramycin
	Tigecycline[c]	Ticarcillin/clavulnate
	Meropenem	Piperacillin/tazobactam
	Cefepime[c]	Doxycycline
	Ceftazidime/avibactam	Doripenem
	Ceftolozane/tazobactam	
S. maltophilia[b]	TMP-SMX	Chloramphenicol
	Minocycline	Ticarcillin/clavulanate
	Doxycycline	Piperacillin/tazobactam

(*Continued*)

TABLE 31.5 (*Continued*)

Empiric Antibiotic Therapy of Selected MDR Pathogens

Potential MDR Pathogens	Preferred Therapy	Alternate Therapy
	Tigecycline[c]	Levofloxacin
	Polymyxin B	Moxifloxacin
	Ceftazidime/avibactam	Colistin
	Ceftolozane/tazobactam	
	Fosfomycin[b,c]	
B. cepacia[b]	Minocycline	Doxycycline
	TMP-SMX	Chloramphenicol
	Meropenem[c]	Levofloxacin
	Cefepime[c]	Moxifloxacin
	Ceftazidime/avibactam	Ticarcillin/clavulanate
	Ceftolozane/tazobactam	Piperacillin/tazobactam

Source: Cunha, C.B., and Cunha, B.A. (Eds.), *Antibiotic Essentials* (16th ed.), Jay Pee Medical Publishers, New Delhi, India, 2018.

Abbreviations: MDR, multi-drug resistant; CRE, carbapenem resistant Enterobacteriaciae; TMP-SMX, trimethoprim-sulfamethoxazole.

[a] Daptomycin: use 2× the MRSA dose for VRE infections, e.g., for MSSA/MRSA soft tissue infection, use 4 mg/kg/day; for VRE, use 8 mg/kg/day; for MSSA/MRSA bacteremia/endocarditis, use 6 mg/kg/day; and for VRE, use 12 mg/kg/day.

[b] For uncomplicated lower UTIs,

[c] **MDR dosing**
- Amikacin: 1 g (IV) q24h
- Cefepime: 2 g (IV) q8h
- Levofloxacin 750 mg (IV/PO) q24h
- Meropenem: 2 g (IV) q8h
- Tigecycline: 400 mg (IV) × 1 dose, then 200 mg (IV) q24h

If the above situations are eliminated, then the liquid stool in the setting of otherwise-unexplained new onset of acute watery diarrhea should be sent for *C. difficile* testing. In the absence of abdominal findings of colitis, a positive test is diagnostic of CDD. *C. difficile* colitis (CDC) may complicate/follow CDD or may present only with colitis. CDC may be diagnosed by positive *C. difficile* stool test, and may present with new abdominal pain/tender, usually fever >102°F, leukocytosis, and pancolitis on abdominal CT scan. CDC may have a diarrheal component, but usually, there is no diarrhea with *de novo* CDC or new cases preceded by CDD. Another clinical clue to the development of CDC in the setting of CDD is the abrupt cessation of CDD and, in addition, now fever and abdominal pain.

The treatment of CDD differs from CDC in that CDD is a toxin-mediated diarrhea limited to mucosal involvement. In contrast, CDC is an invasive transmural process. For CDD, the preferred initial therapy is oral vancomycin 250–500 mg (PO) q6h without metronidazole (no advantage in adding to oral vancomycin therapy). Alternately, nitanoxazide is highly effective. In contrast, CDC should be treated with agents that penetrate the colon wall, e.g., metronizide and nitanoxazide [2,6].

The previous discussion relates to proper diagnosis and treatment of CDD and CDC. However, prevention should be considered as well. A common misconception is that antibiotics are the cause of CDD. While clindamycin and β-lactams (excluding ceftriaxone) are the most common antibiotics causing CDD. Other drugs also may either cause alone or increase with some antibiotics CDD, e.g., proton pump inhibitors (PPIs). As with antibiotic resistance, clinicians should appreciate the *C. difficile* potential of antibiotics. All things being equal, select the antibiotic with a low *C. difficile* potential. Use monotherapy instead of two or three other unnecessary antibiotics. Avoid the routine use of PPIs in the CCU and hospital. As with resistance, treat with an antibiotic for the shortest duration of therapy needed to cure the infection.

The last important ASP problem in the CCU relates to empiric antibiotic coverage for "fevers and leukocytosis," i.e., malignancies, which are unlikely due to infection. Another major area of antibiotic misuse is in treating drug fevers and non-bacterial infections with empiric antibiotics. In addition, treating non-infectious disorders with fever, e.g., adult Still's disease, is another ASP pitfall encountered daily. From an ASP perspective, if with well-chosen empiric or specific antibiotic therapy, fevers persist, the response should be diagnostic, i.e., search for the source of the fever. Instead, the typical response is to add additional antibiotics that also have no effect on the fever. The usual mistaken assumption in this setting is to assume coverage that is not broad enough or a resistant strain has encouraged drug therapy. In this setting, resistance is rarely the cause [2,5]. Broader spectrum implies that there was a problem with the diagnostic approach and assumptions were made that other unusual pathogens are responsible for the continued fevers. Again, this is another false assumption taking the place of another diagnostic assessment as to the cause of the fever (Tables 31.6 and 31.7).

In summary, the most pressing ASP concerns in the CCU have been briefly reviewed. Clearly, with ASPs in the hospital as well as the CCU, the devil is in the details. Full discussion of these topics is found elsewhere in individual chapters in this book.

TABLE 31.6

Differential Diagnosis of Fevers in the CCU. Unresponsive to Appropriate Antimicrobial Therapy[a]

Infectious Causes	Non-Infectious Causes
• CVC-associated infections[a]	• Thrombophlebitis
• Nosocomial pneumonia	• Hemorrhage
• Nosocomial acute bacterial endocarditis	• Acute myocardial infarction
• Abscesses (undrained/inadequately drained)[a]	• Acute pulmonary embolism/infarction
• *C. difficile* diarrhea/colitis	• Acute pancreatitis
	• Drug fever
	• Gout flare
	• Acute adrenal insufficiency
	• Hematomas

Source: Cunha, C.B., and Cunha, B.A., *Antibiotic Essentials*, 17th ed., Jay Pee Medical Publishers, New Delhi, India, 2020.

[a] Require removal (infected devices) or drainage (abscesses).

TABLE 31.7

Presumed Antibiotic Failure: Differential Diagnosis Approach to Continued Fevers on Appropriate Antimicrobial Therapy

Infectious Causes	Non-Infectious Causes
• **Treating colonization** (not infection)	• **Drug fever**
• **Abscesses** (undrained/inadequately drained)	• **Non-infectious disorders** (SLE flare)
• **Viral infections**	
• **Fungal infections**	

Antibiotic Related
- **Inadequate tissue penetration**
  - Prostate: Cephalosporins, carbapenems (water, not lipid soluble)
  - Synovial fluid: Vancomycin
  - (↓ penetration, large molecule)
  - Device associated (no blood supply)
    - CVC
    - Prosthetic devices
- **Inadequate activity**
  - Urine: Low urine levels (~ CrCl)
  - Suboptimal urine pH for the antibiotic
  - (↓ activity, not urine levels)
  - Lungs: Aminoglycosides
  - (↓ activity, not low lung levels)
- **Suboptimal Dosing**
  - MDR GNB: Higher than usual doses may be needed for relative resistant strains (DD-S)
  - Inadequate tissue perfusion (DM, PVD)
  - Susceptible *in vitro* but ineffective *in vivo*

Source: Cunha, C.B., and Cunha, B.A., *Antibiotic Essentials*, 17th ed., Jay Pee Medical Publishers, New Delhi, India, 2020.

Abbreviations: CVC, central venous catheter, PVD, peripheral vascular disease, MDR, multidrug resistant, GNB, gram-negative bacilli, DD-S, dose-dependent susceptibility.

REFERENCES

1. Cunha CB. Principles of antimicrobial stewardship. In: LaPlante KL, Cunha CB, Morrill HJ, Rice LB, Rice B. Mylonakis E eds. *Antimicrobial Stewardship: Principles and Practice*. London, UK: CABI Press, 2017:1–8.
2. Cunha CB, Cunha, BA (eds.). *Antibiotic Essentials* (17th Ed). New Delhi, India: Jaypee Brothers Medical Publishers Ltd, 2020.
3. Doron S, Davidson LE. Antimicrobial stewardship. *Mayo Clin Proc* 2011;86:1113–1123.
4. Wagner B, Filice GA, Drekonja D, et al. Antimicrobial stewardship programs in inpatient hospital settings: A systematic review. *Infect Control Hosp Epidemiol* 2014;35:1209–1228.
5. MacDougall C, Polk RE. Antimicrobial stewardship programs in health care systems. *Clin Microbiol Rev* 2005;18:638–656.
6. Schechner V, Temkin E, Harbarth S, Carmeli Y, Schwaber MJ. Epidemiological interpretation of studies examining the effect of antibiotic usage on resistance. *Clin Microbiol Rev* 2013;26:289–307.
7. Fraser GL, Stogsdill P, Dickens JD, Jr., Wennberg DE, Smith RP, Jr., Prato BS. Antibiotic optimization. An evaluation of patient safety and economic outcomes. *Arch Intern Med* 1997;157:1689–1694.
8. Cunha BA. Effective antibiotic-resistance control strategies. *Lancet* 2001;357:1307–1308.
9. Ohl CA, Luther VP. Health care provider education as a tool to enhance antibiotic stewardship practices. *Infect Dis Clin North Am* 2014;28:177–93.
10. Cunha CB, Varughese CA, Mylonakis E. Antimicrobial stewardship programs (ASPs): the devil is in the details. *Virulence* 2013;4:147–149.
11. Cunha BA. Antibiotic resistance. *Med Clin North Am* 2000;84:1407–1429.
12. Cunha CB, Cunha BA. *Antibiotic Essentials* (16th ed.). New Delhi, India, Jay Pee Medical Publishers, 2018.

32 Colonization, Infection, and Resistance in the Critical Care Unit

Edward J. Septimus

CONTENTS

Bacterial colonization can occur among both healthy and ill populations. Colonization is most common in body sites such as the nose, skin, and gastrointestinal tract. The body sites of colonization are usually specific to the type of bacteria. *S. aureus* and other commensal gram-positive organisms (e.g., coagulase-negative staphylococci [CNS] most commonly colonize the skin and mucosal membranes of the nose) [1]. Both gram-positive (e.g., *Streptococcus pneumoniae*) and some gram-negative organisms can colonize the pharynx [2,3]. Other organisms, such as enterococci, *C difficile*, and gram-negative organisms (e.g., *Enterobacteriaceae*), commonly colonize the gastrointestinal tract [4].

Bacteria have been part of the normal human microflora or commensal microbiota and usually do not cause signs or symptoms of infection. In general, commensal microbiota protects against infections originating at mucous membranes sites. Evidence is accumulating to indicate the importance of dysbiosis in critical illness, which increases the risk of subsequent infections. The best example of dysbiosis leading to infection appears to be *Clostridium difficile* infections (CDI) [5]. The most important modifiable risk factor is antibiotics, which can reduce or eliminate commensal microbiota, leading to an increased secondary pathogen invasion and support for antibiotic-resistant organisms [6].

Antibiotics are common in the CCU. In an international point-prevalence study, 71% of all CCU patient received antibiotics [7]. In addition, other pharmacological interventions can also impact the risk for infections in CCU patients, including digestive decolonization and gastric acid suppressive agents [2,8]. Certain procedures can disrupt the natural barriers to infection such as endotracheal tubes, urinary catheters, and intravascular devices, allowing for microbial entry. Furthermore, the CCU environment has been shown to be a potential reservoir for microbes, which can be inadvertently transmitted to vulnerable patients through patient contact with the environment or indirectly through contamination of healthcare workers' hands and gloves [9].

Sixty-five percent of all healthcare-associated infections (HAIs) occur in the CCU [10]. In the CCU, colonization with healthcare-associated pathogens such as *Staphylococcus aureus*, enterococci, gram-negative organisms, and *Clostrioides difficile* is associated with increased risk of infection. In addition, hospitalized patients in the CCU are at higher risk of colonization with multidrug-resistant (MDR) pathogens. Infections caused by MDR pathogens are associated with worse patient outcomes, including increased morbidity, mortality, healthcare costs, and increased hospital lengths of stay when compared with infections by more drug-sensitive pathogens [11]. Methicillin-resistant *Staphylococcus aureus* (MRSA), vancomycin-resistant *Enterococcus* (VRE), and MDR gram-negative bacteria (MDR-GN), including extended spectrum beta-lactamase-producing *Enterobacteriaceae* (ESBL), carbapenem-resistant *Enterobacteriaceae* (CRE), MDR *Pseudomonas*, and MDR *Acinetobacter*, have been the most commonly drug-resistant pathogens reported in the United States [12]. In a large point-prevalence study from around the world, MDR-GN now account for 62% of CCU infections [7].

Basic to all organisms discussed is the synergy between infection prevention and antimicrobial stewardship (AS). The use of prevention bundles has been shown to reduce HAI rates. Several studies have demonstrated the impact of catheter insertion and maintenance bundles on central line-associated bloodstream infections (CLABSIs) rates and have shown that CLABSI prevention bundles are effective, sustainable, and cost-effective for both adults and children. Bundles have also been used in successful multifaceted efforts to reduce ventilator-associated pneumonia (VAP), catheter-associated urinary tract infections (CAUTIs), and surgical site infections (SSI) [13]. Lastly, AS programs have been shown to improve patient outcomes, reduce antimicrobial adverse events, and decrease antimicrobial resistance [14,15].

The rest of this chapter will focus on the risk of colonization and infection due five common infections in the CCU: MRSA, VRE, CRE, carbapenem-resistant *Pseudomonas aeruginosa* (PA), and CDI. In addition, suggestions will be made in preventing infections in an CCU setting.

METHICILLIN-RESISTANT *STAPHYLOCOCCUS AUREUS*

MRSA has been identified as a significant pathogen worldwide. In the United States, it is estimated that greater than 94,000 MRSA infections occur annually, leading to almost 20,000 MRSA-related deaths per year [16]. Between 15% and 30% of healthy adults are nasally colonized with methicillin-susceptible *S. aureus* (MSSA), and 1%–3% are nasally colonized with MRSA [17,18]. This is more common among high-risk groups such as CCU patients [19]. In a recent meta-analysis on prevalence and MRSA colonization at admission to CCUs, the authors found that 5.8%–8.3% of CCU patients are nasal carriers of MRSA on admission. This represented an upward trend, especially in the United States. More importantly, MRSA colonization was associated with more than an eight-fold increase in the risk of infection with MRSA during their CCU stay [20]. *S. aureus* colonization at other body sites, including the pharynx, groin, perianal region, and axilla, can also be associated with the development of *S. aureus* infections. HAIs secondary to MRSA remain high. In 2014, 51% of CLABSIs, 43% of SSIs, and 42% of VAPs were due to MRSA [12].

Several articles have been published in the last 5 years on the best approaches to reduce MRSA infections in the CCU setting. The Veterans Affairs study showed a decrease in MRSA transmission and healthcare-associated MRSA infections with the use of active surveillance (AS) and contact precautions for patients who tested positive for MRSA [21].

Recently, several studies have evaluated the use of chlorhexidine (CHG) bathing to decrease HAIs, including MRSA in CCUs. The CHG bathing has been shown to decrease the bioburden of bacteria and yeasts on patients, the hospital environment, and the hands of healthcare workers [22]. In a multicenter cluster-crossover study, Climo et al. reported that daily 2% CHG cloth bathing in the CCU resulted in a 23% reduction of VRE and MRSA acquisition and a 28% reduction in BSIs [23]. In another study of pediatric CCU patients, Milstone et al. found a significant association between 2% CHG cloth bathing and a decline in BSIs compared with standard bathing [24]. The REDUCE MRSA study was a pragmatic cluster randomized trial of 74 adult CCUs to evaluate three MRSA prevention interventions: Arm 1 implemented MRSA screening and isolation; arm 2 included screening, isolation, and targeted decolonization of MRSA carriers with CHG bathing and nasal mupirocin; and arm 3 did not screen any patients, but instead, all patients were decolonized with CHG cloth bathing and nasal mupirocin (universal decolonization). Universal decolonization was found to be associated with the greatest decrease in all-cause BSIs, not just MRSA (44%; p = 0.001) and rates of MRSA clinical cultures (37%; p = 0.01) [25].

In a follow-up cost analysis, universal decolonization was estimated to save $171,000 for every 1000 admissions [26]. In 2017, Whittington et al. performed a cost-effectiveness analysis on recommendations for MRSA prevention in adult CCUs. Three strategies were evaluated: Universal decolonization, targeted decolonization, and screen and isolate. Like the Huang et al. study, the authors found that universal decolonization is less costly and more effective [27]. This has led to a shift from a vertical approach targeting a single organism to a horizontal approach to reduce infections from all pathogens [28]. The CHG bathing aligns with this horizontal approach and should be the standard of care in the CCU. In CCUs with high rates of MRSA, universal decolonization (CHG plus mupirocin) should be considered.

VANCOMYCIN-RESISTANT *ENTEROCOCCUS*

Enterococci have become a leading cause of HAIs [29]. VRE now accounts for over 30% of enterococcal infections, with the clear majority being *Enterococcus faecium* [30]. Once a patient becomes colonized with VRE, the risk of developing a subsequent bloodstream infection with the same VRE-colonizing strain appears to increase [31].

There are several risk factors associated with increased VRE colonization and/or infection. Administration of broad-spectrum antimicrobial therapy, especially vancomycin and cephalosporins, has consistently been reported to increase colonization with VRE. In a perspective study conducted for 126 adult CCU patients in 60 hospitals, investigators found that vancomycin and cephalosporins were associated with higher prevalence of VRE rates after controlling for CCU type [32]. Other risk factors include hospitalization longer than 72 hours, previous stay in the CCU, renal failure, transplant recipient, immunosuppression, and resident in a long-term facility [33].

Colonization pressure in hospitals can result in increased transmission [34]. The hospital environment can be heavily colonized with VRE. Transmission of VRE from environmental surfaces to hands or gloves of healthcare professionals (HCPs) has been well-documented [35]. Exposure to contaminated surfaces, even after routine disinfection, can be associated with VRE acquisition. Hospitalization in a room previously occupied by a patient colonized with VRE can also be associated with increased risk of VRE acquisition [36].

Ziakas and colleagues published a meta-analysis to determine the burden and significance of VRE colonization in the CCU. They found that 10.6% of patients admitted to the CCU were colonized with VRE on admission and a similar percentage acquired VRE during their CCU stay. In addition, they found colonization on admission to be a major determinant of VRE dynamics in the CCU, and the risk of VRE-related infections was related to colonization [37]. In another study, VRE colonization in the CCU was associated with increased mortality, length of stay, and costs compared with a matched hospital population [38]. Lastly, two meta-analyses have evaluated the mortality of patients with bacteremia with VRE compared with those with vancomycin-susceptible enterococci (VSE). Both studies concluded that patients with bacteremia with VRE were more than twice as likely to die compared with patients with VSE bacteremia, emphasizing that the development of vancomycin resistance is a poor prognostic sign in critically ill patients [39,40].

Prevention of infections with VRE requires a multidisciplinary approach starting with prevention of HAIs using evidence-based interventions, with a focus on prevention of CLABSIs and CAUTIs—the two HAIs most commonly associated with enterococci [30]. Hospital Infection Control Practices Advisory Committee of the Centers for Disease Control and Prevention (CDC) in 2006 published recommendations to prevent transmission of MDR organisms, including VRE [41]. Since VRE is primarily transmitted from patient to patient via the hands of HCP, hand hygiene remains the most important means of preventing the spread of VRE within the hospital [42].

Contact precaution using private rooms has been recommended for patients colonized or infected with VRE. Wearing gown and gloves when entering a patient room and removing them with hand hygiene prior to exiting the room may decrease VRE transmission. In one study in a medical CCU, gowns and gloves were used in two time periods, while gloves alone were used in a time period between the other two. During the gown period, 59 patients acquired VRE (9.1 cases per 1000 medical intensive care [MICU] days), and during the no-gown period, 73 patients acquired VRE (19.6 cases per 1000 MICU days; p < 0.01) [43].

Active surveillance for VRE by obtaining from rectal swabs or stool samples on admission and then weekly has been suggested for patients at high risk. Active surveillance has been effective in reducing transmission of VRE in outbreak settings [44,45] or in high-risk patients (hematology-oncology, transplant, and intensive care) [46.47].

Unfortunately, no effective treatment for decolonization of patients with VRE has been found [48,49]. CHG bathing, however, has been shown to be useful in reducing enterococcal colonization and infection in CCU settings [22,23]. Judicious use of antimicrobial drugs, especially vancomycin and cephalosporins, has been suggested, but it is unclear if this alone impacts VRE rates.

CARBAPENEM-RESISTANT *ENTEROBACTERIACEAE*

Carbapenem-resistant *Enterobacteriaceae* (CRE), particularly *Klebsiella pneumoniae* (KP), have emerged as an important cause of HAIs. KP carbapenemase (KPC)-producing *Enterobacteriaceae* have been identified in over 40 US states and in more than 25 countries. Data from the CDC indicated that in 2014, 2.8%–12% of *Enterobacteriaceae* HAIs were due to CRE [50]. Risk factors for CRE acquisition and infection include CCU stay, prior antimicrobial therapy, colonization pressure, and certain underlying medical conditions [51,52]. Initial studies have shown that mortality with CRE infections were 3.7–6.5 times greater than infections caused by carbapenem-susceptible strains [51,53].

Studies using active surveillance testing to identify asymptomatic gastrointestinal CRE carriage have reported rates between 2% and 39% in CCU patients [54,55]. Swaminathan and colleagues demonstrated that the burden of CRE is underappreciated when using clinical cultures alone to identify carriers; in their study, only 32% of CRE carriers would have been detected if they solely relied on clinical cultures [52]. Carriers can be a source for transmission as well as at increased risk for developing a future CRE infection [54]. Dickstein et al. reported a retrospective matched cohort study comparing the incidence of invasive infections in CRE-colonized patients and matched non-carriers in the CCU. Colonized patients with CRE had over a two-fold increased risk of infection by the colonizing strain [56].

Several measures have been recommended to decrease CRE transmission and infections in the CCU. Hand hygiene remains the foundation to prevent patient-to-patient transmission. Unfortunately, compliance remains inadequate. Therefore, hand hygiene alone is unlikely to reduce transmission, and as with VRE and MRSA, a multifaceted approach is necessary, starting with prevention of HAIs using evidence-based interventions.

Since there is a direct relationship between colonization pressure and healthcare CRE transmission, infection prevention guidelines recommend contact precautions: For all patients either colonized or infected with CRE, use dedicated staff, rooms, and equipment [57]. Environmental cleaning and disinfection have been shown to reduce infections caused by VRE and *C. difficile*. The evidence for CRE is less convincing due to shorter environmental survival time [58]. However, during CRE outbreaks, cleaning of the environment, especially high-touch surfaces, may assist in reducing transmission [59].

Nonetheless, it is recommended that rooms occupied by patients with CRE should be cleaned and disinfected at least once per day and that dedicated single-patient equipment should be used. Some also recommend cleaning high touch areas every shift.

Following patient discharge, the room should undergo a terminal cleaning procedure [60].

Active surveillance has been advocated to identify patients who are asymptomatic but may serve as a reservoir for transmission. Active surveillance has been shown to decrease colonization pressure and limit spread of CRE [61]. In addition, since CRE colonization is a risk factor for CRE infection, active surveillance may identify patients at risk for CRE infections and reduce the delay in ordering appropriate antimicrobial therapy.

Several recent studies have examined the role of selective digestive decontamination (SDD) and selective oropharyngeal decontamination (SOD) in reducing colonization, infections, and outbreaks caused by MDR gram-negative bacteria, including CRE. Several trials have evaluated the impact of SDD and SOD, specifically on CRE carriage and infection, with conflicting results.

Saidel-Odes et al. performed a blinded RCT comparing placebo with oral gentamicin and oral polymyxin gel plus oral solutions of gentamicin and polymyxin for 7 days to eradicate carbapenem-resistant *Klebsiella pneumoniae* (CRKP) oropharyngeal and gastrointestinal carriage. After 2 weeks, the proportion of rectal cultures that were negative for CRKP was significantly improved in the intervention group. However, colonization rates later increased at 6 weeks. Secondary resistance to gentamicin or colistin was not observed in any of the SDD-treated patients [62].

In another study, non-absorbable oral antibiotics were administered for up to 60 days or until decolonization was documented in patients colonized with CRE. Oral gentamicin or oral colistin was used based on the susceptibility of the isolate. Patients with isolates sensitive to both colistin and gentamicin were randomized to receive either colistin or gentamicin or both. Patients with isolates resistant to both agents were not provided with SDD but were followed to document spontaneous clearance of CRE. Eradication rates in the three treatment groups (gentamicin, colistin, or both) were 42%, 50%, and 37.5%, respectively, each significantly higher than the 7% spontaneous clearance in the control group (P 0.001, P 0.001, and P 0.004, respectively). Mortality in patients who achieved eradication (either spontaneously or by SDD) was significantly lower than that in patients where eradication failed (17% versus 49%, respectively; P 0.002). However, secondary resistance developed in 7 of the 50 SDD-treated patients, gentamicin resistance in 6 of 26 gentamicin-treated patients, and colistin resistance in 1 of 16 colistin-treated patients [63].

The CHG bathing has been studied to see if it can reduce infections with several gram-negatives, including CRE. The best trials have been performed in long-term acute care hospitals (LTACH). A study of LTACH patients assessed whether the use of daily 2% CHG bathing cloths was associated with lower *Klebsiella pneumoniae* carbapenemase-producing *Enterobacteriaceae* (KPC) skin colonization. That study reported that CHG bathing was associated with decreased KPC skin colonization [64]. A follow-up using a stepped-wedge study of LTACHs tested whether an intervention, which included screening for KPC rectal colonization, contact precautions, and daily CHG bathing, would reduce KPC colonization and infection. It was concluded that the intervention was associated with reductions in KPC colonization, blood culture contamination, and BSIs due to all causes [65].

A new promising intervention to eliminate CRE colonization in the GI tract may be fecal microbiota transplantation (FMT). Lagier et al. reported on a patient colonized by CRE who was successfully decolonized with FMT [66]. Further studies are needed to evaluate the safety and efficacy of FMT in eradicating GI colonization with CRE.

Lastly, AS has become part of a strategy to combat antimicrobial resistance for MDROs, including CRE, and should be part of a multifaceted program.

Antimicrobial exposure is the strongest predictor associated with CRE acquisition [67]. Antimicrobials, including carbapenems, fluoroquinolones, and metronidazole, have been identified as possible risk factors for CRE [68]. The AS program should include diagnostic stewardship, de-escalation, and appropriate duration of therapy.

PSEUDOMONAS AERUGINOSA

PA is a leading cause of HAIs in the CCU, especially ventilator-associated pneumonia (VAP) and hospital-associated pneumonia (HAP). PA colonization usually precedes infection. Colonization may be endogenous or exogenous. Intestinal colonization is considered the most important reservoir for endogenous infection. Patients may also become colonized from contaminated reservoirs or by cross-contamination [69,70]. Gomez-Zorrilla found the probability of PA infection 14 days after CCU admission was 26% for carriers versus only 5% for non-carriers (p < 0.001). In addition, 87% of those who developed an infection with PA had the same genotyping as the initial rectal strain from admission [71]. In a separate study, patients who screened positive for PA on admission had an increased risk of infection compared with patients who were not colonized on admission. There was a 50%–70% likelihood that subsequent clinical infection was similar to strain cultured on admission [72].

Venier et al. published results on a five-month prospective multicenter study in 10 French CCUs. Adult patients hospitalized in the CCU for ≥24 hours were screened on admission, weekly, and before discharge. For patients with PA on admission, 15% acquired PA during their stay in the CCU. Results of multivariate analysis showed that independent risk factors for PA acquisition were older age, history of prior PA infection or colonization, longer duration on mechanical ventilation, and longer days on antimicrobial therapy for antibiotics inactive against PA. For CCU factors, positive tap water in a patient's room and cumulative ward level of nursing workload were associated with higher acquisition for PA [73].

Prevention of infection in the CCU depends on consistent application of evidenced practices, including hand hygiene; environmental cleaning and disinfections, especially water-borne sources [74,75]; contact precautions for MDR-PA; and AS, which has a major role in controlling MDR-PA [76]. There is no evidence for routine screening in endemic settings. Active surveillance should only be reserved for outbreaks or for significant increases from baseline. Decolonization using SDD or SOD has had some limited success, but emergence of resistance remains a concern.

C. DIFFICILE INFECTION

CDI is now the most common HAI in the United States [77]. It has been estimated that more than 450,000 infections and 29,000 deaths per year are caused by *Clostridioides difficile* in the United States, and CDI is projected to increase in the future [78]. There is increasing recognition of the importance of asymptomatic *C difficile* carriers as the source of transmission and infection. Studies have shown that 4%–15% of asymptomatic adults are colonized with toxigenic *C difficile* on admission [79]. In one study, the investigators were able to show that 20% of new CDI were transmitted from asymptomatic carriers [80]. In addition, asymptomatic carriers are six times more likely to develop CDI compared with non-carriers [81].

Guidance for prevention of CDI in acute-care hospital settings was published in 2014 by the Society for Healthcare Epidemiology of America and the Infectious Diseases Society of America [82]. Antibiotic use is the most widely recognized and modifiable risk factor for CDI. Use of broad-spectrum antibiotics such as fluoroquinolones, third-generation cephalosporins, clindamycin, and carbapenem are associated with a higher risk of CDI [83]. More recently, proton pump inhibitors (PPIs) have been evaluated as the possible risk factors for CDI [8]. PPIs are commonly prescribed in the CCU setting. Other established risk factors include advanced age, hospitalization, severe illness, gastrointestinal surgery, cancer chemotherapy, hematopoietic stem cell transplantation, and inflammatory bowel disease [84].

HCP should perform hand hygiene by washing hands with soap and water, following care of patients with suspected or proven CDI; use of alcohol-based hand rub (ABHR) is not adequate, because ABHR does not eradicate *C. difficile* spores [85]. Patients with suspected or proven CDI should be placed on contact precautions, including assignment to a single room with dedicated toileting facilities. Gloves and gowns should be donned upon room entry and removed prior to exiting the room.

Multiple studies have demonstrated that implementing ASP programs that target high-risk antibiotics is associated with significant decreases in CDI rates [86,87]. With recent publications around PPIs, appropriate use of PPIs, especially in the CCU, appears prudent.

The potential for enhanced environmental cleaning has also been recognized as a preventive strategy. Studies have shown both symptomatic and asymptomatic patients can shed *C. difficile* in the environment. Patients in rooms previously occupied by CDI patients have been shown to be at increased risk of CDI [88]. *C. difficile* spores can survive on dry surfaces for up to several months, and routine disinfection with standard quaternary ammonium products does not eliminate *C. difficile* spores. Disinfection of clinical areas where patients with CDI are treated requires use of a sporicidal agent.

Another option involves no-touch technologies such as hydrogen peroxide vapor of ultraviolet (UV) light decontamination. Two well-done studies have recently been published. The first was from investigators at Duke. This was a cluster-randomized crossover trial of UV terminal room cleaning in nine hospitals. The rooms of patients with *C. difficile* were cleaned with bleach with and without UV light at discharge. The addition of UV did not change the rate of CDI [89]. Compliance with routine cleaning was very high. A second study was conducted by investigators at the University of Pennsylvania. They added UV light to terminal cleaning with bleach for patients with CDI. The CDI rate dropped by 25% on intervention units and increased 16% on nonintervention units [90].

Another strategy to prevent transmission from asymptomatic carriers is active surveillance, followed by placing positive patients in contact precautions. Longtin et al., in their paper, reported screening all inpatients on admission for *C. difficile*. Carriers were placed in contact precautions until

discharged. They observed a decrease in CDI rates from 6.39 to 3 cases per 10,00 patient-days [79]. Modeling has shown that screening and isolation of asymptomatic carriers could decrease hospital-onset CDI by 10%–25% and hospital-onset colonization by over 40% [91,92].

Lastly, probiotics have been proposed as an adjunctive measure in the prevention of CDI. Johnson et al. reviewed the literature from 1976 to 2010 and found 11 studies where adult patients who received antibiotics were randomized to receive either a probiotic or placebo and in which CDI was a measured outcome. They then selected for meta-analysis those probiotics with at least two randomized, controlled trials for inclusion. Only two probiotics, *Saccharomyces boulardii* and the combination of *L. acidophilus* CL1285, *L. casei* LBC80R, and *L. rhamnosus* CLR2 (Bio-K+) were selected as qualified. Overall, there were fewer cases of CDI in those receiving a probiotic, especially those on Bio-K+, than those in the placebo group [93]. Probiotics started within 2 days of antimicrobial start produced a greater reduction of CDI rates than probiotics started after 2 days [94]. Probiotics are not appropriate for immunosuppressed patients and perhaps for patient with central lines, due to risk of probiotic-associated bacteremia and fungemia [95,96].

CONCLUSIONS

Implementing the infection prevention recommendations, combined with a robust ASP, will lead to improvements in hospitals' infection rates, will lower healthcare costs, and, most importantly, will enhance the quality of healthcare for our patients. Given the complexity of managing the multiplicity of epidemiologically important pathogens across heterogeneous healthcare settings, especially in the CCU, Septimus and colleagues recommend (1) using robust quality-improvement methods to ensure reliable performance of basic infection prevention practices known to mitigate transmission of MDROs and the infections they cause; (2) ensuring adherence to evidence-based, universally applied HAI prevention strategies, including hand hygiene, AS, and adequate environmental cleaning; (3) applying other evidence-based, horizontal strategies such as CHG bathing in settings where benefits are likely to outweigh risks and costs; and (4) using active surveillance and other vertical approaches selectively when outbreaks occur with specific pathogens [28].

REFERENCES

1. Wertheim HF, Melles DC, Vos MC, et al. The role of nasal carriage in *Staphylococcus aureus* infections. *Lancet Infect Dis* 2005;5(12):751–762.
2. Oostdijk EA, de Smet AM, Blok HE, et al. Ecological effects of selective decontamination on resistant gram-negative bacterial colonization. *Am J Respir Crit Care Med* 2010;181(5):452–457.
3. Liberati A, D'Amico R, Pifferi S, et al. Antibiotic prophylaxis to reduce respiratory tract infections and mortality in adults receiving intensive care. *Cochrane Database Syst Rev* 2009;(4):CD000022.

4. Buffie CG, Pamer EG. Microbiota-mediated colonization resistance against intestinal pathogens. *Nat Rev Immunol* 2013;13(11):790–801.

5. Leffler DA, Lamont JT. *Clostridium difficile* infection. *N Engl J Med* 2015;372(16):1539–1548.

6. Modi SR, Collins JJ, Relman DA. Antibiotics and the gut microbiota. *J Clin Invest* 2014;124(10):4212–4218.

7. Vincent JL, Rello J, Marshall J, et al. International study of the prevalence and outcomes of infection in intensive care units. *JAMA* 2009;302(21):2323–2329.

8. Kwok CS, Arthur AK, Anibueze CI, Singh S, Cavallazzi R, Loke YK. Risk of *Clostridium difficile* infection with acid suppressing drugs and antibiotics: Meta-analysis. *Am J Gastroenterol* 2012;107(7):1011–1019.

9. Han JH, Sullivan N, Leas BF, et al. Cleaning hospital room surfaces to prevent health care-associated infections: A technical brief. *Ann Intern Med* 2015;163(8):598–607.

10. Ziakas PD, Zacharioudakis IM, Zervou FN, Mylonakis E. Methicillin-resistant *Staphylococcus aureus* prevention strategies in the ICU: A clinical decision analysis. *Crit Care Med* 2015;43(2):382–393.

11. Cosgrove SE. The relationship between antimicrobial resistance and patient outcomes: Mortality, length of hospital stay, and health care costs. *Clin Infect Dis* 2006;42(Suppl 2):S82–S89.

12. Weiner LM, Webb AK, Limbago B, et al. Antimicrobial-resistant pathogens associated with healthcare-associated infections: Summary of data reported to the national healthcare safety network at the centers for disease control and prevention, 2011–2014. *Infect Control Hosp Epidemiol* 2016;37(11):1288–1301.

13. Septimus E, Yokoe DS, Weinstein RA, et al. Maintaining the momentum of change: The role of the 2014 updates to the compendium in preventing healthcare-associated infections. *Infect Control Hosp Epidemiol* 2014;35(5):460–463.

14. Dodds Ashley ES, Kaye KS, DePestel DD, Hermsen ED. Antimicrobial stewardship: Philosophy versus practice. *Clin Infect Dis* 2014;59(Suppl 3):S112–S121.

15. Kelly AA, Jones MM, Echevarria KL, et al. A report of the efforts of the veterans health administration national antimicrobial stewardship initiative. *Infect Control Hosp Epidemiol* 2017;38(5):513–520.

16. Klevens RM, Morrison MA, Nadle J, et al. Invasive methicillin-resistant *Staphylococcus aureus* infections in the United States. *JAMA* 2007;298(15):1763–1771.

17. VandenBergh MF, Yzerman EP, van Belkum A, et al. Follow-up of *Staphylococcus aureus* nasal carriage after 8 years: Redefining the persistent carrier state. *J Clin Microbiol* 1999;37(10):3133–3140.

18. Graham PL, 3rd, Lin SX, Larson EL. A US population-based survey of *Staphylococcus aureus* colonization. *Ann Intern Med* 2006;144(5):318–325.

19. Sim BL, McBryde E, Street AC, Marshall C. Multiple site surveillance cultures as a predictor of methicillin-resistant *Staphylococcus aureus* infections. *Infect Control Hosp Epidemiol* 2013;34(8):818–824.

20. Ziakas PD, Anagnostou T, Mylonakis E. The prevalence and significance of methicillin-resistant *Staphylococcus aureus* colonization at admission in the general ICU Setting: A meta-analysis of published studies. *Crit Care Med* 2014;42(2):433–444.

21. Jain R, Kralovic SM, Evans ME, et al. Veterans affairs initiative to prevent methicillin-resistant *Staphylococcus aureus* infections. *N Engl J Med* 2011;364(15):1419–1430.

22. Vernon MO, Hayden MK, Trick WE, et al. chlorhexidine gluconate to cleanse patients in a medical intensive care unit: The effectiveness of source control to reduce the bioburden of vancomycin-resistant enterococci. *Arch Intern Med* 2006;166(3):306–312.

23. Climo MW, Yokoe DS, Warren DK, et al. Effect of daily chlorhexidine bathing on hospital-acquired infection. *N Engl J Med* 2013;368(6):533–542.

24. Milstone AM, Elward A, Song X, et al. Daily chlorhexidine bathing to reduce bacteraemia in critically ill children: A multicentre, cluster-randomised, crossover trial. *Lancet* 2013;381(9872):1099–1106.

25. Huang SS, Septimus E, Kleinman K, et al. Targeted versus universal decolonization to prevent ICU infection. *N Engl J Med* 2013;368(24):2255–2265.

26. Huang SS, Septimus E, Avery TR, et al. Cost savings of universal decolonization to prevent intensive care unit infection: Implications of the REDUCE MRSA trial. *Infect Control Hosp Epidemiol* 2014;35(Suppl 3):S23–S31.

27. Whittington MD, Atherly AJ, Curtis DJ, et al. Recommendations for methicillin-resistant *Staphylococcus aureus* prevention in adult ICUs: A cost-effectiveness analysis. *Crit Care Med* 2017;45(8):1304–1310.

28. Septimus E, Weinstein RA, Perl TM, Goldmann DA, Yokoe DS. Approaches for preventing healthcare-associated infections: Go long or go wide? *Infect Control Hosp Epidemiol* 2014;35(7):797–801.

29. Hidron AI, Edwards JR, Patel J, et al. NHSN annual update: Antimicrobial-resistant pathogens associated with healthcare-associated infections: Annual summary of data reported to the National Healthcare Safety Network at the Centers for Disease Control and Prevention, 2006–2007. *Infect Control Hosp Epidemiol* 2008;29(11):996–1011.

30. Sievert DM, Ricks P, Edwards JR, et al. Antimicrobial-resistant pathogens associated with healthcare-associated infections: Summary of data reported to the National Healthcare Safety Network at the Centers for Disease Control and Prevention, 2009–2010. *Infect Control Hosp Epidemiol* 2013;34(1):1–14.

31. Murray BE. Vancomycin-resistant enterococcal infections. *N Engl J Med* 2000;342(10):710–721.

32. Fridkin SK, Edwards JR, Courval JM, et al. The effect of vancomycin and third-generation cephalosporins on prevalence of vancomycin-resistant enterococci in 126 US adult intensive care units. *Ann Intern Med* 2001;135(3):175–183.

33. Furtado GH, Mendes RE, Pignatari AC, Wey SB, Medeiros EA. Risk factors for vancomycin-resistant *Enterococcus faecalis* bacteremia in hospitalized patients: An analysis of two case-control studies. *Am J Infect Control* 2006;34(7):447–451.

34. Cohen MJ, Adler A, Block C, et al. Acquisition of vancomycin-resistant enterococci in internal medicine wards. *Am J Infect Control* 2009;37(2):111–116.

35. Ray AJ, Hoyen CK, Taub TF, Eckstein EC, Donskey CJ. Nosocomial transmission of vancomycin-resistant enterococci from surfaces. *JAMA* 2002;287(11):1400–1401.

36. Huang SS, Datta R, Platt R. Risk of acquiring antibiotic-resistant bacteria from prior room occupants. *Arch Intern Med* 2006;166(18):1945–1951.

37. Ziakas PD, Thapa R, Rice LB, Mylonakis E. Trends and significance of VRE colonization in the ICU: A meta-analysis of published studies. *PLOS ONE* 2013;8(9):e75658.

38. Jung E, Byun S, Lee H, Moon SY, Lee H. Vancomycin-resistant *Enterococcus* colonization in the intensive care unit: Clinical outcomes and attributable costs of hospitalization. *Am J Infect Control* 2014;42(10):1062–1066.

39. Salgado CD, Farr BM. Outcomes associated with vancomycin-resistant enterococci: A meta-analysis. *Infect Control Hosp Epidemiol* 2003;24(9):690–698.

40. DiazGranados CA, Zimmer SM, Klein M, Jernigan JA. Comparison of mortality associated with vancomycin-resistant and vancomycin-susceptible enterococcal bloodstream infections: A meta-analysis. *Clin Infect Dis* 2005;41(3):327–333.

41. Centers for Disease Control and Prevention. Management of multidrug-resistant organisms in healthcare settings, 2006. Available at: www.cdc.gov/ncidod/dhqp/pdf/ar/mdroGuideline2006.pdf. Accessed on December 5, 2017.

42. Muto CA, Jernigan JA, Ostrowsky BE, et al. SHEA guideline for preventing nosocomial transmission of multidrug-resistant strains of *Staphylococcus aureus* and enterococcus. *Infect Control Hosp Epidemiol* 2003;24(5):362–386.

43. Puzniak LA, Leet T, Mayfield J, Kollef M, Mundy LM. To gown or not to gown: The effect on acquisition of vancomycin-resistant enterococci. *Clin Infect Dis* 2002;35(1):18–25.

44. Calfee DP, Giannetta ET, Durbin LJ, Germanson TP, Farr BM. Control of endemic vancomycin-resistant *Enterococcus* among inpatients at a university hospital. *Clin Infect Dis* 2003;37(3):326–332.

45. Mascini EM, Troelstra A, Beitsma M, et al. Genotyping and preemptive isolation to control an outbreak of vancomycin-resistant *Enterococcus faecium*. *Clin Infect Dis* 2006;42(6):739–746.

46. Perencevich EN, Fisman DN, Lipsitch M, et al. Projected benefits of active surveillance for vancomycin-resistant enterococci in intensive care units. *Clin Infect Dis* 2004;38(8):1108–1115.

47. Hachem R, Graviss L, Hanna H, et al. Impact of surveillance for vancomycin-resistant enterococci on controlling a bloodstream outbreak among patients with hematologic malignancy. *Infect Control Hosp Epidemiol* 2004;25(5):391–394.

48. Hachem R, Raad I. Failure of oral antimicrobial agents in eradicating gastrointestinal colonization with vancomycin-resistant enterococci. *Infect Control Hosp Epidemiol* 2002;23(1):43–44.

49. Mondy KE, Shannon W, Mundy LM. Evaluation of zinc bacitracin capsules versus placebo for enteric eradication of vancomycin-resistant *Enterococcus faecium*. *Clin Infect Dis* 2001;33(4):473–476.

50. Weiner LM, Fridkin SK, Aponte-Torres Z, et al. Vital signs: Preventing antibiotic-resistant infections in hospitals—United States, 2014. *MMWR Morb Mortal Wkly Rep* 2016;65(9):235–241.

51. Schwaber MJ, Klarfeld-Lidji S, Navon-Venezia S, et al. Predictors of carbapenem-resistant *Klebsiella pneumoniae* acquisition among hospitalized adults and effect of acquisition on mortality. *Antimicrob Agents Chemother* 2008;52(3):1028–1033.

52. Swaminathan M, Sharma S, Poliansky Blash S, et al. Prevalence and risk factors for acquisition of carbapenem-resistant *Enterobacteriaceae* in the setting of endemicity. *Infect Control Hosp Epidemiol* 2013;34(8):809–817.

53. Patel G, Huprikar S, Factor SH, Jenkins SG, Calfee DP. Outcomes of carbapenem-resistant *Klebsiella pneumoniae* infection and the impact of antimicrobial and adjunctive therapies. *Infect Control Hosp Epidemiol* 2008;29(12):1099–1106.

54. Calfee D, Jenkins SG. Use of active surveillance cultures to detect asymptomatic colonization with carbapenem-resistant *Klebsiella pneumoniae* in intensive care unit patients. *Infect Control Hosp Epidemiol* 2008;29(10):966–968.

55. Bratu S, Landman D, Haag R, et al. Rapid spread of carbapenem-resistant *Klebsiella pneumoniae* in New York City: A new threat to our antibiotic armamentarium. *Arch Intern Med* 2005;165(12):1430–1435.

56. Dickstein Y, Edelman R, Dror T, et al. Carbapenem-resistant *Enterobacteriaceae* colonization and infection in critically ill patients: A retrospective matched cohort comparison with non-carriers. *J Hosp Infect* 2016;94(1):54–59.

57. Friedman ND, Carmeli Y, Walton AL, Schwaber MJ. Carbapenem-resistant *Enterobacteriaceae*: A strategic roadmap for infection control. *Infect Control Hosp Epidemiol* 2017;38(5):580–594.

58. Weber DJ, Anderson D, Rutala WA. The role of the surface environment in healthcare-associated infections. *Curr Opin Infect Dis* 2013;26(4):338–344.

59. Ciobotaro P, Oved M, Nadir E, Bardenstein R, Zimhony O. An effective intervention to limit the spread of an epidemic carbapenem-resistant *Klebsiella pneumoniae* strain in an acute care setting: From theory to practice. *Am J Infect Control* 2011;39(8):671–677.

60. Dancer SJ. Hospital cleaning in the 21st century. *Eur J Clin Microbiol Infect Dis* 2011;30(12):1473–1481.

61. Schwaber MJ, Carmeli Y. An ongoing national intervention to contain the spread of carbapenem-resistant *Enterobacteriaceae*. *Clin Infect Dis* 2014;58(5):697–703.

62. Saidel-Odes L, Polachek H, Peled N, et al. A randomized, double-blind, placebo-controlled trial of selective digestive decontamination using oral gentamicin and oral polymyxin E for eradication of carbapenem-resistant *Klebsiella pneumoniae* carriage. *Infect Control Hosp Epidemiol* 2012;33(1):14–19.

63. Oren I, Sprecher H, Finkelstein R, et al. Eradication of carbapenem-resistant *Enterobacteriaceae* gastrointestinal colonization with nonabsorbable oral antibiotic treatment: A prospective controlled trial. *Am J Infect Control* 2013;41(12):1167–1172.

64. Lin MY, Lolans K, Blom DW, et al. The effectiveness of routine daily chlorhexidine gluconate bathing in reducing *Klebsiella pneumoniae* carbapenemase-producing *Enterobacteriaceae* skin burden among long-term acute care hospital patients. *Infect Control Hosp Epidemiol* 2014;35(4):440–442.

65. Hayden MK, Lin MY, Lolans K, et al. Prevention of colonization and infection by *Klebsiella pneumoniae* carbapenemase-producing *Enterobacteriaceae* in long-term acute-care hospitals. *Clin Infect Dis* 2015;60(8):1153–1161.

66. Lagier JC, Million M, Fournier PE, Brouqui P, Raoult D. Faecal microbiota transplantation for stool decolonization of OXA-48 carbapenemase-producing *Klebsiella pneumoniae*. *J Hosp Infect* 2015;90(2):173–174.

67. Marchaim D, Chopra T, Bhargava A, et al. Recent exposure to antimicrobials and carbapenem-resistant *Enterobacteriaceae*: the role of antimicrobial stewardship. *Infect Control Hosp Epidemiol* 2012;33(8):817–830.

68. Schechner V, Kotlovsky T, Tarabeia J, et al. Predictors of rectal carriage of carbapenem-resistant *Enterobacteriaceae* (CRE) among patients with known CRE carriage at their next hospital encounter. *Infect Control Hosp Epidemiol* 2011;32(5):497–503.

69. Bonten MJ, Bergmans DC, Speijer H, Stobberingh EE. Characteristics of polyclonal endemicity of *Pseudomonas aeruginosa* colonization in intensive care units. Implications for infection control. *Am J Respir Crit Care Med* 1999;160(4):1212–1219.

70. Trautmann M, Halder S, Hoegel J, Royer H, Haller M. Point-of-use water filtration reduces endemic *Pseudomonas aeruginosa* infections on a surgical intensive care unit. *Am J Infect Control* 2008;36(6):421–429.

71. Gomez-Zorrilla S, Camoez M, Tubau F, et al. Prospective observational study of prior rectal colonization status as a predictor for subsequent development of *Pseudomonas aeruginosa* clinical infections. *Antimicrob Agents Chemother* 2015;59(9):5213–5219.

72. Cohen R, Babushkin F, Cohen S, et al. A prospective survey of *Pseudomonas aeruginosa* colonization and infection in the intensive care unit. *Antimicrob Resist Infect Control* 2017;6:7.

73. Venier AG, Leroyer C, Slekovec C, et al. Risk factors for *Pseudomonas aeruginosa* acquisition in intensive care units: A prospective multicentre study. *J Hosp Infect* 2014;88(2):103–108.

74. Rogues AM, Boulestreau H, Lasheras A, et al. Contribution of tap water to patient colonisation with *Pseudomonas aeruginosa* in a medical intensive care unit. *J Hosp Infect* 2007;67(1):72–78.

75. Kossow A, Kampmeier S, Willems S, et al. Control of multidrug-resistant *Pseudomonas aeruginosa* in allogeneic hematopoietic stem cell transplant recipients by a novel bundle including remodeling of sanitary and water supply systems. *Clin Infect Dis* 2017;65(6):935–942.

76. Pakyz AL, Oinonen M, Polk RE. Relationship of carbapenem restriction in 22 university teaching hospitals to carbapenem use and carbapenem-resistant *Pseudomonas aeruginosa*. *Antimicrob Agents Chemother* 2009;53(5):1983–1986.

77. Magill SS, Edwards JR, Bamberg W, et al. Multistate point-prevalence survey of health care-associated infections. *N Engl J Med* 2014;370(13):1198–1208.

78. Lessa FC, Mu Y, Bamberg WM, et al. Burden of *Clostridium difficile* infection in the United States. *N Engl J Med* 2015;372(9):825–834.

79. Longtin Y, Paquet-Bolduc B, Gilca R, et al. Effect of detecting and isolating *Clostridium difficile* carriers at hospital admission on the incidence of *C difficile* infections: A quasi-experimental controlled study. *JAMA Intern Med* 2016;176(6):796–804.

80. Blixt T, Gradel KO, Homann C, et al. Asymptomatic carriers contribute to nosocomial *Clostridium difficile* infection: A cohort study of 4508 patients. *Gastroenterology* 2017;152(5):1031–1041 e1032.

81. Zacharioudakis IM, Zervou FN, Pliakos EE, Ziakas PD, Mylonakis E. Colonization with toxinogenic *C. difficile* upon hospital admission, and risk of infection: A systematic review and meta-analysis. *Am J Gastroenterol* 2015;110(3):381–390; quiz 391.

82. Dubberke ER, Carling P, Carrico R, et al. Strategies to prevent *Clostridium difficile* infections in acute care hospitals: 2014 update. *Infect Control Hosp Epidemiol* 2014;35(6):628–645.

83. Lawes T, Lopez-Lozano JM, Nebot CA, et al. Effect of a national 4C antibiotic stewardship intervention on the clinical and molecular epidemiology of *Clostridium difficile* infections in a region of Scotland: A non-linear time-series analysis. *Lancet Infect Dis* 2017;17(2):194–206.

84. Loo VG, Bourgault AM, Poirier L, et al. Host and pathogen factors for *Clostridium difficile* infection and colonization. *N Engl J Med* 2011;365(18):1693–1703.

85. Jabbar U, Leischner J, Kasper D, et al. Effectiveness of alcohol-based hand rubs for removal of *Clostridium difficile* spores from hands. *Infect Control Hosp Epidemiol* 2010;31(6):565–570.

86. Aldeyab MA, Kearney MP, Scott MG, et al. An evaluation of the impact of antibiotic stewardship on reducing the use of high-risk antibiotics and its effect on the incidence of *Clostridium difficile* infection in hospital settings. *J Antimicrob Chemother* 2012;67(12):2988–2996.

87. Valiquette L, Cossette B, Garant MP, Diab H, Pepin J. Impact of a reduction in the use of high-risk antibiotics on the course of an epidemic of *Clostridium difficile*-associated disease caused by the hypervirulent NAP1/027 strain. *Clin Infect Dis* 2007;45(Suppl 2):S112–S121.

88. Sethi AK, Al-Nassir WN, Nerandzic MM, Bobulsky GS, Donskey CJ. Persistence of skin contamination and environmental shedding of *Clostridium difficile* during and after treatment of *C. difficile* infection. *Infect Control Hosp Epidemiol* 2010;31(1):21–27.

89. Anderson DJ, Chen LF, Weber DJ, et al. Enhanced terminal room disinfection and acquisition and infection caused by multidrug-resistant organisms and *Clostridium difficile* (the benefits of enhanced terminal room disinfection study): A cluster-randomised, multicentre, crossover study. *Lancet* 2017;389(10071):805–814.

90. Pegues DA, Han J, Gilmar C, McDonnell B, Gaynes S. Impact of ultraviolet germicidal irradiation for no-touch terminal room disinfection on *Clostridium difficile* infection incidence among hematology-oncology patients. *Infect Control Hosp Epidemiol* 2017;38(1):39–44.

91. Grigoras CA, Zervou FN, Zacharioudakis IM, Siettos CI, Mylonakis E. Isolation of *C. difficile* carriers alone and as part of a bundle approach for the prevention of *Clostridium difficile* infection (CDI): A mathematical model based on clinical study data. *PLOS ONE* 2016;11(6):e0156577.

92. Lanzas C, Dubberke ER. Effectiveness of screening hospital admissions to detect asymptomatic carriers of *Clostridium difficile*: A modeling evaluation. *Infect Control Hosp Epidemiol* 2014;35(8):1043–1050.

93. Johnson S, Maziade PJ, McFarland LV, et al. Is primary prevention of *Clostridium difficile* infection possible with specific probiotics? *Int J Infect Dis* 2012;16(11):e786–e792.

94. Shen NT, Maw A, Tmanova LL, et al. Timely use of probiotics in hospitalized adults prevents *Clostridium difficile* infection: A systematic review with meta-regression analysis. *Gastroenterology* 2017;152(8):1889–1900, e1889.

95. Munoz P, Bouza E, Cuenca-Estrella M, et al. *Saccharomyces cerevisiae* fungemia: An emerging infectious disease. *Clin Infect Dis* 2005;40(11):1625–1634.

96. Cassone M, Serra P, Mondello F, et al. Outbreak of *Saccharomyces cerevisiae* subtype boulardii fungemia in patients neighboring those treated with a probiotic preparation of the organism. *J Clin Microbiol* 2003;41(11):5340–5343.

33 Rapid Infectious Diseases Diagnostics in the Critical Care Unit

Bronwen Garner and Kimberly Hanson

CONTENTS

CLINICAL PERSPECTIVE

Rapid diagnostic assays for infectious diseases have the potential to improve patient outcomes by informing targeted treatment for individual patients as well as guiding broader antimicrobial stewardship efforts. Unnecessary antibiotic use is associated with excess drug toxicity, *Clostridioides difficile* infection, the development of antibiotic resistance, and higher medical costs due to prolonged hospital stays [1]. Making a specific microbiologic diagnosis is essential for both de-escalation of broad-spectrum empiric therapy as well as optimal treatment of both antibiotic-susceptible and -resistant organisms. Additionally, rapid diagnosis can inform infection control measures. In this chapter, we will review US Food and Drug Administration (FDA)-cleared rapid diagnostic assays, with a focus on new tests for lower respiratory tract infection (LRTI) and bloodstream infection (BSI) in adult patients. The classification of "rapid" in this review varies widely by technology and is benchmarked relative to the classic laboratory methods. Some rapid tests are culture independent and designed to be applied directly to specimens, with results generated in minutes to hours. Alternatively, other assays require pre-amplification of organisms in culture. Although these tests are relatively fast (i.e., organism identification

and/or antimicrobial susceptibility results within hours), the upfront culture requirement still requires days. Additionally, host biomarkers such as procalcitonin (PCT) are complimentary approaches to pathogen-based tests. We will discuss how selected rapid technologies work, the potential benefits, and pitfalls of each, as well as review current evidence to support their use in clinical practice.

PNEUMONIA

Despite major advances in supportive care, severe pneumonia remains one of the most common diagnoses leading to critical care unit (CCU) admission and hospital death. A variety of different pathogen-specific assays are available to assist in the etiologic diagnosis of pneumonia. Testing is useful because a specific cause of pneumonia cannot be established with clinical signs, symptoms, and chest imaging alone. Additionally, biomarkers may help separate patients with bacterial lung infection from those with viral disease or other non-infectious causes of pulmonary infiltrates. This section will review the use of urine antigen testing, nucleic acid amplification testing (NAAT) for respiratory viruses and bacteria, and the use of PCT.

URINE ANTIGEN TESTS

Detection of bacterial antigens in urine is a potentially rapid and non-invasive approach for evaluating suspected pneumonia. Bacterial cell wall components may translocate out of the lung parenchyma and into the bloodstream in the setting of invasive infection. Organism derived proteins in the peripheral circulation are then filtered by the kidney and concentrated in the urine. Urine antigen tests (UATs) are immunoassays that use antibodies to capture and detect bacterial proteins. Immunoassays may be designed as enzyme immunoassays (EIAs) or lateral-flow immunoassays (LFAs). The latter are also referred to as immunochromatographic assays. Current UATs are designed to detect *Legionella pneumophila* and *Streptococcus pneumoniae*.

LEGIONELLA PNEUMOPHILA

L. pneumophila exists as three serotypes, with serotype 1 causing 80% of disease [2–5]. Available *Legionella* UATs only target serotype 1, which has important implications for immunocompromised patients and other settings where non-pneumophila species or serotypes 2 or 3 are important agents of disease. Commercially available *Legionella* UATs utilize either EIA methods or LFA methods, but a College of American Pathologists (CAP) survey in 2013 reported that 95% of clinical laboratories were using an LFA [2,5]. The LFAs have the benefit of simplicity for near-patient testing, with a sensitivity that is generally comparable to laboratory-based EIA methodologies.

There are five FDA-cleared *Legionella* UATs in the United States: Alere BinaxNOW, Binax, SAS, Bartels, and Meridian Tru (fda.gov). In a recent meta-analysis of 32 studies, the pooled sensitivity and specificity of *Legionella* UAT were 74% and 99%, respectively [4]. However, LFAs reportedly perform slightly better, with a sensitivity of 90%–97% and a specificity of 95%–100%. Reported EIA sensitivity is 87%–95%, with a specificity of 86%–91% [6–10]. Urine concentration and incubation for an additional 60 minutes beyond the manufacturer's recommended protocol may increase the sensitivity, without decreasing specificity [6–8]. For the EIA tests, concentrating the urine will improve Binax sensitivity, whereas Bartels performs better on non-concentrated specimens [9,10]. Knowing what assay the clinical laboratory performs and whether the lab performs specimen concentration may be useful for interpreting patient test results. It is also important to note that urine antigens can persist and remain detectable for months after a treated infection [11]. Thus, follow-up testing to gauge response is not recommended, and interpretation of positive results should include a careful assessment of the patient's recent medical history.

STREPTOCOCCUS PNEUMONIAE

Only one *S. pneumoniae* UAT, the BinaxNOW (Abbott), is FDA approved and uses antibodies directed at the pneumococcal C-polysaccharide protein. Urine and cerebrospinal fluid are both acceptable specimens for testing, and turnaround time is approximately 15 minutes. Per the package insert [12], the BinaxNOW detects 23 pneumococcal serotypes, with a clinical sensitivity and specificity ranging from 86% to 90% and 71% to 94%, respectively. Cross-reactivity with closely related *Streptococcus mitis* is expected, and false positives from recent pneumococcal vaccination (within 5 days) are also a theoretic possibility. The severity of illness affects LFA performance. Studies using positive *Streptococcus* culture from sputum, pleural fluid, or blood as the diagnostic gold standard for comparison report the best LFA test performance [13–24].

RESPIRATORY VIRUS MOLECULAR DIAGNOSTICS

Identification of a respiratory virus as a cause of illness has significant implications for patient management. However, it is impossible for clinicians to differentiate between bacterial and viral LRTIs based on signs and symptoms alone. Although the presence of lobar consolidation on a chest radiograph is suggestive of bacterial pneumonia, interstitial infiltrates can be more difficult to interpret and may be present in a variety of viral and non-infectious diseases. Additionally, coinfection with bacterial and viral pathogens is possible. NAATs have revolutionized the diagnosis of respiratory viral illnesses, owing to their speed and high-level sensitivity and specificity. NAAT is now preferred to rapid viral antigen testing, direct fluorescent antibody staining, and viral culture for critically ill adult patients with suspected pneumonia.

SINGLEPLEX ASSAYS

There are a multitude of assays that target a single pathogen (i.e., singleplex tests), and these assays are widely used during respiratory viral season. Additionally, many of these assays are rapid NAAT tests that are Clinical Laboratory Improvement Amendments (CLIA) waived [25]. CLIA waiver means that the testing procedure is of low complexity, and therefore, non-laboratory personnel can be performed at the point of care. Several CLIA-waived assays are commercially available for the detection of influenza and/or respiratory syncytial virus (RSV). These tests include Alere i (Abbot Chicago, IL), cobas Liat (Roche Pleasanton, CA), FilmArray Respiratory EZ panel (BioFire Salt Lake City, UT), Accula (Mesa Biotech San Diego, CA), and Xpert Xpress (Cephied Sunnyvale, CA). The tests are based on a variety of different NAAT chemistries (Table 33.1) and achieve greater sensitivity (91%–95%) than is possible with rapid antigen detection, as well as uniformly high specificity (>98%) [26]. Patients admitted to the CCU during respiratory virus season may have already had a CLIA waived or laboratory-based test performed. If not, singleplex testing for influenza A and B, with/or without RSV, may make the most economic sense for immunocompetent adults during the influenza season. Rapid influenza testing has established benefits, including driving increased antiviral use in patients at risk for complications [27,28] as well as potentially

TABLE 33.1

Commercially Available Multiplex Panels Targeting Respiratory Viruses

Panel	FilmArray	Verigene	x-Tag RVP	x-TAG RVP Fast	NxTAG-RPP	eSensor RVP	ePlex
Platform	FilmArray	Verigene	Luminex	Luminex	Luminex	eSensor XT	ePlex
Method	PCR[a]	Microarray[a]	Fluorescent Bead Array	Fluorescent Bead Array	PCR/Bead Hybridization	Microarray Hybridization	Electrowetting
Target pathogen							
Adenovirus	X	X	X	X	X	X	X
Coronavirus					X		X
Coronavirus HKU1	X			X	X		
Coronavirus NL63	X			X	X		
Coronavirus 229E	X			X	X		
Coronavirus OC43	X			X	X		
Human bocavirus					X		
Human metapneumovirus	X	X	X	X	X	X	X
Influenza A (flu A) virus	X	X	X	X	X	X	X
Flu A subtype H1	X	X	X	X	X	X	X
Flu A subtype H3	X	X	X	X	X	X	X
Subtype 2009 H1N1	X					X	X
Influenza B	X	X	X	X	X	X	X
Parainfluenza virus 1	X	X	X		X	X	X
Parainfluenza virus 2	X	X	X		X	X	X
Parainfluenza virus 3	X	X	X		X	X	X
Parainfluenza virus 4	X	X			X		X
Respiratory syncytial virus (RSV)	X			X			
RSV A		X	X		X	X	X
RSV B		X	X		X	X	X
Rhinovirus/enterovirus	X	X	X	X	X	X	X
Chlamydophila pneumoniae	X				X		X
Mycoplasma pneumoniae	X				X		X
Bordatella pertussis	X	X					
Bordatella parapertussis/ bronchiseptica		X					
Bordatella holmseii		X					
Turnaround time	1 h	2–3 h	8 h	6 h	4 h	6 h	1.5 h

See also: www.fda.gov.

[a] Full methodology described in text.

Multiplex Assays

Respiratory Virus Panels

The widespread use of multiplex respiratory virus panels (RVPs) has shed light onto the significance of respiratory viruses as a major cause of morbidity and mortality among critically ill adult patients. In addition to influenza viruses, human metapneumovirus, parainfluenza viruses (PIV), rhinoviruses, and coronaviruses have all been associated with severe LRTI in immunocompetent adults and the elderly [29,30]. Viral and bacterial coinfection has also been linked to more severe community-acquired pneumonia (CAP) and longer hospitalization than with a bacterial etiology alone [31].

Seven large FDA-cleared RVPs are currently available (Table 33.1) [32]. The panels vary in terms of the number of organisms detected, laboratory complexity, and turnaround

decreasing mortality through earlier administration of treatment. When influenza is known to be circulating in the community, antiviral therapy should not be delayed while awaiting test results.

time to results, but all are intended for use with nasal and/or oropharyngeal (NP/OP) swabs. Clinical laboratories must perform separate validations of test performance to offer testing, using specimens collected from the lower respiratory tract. This is important because lower respiratory tract specimens such as bronchoalveolar lavage fluid (BAL) may be required to confirm whether a virus detected in an NP sample is also the cause of lower tract disease. In addition, viral replication localized to the lower tract is possible, and physicians should consider this [33] when the clinical suspicion for viral LRTI remains high but swab testing from the upper tract is negative.

Test characteristics of current RVPs will vary by individual analyte, platform, duration of symptoms, and host. In terms of test-specific differences, it is essential that CCU providers know which panel, if any, their laboratory is performing and understand potential issues with individual targets within the panel. The sensitivity and specificity of influenza and adenovirus targets, for example, have been shown to vary significantly across assays [34,35]. Additionally, sensitivity for influenza may vary seasonally as a result of genetic shift and drift [33]. Clinical factors affecting test sensitivity are also important and are largely related to virus load, which varies depending on when the specimen is collected during the course of illness as well as by patient population. The burden of organism is typically highest early in infection and lowest in elder patients as compared with other age groups. These factors must be considered when interpreting negative test results.

Testing for a wide array of viral pathogens simultaneously has theoretic benefits, but to date, the impact of multiplex RVP testing on patient outcomes in the CCU has not been systematically evaluated. Multiplex testing makes obvious sense for immunocompromised patients given the breath of viruses that can cause severe LRTI in this population. Furthermore, rapid multiplexed detection can also help to reduce unnecessary antibiotic use, decrease ancillary testing, and shorten length of hospital stay for hospitalized patients and/or those presenting to the emergency department [36–38]. The impact of detecting viruses other than influenza on clinical care decisions, however, has not been definitively established in adult populations. In one randomized study, there was a trend toward higher rates of discharge from the emergency department for adults who tested positive for non-influenza viruses [36]. In contrast, other groups have observed that positivity for respiratory viruses other than influenza does not correlate with reduced resource utilization or fewer antibiotics [39]. Adult providers are often unwilling to stop antibiotics when a virus other than influenza is detected, and this decision may be especially difficult in a critically ill patient with pulmonary infiltrates. This situation, however, represents an opportunity for careful reassessment of the need for antibiotics and may be one where use of a host biomarker such as PCT could be useful.

Despite the potential benefits, multiplex RVP testing also has its limitations. These assays are more expensive than singleplex tests, and there is limited cost-effectiveness data

to support a panel-based approach for all adult patients. An additional drawback is that some RVPs may have a lower sensitivity for individual targets than do singleplex polymerase chain reactions (PCRs) or culture. The FilmArray, for example, has been shown to have decreased sensitivities for detection of adenovirus, H1/2009 A influenza virus, and influenza B virus relative to well-designed laboratory-developed singleplex tests [40]. Additionally, the significance of multiple target detection from multiplex panels (i.e., viral coinfections) remains unclear and can be confusing for clinicians.

Bacterial Pathogen Panels

Rapid initiation of effective antimicrobials improves outcomes for patients with hospital-acquired and ventilator-associated pneumonia (VAP) [41,42]. Selecting effective empiric treatment is a constant challenge in an era of multidrugresistant nosocomial infections. Conventional diagnostics for pneumonia rely on culture and phenotypic susceptibility testing, the results of which are relatively slow (i.e., 48–72 hours minimum) and insensitive, especially in patients who have received antibiotics prior to specimen collection. Molecular detection methods have potential to be more rapid and detect mutations associated with antibiotic resistance.

In April 2018, the FDA approved the first multiplex PCR panel targeting bacterial pneumonia pathogens and associated resistance mutations. The Unyvero pneumonia panel (Curetis, Holzgerlingen Germany) identifies 20 bacteria, 39 genetic resistance markers, and 1 fungus (*Pneumocystis jirovecii*) within 4–5 hours and is currently labeled for use on tracheal aspirates [43]. Detected organisms cover the spectrum of common community-acquired pathogens as well as those encountered in a hospital setting.

The investigators have not yet published the clinical trial supporting FDA approval of the Unyvero pneumonia panel; however, two older studies evaluated the performance of a prototype device in hospitalized patients with severe LRTI [44,45]. In both studies, the multiplex PCR detected more putative pathogens than culture, and the authors did not assess agreement between the resistance markers and phenotypic susceptibility. Overall, the optimized prototype had a sensitivity of 79% and specificity of 97% versus culture for organisms included in the panel [45]. Shulte et al. also attempted to resolve discrepancies between culture and the multiplex panel, with just over half of the multiplex-positive/culture-negative results being confirmed by organism-specific PCR and DNA sequencing Additionally, the authors found 72% (36/50) false-negative multiplex PCR results that they confirmed with reference testing [45]. Resolving differences between culture and molecular methods can be difficult, in part because molecular assays can detect non-viable organisms. Although neither method can separate airway commensals from invasive pathogens, the molecular test may also have detected some organisms that would normally be lumped into the category of "normal respiratory flora" when no single organism was predominant on the culture plate. Alternatively, culture is likely more sensitive than multiplex testing for live bacteria, as not all resistance mechanisms are known, and the presence of a resistance gene does not always mean that it is being expressed. Thus, molecular diagnostics for bacteria cannot replace culture or phenotypic susceptibility testing. It is likely that additional assays will be FDA cleared in the near future. Well-designed clinical studies will be required to determine test performance in "real-life" practice as well as to establish optimal use and cost-effectiveness.

USE OF PROCALCITONIN FOR ACUTE RESPIRATORY INFECTIONS

Procalcitonin (PCT) is a peptide precursor of the hormone calcitonin that also acts as a mediator in inflammatory responses. In healthy individuals, thyroid C cells produce PCT and then convert it to calcitonin before entering the systemic circulation. PCT production can also occur outside of the thyroid, simulated by the cytokines interleukin (IL)-1, IL-6, and tumor necrosis factor-alpha, as well as bacterial lipopolysaccharide. Because non-thyroidal tissue lacks the ability to convert PCT to calcitonin, the pre-hormone enters the systemic circulation and becomes detectable at higher serum concentrations than are seen in healthy subjects (i.e., normal "healthy" range <0.05 ng/mL). PCT levels are highest in patients with acute bacterial sepsis and may be elevated due to other processes that stimulate cytokine production, such as massive trauma, malaria, fungal infections, Addisonian crisis, and graft-versus-host disease. In contrast, autoimmune conditions and viral infections do not affect PCT levels. Interferon gamma actually downregulates PCT, which may explain why the peptide does not increase with viral infections. Recently, multiple authors have published several excellent reviews on the biology and use of PCT in clinical care [46–49].

Procalcitonin is a potentially useful marker of early systemic bacterial infection because levels start to rise within 3–4 hours of exposure and peak within 6–24 hours, which is earlier than other acute-phase reactants such as C-reactive protein (CRP) and erythrocyte sedimentation rate (ESR) [48]. Additionally, serum PCT concentrations generally rise and fall in a pattern that is consistent with bacterial infection, response to therapy, and severity of illness [50]. Table 33.2 lists the FDA-cleared PCT assays along with their respective reportable ranges and turnaround time to results. Currently, the VIDAS BRAHMS PCT assay (bioMerieux, Marcy-l'Etoile, France) and the BRAHMS PCT Sensitive Kryptor (Thermo Fisher Scientific, Waltham, MA) have FDA-cleared indications for initiating or discontinuing antibiotics in patients with LRTIs and for discontinuing antibiotics in patients with sepsis. Recommended algorithms for PCT as a guide for antibiotic prescribing in adult patients have been established and are illustrated in Figures 33.1 and 33.2 [51,52].

In general, the sensitivity and specificity of PCT for the diagnosis acute bacterial pneumonia is better than other inflammatory markers such as CRP. A recent meta-analysis

TABLE 33.2
The FDA-Cleared PCT Assays

Assay (Manufacturer)	Reportable Range	Turnaround Time
Liaison BRAHMS PCT II Gen (DiaSorin)	0.02–100 ng/mL	16 min
Lumipulse G BRAHMS PCT (Fujirebio)	0.02–100 ng/mL	30 min
ARCHITECHT BRAHMS PCT (Fisher)	0.02–100 ng/mL	22 min
BRAHMS PCT sensitive KRYPTOR (BRAHMS GmbH)	0.02–5000 ng/mL	19 min
Diazyme Procalcitonin assay (Diazyme)[a]	0.2 µg/L–52 ng/mL	10 min
VIDAS BRAHMS PCT (BioMerieux)	0.05–200 ng/mL	20 min
Elecsys BRAHMS PCT (Roche)	0.02–100 ng/mL	18 min

[a] Use on Olympus AU400 chemistry analyzer.

summarized the clinical impact of PCT-guided antibiotic decision making, specifically for adults with LRTI across a variety of healthcare settings, including the CCU. LRTIs included acute bronchitis, exacerbations of chronic obstructive pulmonary disease (COPD), and CAP but excluded studies focused on VAP [53]. A total of 11 randomized controlled trials involving 4090 subjects were included in the analysis. All studies used the 0.25 ng/mL cutoff, below which antibiotic treatment was discouraged, and additional triggers generally mirrored Figure 33.1. Overall, subjects who had PCT-guided treatment had lower odds of antibiotic initiation (odds ratio 0.26 [95% CI: 013–0.52]) and shorter mean antibiotic use (weighted mean difference −2.15 days [95% CI: −3.30 to −0.99]) compared with those subjects who managed with routine care alone. Additionally, there was no adverse impact on mortality or length of hospital stay.

A number of patient-level systematic reviews from the same group of authors have reported similar findings in terms of the impact of PCT-driven prescribing decisions on reduced antibiotic usage as well as reduced morbidity and mortality for acute respiratory infections [54,55]. Reasons for reduced mortality with the use of PCT are unclear but may be related to reductions in antibiotic-associated toxicities and/or earlier diagnosis and treatment of other conditions when PCT values are low. Unfortunately, small patient numbers in subgroup analyses limit evaluation of PCT in CCU patients with CAP or severe exacerbation of COPD. Additionally, no prospective randomized study has ever compared outcomes among patients with VAP managed with clinical criteria plus PCT versus clinical criteria alone.

Procalcitonin is not a substitute for sound medical judgment. In critically ill patients with a high pre-test probability for pneumonia, physicians should initiate antibiotics despite low initial PCT levels. In this scenario, physicians

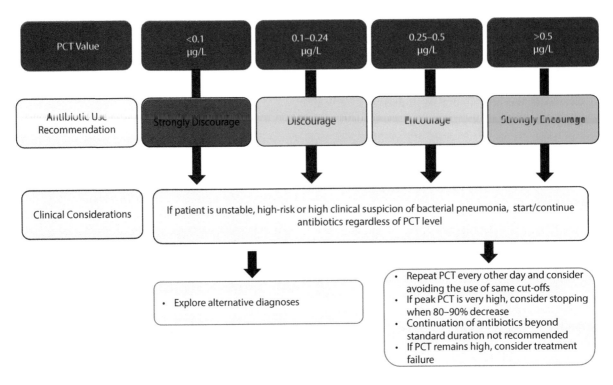

FIGURE 33.1   Example procalcitonin (PCT) algorithm lower respiratory tract infections.

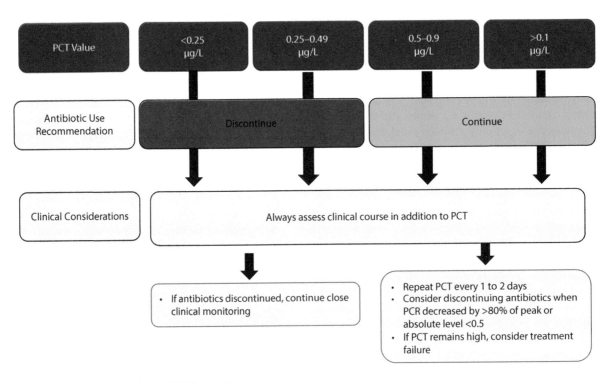

FIGURE 33.2   Example procalcitonin (PCT) algorithm sepsis.

could still monitor PCT to assess treatment response and should prompt exploration of alternative diagnoses. It is also important to recognize that patients with atypical pathogens, such as *Mycoplasma pneumoniae* and *Chlamydophila pneumoniae*, or localized abscess or empyema may have

low PCT levels [56,57] Furthermore, most studies excluded immunocompromised patients, which also limit the generalizability of meta-analysis results to this population. An additional limitation is the variability in protocols and investigator adherence to antibiotic-stopping rules across trials. Intensive care unit studies have mainly used PCT to stop antibiotics when levels decreased to below 0.1–0.5 ng/mL or by at least 80%–90% of its peak level. In the emergency department and primary care trials, providers used PCT cutoff of 0.25 ng/mL cutoff to start and stop antibiotics. These differences have implications for syndrome-specific algorithms. Additionally, adherence to the algorithm, which is likely better in a clinical trial than in "real-life," will also impact the potential benefits derived from PCT testing [58].

SUMMARY OF RECOMMENDATIONS FOR DIAGNOSTIC USE IN THE CCU

COMMUNITY-ACQUIRED PNEUMONIA

For patients admitted to the CCU with CAP, current guidelines recommend obtaining blood and sputum or endotracheal suction (for intubated patients) specimens for culture along with UAT for *Legionella* and *S. pneumonia* [59]. Of note, the Infectious Diseases Society of America committee published CAP recommendations in 2007, and an update is currently underway [59]. The committee did not address the use of additional methodologies, including multiplex NAAT and/or PCT in the 2007 CAP document. We recommend multiplex RVPs be considered for critically ill patients during respiratory virus season, especially when first-line influenza testing is negative, and for all significantly immunocompromised hosts [60]. Lastly, available evidence supports the use of PCT in conjunction with clinical assessment for safely de-escalating antibiotics in immunocompetent adults with LRTI, but antibiotics should not be withheld from patients with CAP [61] or severe exacerbations of chronic obstructive lung disease [62] based on low PCT.

VENTILATOR-ASSOCIATED AND HOSPITAL-ACQUIRED PNEUMONIA

Guidelines for the management of adults with VAP or HAP are relatively recent (2016) but still predate the availability of new multiplex PCR panels targeting bacterial pathogens [59]. Because of the growing incidence of multidrug-resistant organisms in the hospital, standard care for patients with suspected HAP/VAP is also to collect respiratory tract secretions and blood for culture. The role that multiplex bacterial panels should play requires further study, and their routine use cannot be recommended at this time. Lastly, it is recommended to use clinical criteria alone, rather than using serum PCT plus clinical criteria, to decide whether or not to initiate antibiotic therapy. PCT, however, may be useful as an aid in antibiotic de-escalation decisions.

Bloodstream Infection

Standard clinical care is to immediately initiate empiric broad spectrum antibiotic therapy, after blood is collected for culture, in patients suspected to have sepsis. In fact, the surviving sepsis campaign guidelines recommend administration of empiric broad spectrum antibiotics as soon as possible, and within 1 hour maximum, from recognition of severe sepsis or septic shock [63]. In the guidelines, physicians should continue until they identify the etiological agent of sepsis and antimicrobial susceptibility test (AST) results are available to tailor therapy. Unfortunately, empiric antimicrobial treatment choices are often inadequate or excessively broad in a significant proportion of patients [64]. Ineffective empiric choices are associated with increased mortality [65]. Thus, new technologies that more quickly and accurately identify a microbial cause of sepsis are important tools for the intensivist. In this section, we focus our review on new approaches to the rapid diagnosis of BSI. Blood cultures remain the diagnostic gold standard for BSI, and there are new complementary tools that can be applied to pure organism isolates, positive blood culture bottle aliquots, or directly to whole blood for more rapid organism detection.

Matrix-Assisted Laser Desorption Ionization Time-of-Flight Mass Spectroscopy

Matrix-assisted laser desorption ionization time-of-flight mass spectroscopy (MALDI-TOF MS) has revolutionized the identification of microorganisms in the clinical laboratory. This technology uses a small amount of pure organism growth taken from solid or broth culture media and spotted onto a target plate. Matrix, which is critical for protein ionization, is added to the sample spot, and then, the target plate is allowed to dry. After drying, the target plate gets loaded onto the MS instrument, where each sample is vaporized using a laser pulse. An electric field directs and accelerates the ionized particles down a "time-of-flight" tube. The time it takes for the ionized particles to reach the detector at the end of the tube is directly proportional to a molecule's mass and charge. The mass to charge ratio of detected proteins creates a spectral fingerprint that is compared to a reference database of known organism patterns. This entire process takes about 10–30 minutes.

MALDI-TOF MS is generally more accurate than phenotypic identification methods (i.e., morphology and biochemical analysis). In addition, the process significantly speeds time to identification relative to classical methods and is cost-effective for the clinical laboratory [66]. There are two FDA-cleared MALDI-TOF MS platforms available in the United States (MALDI Biotyper [Bruker; Billerica, MA] and VITEK MS [bioMerieux; Marcy l'Etoile France]), each with proprietary databases and algorithms for assigning organism identification. The Bruker system in FDA cleared for the identification of common bacteria and yeast, while the bioMerieux instrument has FDA-cleared protocols for bacterial, yeast, mycobacteria, and filamentous fungi. It is important to recognize, however, that there are some organisms that cannot be definitively identified by MALDI, either because of close phylogenetic relationships or as a result of limited representation in available databases. Additionally, MALDI identifications still need to be matched to phenotypic characteristics and expected antibiotic susceptibility patterns.

From a laboratory perspective, MALDI-TOF MS identifies bacteria and yeast on average 1.45 days earlier than traditional methods and can reduce labor and reagent costs on the order of $100,000 [67]. In addition to the laboratory workflow benefits, more rapid organism identification from pure culture can also translate into improved patient outcomes. In a single-center study of 245 patients with BSI, MALDI-TOF MS combined with antibiotic stewardship significantly decreased time to effective therapy (−9.7 hours), reduced length of CCU stay (−6.6 days), and there was a trend toward reduced mortality relative to routine testing with a laboratory report of results only [68].

Organism Identification in Positive Blood Culture Aliquots

A variety of technologies have been used to detect microorganisms growing in blood culture bottle broth. For this approach, an aliquot of blood is taken from the bottle at the time the culture flags positive for growth, and a gram stain confirms the presence of a microorganism. Both single-organism and multiplex molecular methods, including protein nucleic acid (PNA), fluorescence in situ hybridization (FISH), multiplex PCR, and microarray technologies, are available to detect the most common BSI organisms. Although MALDI-TOF MS procedures can be adapted for use with positive blood culture aliquots [69–72], only testing from pure culture is currently FDA cleared.

PNA FISH

PNA FISH was one of the first methodologies used for rapid nucleic acid identification from blood culture bottles. The key reagent is a species-specific DNA probe that targets pathogen ribosomal RNA and can be applied to a smear of blood taken from the culture bottle. The probe is labeled with a fluorescent molecule that allows the technologist to visualize color fluorescence under a fluorescent microscope. Test characteristics are dependent upon technician expertise, and therefore, the results are subject to inter-reader variability. Commercially available assays (Table 33.3) differentiate between coagulase-negative *Staphylococcus* species (CoNS) and *Staphylococcus aureus*, *Enterococcus faecalis*, and other *Enterococcus* spp.; three gram-negative rods (*E. coli*, *K. pneumonia*, and *P. aeruginosa*); as well as group six *Candida* common species, according to likely fluconazole susceptibility (*C. albicans*, *C. parapsilosis*, *C. glabrata*, *C. krusei*, and *C. tropicalis*).

A number of studies have shown that PNA FISH testing reduces time from positive culture to pathogen identification, and when these results are applied in conjunction with an antimicrobial stewardship program, it can ensure correct antimicrobial therapy, improve patient outcomes, and decrease hospital costs (Table 33.3). Specifically, rapid differentiation of CoNS from *S. aureus* has established benefits. Forrest et al. retrospectively evaluated the impact of rapidly identifying CoNS when gram-positive cocci in clusters were observed on the blood culture gram stain and reported that length of hospital stay could be decreased with a cost savings of about $4000 when the results were acted on with the help of an antibiotic stewardship team [73]. Additionally, in a prospective study by Ly et al., active physician notification of positive *S. aureus* PNA FISH results decreased mortality and reduced cost by almost $20,000 per patient, likely as a result of decreased time to optimal antibiotic therapy [74]. Without active physician notification, PNA FISH testing for *S. aureus* may have no benefit [75]. PNA FISH for *C. albicans* also has similar economic benefits via reduced echinocandin use [76].

SINGLE-PATHOGEN PLATFORMS

The GeneOhm StaphSR (BD, Sparks MD) and Xpert MRSA/SA (Cephied, Sunnyvale CA) are the two FDA-cleared real time PCR assays for *S. aureus* and methicillin-resistant *S. aureus* (MRSA) from positive blood cultures. Both tests function similarly, with a clinical accuracy of >97% for detection of *S. aureus* and differentiation of methicillin-resistance via *mecA* gene detection [77–79]. Similar to PNA FISH studies, rapid differentiation of MRSA in patients with *S. aureus* bacteremia has the potential to impact clinical outcomes. In a single-center study including 156 patients with *S. aureus* bacteremia, median time to de-escalation from empiric vancomycin to targeted nafcillin or cefazolin in patients with methicillin-susceptible *S. aureus* was 1.7 days faster with rapid testing and pharmacist intervention [80]. Additionally, length of hospital stay was reduced by 6.2 days (p = 0.07) and mean hospital costs were $21,387 less than the time period before rapid testing with stewardship.

MULTIPLEX PLATFORMS

Two FDA-approved multiplex panels provide rapid identification combined with limited resistance gene detection from blood culture aliquots (Table 33.3). Current assays (Verigene gram-positive blood culture test [BC-GP], Verigene gram-negative blood culture test [BC-GN] both from Luminex [Northbrook IL], and the FilmArray Blood Culture Identification Panel or BCID [Biofire Diagnostics, Salt Lake City UT]) are fully automated and produce results in approximately 1–2 hours. The FilmArray platform is a closed, multiplex PCR system that integrates sample preparation, nucleic acid amplification, organism detection, and analysis of 27 targets, including gram-positive and gram-negative bacteria, selected bacterial drug-resistance genes, plus identification of the five most common *Candida* species. The Verigene platform performs automated nucleic acid extraction, followed by target detection, using hybridization on to a microarray containing complementary nucleic acid targets. The Verigene system has two cartridges, a gram-positive and a gram-negative microarray, which are selected based on the Gram stain morphology observed from the blood culture bottle [32,79].

There is a robust literature comparing the accuracy of the aforementioned multiplex panels to conventional identification methods. Overall, available systems are highly accurate for speciation (i.e., 87%–97% correct identifications) compared with standard methods [81,82]. Clinically, multiplex platforms affect antibiotic use. Ultimately, a significant

TABLE 33.3

Molecular Assays for Organism Detection Using Positive Blood Culture Aliquots

Panel	FilmArray BCID	Verigene Gram-Positive	PNA FISH
Platform	FilmArray	Verigene	Vendor Dependent
Method	PCR[a]	Microarray[a]	Nucleic Acid Hybridization to Target Organism DNA
Gram-Positive Organism			
Staphylococcus spp.	X	X	X
Staphylococcus aureus	X	X	X
Staphylococcus epidermidis		X	
Staphylococcus lugdunensis		X	
Streptococcus spp.	X	X	
Streptococcus agalactiae	X	X	
Streptococcus pyogenes	X	X	
Streptococcus pneumoniae	X	X	
Streptococcus anginosus		X	
Enterococcus spp.	X		X
Enterococcus faecalis		X	X
Enterococcus faecium		X	
Listeria spp.		X	
Listeria monocytogenes	X		
Resistance genes			
mecA	X	X	
vanA	X	X	
vanB	X	X	
Gram-Negative Organism	**FilmArray BCID**	**Verigene Gram-Negative**	**PNA FISH**
Klebsiella oxytoca	X	X	
Klebsiella pneumoniae	X	X	X
Serratia marcescens	X		
Proteus spp.		X	
Acinetobacter spp.		X	
Acinetobacter baumannii	X		
Haemophilus influenzae	X	X	
Neisseria meningitis	X	X	
Pseudomonas aeruginosa	X	X	X
Enterobacteriaceae	X		
Escherichia coli	X	X	X
Enterobacter spp.		X	
Enterobacter cloacae complex	X		
Citrobacter spp.		X	
Resistance genes			
bla$_{KPC}$	X	X	
bla$_{NDM}$		X	
bla$_{OXA}$		X	
bla$_{VIM}$		X	
bla$_{IMP}$		X	
bla$_{CTX-M}$		X	
Yeast	**FilmArray BCID**	**Verigene**	**PNA FISH**
Candida albicans	X		X[b]
Candida glabrata	X		X[c]
Candida krusei	X		X[c]
Candida parapsilosis	X		X[b]
Candida tropicalis	X		X

[a] Methodology previously described in text.

[b] Cannot differentiate between *C. albicans* and *C. parapsilosis*, unless paired with *C. albicans*-specific assay.

[c] Cannot differentiate between *C. glabrata* and *C. krusei*, unless paired with *C. glabrata*-specific assay.

decrease in inappropriate or unnecessary antimicrobial use occurs when rapid identification couples with an active antimicrobial stewardship intervention [32,66]. Most studies, however, are not powered to demonstrate a mortality benefit or influence on hospital or CCU length of stay. Additionally, use of a multiplex molecular panel may be of incremental benefit when a laboratory is already using MALDI-TOF MS for rapid organism identification from culture.

As with all tests, multiplex panels have some important limitations. All current platforms perform better with monomicrobial than with polymicrobial BSIs, because they often cannot detect all organisms in a mixed infection [83–85]. Additionally, multiplex panels cannot link resistance determinants to a specific organism in a mixed infection (e.g., assignment of a mecA gene to S. aureus in a mixed culture also containing CoNS). Because the FilmArray system uses nucleic acid amplification, it may also detect DNA contaminants and/or non-viable bacteria in the blood culture bottle. Although the bottle is technically sterile, detection of *Candida*, *Proteus*, and *Pseudomonas* DNA in specimens that never grow these organisms can be misleading. Therefore, the correlation of multiplex results with the Gram stain is absolutely essential. Finally, although these panels detect the most common causes of BSI, local epidemiology may differ. The spectrum of targeted pathogens in current panels may be most useful in general medical or surgical CCUs, as opposed to units in cancer hospitals or transplant centers that encounter a more diverse group of pathogens.

RAPID ANTIMICROBIAL SUSCEPTIBILITY TESTING

Traditional identification and antimicrobial susceptibility testing (AST) results for the most common organisms causing BSIs typically take longer than 48 hours to obtain [86]. The molecular assays for rapid organism identification from positive blood culture aliquots also detect a few resistance genes such as mecA, VanA/B, CTX-M, and selected carbapenemase genes. However, these targets provide limited information, especially for gram-negative pathogens such as *Pseudomonas*, *Acinetobacter*, and the *Enterobacteriaceae*. A new FDA-cleared platform called the Accelerate Pheno System (Accelerate Diagnostics, Tucson AZ) automates FISH-based organism identification of common bacteria and yeast, combined with morphokinetic analysis of bacterial cells growing in the presence of various antibiotics to calculate a minimum inhibitory concentration (MIC). The instrument produces organism identification results within 90 minutes and AST in approximately 7 hours as well as generates a "monomicrobial" call, indicating that only one organism is present. A number of studies have evaluated Accelerate test performance [87–90]. Overall, sensitivity and specificity for identification of organisms contained in the FISH panel have ranged from 95% to 100% and 99%, respectively. Additionally, categorical agreement (i.e., susceptible, intermediate, or resistant per current Clinical and Laboratory Standards Institute [CLSI] breakpoints) compared with standard phenotypic AST has been generally good (~95%).

It is clear that Accelerate speeds time to results and may reduce "hands on time" in the clinical laboratory [90]. However, in its current format, Accelerate cannot replace standard AST methods. Routine testing is required for all off-panel organisms or drugs, to resolve discrepancies or invalid Accelerate results and to match Accelerate results to the Gram stain results. Other considerations for the clinical laboratory are the relatively high price or kits and the instrument with a limitation of only running one blood culture sample per unit at any given time (although the system can integrate up to four individual units). Prospective studies are required to know whether the addition of rapid AST to rapid identification procedures with/or without resistance gene detection can improve patient outcomes in the CCU.

ORGANISM DETECTION DIRECTLY FROM BLOOD

T2CANDIDA

Candida is the third most common cause of BSI in the CCU [91]. The incidence of invasive candidiasis (IC), however, may vary widely based on clinical and host-associated risk factors for disease. A large epidemiologic study carried out in patients who stayed at least 4 days in one of 12 participating medical and surgical CCUs observed a candidemia prevalence of 3% across general critical care settings [92]. However, patients with multiple IC risk factors fulfilling prediction rule criteria have a higher prevalence (~10%) [93,94], and rates of intra-abdominal candidiasis may be exceptionally high (~30%) in surgical CCU patients with biliary leaks or gastro/duodenal perforation [95,96]. The overall mortality due to IC in CCU patients is comparable a those with severe sepsis and septic shock. Blood culture remains the diagnostic standard for *Candida* BSI but has a poor sensitivity as a result of the generally low numbers of yeast cells circulating in the blood [97]. Additionally, average time to culture positivity ranges from 2–5 days, and delays in antifungal treatment are directly associated with increased mortality [98].

T2 magnetic resonance (T2MR) is a culture-independent technology applied directly to whole blood specimens. The T2Candida test (T2 Biosystems, Lexington, MA) integrates whole cell organism concentration coupled with multiplex PCR to amplify and detect DNA from the five most common *Candida* species. Complementary oligonucleotides bound to paramagnetic nanoparticles are used to capture the amplified DNA of interest, and when specific DNA amplicons are present in a specimen, the nanoparticles agglomerate, causing a change in the aqueous environment around the particles that is detected using magnetic resonance [99]. The method is highly sensitive (limit of detection as low as 1 CFU/mL), with results reported qualitatively for *C. albicans*/*C. parapsilosis*, *C. tropicalis*, and/or *C. glabata*/*C. krusei* in approximately 3–5 hours [100].

In the prospective clinical trial that supported FDA approval of the assay, T2Candida had an overall sensitivity of 91% and specificity of 98% for candidemia [101]. A follow-up study also showed that prior antifungal exposure and neutropenia were independently associated with T2-positive/culture-negative results [102]. Ostrosky-Zeichner et al. evaluated T2Candida test performance in the CCU specifically [92]. Assuming a prevalence of 3%, the authors calculated a positive predictive value (PPV) of close to 80% and negative predictive value (NPV) of 99.7% [92,99,101]. Thus, the test may be most useful for withholding or stopping antifungal therapy when the prevalence of disease is in an "average ICU patient with sepsis" range. A pair of recent studies from Spain also showed that a positive test may have prognostic value [103,104]. Positive T2Candida result within the first 5 days of a positive blood culture was an independent risk factor for higher attributable mortality and/or the development of a complicated infection (odds ratio 36.5) [105]. Similarly, a positive baseline T2Candida after initiation of empirical therapy was an independent risk factor for poor outcomes (odds radio 26.4) [103].

The T2Candida test represents an exciting development in the fungal diagnostics landscape, but there are some associated drawbacks. The technology is still relatively new and remains quite expensive. Mylonakis et al. classified 10% of test results as "invalid" due to technical run failures [101], which, if not corrected, could have substantial associated cost and frustration. Additionally, finding the sweet spot of prevalence for optimal use may not be straightforward and additional studies are required to define test characteristics for other forms of *Candida* infection such as intra-abdominal candidiasis. If physicians do not interpret test results properly, especially the T2Candida-positive/culture-negative results, there may be unintended consequences for stewardship and nosocomial infection reporting. It is also important to note that T2 is not a substitute for culture. Organism isolation is still required to perform susceptibility testing, and the current assay does not detect all possible *Candida* species.

SELECTED BIOMARKERS

(1,3)-Beta-D-Glucan

Patients with invasive fungal infections often have detectable (1,3)-beta-D-glucan (BDG) levels, using the limulus amebocyte lysate reaction [106]. BDG is a cell wall polysaccharide found in many medically important fungi, including *Candida*, *Aspergillus*, and *Pneumocystis*; notable exceptions are *Cryptococcus*, *Mucorales*, and the yeast form of *Blastomyces*. The Fungitell test (Associates of Cape Cod, Falmouth, MA) is currently the only FDA-cleared BDG assay in the United States and produces quantitative results in about 2–3 hours.

The majority of BDG studies have focused on serial surveillance, with testing performed either once or twice a week for the early diagnosis of invasive *Candida* infection in at-risk patients. Multiple CCU studies have reported earlier diagnosis using BDG monitoring (3–6 days sooner) as compared with culture-based on symptoms [107,108]. A number of systematic reviews have also summarized BDG test characteristics. The pooled sensitivity and specificity of BDG were approximately 75%–80% and 80%–85%, respectively [109,110]. Requiring two sequential positive tests to define a true positive result may increase specificity [108,111], but in general, the PPV and specificities of BDG are lower in the critical care setting than has been reported for hematology/oncology patients. Like T2Candida, the prevalence of invasive *Candida* infections in a given CCU will impact the predictive values of the BDG test. Figure 33.3 graphs predictive values for BDG and T2Candida as a function of prevalence and estimated assay sensitivity and specificity. Again, for a "typical" CCU patient with a pre-test probability on the order of 3%, repeatedly negative BDG results may be useful for stopping empiric treatment and thus reducing unnecessary antifungal use. This potential benefit was demonstrated in a prospective study of 198 critically ill adult patients with signs and symptoms of sepsis and a *Candida* score ≥3 [112]. In this study, there were 47 cases of candidemia, and all of these subjects had a positive BDG test. However, a total of 63 patients tested positive for BDG and were treated. Posteraro et al. observed that physicians eventually stopped antifungal therapy for the 16 false-positive cases once IC was ruled out. The authors also observed avoidance of antifungal therapy in approximately 73% of potentially treatable patients based in part on negative BDG results, and they observed shorter treatment in another 20% of cases. Overall, the BDG negative group received less antifungal therapy than did the positive group (10 days vs. 5 days; p = 0.04), without impacting outcome.

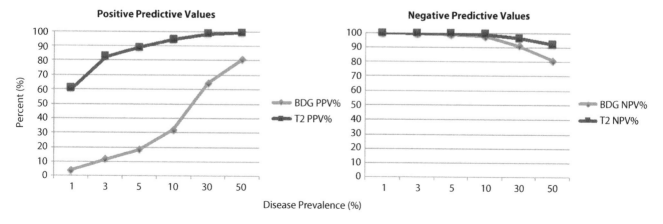

FIGURE 33.3 Predictive value of fungal diagnostics.

There are several important limitations of the BDG test that must also be mentioned. First, the test is a pan-fungal marker that does not identify the presence of a specific fungal pathogen. In addition, multiple blood products, some antibiotics, and/or gram-positive BSIs, hemodialysis/hemofiltration, enteral nutrition, gastrointestinal disruption, and use of gauze products during surgery have all been linked to false-positive glucan results [109,111,113–115]. Many of these are common occurrences in the CCU. Lastly, although the test can be automated [116], the FDA-approved Fungitell protocol is a cumbersome manual process. Many laboratories may elect to send testing out to a reference laboratory or perform batched testing only on certain days, which significantly delays turnaround time to results.

USE OF PROCALCITONIN IN CRITICAL ILLNESS AND SEPSIS

Multiple randomized controlled trials have examined PCT for antibiotic de-escalation in the CCU, and these studies have been recently been review elsewhere [46,47]. When compared with standard care, PCT monitoring reduced median durations of antibiotic therapy on the order of 1.7–3.8 days across trials, without affecting mortality or CCU length of stay. Additionally, a large propensity score-matched analysis investigated the impact of one to two PCT determinations ordered day 1 of CCU admission. PCT utilization was associated with significantly decreased total hospital and CCU length of stay, lower hospital costs, and lower total antibiotic exposure [117].

Despite the strength of the PCT sepsis literature, the same limitations discussed in the LRTI section apply here. Additionally, an important consideration in septic patients is that reduced glomerular filtration may affect PCT clearance, and, as a result, PCT may be artificially elevated during periods of renal impairment [118]. The optimal strategy for implementing PCT algorithms in CCU sepsis protocols has not been established. Whether stewardship team intervention is essential to realizing the potential benefits, as has been shown for other rapid BSI diagnostics, has also not been rigorously studied in a prospective fashion.

RECOMMENDATIONS FOR RAPID BLOODSTREAM INFECTION DIAGNOSTICS IN THE CCU

Rapid diagnostics for bacteria and yeast in patients with BSI have consistently been shown to reduce time to organism identification relative to standard culture methods. Faster time to optimal antimicrobial therapy can be achieved based on rapid identification when the testing is paired with an antibiotic stewardship team intervention. At a minimum, the use of MALDI-TOF MS for organism identification is recommended, whenever resources allow. The instruments themselves are quite expensive, but the cost can be offset by savings in labor, reagents, and potentially reduced antimicrobial costs to the pharmacy. Whether rapid phenotypic susceptibility testing can further improve outcomes, particularly for gram-negative infections, requires further study. The utility of T2MR and BDG for candidemia largely depends on the prevalence of disease. In general, in medical and surgical CCUs, the incorporation of T2MR or BDG surveillance into diagnostic algorithms is most beneficial when restricted to situations where the positive or negative predictive values of the test differ in a clinically meaningful way from the pretest probability for IC. Lastly, current evidence supports use of PCT testing algorithms, along with clinical criteria and pathogen-based diagnostics, to help guide early antibiotic discontinuation decisions in adult CCU patients with sepsis or septic shock who have stabilized.

SUMMARY AND CONCLUSIONS

Major recent advances in diagnostic technologies have enabled more rapid and accurate diagnosis of a number of important infectious diseases. Decreasing the time it takes for LRTI and BSI microorganism identification, with or without a rapid AST, is considered likely to improve patient outcomes and reduce healthcare costs by reducing time to targeted antimicrobial therapy. Additionally, serum biomarkers used in conjunction with clinical signs/symptoms plus pathogen-specific testing have the potential to reduce unnecessary antimicrobial use. It is important to note, however, that most of the studies included in this review were conducted in large university or tertiary care centers. Implementation of the rapid testing discussed in this chapter will likely be affected by many local factors, including available resources and space, staff expertise, specimen volume, budgetary constraints, and the ability to provide active notification of test results to physicians or pharmacists to ensure early appropriate interventions. Antibiotic stewardship team involvement is essential for realizing the potential power of rapid diagnostics, but these types of staff members may not be readily available in all hospitals. Additionally, many studies came from single centers and included relatively small numbers of CCU patients. Going forward, additional high-quality studies are required to definitively establish the cost-effectiveness of the new technologies reviewed here. Educational campaigns conducted by clinical and laboratory stakeholders may also help to assure that rapid testing is optimally utilized, with the goal of improving patient care.

REFERENCES

1. Tamma PD, Avdic E, Li DX, Dzintars K, Cosgrove SE. Association of adverse events with antibiotic use in hospitalized patients. *JAMA Intern Med* 2017;177(9):1308–1315.
2. Couturier MR, Graf EH, Griffin AT. Urine antigen tests for the diagnosis of respiratory infections: Legionellosis, histoplasmosis, pneumococcal pneumonia. *Clin Lab Med* 2014;34(2):219–36.
3. Pierre DM, Baron J, Victor LY, Stout JE. Diagnostic testing for legionnaires' disease. *Ann Clin Microbiol Antimicrob* 2017;16(1):59.

4. Shimada T, Noguchi Y, Jackson JL, et al. Systematic review and metaanalysis: Urinary antigen tests for legionellosis. *Chest* 2009;136(6):1576–1585.

5. Mercante JW, Winchell JM. Current and emerging *Legionella* diagnostics for laboratory and outbreak investigations. *Clin Microbiol Rev* 2015;28(1): 95–133.

6. Helbig JH, Uldum SA, Lück PC, Harrison TG. Detection of *Legionella pneumophila* antigen in urine samples by the BinaxNOW immunochromatographic assay and comparison with both binax *Legionella* urinary enzyme immunoassay (EIA) and biotest *Legionella* urin antigen EIA. *J Med Microbiol* 2001;50(6):509–516.

7. Bruin JP, Diederen BM. Evaluation of meridian TRU *Legionella*(R), a new rapid test for detection of *Legionella pneumophila* serogroup 1 antigen in urine samples. *Eur J Clin Microbiol Infect Dis* 2013;32(3):333–334.

8. Diederen BM, Peeters MF. Evaluation of the SAS *Legionella* test, a new immunochromatographic assay for the detection of *Legionella pneumophila* serogroup 1 antigen in urine. *Clin Microbiol Infect* 2007;13(1):86–88.

9. Dominguez J, Galı N, Blanco S, et al. Assessment of a new test to detect *Legionella* urinary antigen for the diagnosis of legionnaires' disease. *Diagn Microbiol Infect Dis* 2001;41(4):199–203.

10. de Ory F. Evaluation of a new ELISA (Bartels) for detection of *Legionella pneumophila* antigen in urine. *Enferm Infecc Microbiol Clin* 2002;20(3):106–109.

11. Reller LB, Weinstein MP, Murdoch DR. Diagnosis of *Legionella* infection. *Clin Infect Dis* 2003;36(1):64–69.

12. Alere BinaxNOW *Streptococcus pneumoniae* Antigen Card.

13. Dominguez J, Gal N, Blanco S, et al. Detection of *Streptococcus pneumoniae* antigen by a rapid immunochromatographic assay in urine samples. *Chest* 2001;119(1):243–249.

14. Murdoch DR, Laing RT, Mills GD, et al. Evaluation of a rapid immunochromatographic test for detection of *Streptococcus pneumoniae* antigen in urine samples from adults with community-acquired pneumonia. *J Clin Microbiol* 2001;39(10):3495–3498.

15. Gutierrez F, Mar M, Rodríguez JC, et al. Evaluation of the immunochromatographic Binax NOW assay for detection of *Streptococcus pneumoniae* urinary antigen in a prospective study of community-acquired pneumonia in Spain. *Clin Infect Dis* 2003;36(3):286–292.

16. Marcos MA, de Anta MJ, De La Bellacasa JP, et al. Rapid urinary antigen test for diagnosis of pneumococcal community-acquired pneumonia in adults. *Eur Respir J* 2003;21(2):209–214.

17. Roson B, Fernández-Sabé N, Carratala J, et al. Contribution of a urinary antigen assay (Binax NOW) to the early diagnosis of pneumococcal pneumonia. *Clin Infect Dis* 2004;38(2):222–226.

18. Stralin K, Kaltoft MS, Konradsen HB, Olcén P, Holmberg H. Comparison of two urinary antigen tests for establishment of pneumococcal etiology of adult community-acquired pneumonia. *J Clin Microbiol* 2004;42(8):3620–3625.

19. Guchev IA, Yu VL, Sinopalnikov A, et al. Management of non-severe pneumonia in military trainees with the urinary antigen test for *Streptococcus pneumoniae*: An innovative approach to targeted therapy. *Clin Infect Dis* 2005;40(11):1608–1616.

20. Briones ML, Blanquer J, Ferrando D, Blasco ML, Gimeno C, Marín J. Assessment of analysis of urinary pneumococcal antigen by immunochromatography for etiologic diagnosis of community-acquired pneumonia in adults. *Clin Vaccine Immunol* 2006;13(10):1092–1097.

21. Genne D, Siegrist HH, Lienhard R. Enhancing the etiologic diagnosis of community-acquired pneumonia in adults using the urinary antigen assay (Binax NOW). *Int J Infect Dis* 2006;10(2):124–128.

22. Boulware DR, Daley CL, Merrifield C, Hopewell PC, Janoff EN. Rapid diagnosis of pneumococcal pneumonia among HIV-infected adults with urine antigen detection. *J Infect* 2007;55(4):300–309.

23. Smith MD, Sheppard CL, Hogan A, et al. Diagnosis of *Streptococcus pneumoniae* infections in adults with bacteremia and community-acquired pneumonia: Clinical comparison of pneumococcal PCR and urinary antigen detection. *J Clin Microbiol* 2009;47(4):1046–1049.

24. Sorde R, Falcó V, Lowak M, et al. Current and potential usefulness of pneumococcal urinary antigen detection in hospitalized patients with community-acquired pneumonia to guide antimicrobial therapy. *Arch Intern Med* 2011;171(2):166–172.

25. Azar MM, Landry ML. Detection of influenza A and B viruses and respiratory syncytial virus using CLIA-waived point-of-care assays: A paradigm shift to molecular tests. *J Clin Microbiol* 2018;56(7):e00367–18.

26. Merckx J, Wali R, Schiller I, et al. Diagnostic accuracy of novel and traditional rapid tests for influenza infection compared with reverse transcriptase polymerase chain reaction: A systematic review and meta-analysis. *Ann Intern Med* 2017;167(6):394–409.

27. Bonner AB, Monroe KW, Talley LI, Klasner AE, Kimberlin DW. Impact of the rapid diagnosis of influenza on physician decision-making and patient management in the pediatric emergency department: Results of a randomized, prospective, controlled trial. *Pediatrics* 2003;112(2):363–367.

28. Falsey AR, Murata Y, Walsh EE. Impact of rapid diagnosis on management of adults hospitalized with influenza. *Arch Intern Med* 2007;167(4):354–360.

29. Ahn MY, Choi SH, Chung JW, Kim HR. Utilization of the respiratory virus multiplex reverse transcription-polymerase chain reaction test for adult patients at a Korean tertiary care center. *Korean J Intern Med* 2015;30(1):96–103.

30. Ruuskanen O, Lahti E, Jennings LC, Murdoch DR. Viral pneumonia. *Lancet* 2011;377(9773):1264–1275.

31. Voiriot G, Visseaux B, Cohen J, et al. Viral-bacterial coinfection affects the presentation and alters the prognosis of severe community-acquired pneumonia. *Crit Care* 2016;20(1):375.

32. Ramanan P, Bryson AL, Binnicker MJ, Pritt BS, Patel R. Syndromic panel-based testing in clinical microbiology. *Clin Microbiol Rev* 2018;31(1):e00024–17.

33. Stellrecht KA, Nattanmai SM, Butt J, et al. Effect of economic drift of influenza PCR tests. *J Clin Virol* 2017(93):25–29.

34. Popowitch EB, O'Neill SS, Miller MB. Comparison of the Biofire FilmArray RP, Genmark eSensor RVP, Luminex xTAG RVPv1, and Luminex xTAG RVP fast multiplex assays for detection of respiratory viruses. *J Clin Microbiol* 2013;51(5):1528–1533.

35. Doern CD, Lacey D, Huang R, Haag C. Evaluation and implementation of FilmArray version 1.7 for improved detection of adenovirus respiratory tract infection. *J Clin Microbiol* 2013;51(12):4036–4039.

36. Rappo U, Schuetz AN, Jenkins SG, et al. Impact of early detection of respiratory viruses by multiplex PCR assay on clinical outcomes in adult patients. *J Clin Microbiol* 2016;54(8):2096–2103.

37. Subramony A, Zachariah P, Krones A, Whittier S, Saiman L. Impact of multiplex polymerase chain reaction testing for respiratory pathogens on healthcare resource utilization for pediatric inpatients. *J Pediatr* 2016;173:196–201 e2.

38. Rogers BB, Shankar P, Jerris RC, et al. Impact of a rapid respiratory panel test on patient outcomes. *Arch Pathol Lab Med* 2015;139(5):636–641.

39. Semret M, Schiller I, Jardin BA, Frenette C, Loo VG, Papenburg J, McNeil SA, Dendukuri N. Multiplex respiratory virus testing for antimicrobial stewardship: A prospective assessment of antimicrobial use and clinical outcomes among hospitalized adults. *J Infect Dis* 2017;216(8):936–944.

40. Popowitch EB, Miller MB, Performance characteristics of expert Flu/RSV XC assay. *J Clin Microbiol* 2015;53(8):2720–2721.

41. Kuti EL, Patel AA, Coleman CI. Impact of inappropriate antibiotic therapy on mortality in patients with ventilator-associated pneumonia and bloodstream infection: A meta-analysis. *J Crit Care* 2008;23(1):91–100.

42. Iregui M, Ward S, Sherman G, Fraser VJ, Kollef MH. Clinical importance of delays in the initiation of appropriate antibiotic treatment for ventilator-associated pneumonia. *Chest* 2002;122(1):262–268.

43. Curetis - Unyvero pneumonia panel.

44. Jamal W, Al Roomi E, AbdulAziz LR, Rotimi VO. Evaluation of curetis unyvero, a multiplex PCR-based testing system, for rapid detection of bacteria and antibiotic resistance and impact of the assay on management of severe nosocomial pneumonia. *J Clin Microbiol* 2014;52(7):2487–2492.

45. Schulte B, Eickmeyer H, Heininger A, et al. Detection of pneumonia associated pathogens using a prototype multiplexed pneumonia test in hospitalized patients with severe pneumonia. *PLOS ONE* 2014;9(11):e110566.

46. Covington EW, Roberts MZ, Dong J. Procalcitonin monitoring as a guide for antimicrobial therapy: A review of current literature. *Pharmacotherapy* 2018;38(5):569–581.

47. Rhee C. Using procalcitonin to guide antibiotic therapy. *Open Forum Infect Dis* 2017;4(1):ofw249.

48. Markanday A. Acute phase reactants in infections: Evidence-based review and a guide for clinicians. *Open Forum Infect Dis* 2015;2(3):ofv098.

49. Gilbert DN. Use of plasma procalcitonin levels as an adjunct to clinical microbiology. *J Clin Microbiol* 2010;48(7):2325–2329.

50. Reynolds SC, Shorr AF, Muscedere J, Jiang X, Heyland DK. Longitudinal changes in procalcitonin in a heterogeneous group of critically ill patients. *Crit Care Med* 2012;40(10):2781–2787.

51. Sager R, Kutz A, Mueller B, Schuetz P. Procalcitonin-guided diagnosis and antibiotic stewardship revisited. *BMC Med* 2017;15(1):15.

52. Schuetz P, Chiappa V, Briel M, Greenwald JL. Procalcitonin algorithms for antibiotic therapy decisions: A systematic review of randomized controlled trials and recommendations for clinical algorithms. *Arch Intern Med* 2011;171(15):1322–1331.

53. Hey J, Thompson-Leduc P, Kirson NY, et al. Procalcitonin guidance in patients with lower respiratory tract infections: A systematic review and meta-analysis. *Clin Chem Lab Med* 2018;56(8):1200–1209.

54. Schuetz P, Muller B, Christ-Crain M, et al. Procalcitonin to initiate or discontinue antibiotics in acute respiratory tract infections. *Cochrane Database Syst Rev* 2017;10:CD007498.

55. Schuetz P, Wirz Y, Sager R, et al. Effect of procalcitonin-guided antibiotic treatment on mortality in acute respiratory infections: A patient level meta-analysis. *Lancet Infect Dis* 2018;18(1):95–107.

56. Masia M, Gutiérrez F, Padilla S, et al. Clinical characterisation of pneumonia caused by atypical pathogens combining classic and novel predictors. *Clin Microbiol Infect* 2007;13(2):153–161.

57. Kasamatsu Y, Yamaguchi T, Kawaguchi T, et al. Usefulness of a semi-quantitative procalcitonin test and the A-DROP Japanese prognostic scale for predicting mortality among adults hospitalized with community-acquired pneumonia. *Respirology* 2012;17(2):330–336.

58. Dusemund F, Bucher B, Meyer S, et al. Influence of procalcitonin on decision to start antibiotic treatment in patients with a lower respiratory tract infection: insight from the observational multicentric ProREAL surveillance. *Eur J Clin Microbiol Infect Dis* 2013;32(1):51–60.

59. Mandell LA, Wunderink RG, Anzueto A, et al. Infectious diseases society of America/American thoracic society consensus guidelines on the management of community-acquired pneumonia in adults. *Clin Infect Dis* 2007;44(Suppl 2):S27–S72.

60. Manuel O, Estabrook M, A.S.T.I.D.C.o. Practice, RNA respiratory viruses in solid organ transplantation. *Am J Transplant* 2013;13(Suppl 4):212–219.

61. Kamat IS, Ramachandran V, Eswaran H, Abers MS, Musher DM. Low procalcitonin, community acquired pneumonia, and antibiotic therapy. *Lancet Infect Dis* 2018;18(5):496–497.

62. Daubin C, Valette X, Thiollière F, et al. Procalcitonin algorithm to guide initial antibiotic therapy in acute exacerbations of COPD admitted to the ICU: A randomized multicenter study. *Intensive Care Med* 2018;44(4):428–437.

63. Rhodes A, Evans LE, Alhazzani W, et al. Surviving sepsis campaign: International guidelines for management of sepsis and septic shock: 2016. *Intensive Care Med* 2017;43(3):304–377.

64. Zubert S, Funk DJ, Kumar A. Antibiotics in sepsis and septic shock: Like everything else in life, timing is everything. *Crit Care Med* 2010;38(4):1211–1212.

65. Cheong HS, Kang CI, Wi YM, et al. Inappropriate initial antimicrobial therapy as a risk factor for mortality in patients with community-onset *Pseudomonas aeruginosa* bacteraemia. *Eur J Clin Microbiol Infect Dis* 2008;27(12):1219–1225.

66. Buehler SS, Madison B, Snyder SR, et al. Effectiveness of practices to increase timeliness of providing targeted therapy for inpatients with bloodstream infections: A laboratory medicine best practices systematic review and meta-analysis. *Clin Microbiol Rev* 2016;29(1):59–103.

67. Tan KE, Ellis BC, Lee R, et al. Prospective evaluation of a matrix-assisted laser desorption ionization-time of flight mass spectrometry system in a hospital clinical microbiology laboratory for identification of bacteria and yeasts: A bench-by-bench study for assessing the impact on time to identification and cost-effectiveness. *J Clin Microbiol* 2012;50(10):3301–3308.

68. Huang AM, Newton D, Kunapuli A, et al. Impact of rapid organism identification via matrix-assisted laser desorption/ionization time-of-flight combined with antimicrobial stewardship team intervention in adult patients with bacteremia and candidemia. *Clin Infect Dis* 2013;57(9):1237–1245.

69. Romero-Gomez MP, Muñoz-Velez M, Gómez-Gil R, Mingorance J. Evaluation of combined use of MALDI-TOF and Xpert((R)) MRSA/SA BC assay for the direct detection of methicillin resistance in *Staphylococcus aureus* from positive blood culture bottles. *J Infect* 2013;67(1):91–92.

70. Yonezawa T, Watari T, Ashizawa K, et al. Development of an improved rapid BACpro(R) protocol and a method for direct identification from blood-culture-positive bottles using matrix-assisted laser desorption ionization time-of-flight mass spectrometry. *J Microbiol Methods* 2018;148:138–144.

71. Sharma M, Gautam V, Mahajan M, et al. Direct identification by matrix-assisted laser desorption ionization-time of flight mass spectrometry (MALDI-TOF MS) from positive blood

culture bottles: An opportunity to customize growth conditions for fastidious organisms causing bloodstream infections. *Indian J Med Res* 2017;146(4):541–544.

72. Mauri C, Principe L, Bracco S, et al. Identification by mass spectrometry and automated susceptibility testing from positive bottles: A simple, rapid, and standardized approach to reduce the turnaround time in the management of blood cultures. *BMC Infect Dis* 2017;17(1):749.

73. Forrest GN, Mehta S, Weekes E, et al. Impact of rapid in situ hybridization testing on coagulase-negative staphylococci positive blood cultures. *J Antimicrob Chemother* 2006;58(1):154–158.

74. Ly T, Gulia J, Pyrgos V, Waga M, Shoham S. Impact upon clinical outcomes of translation of PNA FISH-generated laboratory data from the clinical microbiology bench to bedside in real time. *Ther Clin Risk Manag* 2008;4(3):637–640.

75. Holtzman C, Whitney D, Barlam T, Miller NS. Assessment of impact of peptide nucleic acid fluorescence in situ hybridization for rapid identification of coagulase-negative staphylococci in the absence of antimicrobial stewardship intervention. *J Clin Microbiol* 2011;49(4):1581–1582.

76. Forrest GN, Mankes K, Jabra-Rizk MA, et al. Peptide nucleic acid fluorescence in situ hybridization-based identification of candida albicans and its impact on mortality and antifungal therapy costs. *J Clin Microbiol* 2006;44(9):3381–3383.

77. Stamper PD, Cai M, Howard T, Speser S, Carroll KC. Clinical validation of the molecular BD GeneOhm StaphSR assay for direct detection of *Staphylococcus aureus* and methicillin-resistant *Staphylococcus aureus* in positive blood cultures. *J Clin Microbiol* 2007;45(7):2191–2196.

78. Buchan BW, Allen S, Burnham CA, et al. Comparison of the next-generation Xpert MRSA/SA BC assay and the GeneOhm StaphSR assay to routine culture for identification of *Staphylococcus aureus* and methicillin-resistant *S. aureus* in positive-blood-culture broths. *J Clin Microbiol* 2015;53(3):804–809.

79. Rubach MP, Hanson KE. ID learning unit-diagnostics update: Current laboratory methods for rapid pathogen identification in patients with bloodstream infections. *Open Forum Infect Dis* 2015;2(4):ofv174.

80. Bauer KA, West JE, Balada-Llasat JM, et al. An antimicrobial stewardship program's impact with rapid polymerase chain reaction methicillin-resistant *Staphylococcus aureus/S. aureus* blood culture test in patients with *S. aureus* bacteremia. *Clin Infect Dis* 2010;51(9):1074–1080.

81. Ward C, Stocker K, Begum J, et al. Performance evaluation of the Verigene(R) (Nanosphere) and FilmArray(R) (BioFire(R)) molecular assays for identification of causative organisms in bacterial bloodstream infections. *Eur J Clin Microbiol Infect Dis* 2015;34(3):487–496.

82. Bhatti MM, Boonlayangoor S, Beavis KG, Tesic V. Evaluation of FilmArray and verigene systems for rapid identification of positive blood cultures. *J Clin Microbiol* 2014;52(9):3433–3436.

83. Southern TR, VanSchooneveld TC, Bannister DL, et al. Implementation and performance of the BioFire FilmArray(R) blood culture identification panel with antimicrobial treatment recommendations for bloodstream infections at a midwestern academic tertiary hospital. *Diagn Microbiol Infect Dis* 2015;81(2):96–101.

84. Altun O, Almuhayawi M, Ullberg M, Özenci V. Clinical evaluation of the FilmArray blood culture identification panel in identification of bacteria and yeasts from positive blood culture bottles. *J Clin Microbiol* 2013;51(12):4130–4136.

85. Aitken SL, Hemmige VS, Koo HL, et al. Real-world performance of a microarray-based rapid diagnostic for Gram-positive bloodstream infections and potential utility for antimicrobial stewardship. *Diagn Microbiol Infect Dis* 2015;81(1):4–8.

86. van Belkum A, Dunne WM Jr. Next-generation antimicrobial susceptibility testing. *J Clin Microbiol* 2013;51(7):2018–2024.

87. Marschal M, Bachmaier J, Autenrieth I, et al. Evaluation of the accelerate pheno system for fast identification and antimicrobial susceptibility testing from positive blood cultures in bloodstream infections caused by gram-negative pathogens. *J Clin Microbiol* 2017;55(7):2116–2126.

88. Lutgring JD, Bittencourt C, TeKippe EM, et al. Evaluation of the accelerate pheno system: Results from two academic medical centers. *J Clin Microbiol* 2018;56(4):e01672–17.

89. Pancholi P, Carroll KC, Buchan BW et al. Multicenter evaluation of the accelerate PhenoTest BC kit for rapid identification and phenotypic antimicrobial susceptibility testing using morphokinetic cellular analysis. *J Clin Microbiol* 2018;56(4):e01329–17.

90. Charnot-Katsikas A, Tesic V, Love N, et al. Use of the accelerate pheno system for identification and antimicrobial susceptibility testing of pathogens in positive blood cultures and impact on time to results and workflow. *J Clin Microbiol* 2018;56(1):e01166–17.

91. King JM, Kulhankova K, Stach CS, Vu BG, Salgado-Pabón W. Phenotypes and virulence among *Staphylococcus aureus* USA100, USA200, USA300, USA400, and USA600 clonal lineages. *mSphere* 2016;1(3):e00071–16.

92. Ostrosky-Zeichner L, Sable C, Sobel J, et al. Multicenter retrospective development and validation of a clinical prediction rule for nosocomial invasive candidiasis in the intensive care setting. *Eur J Clin Microbiol Infect Dis* 2007;26(4):271–276.

93. Fernandez-Ruiz M, Aguado JM, Almirante B, et al. Initial use of echinocandins does not negatively influence outcome in Candida parapsilosis bloodstream infection: A propensity score analysis. *Clin Infect Dis* 2014;58(10):1413–1421.

94. Playford EG, Lipman J, Jones M, et al. Problematic dichotomization of risk for intensive care unit (ICU)-acquired invasive candidiasis: Results using a risk-predictive model to categorize 3 levels of risk from a multicenter prospective cohort of Australian ICU patients. *Clin Infect Dis* 2016;63(11):1463–1469.

95. Tissot F, Lamoth F, Hauser PM, et al. β-glucan antigenemia anticipates diagnosis of blood culture-negative intraabdominal candidiasis. *Am J Respir Crit Care Med* 2013;188(9):1100–1109.

96. Leon C, Ruiz-Santana S, Saavedra P, et al. A bedside scoring system ("Candida score") for early antifungal treatment in nonneutropenic critically ill patients with Candida colonization. *Crit Care Med* 2006;34(3):730–737.

97. Pfeiffer CD, Samsa GP, Schell WA, et al. Quantitation of Candida CFU in initial positive blood cultures. *J Clin Microbiol* 2011;49(8):2879–2883.

98. Garey KW, Rege M, Pai MP, et al. Time to initiation of fluconazole therapy impacts mortality in patients with candidemia: A multi-institutional study. *Clin Infect Dis* 2006;43(1):25–31.

99. Neely LA, Audeh M, Phung NA, et al. T2 magnetic resonance enables nanoparticle-mediated rapid detection of candidemia in whole blood. *Sci Transl Med* 2013;5(182):182ra54.

100. Beyda ND, Alam MJ, Garey KW. Comparison of the T2Dx instrument with T2Candida assay and automated blood culture in the detection of Candida species using seeded blood samples. *Diagn Microbiol Infect Dis* 2013;77(4):324–326.

101. Mylonakis E, Clancy CJ, Ostrosky-Zeichner L, et al. T2 magnetic resonance assay for the rapid diagnosis of candidemia in whole blood: A clinical trial. *Clin Infect Dis* 2015;60(6):892–899.

102. Clancy CJ, Pappas PG, Vazquez J, et al. Detecting infections rapidly and easily for candidemia trial, Part 2 (DIRECT2): A prospective, multicenter study of the T2Candida panel. *Clin Infect Dis* 2018;66(11):1678–1686.

103. Munoz P, Vena A, Machado M, et al. T2MR contributes to the very early diagnosis of complicated candidaemia. A prospective study. *J Antimicrob Chemother* 2018;73(suppl_4):iv13–iv19.

104. Patch ME, Weisz E, Cubillos A, Estrada SJ, Pfaller MA. Impact of rapid, culture-independent diagnosis of candidaemia and invasive candidiasis in a community health system. *J Antimicrob Chemother* 2018;73(suppl_4):iv27–iv30.

105. Munoz P, Vena A, Machado M, et al. T2Candida MR as a predictor of outcome in patients with suspected invasive candidiasis starting empirical antifungal treatment: A prospective pilot study. *J Antimicrob Chemother* 2018;73(suppl_4):iv6–iv12.

106. Ostrosky-Zeichner L, Alexander BD, Kett DH, et al. Multicenter clinical evaluation of the (1–3) beta-D-glucan assay as an aid to diagnosis of fungal infections in humans. *Clin Infect Dis* 2005;41(5):654–659.

107. Posteraro B, De Pascale G, Tumbarello M, et al. Early diagnosis of candidemia in intensive care unit patients with sepsis: A prospective comparison of (1→3)-beta-D-glucan assay, Candida score, and colonization index. *Crit Care* 2011;15(5):R249.

108. Mohr JF, Sims C, Paetznick V, et al. Prospective survey of (1→3)-beta-D-glucan and its relationship to invasive candidiasis in the surgical intensive care unit setting. *J Clin Microbiol* 2011;49(1):58–61.

109. Lu Y, Chen YQ, Guo YL, et al. Diagnosis of invasive fungal disease using serum (1→3)-beta-D-glucan: A bivariate meta-analysis. *Intern Med* 2011;50(22):2783–2791.

110. Karageorgopoulos DE, Vouloumanou EK, Ntziora F, et al. β-D-glucan assay for the diagnosis of invasive fungal infections: A meta-analysis. *Clin Infect Dis* 2011;52(6):750–770.

111. Hanson KE, Pfeiffer CD, Lease ED, et al. β-D-glucan surveillance with preemptive anidulafungin for invasive candidiasis in intensive care unit patients: A randomized pilot study. *PLOS ONE* 2012;7(8):e42282.

112. Posteraro B, Tumbarello M, De Pascale G, et al. (1,3)-beta-d-glucan-based antifungal treatment in critically ill adults at high risk of candidaemia: An observational study. *J Antimicrob Chemother* 2016;71(8):2262–2269.

113. Kanamori H, Kanemitsu K, Miyasaka T, et al. Measurement of (1-3)-beta-D-glucan derived from different gauze types. *Tohoku J Exp Med* 2009;217(2):117–121.

114. Alexander BD, Smith PB, Davis RD, Perfect JR, Reller LB. The (1,3){beta}-D-glucan test as an aid to early diagnosis of invasive fungal infections following lung transplantation. *J Clin Microbiol* 2010;48(11):4083–4088.

115. Albert O, Toubas D, Strady C, et al. Reactivity of (1→3)-beta-d-glucan assay in bacterial bloodstream infections. *Eur J Clin Microbiol Infect Dis* 2011;30(11):1453–1460.

116. Pruller F, Wagner J, Raggam RB, et al. Automation of serum (1→3)-beta-D-glucan testing allows reliable and rapid discrimination of patients with and without candidemia. *Med Mycol* 2014;52(5):455–461.

117. Balk RA, Kadri SS, Cao Z, et al. Effect of procalcitonin testing on health-care utilization and costs in critically ill patients in the United States. *Chest* 2017;151(1):23–33.

118. Heredia-Rodriguez M, Bustamante-Munguira J, Fierro I, et al. Procalcitonin cannot be used as a biomarker of infection in heart surgery patients with acute kidney injury. *J Crit Care* 2016;33:233–239.

34 Antibiotic Therapy of Multidrug Resistant Organisms in the Critical Care Unit

Burke A. Cunha

CONTENTS

CLINICAL PERSPECTIVE

Multidrug resistant (MDR) organisms may be defined as being resistant to three or more different antibiotic classes. Some MDR organisms have always been MDR, i.e., among gram-positive organisms, methicillin-resistant *S. aureus* (MRSA) has always been MDR. Among gram-negative bacilli (GNB), *Acinetobacter* spp. have always been MDR.

The concern, of course, is emerging on new MDR, particularly among aerobic GNB. The determinants of antibiotic resistance include the "resistance potential" of the antibiotic, which is independent of antibiotic class, volume, or duration of use; thus, antibiotics may be considered as "low resistance potential" antibiotics, i.e., those antibiotics not associated with widespread resistance problems with high volume/prolonged use. There has been and will be no resistance to worldwide extensive prolonged use with several "low resistance potential" antibiotics, e.g., ceftriaxone. In contrast, "high resistance potential" antibiotics are those that even with minimal use have been associated with resistance to one or two (but not all other) species, e.g., ceftazidime, a "high resistance potential" antibiotic has resistance problems with *P. aeruginosa* but not other GNB organisms in its spectrum. Resistance problems in the critical care unit (CCU) and hospital may be made worse by prolonged high-volume use of "high resistance potential" antibiotics, particularly to treat colonization and not infection [1–6] (Table 34.1).

Infection control (IC) measures are critical in limiting the spread of MDR organisms in the CCU as well as the hospital. IC measures aside, well-selected antibiotic therapy, with "low resistance potential" optimally dosed, and used for the shortest possible duration to effect cure are the cornerstones of optimal therapy with minimal resistance potential is the preferred antibiotic stewardship program (ASP) approach.

SUSCEPTIBILITY TESTING

The clinician should recognize and appreciate the importance of differentiating high-grade/absolute resistance from relative resistance, also known as "dose-dependent susceptibility" (DDS), i.e., organisms with minimal inhibitory concentration (MICs) just above the resistance breakpoint, depending on the site of infection, may be susceptible, even though reported as "resistant." For example, if a *P. aeruginosa* strain in respiratory secretions is reported as "resistant" to meropenem (with an MIC $\geq$ 8 mcg/mL), it may, in fact, be "susceptible" to high-dose meropenem, e.g., 2 g (IV) q8h. Also, if the isolate is from urine, it will be susceptible using standard dosing 1 g (IV) q8h, since meropenem is concentrated in the urine to above serum levels (with good renal function). For these reasons, the treatment of "penicillin- resistant" *S. pneumoniae* (MIC >2 µg/mL) is easily eradicated from body sites with usual doses (1 g (IV) q24h) and from the CSF with "meningeal doses 2 g (IV) q12h" [7–11] (Table 34.2).

TABLE 34.1
Antibiotic Resistance Potential

"High Resistance Potential" Antibiotics (*Antibiotics to Avoid*)

IV Antibiotics	PO Antibiotics
Ciprofloxacin	Gentamicin or tobramycin
Organism often resistant: *E. coli*	Organism often resistant: *P. aeruginosa*
TMP-SMX	Ceftazidime
Organism often resistant: *E. coli*	Organism often resistant: *P. aeruginosa*
Imipenem	Ciprofloxacin
Organism often resistant: *P. aeruginosa*	Organism often resistant: *E. coli*
	TMP-SMX
	Organism often resistant: *E. coli*

"Low Resistance Potential" Antibiotics (*Preferred Antibiotics*)

IV Antibiotics		PO Antibiotics	
Meropenem	Levofloxacin	Doxycycline	Nitrofurantoin[a]
Amikacin	Aztreonam	Minocycline	Methenamine salts[a]
Ceftriaxone	Cefepime	Levofloxacin	Fosfomycin[a]
Doxycycline	Colistin		
Tigecycline	Polymyxin B		

Source: Cunha, B.A., *Med. Clin. North Am.*, 84, 1407–1429, 2000; Cunha, B.A., *Lancet*, 357, 1307–1308, 2001; Cunha, C.B. and Cunha, B.A. (eds.), *Antibiotic Essentials*, 17th ed., Jay Pee Medical Publishers, New Delhi, India, 2020.
Abbreviation: TMP-SMX, Trimethoprim-sulfamethoxazole.
[a] For uncomplicated lower UTIs.

TABLE 34.2
Susceptibilities of "Ampicillin Resistant *E. coli*" Tested in Broth at Serum pH Compared with Human Urine at Achievable Urinary Concentrations and Urinary pH

Oral Antibiotics	Broth at pH 7.4		Urine at pH 6.0[a]	
	% Susceptible	% Resistant	% Susceptible	% Resistant
Ampicillin	0% (0/25)	(25/25) **100%**	64% (16/25)	(9/25) **36%**
Amoxicillin	28% (7/25)	(18/25) **72%**	100% (25/25)	(0/25) **0%**
Doxycycline	40% (10/25)	(15/25) **60%**	76% (19/25)	(6/25) **24%**

Source: Ristuccia, P.A. et al., *Adv. Ther.*, 3, 163–167, 1986.
[a] Tested at urinary concentrations in human heat-treated urine to remove thermolabile anti-bacterial activity.

MDR COLONIZATION IN THE CCU

The treatment of MDR GNB in the CCU should be based on clinical site correlation, i.e., relevance of the isolate to infection at the body site cultured. Second, if colonization of the site is ruled out, then select for treatment with a high degree of activity against the pathogen and a "low resistance potential" antibiotic. The antibiotic should be optimally dosed based on MIC of the organism and pharmacokinetic considerations relative to body site. Given these important clinical and ASP considerations, the most common error in "covering" MDR GNB is in failing to correlate the clinical significance of the organism with the body site from which it was cultured. Importantly, culture results should not be routinely "covered," unless deemed clinically relevant to the patient, i.e., clinical correlation of the isolate and the body site. As a rule, only infection, not colonization, should be treated. Needlessly, treating colonizing organisms is the major resistance problem in the CCU and elsewhere in the hospital. There are several approaches to this problem. First, does the isolate cause infection at the body site cultured? Are multiple isolates in cultures from the same site in infections that are monomicrobial, not polymicrobial? [10]

RESPIRATORY SECRETION COLONIZATION VS. NOSOCOMIAL PNEUMONIA

Examples of clinical correlation include MRSA cultured from respiratory secretions in ventilated patients. MRSA rarely causes CAP in those with concomitant influenza pneumonia but is not a cause of nosocomial pneumonia. Therefore, the culture of MRSA from respiratory secretions in ventilated patients (unless accompanied by new high spiking fevers, cyanosis, rapidly cavitating infiltrates, and elastin fibers in respiratory secretions) is diagnostic of MRSA airway colonization not VAP. Furthermore, culture site organisms are not reflective of pathogens from the site of infection and are necessarily misleading. The organisms causing VAP are *P. aeruginosa* or one of the aerobic GNB respiratory pathogens. Treatment, as short as is clinically effective, that is optimally dosed should be with a "low resistance potential" antibiotic with a high degree of anti-*P. aeruginosa* activity, e.g., meropenem and cefepime [10,12].

WOUND COLONIZATION VS. INFECTION

A common problem in the CCU is that of sacral decubitus ulcers with underlying chronic osteomyelitis (stage III/IV). From the ulcer, multiple organisms are often cultured (*S. maltophilia*, *B. cepacia*, VRE, and *E. agglomerans*) and "covered." First, chronic osteomyelitis is a monomicrobial process, not polymicrobial. Second, in chronic osteomyelitis, the (site-clinical correlation) infection is in the bone, not the skin ulcer. The organisms cultured from the skin are not reflective of the pathogen in bone, Therefore, first, the clinical problem is that of colonization (skin) vs. infection (bone).

The pathogens causing sacral chronic osteomyelitis are well-known. Since aseptic acquired bone biopsy cultures obtained from the operating room (OR) is usually not feasible, appropriate empiric coverage should be directed against the usual bone pathogens, e.g., MSSA and MRSA, with an antibiotic that has the appropriate spectrum and a "low resistance potential," e.g., ceftaroline and tigecycline. Trying to treat chronic osteomyelitis based on unrelated sacral ulcer cultures is not good clinically or from an ASP perspective. Clinical correlation again is the optimumal decision-making tool. Since polymicrobial isolates from any site suggest a poor specimen, cultures of each clinical correlation (*vide supra*), e.g., neither *S. maltophilia*, VRE, and *B. cepacia*, nor *E. agglomerans* alone or together, are osteomyelitis pathogens [10].

URINE COLONIZATION VS. URINARY TRACT INFECTION

The most common CCU colonization vs. infection problem is that of MDR organism cultured from the urine in patients with indwelling urinary catheters, i.e., catheter-associated bacteriuria (CAB) [13].

Colonization of urine with an indwelling urinary catheter is a function of time/aseptic technique. Containment of MDR GNB spread from patient to patient in the CCU depends on effective IC measures. Most cases of CAB in immunocompetent hosts represent colonization and should not be treated. Treating colonization is one of the primary drivers of MDR in the CCU.

The clinical approach begins with clinical correlation, i.e., assessing the degree/intensity of pyuria with the urine colony count. Urinalysis (UA) with microscopic (not dipstick UA) with minimal pyuria (<10 WBC/hpf) indicates colonization (CAB), regardless of urine colony count, and such patients should not be treated. If the pyuria is intense, the indwelling urinary catheter should be removed/replaced and the UA/UC repeated and re-assessed in 24 hours. Urinary catheter replacement is often "curative" of itself. If pyuria >10 WBC/hpf persists, treatment should be considered, especially in compromised hosts that may be prone to urosepsis, e.g., diabetes mellitus (DM) [10] (Tables 34.3 and 34.4).

TABLE 34.3
Pharmacokinetic/Pharmacodynamic Considerations

Antibiotics		Optimal Dosing Strategies
Concentration-Dependent Antibiotics (Cmax:MIC)		
• Quinolones	• Doxycycline	**Use highest effective dose without toxicity**
• Aminoglycosides	• Tigecycline	
• Vancomycin (if MIC >1 µg/mL, use 2 g (IV) q12h)	• Polymyxin B	
	• Colistin	
Time-Dependent Antibiotics (T > MIC)		
• PCN: maintain concentrations > MIC for >60% of the dosing interval		**Use high doses (which increase serum concentrations, which also increase T > MIC for more of the dosing interval)**
• β-lactams: maintain concentrations > MIC for >75% of the dosing interval		
• Carbapenems: maintain concentrations > MIC for >40% of the dosing interval		
• Vancomycin (if MIC <1 µg/mL, use 1 g (IV) q12h)		

Source: Cunha, C.B. and Cunha, B.A. eds., *Antibiotic Essentials*, 16th ed., Jay Pee Medical Publishers, New Delhi, India, 2017.

Abbreviations: Cmax, peak serum concentration; T, time.

TABLE 34.4

Clinical Approach to the Therapy of MDR Gram-Negative Acute Uncomplicated Cystitis Using Decreased Intensity of Pyuria as a Predictor of Effectiveness

Marked Decrease in Intensity of Pyuria (TTNC <2 days) **is Predictive of Eradication of Bacteriuria**
- *Complete therapy with antibiotic selected*
- Normal hosts: 3 days
- Compromised hosts: 3–5 days

Mild-Moderate Decrease in Intensity of Pyuria is Predictive of Delayed Eradication of Bacteriuria (TTNC >2 days)
- If the antibiotic being used has optimal activity in an *alkaline urine* (pH >6) but urinary pH is acid (pH = 5–6), retreat with an antibiotic with optimal activity in an *alkaline urine* or alkalinize the urine (sodium bicarbonate).
- If the antibiotic has optimal activity in an *acid urine* (pH = 5–6) but urine pH is alkaline (pH >6), retreat with an antibiotic with optimal activity in an acid urine or acidify the urine (ascorbic acid).

No Decrease in Intensity of Pyuria after 2 days is Predictive of Treatment Failure
- Discontinue antibiotic.
- *Retreat with another antibiotic* with inherent activity against the uropathogen that achieves high urinary concentrations.

Source: Cunha, C.B. and Cunha, B.A. eds., *Antibiotic Essentials*, 16th ed., Jay Pee Medical Publishers, New Delhi, India, 2017; Cunha, B.A., *Eur. J. Clin. Micro. & Inf. Dis.*, 35, 521–526, 2016.

Abbreviation: TTNC, time to negative culture.

TABLE 34.5

Pharmacokinetic and Microbiological Parameters of Selected Oral Antibiotics Useful in the Therapy of MDR Uropathogens

Nitrofurantoin	Doxycycline	Fosfomycin
• Usual dose = 100 mg	• Usual dose = 100 mg	• Usual dose = 3 g
Peak serum levels = 1 µg/mL	**Peak serum levels = 4 µg/mL**	**Peak serum levels = 26 µg/mL**
• Serum half-life ($t_{1/2}$) = 0.5 hours	• Serum half-life ($t_{1/2}$) = 20 hours	• Serum half-life ($t_{1/2}$) = 5.7 hours
• Bioavailability = 80%	• Bioavailability = 93%	• Bioavailability = 37%
• PD = Concentration-dependent kinetics	• PD = Concentration-dependent kinetics	• PD = Concentration-dependent kinetics
• Excreted (unchanged) in the urine = 25%	• Excreted (unchanged) in the urine = 48%	• Excreted (unchanged) in the urine = 60%
Urine levels = 100 µg/mL[a]	**Urine levels = 300 µg/mL[a]**	**Urine levels = 1000 µg/mL[a]**
Optimal urinary pH = Acid urine (pH = 5–6)	**Optimal urinary pH = Acid urine (pH = 5–6)**	**Optimal urinary pH = Acid urine (pH = 5–6)**
Urinary spectrum	**Urinary spectrum**	**Urinary spectrum**
• *E. coli*[b]	• *E. coli*[b]	• *E. coli*[b]
• *Klebsiella* sp.[c]	• *Klebsiella* sp.[c]	• *Klebsiella* sp.[c]
• *Enterobacter* sp.[c]	• *Enterobacter* sp.[c]	• *Enterobacter* sp.[c]
	• *Pseudomonas aeruginosa*[c]	• *Serratia marcescens*[c]
		• *Proteus* sp.
		• *Pseudomonas aeruginosa*[c]

Source: Cunha, C.B. and Cunha, B.A. eds., *Antibiotic Essentials*, 16th ed., Jay Pee Medical Publishers, New Delhi, India, 2017; Cunha, B.A., *Eur. J. Clin. Micro. & Inf. Dis.*, 35, 521–526, 2016.

Abbreviation: PD, pharmacodynamic.

[a] With adequate renal function.
[b] Including ESBL + strains.
[c] Including MDR strains.

If MDR GNB cystitis is present (moderate/intense pyuria *plus* >10⁶ urine colony count), treatment with a "low resistance potential" antibiotic is indicated. Fortunately, most CCU patients have sufficient renal function that results in urinary antibiotic levels much greater than that in serum. Therefore, many MDR uropathogens that tested "resistant" at serum concentrations, causing area under the curve (AUC), may be treated with oral antibiotics, e.g., doxycycline, nitrofurantoin, and fosfomycin. At high urinary levels, organisms reported as "resistant" (to serum levels) may be effective against some MDR uropathogens in the urine [14–27] (Table 34.5).

OPTIMAL THERAPY FOR MDR INFECTIONS IN THE CCU

In summary, treat only infection, not colonization. For clinical relevance, isolates cultured from the body site should be clinically correlated to the site of infection. Clinically, if the treatment of MDR organisms is warranted, then select a "low resistance potential" antibiotic, dosed optimally based on pharmacokinetic/pharmacodynamic (PK/PD) considerations, while taking into account achievable antibiotics concentrations at the site of infection, e.g., serum, respiratory secretions, and urine. Treat for the shortest duration that will effect clinical cure [28–31] (Table 34.6). The optimal clinical approach in the CCU is not to treat colonization but treat infections with optimal antibiotic monotherapy. Optimal therapy means using "low resistance potential" antibiotics at full dose and at higher-than-usual doses for DDS pathogens or those that are difficult to penetrate tissue for the shortest

period of time to eradicate the infection [32–41]. Importantly, in those situations where antibiotic therapy is not primary therapy ineffective, e.g., abscesses, device-related infected source control is essential for cure.

CONCLUSION

The three cardinal principles of antibiotic therapy of MDR organisms in the CCU are (1) source control, i.e., device-related infection or undrained abscesses cannot be cured with antibiotic therapy alone. (2) Avoid treating colonization, i.e., do not "cover" all cultured isolates, as treating colonization is ineffective and

TABLE 34.6

Empiric Antibiotic Therapy of Selected MDR Pathogens

Potential MDR Pathogens	Preferred Therapy	Alternate Therapy
MRSA	Tigecycline	Clindamycin
	Minocycline	(CA-MRSA)
	Ceftaroline	Doxycycline
	Quinupristin/dalfopristin	(CA-MRSA)
	Linezolid	TMP-SMX
	Daptomycin	(CA-MRSA)
	Vancomycin	
VRE	Tigecycline	Chloramphenicol
	Minocycline	
	Quinupristin/dalfopristin	
	Daptomycin[a]	
	Linezolid	
	Nitrofurantoin[b]	
	Fosfomycin[b]	
Klebsiella	Meropenem[c]	Levofloxacin
	Cefepime[c]	Moxifloxacin
	Amikacin[c]	Colistin
	Aztreonam	Doxycycline
	Tigecycline[c]	
	Polymyxin B	
	Nitrofurantoin[b]	
	Fosfomycin[b]	
Enterobacter	Ceftriaxone	Second-generation cephalosporins
	TMP-SMX	Ticarcillin/clavulanate
	Cefepime[c]	Piperacillin/tazobactam
	Meropenem[c]	Levofloxacin
	Amikacin	Moxifloxacin
	Aztreonam	Colistin
	Polymyxin B	
	Tigecycline[c]	
	Ceftazidime/Avibactam	
	Ceftolozane/Tazobactam	
	Nitrofurantoin[b]	
	Fosfomycin[b]	
Serratia	Ceftriaxone	Second-generation cephalosporins
	Cefepime[c]	Piperacillin/tazobactam
	TMP-SMX	Levofloxacin[c]
	Meropenem[c]	Moxifloxacin
	Amikacin[c]	Colistin
	Aztreonam	
	Polymyxin B	
	Tigecycline[c]	

(Continued)

TABLE 34.6 (*Continued*)
Empiric Antibiotic Therapy of Selected MDR Pathogens

Potential MDR Pathogens	Preferred Therapy	Alternate Therapy
	Ceftazidime/avibactam	
	Ceftolozane/tazobactam	
	Fosfomycin[b]	
P. aeruginosa (Meropenem susceptible)	Meropenem[c]	Gentamicin
	Aztreonam	Tobramycin
	Amikacin[c]	Piperacillin/tazobactam
	Ciprofloxacin	Cefoperazone
	Levofloxacin[c]	Doripenem
	Polymyxin B	Colistin
	Doxycycline[b]	
	Fosfomycin[b]	
P. aeruginosa (Meropenem resistant)	Doripenem	Colistin
	Polymyxin B	
	Amikacin[c]	
	Ceftazidime/avibactam	
	Ceftolozane/Tazobactam	
	Meropenem/Verobactam	
CRE[b]	Tigecycline[c]	Colistin
	Ceftazidime/Avibactam	Aztreonam
	Meropenem/Verobactam	
	Polymyxin B	
	Nitrofurantoin[c]	
	Fosfomycin[c]	
Acinetobacter[b]	TMP-SMX	Aztreonam
	Amikacin[c]	Gentamicin
	Minocycline	Tobramycin
	Tigecycline[c]	Ticarcillin/clavulnate
	Meropenem	Piperacillin/tazobactam
	Cefepime[c]	Doxycycline
	Ceftazidime/avibactam	Doripenem
	Ceftolozane/tazobactam	
S. maltophilia[b]	TMP-SMX	Chloramphenicol
	Minocycline	Ticarcillin/clavulanate‴
	Doxycycline	Piperacillin/tazobactam‴
	Tigecycline[c]	Levofloxacin
	Polymyxin B	Moxifloxacin
	Ceftazidime/avibactam	Colistin
	Ceftolozane/tazobactam	
	Fosfomycin[b,c]	
B. cepacia[b]	Minocycline	Doxycycline
	TMP-SMX	Chloramphenicol
	Meropenem[c]	Levofloxacin
	Cefepime[c]	Moxifloxacin
	Ceftazidime/avibactam	Ticarcillin/clavulanate
	Ceftolozane/tazobactam	Piperacillin/tazobactam

Source: Cunha, C.B. and Cunha, B.A. eds., *Antibiotic Essentials*, 16th ed., Jay Pee Medical Publishers, New Delhi, India, 2017; Cunha, B.A., *Eur. J. Clin. Micro. & Inf. Dis.*, 35, 521–526, 2016.

[a] Daptomycin: Use 2x the MRSA dose for VRE infections, e.g., MSSA/MRSA soft tissue infection, use 4 mg/kg/day; for VRE, use 8 mg /kg/day. For MSSA/MRSA bacteremia/endocarditis, use 6 mg/kg/day; for VRE, use 12 mg/kg/day.

[b] For uncomplicated lower UTIs.

[c] MDR dosing
- Amikacin: 1 g (IV) q24h
- Cefepime: 2 g (IV) q8h
- Levofloxacin 750 mg (IV/PO) q24h
- Meropenem: 2 g (IV) q8h
- Tigecycline: 400 mg (IV) × 1 dose, then 200 mg (IV) q24h

predisposes to further MDR problems. (3) Treat MDR pathogens for the shortest duration needed to eliminate the infection, and use doses at the high end of the therapeutic range to prevent more resistance and treat relatively resistant (dose-dependent susceptibility) organisms while avoiding toxicity.

REFERENCES

1. Cunha BA. Antibiotic resistance: A historical perspective. *Semin Res Crit Care Med* 2000;21:3–8.
2. Cunha BA. Antibiotic resistance. *Med Clin N Amer* 2000;84:1407–1429.
3. Cunha BA. Effective antibiotic-resistance control strategies. *Lancet* 2001;357:1307–1308.
4. Cunha BA. Strategies to control antibiotic resistance. *Semin Respir Infect* 2002;17:250–258.
5. Cunha CB, Cunha BA. (eds.). *Antibiotic Essentials* (16th ed.). New Delhi, India: Jay Pee Medical Publishers, 2017:1–15, 103–106,596–599,619–620,657–658.
6. Denny KJ, Cotta MO, Parker Sl, Roberts JA, Lipman J. The use and risks of antibiotics in cirtically ill patients. *Xpert Opin Drug Saf* 2016;15:667–678.
7. Cunha BA. Problems arising in antimicrobial therapy due to false susceptibility testing. *J Chemother* 1997;1:25–35.
8. Doern GV, Brecher SM. The clinical predictive value (or lack thereof) of the results of in vitro antimicrobial susceptibility tests. *J Clin Micro* 2011;49:S11–S14.
9. Washington JA. Discrepancies between in vitro activity and in vivo response to antimicrobial agents. *Diagn Micro Inf Dis* 1983;1:25–31.
10. Cunha BA. Tigecycline dosing is critical in preventing tigecycline resistance because relative resistance is, in part, concentration dependent. *Clin Microbiol Infect* 2015;21:e39–e40.
11. Park KH, Chong YP, Kim SH, et al. Impact of revised board-spectrum cephalosporin clinical and laboratory standards institute breakpoints on susceptibility in enterobacteriaceae producing AmpC β-Lactamase. *Infect Chemo* 2017;49:62–67.
12. Cunha BA. *Pneumonia Essentials* (3rd ed.). Sudbury, MA: Jones & Bartlett Publishers, 2010.
13. Trevine SE, Babcock HM, Henderson JP, et al. Perceptions and behaviors of infectious disease physicians when managing urinary tract infections due to MDR organisms. *J Antimicrob Chemo* 2015;70:3397–3400.
14. Stamey TA, Govan DE, Palmer JM. The localization and treatment of urinary tract infections: The role of bactericidal urine levels as opposed to serum levels. *Medicine* 1965;44:1–36.
15. Musher DM, Minuth JN, Thorsteinsson SB, Holmes T. Effectiveness of achievable urinary concentrations of tetracyclines against "tetracycline-resistant" pathogenic bacteria. *J Infect Dis* 1975;131:S40–S44.
16. Stamey TA, Fair WR, Timothy MM, et al. Serum versus urinary antimicrobial concentration in cure of urinary tract infections. *N Engl J Med* 1974;291:1159.
17. Frimodt-Moller. Correlation between pharmacokinetic/pharmacodynamic parameters and efficacy for antibiotics in the treatment of urinary tract infection. *Int J Antimicrob Agents* 2002;19:546–553.
18. Cunha BA. Predicting in vivo effectiveness from in vitro susceptibility: A step closer to performing testing of uropathogens in human urine. *Scand J Infect Dis* 2012;44:714–715.
19. Cunha BA. Oral doxycycline for non-systemic urinary tract infections (UTIs) due to *P. aeruginosa* and other gram negative uropathogens. *Eur J Clin Micro Infect Dis* 2012;31:2865–2868.
20. Khoshnood S, Heidary M, Mirnejad R, Bahramian A, Sedighi M, Mirzaei H. Drug-resistant gram-negative uropathogens: A review. *Biomed Pharm* 2017;94:982–994.
21. Comer JB, Ristuccia PA, Digamon M, Cunha BA. Antibiotic pharmacokinetics in urine. In: Ristuccia AM, Cunha BA eds. *Antimicrobial Therapy*. New York: Raven Press, 1984:487–488.
22. Cunha BA, Comer JB. Pharmacokinetic considerations in the treatment of urinary tract infections. *Conn Med* 1979;43:347–353.
23. Breteler KK, Rentenaar RJ, Verkaart G, Sturm PDJ. Performance and clinical significance of direct antimicrobial susceptibility testing on urine from hospitalized patients. *Scand J Infect Dis* 2011;43:771–776.
24. Ristuccia PA, Jonas M, Cunha BA. Antibiotic susceptibility of ampicillin resistant *E. coli* in urine to antibiotics at urinary concentration. *Adv Ther* 1986;3:163–167.
25. Cunha BA, Giuga J, Gerson S. Predictors of ertapenem therapeutic efficacy in the treatment of urinary tract infections in hospitalized adults: The importance of renal insufficiency and urinary pH. *Eur J of Clin Micro & Inf Dis* 2016;35: 673–679.
26. Cunha BA. An infectious disease and pharmacokinetic perspective on oral antibiotic treatment of uncomplicated urinary tract infections due to multidrug resistant gram negative uropathogens: The importance of urinary antibiotic concentrations and urinary pH. *Eur J of Clin Micro & Inf Dis* 2016;35:521–526.
27. Yang L, Wang K, Li H, Denstedt JD, Cadieux PA. The influence of urinary pH on antibiotic efficacy against bacterial uropathogens. *Urology* 2014;84:713.e1–e7.
28. Cunha BA, Domenico PD, Cunha CB. Pharmacodynamics of doxycycline. *Clin Micro Infect Dis* 2000;6:270–273.
29. Cunha BA, Schoch P, Hage J. Oral therapy of catheter associated bacteriuria (CAB) in the era of antibiotic resistance: Nitrofurantoin revisited. *J Chemother* 2012;24:122–124.
30. Cunha BA. Multidrug-resistant gram-negative bacilli causing urinary tract infections: Clinical considerations. *J Chemother* 2011;23:171–174.
31. Lehmann C, Berner R, Bogner JR, et al. The "Choosing Wisely" initiative in infectious diseases. *Infection* 2017;45:263–268.
32. Cunha BA. Single daily high dose tigecycline therapy of a multidrug resistant *Klebsiella pneumoniae* and *Enterobacter aerogenes* nosocomial urinary tract infection. *J Chemother* 2007;19:753–754.
33. Cunha BA. Pharmacokinetic considerations regarding tigecycline for multidrug-resistant *Klebsiella pneumoniae* or MDR *Acinetobacter baumanni* urosepsiis. *J Clin Microbiol* 2009;47:1613.
34. Brust K, Evans A, Phemmons R. Favorable outcome in the treatment of carbapenem-resistant enterobacteriaceae urinary tract infection with high dose tigecycline. *J Antimicrob Chemother* 2014;69:2875–2876.
35. Brust K, Evans A, Plammons R. Tigecycline in treatment of multidrug resistant gram negative bacillus urinary tract infections: A systematic review. *J Antimicrob Chemother* 2014;69:2606–2610.
36. Bassetti M, Peghin M, Pecori D. The management of multidrug-resistant enterobacteriaceae. *Curr Opin Infect Dis* 2016;29:583–594.
37. Parker SL, Sime FB, Roberts JA. Optimizing dosing of antibiotics in critically ill patients. *Curr Opin Infect Dis* 2015;28:497–404.
38. Cotta MO, Roberts JA, Lipman J. Antibiotic dose optimization in critically Ill patients. *Med Intensiva* 2015;39:563–572.

39. Sime FB, Roberts MS, Roberts JA. Optimization of dosing regimens and dosing in special populations. *Clin Microbiol Infect* 2015;21:886–893.

40. Tangden T, Ramos Martin V, Felton TW, et al. The role of infection models and PK/PD modeling for optimising care of critically Ill patients with severe infections. *Int Care Med* 2017;43:1021–1032.

41. Roberts JA, Taccone FS, Lipman J. Understanding PK/PD. *Int Care Med* 2016;42:1797–1800.

35 Antibiotic Therapy in the Penicillin-Allergic Patient in the Critical Care Unit

Burke A. Cunha

CONTENTS

CLINICAL PERSPECTIVE

Empiric antimicrobial therapy is a necessity in the critically ill patient with a life-threatening infectious disease. Several factors go into antibiotic selection, including (i) spectrum of activity against the presumed pathogens, which is related to the source of infection or organ system involved; (ii) pharmacokinetic (PK) and pharmacodynamic (PD) considerations, which affect dosing and concentration in the organ source of sepsis; and (iii) the resistance potential of the antibiotic. Although rapid eradication of infection is the immediate priority, antibiotic selection has a subsequent effect on the flora of the critical care unit (CCU) and later may impact on the hospital flora. The fourth consideration is the drug safety, i.e., adverse side effects and drug-drug interactions, as well as the patient's allergic history. The most common problem encountered in treating critically ill patients relates to the question of potential or actual penicillin allergy.

DETERMINING THE TYPE OF PENICILLIN ALLERGY

There are no good clinical data on the incidence of penicillin allergy. Some studies use skin testing to derive the clinical implication of the data. Other studies are based on clinical information, i.e., questioning the patient or relatives regarding the nature of potential penicillin allergy. Often, penicillin allergy is mentioned, but further or detailed question reveals that it is not truly an allergic reaction. Patients, if they are able to respond, are either vague or very clear about the nature of their penicillin allergy. In the CCU, it is often impossible to get an accurate drug allergy history. There is poor correlation between the patient reporting penicillin allergy and subsequent penicillin skin testing. In the CCU, the patient's history is the only piece of information that the clinician has

to work with to make a therapeutic decision regarding the possible penicillin allergy [1–6]. Because β-lactam antibiotics are one of the most commonly used classes of antibiotics, the question of using these agents in patients with penicillin allergy is a daily clinical consideration. The clinical approach to the patient with a potential skin allergy involves determining the nature of the penicillin allergy as well as selecting an agent with an appropriate spectrum relative to the source of the infection. Penicillin allergies may be considered as anaphylactic reactions, i.e., anaphylaxis, laryngospasm, bronchospasm, hypotension, or total body hives, or non-anaphylactic reactions, i.e., drug fever or skin rash. Patients with non-anaphylactoid skin reactions may be safely given β-lactam antibiotics, except for select carbapenems, e.g., meropenem and ertapenem. Patients with a history of an anaphylactic reaction should be treated with an antibiotic of an unrelated class [7–11].

CLINICAL TYPES OF PENICILLIN-ALLERGIC REACTIONS

In the CCU, when urgent antimicrobial therapy is necessary, there is no time for skin testing to rule out or confirm penicillin allergy. Patients who are communicative can indicate, on direct questioning, the nature of their penicillin reaction. Often what is considered a penicillin reaction by the patient is in fact an unrelated non-allergic drug side effect. Patients often report a vague history of penicillin allergy during childhood that has not recurred subsequently; others report that penicillin allergy occurred in relatives, but not themselves. Some patients were told they had a drug fever reaction due to penicillin but did not have a rash (drug rash), and others reported that the reaction to penicillin was limited to a maculopapular rash. Responses to any of these indicate that the patient had a non-anaphylactoid reaction to penicillin.

Patients with drug fever or drug rash due to penicillin may be safely repeatedly given penicillin [12,13]. Hypersensitivity reactions are stereotyped, such that if the patient had a drug fever as the manifestation of penicillin allergy, on re-challenge, the patient would develop drug fever again and not a different/more severe allergic reaction of penicillin allergy. Patients with drug fevers or drug rashes due to penicillin may have a similar non-anaphylactic reaction on re-challenge with penicillin. Alternately, they may have no reaction at all if the β-lactam chosen is antigenetically sufficiently different than the one causing the reaction. Among the second-generation cephalosporins, cefoxitin is the least likely to cross-react with other second-generation cephalosporins [12–14].

ALLERGIC CROSS-REACTIONS BETWEEN PENICILLINS AND β-LACTAMS

When cephalosporins were first introduced, the reported cross-reactivity rate with penicillins was as high as 30%. Subsequently, actual cross allergic reactions were <3%. Many of the cross-reactions initially thought to be between penicillins and cephalosporins were non-specific allergic reactions and not penicillin/cephalosporin cross-reactivity. Patients with a penicillin allergy who have had a non-anaphylactic reaction may be safely given β-lactam antibiotics. In the unlikely event where the patient has a reaction, the patient would develop the same non-anaphylactic reaction, e.g., a drug fever or drug rash, but not anaphylaxis [15–22].

USE OF CARBAPENEMS AND MONOBACTAMS WITH PENICILLIN

ANAPHYLACTIC REACTIONS

With the exceptions of cefoxitin and cefoperazone, allergy to one is likely to result in cross-reactivity with another cephalosporin. Although carbapenems are structurally related to β-lactam antibiotics, from an allergic perspective, they should not be regarded as β-lactam antibiotics. Carbapenems, e.g., meropenem and ertapenem, do not cross-react with other β-lactams. Clinically, carbapenems are frequently used as an alternative to β-lactams antibiotics and do not cross-react with β-lactams. Meropenem, in particular, is safe to use, even in patients with known/suspected history of β-lactam anaphylaxis. With a history of anaphylaxis to penicillin or β-lactams, clinicians can safely use meropenem [23–25].

NON-β-LACTAM ANTIBIOTIC USE WITH PENICILLIN ANAPHYLACTIC REACTIONS

In patients with a history of an anaphylactic reaction, i.e., anaphylaxis, laryngospasm, bronchospasm, hypotension, or total body hives, it is important to select a non-β-lactam antibiotic to avoid further complicating the situation in the CCU. As with non-anaphylactoid penicillin reactions, anaphylactic reactions tend to be stereotyped with repeated exposures. Patients who

develop laryngospasm as the manifestation of their penicillin allergy, on subsequent re-exposure, will repeatedly develop laryngospasm as the manifestation of their anaphylactic reaction. Fortunately, there are many highly effective non-β-lactam antibiotics available and many appropriate non-β-lactam antibiotics to choose from, to treat the life-threatening infections encountered in the CCU (Table 35.1) [22–25].

Antibiotic classes that have no allergic cross-reactivity with β-lactams include the macrolides, tetracyclines, clindamycin, chloramphenicol, trimethoprim-sulfamethoxazole (TMP-SMX), aminoglycosides, metronidazole, polymyxin B, colistin, vancomycin, quinupristin/dalfopristin, linezolid, daptomycin, quinolones, monobactams, and, as previously mentioned, selected carbapenems; e.g., imipenem/cilaslatin has a low but definite potential for cross-reactions with β-lactams,

---

TABLE 35.1

Antimicrobials Safe to Use in Penicillin-Allergic Patients in the CCU

Meropenem	Gentamicin
Ertapenem	Tobramycin
Doripenem	Amikacin
Imipenem[a]	Doxycycline
Aztreonam	Minocycline
Ciprofloxacin	Clindamycin
Levofloxacin	Chloramphenicol
Moxifloxacin	TMP-SMX
Delafloxacin	Rifampin
Vancomycin	Colistin
Quinupristin/dalfopristin	Polymyxin B
Linezolid	Daptomycin
	Tigecycline

[a] Allergic reactions very uncommon.

TABLE 35.2

Clinical Approach to β-Lactam Use in Those with Known or Unknown Reported Reactions to Penicillin

	Nature of Reported Penicillin Allergy	β-Lactams Safe to Use
Non-anaphylactic reactions	Drug fever	First-, second-, third-, and fourth-generation cephalosporins
	Drug rash	Avoid penicillins or cephalosporins
	E. multiforme	Avoid penicillins or cephalosporins
	Steven-Johnson syndrome	Avoid penicillins or cephalosporins
Anaphylactic reactions	Hypotension	Meropenem[a], Ertapenem[a]
	Laryngospasm	
	Bronchospasm	
	Generalized hives	

[a] No/minimal potential for allergic cross reactions.

TABLE 35.3
Antibiotics Safe in Penicillin Allergic Adult Patients in the CCU

Clinical Syndrome	PCN Allergy	Non-PCN Allergic
Acute bacterial meningitis		
H. meningitidis	• Meropenem (meningeal dose)[a]	Ceftriaxone[b]
H. influenzae	• TMP-SMX	
S. pneumoniae	• Chloramphenicol	
MSSA	• Meropenem (meningeal dose)[a]	
Listeria	• Linezolid	Ampicillin
	• Meropenem (meningeal dose)[a]	
Brain abscess (oral anerobes)	• Meropenem (meningeal dose)	Ceftriaxone (meningeal dose)[a]
	• Chloramphenicol	
Severe CAP (typical/atypical pathogens)	• Levofloxacin[d]	Ceftriaxone *plus either*
	• Moxifloxacin	doxycycline *or* azithromycin
	• Doxycycline	
NP/VAP (*P. aeruginosa*)	• Levofloxacin[d]	Cefepime
	• Meropenem	Piperacillin/tazobactam *plus*
	• Aztreonam	amikacin
ABE (MSSA/MRSA)	• Daptomycin	Nafcillin
	• Linezolid	Cefazolin
	• Minocycline	Ceftaroline
	• Vancomycin	
Cholangitis (*E. coli, Klebsiella*, VSE)	• Meropenem	Piperacillin/tazobactam
	• Tigecycline	
Liver abscess (aerobic GNB, *B. fragilis*)	• Meropenem	Piperacillin/tazobactam
	• Tigecycline	
Intra-abdominal source (aerobic GNB, *B. fragilis*)	• Meropenem	Piperacillin/tazobactam
	• Tigecycline	Cefoxitin
	• Ertapenem	Cefoperazone
	• Moxifloxacin[c]	Ceftizoxime
	• Levofloxacin *plus either* metronidazole *or* clindamycin	
Pelvic source: (aerobic GNB, *B. fragilis*)	• Meropenem	Piperacillin/tazobactam
	• Ertapenem	Cefoxitin
	• Tigecycline	
	• Moxifloxacin	
	• Levofloxacin *plus* metronidazole	
Urosepsis (aerobic GNBs)	• Meropenem	Piperacillin/tazobactam
Group D enterococci	• Vancomycin	Ampicillin
E. faecalis (VSE)	• Linezolid	
	• Meropenem	
E. faecium (VRE)	• Linezolid	
	• Quinupristin/dalfopristin	
Complicated wound infections (GAS, MSSA)	• Tigecycline	Piperacillin/tazobactam
	• Meropenem	Ceftaroline
	• Ertapenem	
	• Moxifloxacin	
	• Delafloxacin	
Necrotizing fasciitis (GAS, MSSA)	• Tigecycline	Piperacillin/tazobactam
	• Meropenem	
	• Ertapenem	
Sepsis (unknown source)	• Meropenem	Piperacillin/tazobactam
	• Tigecycline	

[a]   2 g (IV) q8h.

[b]   2 g (IV) q12h.

[c]   For mild/moderately severe infection.

[d]   750 mg (IV) q24h.

Abbreviations: PCN, penicillin; CAP, community-acquired pneumonia; TMP-SMX, trimethoprim-sulfamethoxazole; MSSA, methicillin-sensitive *Staphylococcus aureus*; MRSA, methicillin-resistant *Staphylococcus aureus*; NP, nosocomial pneumonia; VAP, ventilator associated pneumonia; ABE, acute bacterial endocarditis; VRE, vancomycin-resistant enterococci; VSE, vancomycin-susceptible enterococci; GNB, gram-negative bacilli.

probably due to the cilastatin component. There are no data on doripenem, but meropenem and ertapenem are safe alternatives. In 30 years of clinical experience in infectious disease, the author has never had to resort to penicillin desensitization to treat a patient. There is always an alternative, non-β-lactam antibiotic, which is suitable for virtually every conceivable clinical situation. Although penicillin sensitivity testing/desensitization is a potential consideration in the non-critical ambulatory patients, in the critical care setting, there is no time or need for penicillin testing/desensitization. If there is any question about a penicillin allergy in a non-communicative patient in the CCU, then monotherapy or combination therapy with a non-β-lactam antibiotic is appropriate and safe. The non-β-lactam antibiotics most useful in the CCU for the most common infectious disease syndromes are presented in Tables 35.2 and 35.3 [22,26].

CONCLUSIONS

The incidence of penicillin allergy in the general population has been estimated to be 1%–10%, but no good reliable data exist on the actual incidence of penicillin allergy. Penicillin data derived from penicillin skin testing do not correlate with penicillin reactions in the clinical setting. Many patients reporting penicillin allergy have in fact had reactions to penicillin but not on an allergic basis and are of the non-anaphylactic or anaphylactic variety if they are indeed penicillin reactions. Penicillin reactions may occur after a single exposure to a penicillin or β-lactam antibiotic. From questioning or previous history, patients' penicillin reactions may be classified as anaphylactic or non-anaphylactic. Because the cross-reactivity between β-lactams and penicillin is so low, β-lactam antibiotics may be used in patients who have had a drug fever or a drug rash. Should the patient have an allergic cross-reaction between the β-lactam and the penicillin, the allergic manifestation will be of the same type as experienced previously.

In patients with a history of anaphylactic reactions to β-lactams, it is essential to use a non-β-lactam antibiotic, i.e., a carbapenem (meropenem), quinolone, clindamycin, TMP-SMX, quinupristin/dalfopristin, linezolid, vancomycin, daptomycin, clindamycin, metronidazole, polymyxin B, colistin, aminoglycoside, or tigecycline. As with non-anaphylactic penicillin cross-reactions, anaphylactic reactions to penicillin also tend to be stereotyped and on repeated exposure manifest the same clinical expression as initial allergic response. It is important to remember that although meropenem is structurally a β-lactam, meropenem does not cross-react with those with β-lactam allergies, including those with anaphylactic reactions, as has been shown in a large prospective clinical study [27–33]. Importantly, if meropenem is being used in β-lactam anaphylaxis, there is no rationale for a "test dose," since the anaphylactic reactions are IgE mediated and are not dose dependent [34,35].

Because the therapeutic armamentarium is extensive, it is rarely necessary to desensitize a patient in the CCU when so many antibiotic alternatives are available and safe.

REFERENCES

1. Salkind AR, Cuddy PG, Foxworth JW. Is this patient allergic to penicillin? *JAMA* 2001;285:2498–505.
2. Surtees SJ, Stockton MG, Gietzen TW. Allergy to penicillin: Fable or fact? *Br Med J* 1991;302:1051–1052.
3. Krishna MT, Huissoon AP, Li M, et al. Enhancing antibiotic stewardship by tackling "Spurious" penicillin allergy. *Clin Exp Allergy* 2017;47:1362–1373.
4. Kerr JR. Penicillin allergy: A study of incidence as reported by patients. *Br J Clin Practr* 1994;48:5–7.
5. Solensky R, Earl HS, Gruchalla RS. Penicillin allergy: Prevalence of vague history in skin test-positive patients. *Ann Allergy Asthma Immunol* 2000;85:195–199.
6. Lin RY. A perspective on penicillin allergy. *Arch Intern Med* 1992;152:930–937.
7. Green GR, Rosenblum AH, Sweet LC. Evaluation of penicillin hypersensitivity: Value of clinical history and skin testing with penicilloyl-polylysine and penicillin G: A cooperative prospective study of the penicillin study group of the American Academy of Allergy. *J Allergy Clin Immunol* 1977;60:339–345.
8. Rank MA, Park MA. Anaphylaxis to piperacillin-tazobactam despite a negative penicillin skin test. *Allergy* 2007;62:964–965.
9. Sogn DD, Evans R III, Shepherd GM, et al. Results of the national institute of allergy and infectious disease collaborative clinical trial to test the predictive value of skin testing with major and minor penicillin derivatives in hospitalized adults. *Arch Intern Med* 1992;152:1025–1032.
10. Har D, Solensky R. Penicillin and beta-lactam hypersensitivity. *Immunol Allergy Clin North Am* 2017;47:1292–1297.
11. Levine BB, Zolov DM. Prediction of penicillin allergy by immunological tests. *J Allergy* 1969;43:231–244.
12. Soria A, Autegarden E, Amsler E, Gaouar H, Vial A, Frances C, Autegarden JE. A Clinical decision-making algorithm for penicillin allergy. *Ann Med* 2017;49:710–717.
13. Doern GV, Brecher SM. The clinical predictive value (or lack thereof) of the results of *in vitro* antimicrobial susceptibility tests. *J Clin Micro* 2011;49:S11–S14.
14. Cunha BA, Ristuccia A. The third-generation cephalosporins. *Med Clin North Am* 1982;66:283–291.
15. Anne S, Reisman RE. Risk of administering cephalosporin antibiotics to patients with histories of penicillin allergy. *Ann Allergy Asthma Immunol* 1995;74:167–170.
16. Blanca M, Fernandez J, Miranda A, et al. Cross-reactivity between penicillins and cephalosporins: Clinical and immunological studies. *J Allergy Clin Immunol* 1989;83:381–385.
17. Saxon A, Beall GN, Rohr AS, et al. Immediate hypersensitivity reactions to β-lactam antibiotics. *Ann Intern Med* 1987;107:204–214.
18. Thethi AK, Van Dellen RG. Dilemmas and controversies in penicillin allergy. *Immunol Allergy Clin North Am* 2004;24:445–461.
19. Weiss ME, Adkinson NF. Immediate hypersensitivity reactions to penicillin and related antibiotics. *Clin Allergy* 1988;18:515–540.
20. Kelkar PS, Li JT. Cephalosporin allergy. *N Engl J Med* 2001;345:804–809.
21. Daulat S, Solensky R, Earl HS, et al. Safety of cephalosporin administration to patients with histories of penicillin allergy. *J Allergy Clin Immunol* 2004;113:1220–1222.
22. Novalbos A, Sastre J, Cuesta J, et al. Lack of allergic cross-reactivity to cephalosporins among patients allergic to penicillins. *Clin Exp Allergy* 2001;31:438–443.

23. Cunha BA. Cross allergenicity of penicillin with carbapenems and monobactams. *J Crit Illness* 1998;13:344.

24. Cunha BA. The safety of meropenem in elderly and renally-impaired patients. *Int J Antimicrob Ther* 1998;10:109–117.

25. Cunha BA. Antimicrobial selection in the penicillin-allergic patient. *Drugs Today (Barc)* 2001;37:377–383.

26. Cunha BA. Clinical approach to antibiotic therapy in the penicillin allergic patient. *Med Clin North Am* 2006;90:1257–1264.

27. Sade K, Holtzer I, Levo Y, et al. The economic burden of antibiotic treatment of penicillin-allergic patients in internal medicine wards of a general tertiary care hospital. *Clin Exp Allergy* 2003;33:501–506.

28. Prescott WA, DePestal DD, Eliss JJ, et al. Incidence of carbapenem-associated allergic-type reactions among patients with versus patients without reported penicillin allergy. *Clin Infect Dis* 2004;38:1102–1107.

29. Sodhi M, Axtell SS, Callahan J, et al. Is it safe to use carbapenems in patients with a history of allergy to penicillin? *J Antimicrob Chemother* 2004;54:1155–1157.

30. Romano A, Marinella V, Gueant-Rodriguez R, et al. Tolerability of meropenem in patients with IgE-mediated hypersensitivity to penicillins. *Ann Intern Med* 2007;146:266–269.

31. Linden P. Safety profile of meropenem: An updated review of over 6,000 patients treated with meropenem. *Drug Saf* 2007;30:657–668.

32. Lakhal K, Lortat-Jacob B, Neukirch C, et al. Safe Use of meropenem in a patient with a possible nonimmediate allergy to imipenem. *Pharmacotherapy* 2007;27:1334–1338.

33. Cunha BA, Hamid NS, Krol V, et al. Safety of meropenem in patients reporting penicillin allergy: Lack of allergic cross reactions. *J Chemother* 2008;20:233–237.

34. Cunha BA, Jose A, Hage J. Ertapenem: Lack of allergic reactions in hospitalized adults reporting a history of penicillin allergy. *Int J Anti Agents* 2013;42:585–586.

35. Cunha BA. No need for an initial test dose of meropenem or ertapenem in patients reporting anaphylactic reactions to penicillins. *J Chemother* 2015;27:317–318.

36 Adverse Reactions to Antibiotics in the Critical Care Unit

Diane M. Parente, Cheston B. Cunha, and Michael Lorenzo

CONTENTS

CLINICAL PERSPECTIVE

While similar to many countries in the rates of hospitalization, life expectancy, and causes of mortality in adults per capita, the United States is rather dissimilar in the high utilization of critical care units (CCU) [1,2]. Proportionally, this correlates with a high rate of anti-infective use, with some estimates as high as 71% [3]. While this high rate of anti-infective use is concerning for a variety of reasons, including increased selection pressure for multidrug-resistant organisms and risk of *C. difficile*-associated diarrhea (see Chapter 23), perhaps chief among these concerns to the treating clinician is the deleterious effect of anti-infective-associated adverse events.

The "To Err Is Human" report published in 1999 shed light on the alarming frequency of avoidable medical errors, and since its publication, significant efforts have been undertaken to improve the safety of patient care by reducing medications errors [4]. While some anti-infective-associated adverse events can be the result of a medication error (e.g., acute renal failure due to a patient receiving colistin dosing based on colistin base when the intended dose was based on the salt colistimethate sodium), the unavoidable necessity of anti-infective use in the CCU represents a significant challenge in assuring patient safety, as adverse events may be present even in the most vigilant monitoring and risk mitigation strategies. For this reason, it behooves clinicians in the CCU setting to be familiar with common anti-infective adverse events and be able to recognize such events in a timely manner to avoid undue patient harm [5,6]. The following chapter includes a summary of adverse events seen with anti-infectives commonly utilized in the adult critical care arena. Discussions of adverse events secondary to anti-retrovirals and direct acting antivirals used to treat the human immunodeficiency virus and viral hepatitis are excluded. Similarly, anti-infectives that are unlikely to be used in critically ill patients (e.g., nitrofurantoin and oral cephalosporins) and those unavailable in the US market are excluded. Some of the work included in this chapter is adapted from the work of Granowitz and Brown [7].

DRUG ALLERGIES AND HYPERSENSITIVITY REACTIONS

Allergies can often be difficult to clarify in the critically ill patient who may present obtunded, intubated in the field, or with an altered mental status. For this reason, unless a medication administration record can document the safe receipt of an antibiotic in question, providers may consider allergies from a "worst case scenario" standpoint and avoid drugs that will cause a potentially life-threatening reaction (anaphylactic vs. non-anaphylactic reactions). Both inside and outside the CCU, antibiotic allergies become most relevant when considering β-lactams, particularly penicillin. A penicillin allergy is the most commonly reported drug allergy, with 1 in 10 hospitalized patients carrying such a label [8]. Ultimately, very few of these patients will have a positive reaction to penicillin skin testing. A true penicillin allergy is only found in approximately 1% of the general population, and the avoidance of β-lactams may carry a risk of harm to the patient in a variety of ways [9]. Even in patients with a confirmed history of anaphylaxis to penicillin, roughly 80% of patients will be non-reactive 10 years following the initial allergy, owing to a loss of antibodies over time [10]. While skin testing remains the gold standard for determining the presence of IgE-mediated allergic responses to penicillin (and are increasingly being utilized by antimicrobial stewardship programs), the critically ill patient can often be on medications that can interfere with the interpretation of this test [9]. In patients with a history of anaphylaxis to all β-lactams, aztreonam (unless allergic to ceftazidime), tigecycline, and meropenem can be used safely.

A sound understanding of β-lactam cross-reactivity can often obviate the need for such testing. The immunologically responsible part of the β-lactam is the R-1 side chain, which varies drastically between penicillins and all intravenous cephalosporins [11]. That is to say, most patients can safely receive an intravenous cephalosporin, regardless of the significance or accuracy of the reported penicillin allergy. These patients will experience allergic reactions to cephalosporins at similar rates whether or not a reported penicillin allergy existed in their chart in a retrospective review of almost 65,000 patients receiving over 125,000 courses of cephalosporins [12]. In patients with penicillin allergies (anaphylactic or non-anaphylactic), meropenem can be given without skin testing or a test dose [13–15].

While IgE-mediated reactions to penicillins and the resulting lack of cross-reactivity to intravenous cephalosporins are well researched and evaluated, such data are lacking for many T-cell mediated reactions [8–12,16]. In patients with a history of a severe cutaneous adverse reaction, e.g., drug reactions with eosinophilia and systemic symptoms (DRESS), Stevens-Johnson syndrome, and acute generalized exanthematous pustulosis, to a penicillin or cephalosporin, avoidance of β-lactams is reasonable. However, these patients will likely tolerate carbapenems if such antibiotics are required [16]. While other antibiotics, such as trimethoprim-sulfamethoxazole (sulfa component is responsible for allergy, not trimethoprim alone), or fluoroquinolones, have been known to cause cutaneous reactions, the low incidence of these events overall makes it difficult to implicate any one class as a predominant culprit [16,17].

CARDIOTOXICITY

Perhaps one of the most concerning cardiotoxicities of anti-infectives is a prolongation of the QT interval corrected for the heart rate, or the QTc. However, of the 171 drugs with "known" or "possible" risk of torsades de pointes (TdP) listed at the time of writing, only 14% (24/171) are anti-infectives, with the lion's share of these agents belonging to a single antimicrobial class [18]. Anti-infectives commonly prolong the QTc by one of two ways: Modulation of the human-Ether-a-go-go gene, causing a blockade of outward rectifying potassium channels (I_{kr} channel) in cardiac myocytes or decreasing the clearance of other drugs that display the aforementioned effect. The prolongation of the QTc is often used by clinicians to identify patients that may be at a risk of developing TdP, a potentially life-threating arrhythmia. Assessing the direct impact of an anti-infective on the prolongation of the QTc in critically ill patients can be particularly challenging. The factors that can also contribute to the prolongation of the QTc, such as electrolyte abnormalities, bradyarrhythmias, and use of electrical conduction devices, can commonly be seen in critically ill patients and confound the impact of any one factor on the overall prolongation of the QTc.

One of the most commonly implicated classes of antibiotics in cases of QTc prolongation comprises the fluoroquinolones (moxifloxacin has the greatest QTc prolongation potential). In healthy patient studies, the impact of various fluoroquinolones is minimal, with changes in the QTc ranging from 0 to 11 ms when used at conventional dosing [19]. However, higher doses and use of intravenous fluoroquinolones, both of which may be required in CCU patients, may have a more dramatic effect on QTc prolongation [20,21]. Macrolides are also QTc prolongers, and azithromycin has demonstrated an association with sudden cardiac death when compared with amoxicillin; however, this was not reflected in a similar study with penicillin as the comparator. The QTc prolongation may occur with IV macrolides, resulting in high serum levels, e.g., erythromycin lactobionate, but does not result from IV azithromycin use because of its comparably low serum levels. The population studied in these investigations were largely represented by outpatients, and not reflective of an CCU population, where far less data on the incidence of macrolide induced QTc prolongation exist [22,23]. Azole antifungals represent a known class of QTc prolongers. The azole antifungal class is likely to be used in CCUs, owing to higher rates of invasive candidiasis and frequent care of immunocompromised patients. Importantly, azoles frequently cause drug interactions, thereby increasing the concentration of other QTc prolonging drugs. Azoles are also often used as prophylactic agents in patients with cancer in conjunction with fluoroquinolones. This has been shown to have a dramatic impact on rates of QTc prolongation, with one in five such patients experiencing it [24]. Antibiotics are typically weak blockers of the IKr channel. When modifiable risk factors are addressed appropriately (i.e., correction of hypomagnesemia, hypokalemia, and appropriate renal adjustments of anti-infectives), the risk of QTc prolongation causing a cardiac event is rather low [25]. Additionally, in patients whose baseline QTc is above 500 ms, alternative antibiotics without QTc prolongating potential should be considered. Exceptions to this include the anti-malarial quinidine, which requires routine monitoring of ECGs and is generally reserved for severe cases of malaria in which enteral administration is not feasible. Drug-induced QTc prolongation is additive and may, in combination, exceed 500 ms.

Other notable cardiotoxicities of anti-infectives include itraconazole-induced heart failure, caused by its negative inotropic effects. Clinicians should suspect this in patients with a new onset of symptoms following the start of therapy or a worsening of symptoms in patients with pre-existing heart failure [26]. Rapid infusion of amphotericin B may cause ventricular fibrillation in patients with renal dysfunction, possibly due to potassium load released by amphotericin B lysed cells [27].

DERMATOLOGICAL ADVERSE REACTIONS

In CCU patients, rashes are common and their etiology can be a challenge to determine. Additionally, skin abnormalities in these CCU patients may vary from mild to life threatening. The cause of rash may be due to disease, pressure, or medications. Identifying an offending agent may be difficult because of the large number of medications administered to CCU patients and the difficulties in temporally associating the rash with the initiation of any single agent [7]. Any antimicrobial agent has the potential to cause an allergic rash, but this problem occurs most commonly with β-lactams, sulfonamides, and fluoroquinolones [28].

Factors that should lead the clinician to suspect a serious drug reaction include facial edema, mucosal involvement, palpable or extensive purpura, pruritic, and fever. The presence of eosinophilia is associated with more severe disease. Maculopapular eruptions associated with antibiotics are especially common, usually occurring within 1–2 weeks after starting the offending agent and often becoming generalized and pruritic. The sensitivity of skin testing is low for β-lactam-induced maculopapular rashes. In patients with thrombocytopenia or other coagulopathies, hemorrhage into the skin may modify the appearance of the rash. In patients with penicillin-induced mild or moderately severe maculopapular rashes, it is generally safe to use cephalosporins [29].

Stevens-Johnson syndrome is erythema multiforme with mucosal involvement. The most commonly implicated antibiotics are the aminopenicillins and sulfonamides. Onset is typically 1–3 weeks. The rash can present as maculopapular and/or target lesions [30]. Stevens-Johnson syndrome can involve mucosa of the eyes, mouth, and the genitourinary tract, and up to 25% of cases may only involve the oral mucosa. Diagnosis can be confirmed by skin biopsy with immunofluorescent staining. Infections, e.g., mycoplasma, may cause Stevens-Johnson syndrome. Stevens-Johnson syndrome can evolve into toxic epidermal necrolysis, which carries a morality of 30% [30].

"Red man" syndrome is a transient, non-allergic, reaction to vancomycin, characterized by flushing of the head and neck, typically beginning within an hour of the start of an infusion [31]. Severe cases have been associated with angioedema, hypotension, chest pain, and, rarely, severe cardiac toxicity and death [32–34]. Red man syndrome is more frequently associated with rapid administration (i.e., <30 minutes). Each gram of vancomycin should be infused over at least 60 minutes to avoid red man syndrome. Histamine antagonists may be helpful in preventing or limiting the reaction in patients who require vancomycin and who continue to have red man syndrome despite slow administration of the drug [31,35]. Patients who develop red man syndrome should not be classified as having a vancomycin allergy, as this can be managed by stopping the infusion, administering a histamine antagonist (e.g., diphenhydramine), and then eventually re-starting at a slower rate.

A common problem in the CCU is differentiating between septic and drug-induced (chemical) phlebitis. Chemical phlebitis is associated with temperatures <102°F without shaking chills, while septic phlebitis is associated with temperatures >102°F with shaking chills. Both may be associated with erythema, heat, tenderness, and a "cord" at the peripheral catheter site. Therapy for septic phlebitis is catheter removal. Antibiotics most likely to cause chemical phlebitis include potassium penicillin, cephalosporins, and the streptogramins.

ELECTROLYTE AND GLUCOSE ADVERSE REACTIONS

Intravenous pentamidine can cause dramatic dysglycemias requiring routine monitoring of blood glucose 6–12 times per day [36]. Fluoroquinolones can also cause dysglycemias, in both diabetic and non-diabetic patients [37,38].

Electrolyte abnormalities are common adverse events of parenterally administered anti-infectives. These are due to the electrolyte load carried by the agent or direct toxicity and alterations in electrolyte homeostasis. Sodium is typically the most concerning electrolyte and can lead to edema and heart failure. Alternatively, antibiotics with potassium have negligible effects in patients with normal renal function. The antistaphylococcal penicillins (nafcillin and oxacillin) are also associated with hypokalemia as a result of potassium wasting. Nafcillin and oxacillin act as non-resorbable anions, increasing potassium extraction [39]. This effect is more commonly observed with nafcillin than with oxacillin and can be mitigated by potassium repletion or switching to another antibiotic class [40]. Trimethoprim acts as a potassium-sparing diuretic and can be associated with hyperkalemia. Hyperkalemia is particularly observed in patients receiving high trimethoprim doses for the treatment of *P. jirovecii* pneumonia and in those with renal dysfunction [41]. Amphotericin B can cause hypokalemia and hypomagnesemia, and these factors can be predictive of ensuing nephrotoxicity. Clinicians should replete these electrolytes along with sodium prior to starting therapy with amphotericin B. Continuous repletion of potassium may be required throughout therapy [42,43]. These complications are potentially reduced with liposomal formulations of amphotericin B.

DRUG FEVER

Drug fever is a hypersensitive reaction to a drug without cutaneous manifestations. Approximately 7% of febrile episodes are of drug-induced etiology [44]. In CCU patients, a majority will have fever episodes (without rash) and about half will be of non-infectious etiology [44]. Drug-induced fever is typically a diagnosis of exclusion and should be considered on the differential in patients on agents known to cause fever, e.g., β-lactams, sulfonamides, and amphotericin. An anti-infective-induced fever can occur at any time during therapy, and fever patterns can be characterized as continuous, remittent, intermittent, or a combination thereof. A clue to drug fever is the presence of relative bradycardia. The presentation of fever may coincide with the administration time of the agent.

A patient with drug fever will typically appear clinically well in comparison with what the fever curve would suggest. The presence of otherwise-unexplained peripheral eosinophilia, an elevated erythrocyte sedimentation rate, relative bradycardia, mildly elevated transaminases, and/or cutaneous manifestations of hypersensitivity further favors the diagnosis of drug fever [45,46]. When antibiotic-induced fever is suspected, the offending agent should be discontinued, and an alternative agent should be initiated to complete the course of therapy. On discontinuation of the offending antibiotic, the fever should resolve within 72 hours, provided no rash is present. Drug fevers are not only due to newly prescribed medications. Commonly, the longer a sensitizing drug is continued (weeks–years), the more likely it is the cause of the patients' drug fever.

HEMATOLOGICAL ADVERSE REACTIONS

COAGULATION ABNORMALITIES

Anti-infectives rarely lead to clinically significant bleeding; however, they commonly can cause alterations in the clotting cascade and lead to noticeable changes in coagulation markers. As a result of the N-methylthiotetrazole side chain, some cephalosporins are associated with bleeding; however, these antibiotics are currently unavailable in many countries, and this effect has not been reflected with newer cephalosporins [47,48]. Most bleedings or alterations of clotting pathways seen in available anti-infectives are largely due to drug-drug interactions with vitamin K antagonists, which can be multifactorial in nature and are best exemplified by trimethoprim-sulfamethoxazole.

Highly protein-bound drugs, such as trimethoprim-sulfamethoxazole, can displace warfarin from its binding site, leading to a higher fraction of free active drug available in the bloodstream. Penicillins and cephalosporins also share this effect [49–51]. Trimethoprim-sulfamethoxazole also inhibits the metabolism of warfarin via inhibition of cytochrome p450 enzymes responsible for warfarin metabolism. Azole antifungals interact with these enzymes and cause the same effect [49,52,53]. Finally, trimethoprim-sulfamethoxazole and most antibiotics can cause destruction of gut flora, which is responsible for natural production of vitamin K. This results in a sudden decrease in endogenous vitamin K and subsequent increases in international normalized ratio (INR). Daptomycin can cause an artificial increase in INR independent of warfarin by interference with commercially available tests. This laboratory abnormality does not seem to have any clinical effect

on bleeding risk or intrinsic clotting ability [54,55]. In contrast, dicloxacillin decreases the INR, predisposing patients on vitamin-K antagonists to hypercoagulable events [56].

DRUG-INDUCED NEUTROPENIA

β-lactams [57], vancomycin, flucytosine, trimethoprim sulfamethoxazole [58], and amphotericin B have the potential to cause neutropenia. Anti-infective related neutropenia is typically reversible on discontinuation of the offending agent [7,59,60]. The likelihood of neutropenia is less than 1% with shorter courses of β-lactams [7,60]. While neutropenia with cephalosporins is relatively rare, in a study of 39 patients, up to 18% developed neutropenia on ceftaroline, a fifth-generation cephalosporin [61]. Like other β-lactams, ceftaroline-induced neutropenia typically develops with longer durations of therapy (>2 weeks) and resolves about 7 days after discontinuation of therapy [61,62].

Vancomycin-induced neutropenia usually occurs after over 2 weeks of intravenous treatment [7,63]. Flucytosine is known for causing hematological toxicities (e.g., leukopenia, thrombocytopenia, and myelosuppression), particularly with concentrations greater than 100 mg/L [64]. Bone-marrow depression from flucytosine commonly develops within the first 2–4 weeks of therapy. Appropriate dose reductions based on renal function are necessary to minimize the risk of bone-marrow toxicity. Therapeutic drug monitoring of flucytosine is essential when high doses or prolonged therapy is utilized. Flucytosine peaks should be obtained after three to five doses at 2 hours post-dose. A goal peak of 50–80 mg/L is considered adequate. Peaks greater than 100 mg/L require dose reduction to minimize bone-marrow suppression.

DRUG-INDUCED THROMBOCYTOPENIA

An estimated 10%–25% of thrombocytopenia cases are drug-induced, of which antibiotics are frequently implicated [65]. The rate of thrombocytopenia may be higher in critically ill patients, owing to their complex nature [66]. The most common mechanisms of anti-infective-induced thrombocytopenia are hapten-mediated thrombocytopenia (e.g., β-lactams), "quinine-type" immune thrombocytopenia (e.g., fluoroquinolones and quinine), and myelosuppression (e.g., linezolid) [67].

Linezolid-induced thrombocytopenia is typically associated with durations longer than 10 days. When compared with vancomycin, shorter linezolid durations were not associated with increased rates of thrombocytopenia [68]. In clinical trials, tedizolid was noted to have lower rates of thrombocytopenia. However, post-marketing studies have displayed conflicting results, and the benefit of one over the other remains to be determined [69,70]. While thrombocytopenia induced by β-lactams, specifically piperacillin-tazobactam and fluoroquinolone, is a relatively rare event, they have been identified to have the highest relative risk of thrombocytopenia in critically ill patients [65,71]. Importantly, anti-infective-induced thrombocytopenia is commonly reversible and best managed by prompt identification and discontinuation of the offending agent.

HEPATOTOXICITY

Mildly elevated serum transaminases are common in CCU patients and are relatively common. Abnormalities are generally classified as hepatocellular injury, obstructive, or mixed [72,73]. The majority of antibiotic-induced hepatotoxicity is idiosyncratic and occurs via immunological reaction or in response to hepatotoxic metabolites [74]. Anti-infective induced hepatotoxicity rarely causes severe adverse outcomes, including acute liver failure. Most cases are asymptomatic or transient and resolve with the cessation of the drug. Hepatic adverse reactions may develop immediately, during prolonged therapy, or after completion of therapy with the antibiotic.

Amoxicillin combined with clavulanic acid is a frequent cause of cholestatic hepatotoxicity and is responsible for 13%–23% of drug-induced hepatotoxicity cases [74]. Hepatotoxicity is primarily associated with the clavulanic acid component, and onset typically occurs within 4 weeks of treatment and more commonly after discontinuation of therapy. Cases are associated with prolonged or repeated exposure of amoxicillin/clavulanic acid and older age (>65 years). Most cases are benign, and patients recover within weeks. Cephalosporins are rarely causes of hepatotoxicity; however, prolonged courses (>9 days) of high-dose ceftriaxone can cause biliary sludge formation in approximately 25% of adult patients [74]. Rifampin also commonly causes mild hepatitis that, on occasion, may be severe. Although rare, hepatotoxicity can also be caused by tetracyclines (not usually doxycycline or minocycline), macrolides, quinolones, sulfonamides, clindamycin, azoles, and ganciclovir [7,72].

MUSCULOSKELETAL ADVERSE REACTIONS

Quinupristin/dalfopristin can cause reversible musculoskeletal adverse reactions, including severe, protracted myalgias and rhabdomyolysis. Daptomycin can cause creatine kinase elevation and reversible myalgias. While the mechanism of daptomycin-induced myopathy is unknown, higher doses (>6 mg/kg) and concomitant use of 3-hydroxy-3-methyl-glutaryl-coenzyme A reductase (HMG-CoA) reductase inhibitors (statins) have been associated with increased risk [75–77]. Owing to the potential synergistic myopathic toxicity, evaluation of whether to hold statin therapy while on daptomycin may be considered. However, concurrent statin therapy should not hinder CCU practitioners from daptomycin use when clinically indicated for severe infections. Creatine kinase monitoring is recommended once weekly while on daptomycin, and it should be discontinued if the creatine kinase is greater than 1000 U/L in patients with symptoms of myopathy or greater than 2000 U/L in asymptomatic patients. Quinupristin/dalfopristin can cause severe, protracted arthralgias (9%) and myalgias (6%) typically with higher doses [78].

DRUG-INDUCED NEPHROTOXICITY

The polymyxins (colistin and polymyxin B) have high incidences of nephrotoxicity with polymyxin B, representing a potentially lower risk. In the case of colistin, doses required to achieve serum concentrations capable of even minimal bacterial kill coincide with serum concentrations known to pre-dispose patients to nephrotoxicity [79,80]. Outside of dose and serum concentrations, risk factors for colistin-induced nephrotoxicity are poorly defined. In general, risk factors for anti-infective-induced nephrotoxicity can also be applied to polymyxins, which include, advanced age, use of concomitant nephrotoxins, and obesity [80]. It is worth noting that polymyxin-induced nephrotoxicity is often reversible, and as such, the benefits of aggressive dosing may outweigh the risks [80].

Aminoglycosides represent another class of antibiotics that will likely be used more frequently in the CCU than other wards. For this reason, the incidence of nephrotoxicity in these patients is often cofounded by the degree of illness. Aminoglycoside-induced nephrotoxicity typically manifests as a non-oliguric renal failure, likely caused by tubular necrosis, with a slow rise in serum creatinine and typically reversible injury [81]. Extended interval dosing has reduced the rates of nephrotoxicity compared with traditional multiple daily dosing of aminoglycosides. Once-daily, properly dosed aminoglycoside therapy has virtually eliminated aminoglycoside-induced nephrotoxicity [81,82]. High trough levels are associated with increased incidence of nephrotoxicity. Therapeutic drug monitoring should be applied to ensure that both therapeutic effectiveness (adequate peaks based on indication) and safety (adequate troughs) are achieved [81,83]. Shorter durations of therapy may help to avoid nephrotoxicity, which is often consistent with the empiric use of these agents in the CCU [82].

Vancomycin is one of the most misdiagnosed causes of antibiotic-induced nephrotoxicity in hospitalized patients [84,85]. Vancomycin alone has little nephrotoxic potential when properly dosed. In recent years, significant literature regarding the contributing risk factors and effective mitigation strategies have come to light. Vancomycin troughs of 15–20 mcg/mL have been noted to be significantly associated with increased rates of nephrotoxicity, without notably offering a significant clinical benefit, specifically in patients with severe MRSA infections. (e.g., bacteremia and endocarditis) [86,87]. The reason for this is likely the poor correlation between troughs and pharmacodynamics of vancomycin. An area under the concentration time curve between 400 and 700 has since been linked to the efficacy and safety of vancomycin, respectively [86,88]. Use of intensive pharmacokinetic monitoring may help to decrease the incidence of nephrotoxicity by providing a more exact and individualized method of vancomycin dosing. Reports of vancomycin nephrotoxicity usually involve a concomitant nephrotoxic agent. Pharmacists trained in infectious diseases and critical care commonly have experience in such dosing strategies [89].

Another interesting contributor to vancomycin induced nephrotoxicity is the concomitant use of piperacillin-tazobactam. This combination often represents the backbone of empiric treatment of critically ill patients but carries with it a significantly increased risk of acute kidney injury (AKI). In patients at risk for AKI (e.g., pre-existing renal dysfunction, diabetes, hyper- or hypotension, malignancy, sepsis, hypoalbuminemia, volume depletion, and concomitant use of other nephrotoxic agents), an alternative combination not shown to increase the risk of AKI, such as vancomycin and cefepime, should be considered. Intensivists should note that the increased incidence of nephrotoxicity is commonly seen with durations greater than 3 days of therapy, and it is likely that during this time, sufficient information will be collected to allow for streamlining of the empiric regimen, potentially mitigating this risk [90,91]. Obesity represents another independent risk factor for vancomycin induced nephrotoxicity, with a possible contributor being the general lack of consideration of allometric dosing in obese patients. This leads to large overall exposures of vancomycin in these patients. However, lower doses will likely provide an optimal pharmacodynamic indices [92].

Amphotericin B can cause a renal tubular acidosis (distal or proximal), resulting in increased serum creatinine, along with wasting of potassium and magnesium. This risk is higher with conventional formulations, amphotericin B deoxycholate, and can be mitigated to some degree with the appropriate use of fluid administration and electrolyte replacement [93].

NEUROTOXICITY

DRUG-INDUCED OTOTOXICITY

Ototoxicity is an exceedingly rare and unpredictable event associated with few anti-infectives. Macrolides are associated with rare cases of mild-to-moderate sensorineural hearing loss in patients receiving long courses of therapy for the treatment of non-tuberculosis-mycobacterial infections [94,95]. In most cases, this hearing loss was reversible on discontinuation, and most patients had received greater than 1 month of therapy prior to the identification of ototoxicity [94,95]. Shorter courses are unlikely to result in such events [94–96]. Aminoglycoside toxicity is related to high, prolonged peak levels, not isolated high peaks. Aminoglycosides are possibly the most well-known anti-infective causes of ototoxicity. Of concern, this adverse event, unlike nephrotoxicity, is irreversible and not mitigated through the use of extended interval dosing [97]. There is no correlation to serum concentrations or dosing strategies, and it can occur with as little as one dose. Notably, risk factors include genetic predisposition and longer durations of therapy (>2 weeks) [97–99]. Vestibular toxicity may occur in up to 10% of gentamicin treated patients; however, the risk seems lower with other aminoglycosides [97,98]. Ototoxicity will typically present as a loss of balance and later as loss of high-pitch hearing. Both subtle factors can be extremely difficult to detect in the critically ill patient, particularly if intubated, sedated, and paralyzed. Clinicians should weigh the risks and benefits when considering an aminoglycoside, particularly areas with low resistance rates and availability of less toxic anti-infectives [100,101].

OTHER NEUROTOXICITIES

A wide spectrum of neurological manifestations from delirium to seizures (e.g., non-convulsive status epilepticus) can be caused by penicillins, cephalosporins (cefepime), carbapenems (imipenem, not meropenem or ertapenem), and fluoroquinolones (ciprofloxacin, not levofloxacin or moxifloxacin) [102–105]. The average time to onset is 5 days and ranges from 1 to 10 days [103–105]. β-lactam-induced seizures are thought to result from inhibition of the neurotransmitter γ-aminobutyric acid [106]. Penicillins, particularly benzylpenicillin, and less so ampicillin and piperacillin, have been known to cause neurotoxic effects ranging from encephalopathy, behavioral alterations, and myoclonus to seizures. Patients on piperacillin who progress from altered mental status to seizures not alleviated by anticonvulsant medications may require high-flux hemodialysis for resolution of symptoms. Cefepime-related neurotoxicity (particularly non-convulsive status epilepticus) is increased when the dose is not appropriately adjusted in patients with reduced renal function. Dose adjustments are recommended when the creatinine clearance is less than 60 mL/min. Other cephalosporins with neurotoxic potential (e.g., encephalopathy, myoclonus, and seizures) include cefazolin and ceftazidime [107]. Of the carbapenem class, imipenem/cilstatin has a higher reported incidence of seizures (0.9%–3%) compared with other carbapenems (<0.8%). Patients on carbapenems can experience encephalopathy, headache, myoclonus, or seizures.

Ciprofloxacin use has been associated with central nervous system (CNS) adverse effects, including headache and seizures (1%–2% of recipients) [108]. The incidence is greater in patients with renal insufficiency. Hallucinations, slurred speech, and confusion have been described and generally resolve rapidly once ciprofloxacin is discontinued.

Serotonin toxicity is due to impaired serotonin metabolism and is characterized by agitation, neuromuscular hyperactivity, fever, hypotension, and even death. Linezolid is a weak, reversible inhibitor of monoamine oxidase. Using linezolid in combination with other monoamine oxidase inhibitors can potentially cause serotonin toxicity. A small percentage (<5%) of patients on selective serotonin reuptake inhibitors who are given linezolid develop serotonin toxicity [109–112]. Serotonin toxicity is reversible on discontinuation of the offending agents. Onset and recognition of serotonin toxicity in published cases range from 30 minutes to 21 days from the combination of linezolid and serotonergic agents [113,114]. The average time to symptom resolution is 48 hours and ranges from 2 hours to 9 days. Unlike linezolid, tedizolid does not appear to markedly inhibit monoamine oxidase and, therefore, may not have clinically important interactions with serotonergic agents. However, in phase III clinical trials evaluating tedizolid, patients on serotonergic agents were not included. Hence, clinicians should proceed with caution until more evidence is available when using tedizolid with serotonergic agents.

Neuromuscular blockade is a potential side effect of aminoglycosides, particularly after intraperitoneal administration [102]. Polymyxins may also result in neuromuscular blockade. Characteristic signs occur soon after drug administration and include acute paralysis and apnea. Aminoglycosides and polymyxins should be avoided in patients with myasthenia gravis, owing to exacerbation of neuromuscular weakness. Paresthesias can occur in up to 27% of patients on polymyxins and is more common with intravenous versus intramuscular use (7%) [107]. Polymyxin neurotoxicity is theorized to be dose-dependent, with high binding to brain tissue and increased interaction with neurons. Risk factors for polymyxin-induced neurotoxicity include concomitant administration of narcotics, sedatives, anesthetic agents, corticosteroids, and/or muscle relaxants, which are all commonly used in CCU patients. Polymyxins can also cause peripheral neuropathy, visual disturbances, vertigo, confusion, partial deafness, hallucinations, and seizures.

Trimethoprim-sulfamethoxazole has excellent CNS penetration and has been reported to precipitate aseptic meningitis and psychosis [107]. The neurotoxic effects of trimethoprim-sulfamethoxazole particularly occur in the elderly or those who are immunocompromised. In 30% of patients, voriconazole, an azole antifungal, will cause transient visual changes with the first dose of therapy. These visual disturbances are described as altered light perception, photophobia, blurred vision, or color vision changes in the absence of an abnormality in the fundus oculi [115]. Although the mechanism is unknown, these visual disturbances typically last 30 minutes and are not associated with permanent visual sequelae.

ACKNOWLEDGMENTS

The authors appreciatively acknowledge Drs. Eric V. Granowitz and Richard B. Brown for their work in this chapter published in earlier editions. The authors have no conflicts of interest.

REFERENCES

1. Prin M, Wunsch H. International comparisons of intensive care: Informing outcomes and improving standards. *Curr Opin Crit Care* 2012;18(6):700–706.
2. Wunsch H, Angus DC, Harrison DA, Linde-Zwirble WT, Rowan KM. Comparison of medical admissions to intensive care units in the United States and United Kingdom. *Am J Respir Crit Care Med* 2011;183(12):1666–1673.
3. Vincent JL, Rello J, Marshall J, et al. International study of the prevalence and outcomes of infection in intensive care units. *JAMA* 2009;302(21):2323–2329.
4. Stelfox HT, Palmisani S, Scurlock C, Orav EJ, Bates DW. The "To Err is Human" report and the patient safety literature. *Qual Saf Health Care* 2006;15(3):174–178.
5. Cunha BA. Antibiotic side effects. *Med Clin North Am.* 2001;85:149–185.
6. Ambrose PG, Owens RC, Quintiliani R, et al. Antibiotic use in the critical care unit. *Crit Care Clin.* 1998;14:283–308.
7. Granowitz EV, Brown RB. Adverse reactions to antibiotics in critical care. In: Cunha BA ed. *Infectious Diseases in Critical Care Medicine* (3rd ed.). New York: Informa Healthcare USA, Inc., 2010;51:542–555.
8. Rubin R. Overdiagnosis of penicillin allergy leads to costly, inappropriate treatment. *JAMA* 2018;320(18):1846–1848.
9. Leis JA, Palmay L, Ho G, et al. Point-of-care beta-lactam allergy skin testing by antimicrobial stewardship programs: A pragmatic multicenter prospective evaluation. *Clin Infect Dis* 2017;65(7):1059–1065.
10. Trubiano JA, Adkinson NF, Phillips EJ. Penicillin allergy is not necessarily forever. *JAMA* 2017;318(1):82–83.
11. DePestel DD, Benninger MS, Danziger L, et al. Cephalosporin use in treatment of patients with penicillin allergies. *J Am Pharm Assoc* 2008;48(4):530–540.
12. Macy E, Contreras R. Adverse reactions associated with oral and parenteral use of cephalosporins: A retrospective population-based analysis. *J Allergy Clin Immunol* 2015;135(3):745–52e5.
13. Cunha BA, Hamid NS, Krol V, Eisenstein L. Safety of meropenem in patients reporting penicillin allergy: Lack of allergic cross reactions. *J Chemother* 2008;20:233–237.
14. Cunha BA. No need for an initial test dose of meropenem or ertapenem in patients reporting anaphylactic reactions to penicillins. *J Chemother* 2015;27:317–318.
15. Cunha BA. Meropenem in elderly and renally impaired patients. *Int J Antimicrob Agents* 1999;11:167–177.
16. Lin YF, Yang CH, Sindy H, et al. Severe cutaneous adverse reactions related to systemic antibiotics. *Clin Infect Dis* 2014;58(10):1377–1385.
17. Duong TA, Valeyrie-Allanore L, Wolkenstein P, Chosidow O. Severe cutaneous adverse reactions to drugs. *Lancet* 2017;390(10106):1996–2011.
18. Woosley RL, Romero KA. QTdrugs List. Available at: www.crediblemeds.org. Accessed on October 25, 2018.
19. Tsikouris JP, Peeters MJ, Cox CD, Meyerrose GE, Seifert CF. Effects of three fluoroquinolones on QT analysis after standard treatment courses. *Ann Noninvasive Electrocardiol* 2006;11(1):52–56.
20. Basyigit I, Kahraman G, Ilgazli A, Yildiz F, Boyaci H. The effects of levofloxacin on ECG parameters and late potentials. *Am J Ther* 2005;12(5):407–410.
21. Noel GJ, Goodman DB, Chien S, Solanki B, Padmanabhan M, Natarajan J. Measuring the effects of supratherapeutic doses of levofloxacin on healthy volunteers using four methods of QT correction and periodic and continuous ECG recordings. *J Clin Pharmacol* 2004;44(5):464–473.
22. Ray WA, Murray KT, Hall K, Arbogast PG, Stein CM. Azithromycin and the risk of cardiovascular death. *N Engl J Med* 2012;366(20):1881–1890.
23. Svanstrom H, Pasternak B, Hviid A. Use of azithromycin and death from cardiovascular causes. *N Engl J Med* 2013;368(18):1704–1712.
24. Zeuli JD, Wilson JW, Estes LL. Effect of combined fluoroquinolone and azole use on QT prolongation in hematology patients. *Antimicrob Agents Chemother* 2013;57(3):1121–1127.
25. Abo-Salem E, Fowler JC, Attari M, et al. Antibiotic-induced cardiac arrhythmias. *Cardiovasc Ther* 2014;32(1):19–25.
26. Ahmad SR, Singer SJ, Leissa BG. Congestive heart failure associated with itraconazole. *Lancet* 2001;357(9270):1766–1767.
27. Drutz DJ. Rapid infusion of amphotericin B: Is it safe, effective, and wise? *Am J Med* 1992;93(2):119–121.

28. Iannini P, Mandell L, Felmingham J, Patou G, Tillotson GS. Adverse cutaneous reactions and drugs: A focus on antimicrobials. *J Chemother* 2006;18(2):127–139.

29. Fonacier L, Hirschberg R, Gerson S. Adverse drug reactions to a cephalosporins in hospitalized patients with a history of penicillin allergy. *Allergy Asthma Proc* 2005;26(2):135–141.

30. Roujeau JC, Stern RS. Severe adverse cutaneous reactions to drugs. *N Engl J Med* 1994;331(19):1272–1285.

31. Wallace MR, Mascola JR, Oldfield EC, 3rd. Red man syndrome: Incidence, etiology, and prophylaxis. *J Infect Dis* 1991;164(6):1180–1185.

32. Glicklich D, Figura I. Vancomycin and cardiac arrest. *Ann Intern Med* 1984;101(6):880.

33. O'Sullivan TL, Ruffing MJ, Lamp KC, Warbasse LH, Rybak MJ. Prospective evaluation of red man syndrome in patients receiving vancomycin. *J Infect Dis* 1993;168(3):773–776.

34. Polk RE, Healy DP, Schwartz LB, Rock DT, Garson ML, Roller K. Vancomycin and the red-man syndrome: Pharmacodynamics of histamine release. *J Infect Dis* 1988;157(3):502–507.

35. Sahai J, Healy DP, Garris R, Berry A, Polk RE. Influence of antihistamine pretreatment on vancomycin-induced red-man syndrome. *J Infect Dis* 1989;160(5):876–881.

36. Assan R, Perronne C, Assan D, et al. Pentamidine-induced derangements of glucose homeostasis. Determinant roles of renal failure and drug accumulation. A study of 128 patients. *Diabetes Care* 1995;18(1):47–55.

37. Chou HW, Wang JL, Chang CH, Lee JJ, Shau WY, Lai MS. Risk of severe dysglycemia among diabetic patients receiving levofloxacin, ciprofloxacin, or moxifloxacin in Taiwan. *Clin Infect Dis* 2013;57(7):971–980.

38. Kabbara WK, Ramadan WH, Rahbany P, Al-Natour S. Evaluation of the appropriate use of commonly prescribed fluoroquinolones and the risk of dysglycemia. *Ther Clin Risk Manag* 2015;11:639–647.

39. Qua DC, Tan MJ. Hypokalemia associated with nafcillin treatment. *Infect Dis Clin Pract* 2009;17(2):130–131.

40. Viehman JA, Oleksiuk LM, Sheridan KR, et al. Adverse events lead to drug discontinuation more commonly among patients who receive nafcillin than among those who receive oxacillin. *Antimicrob Agents Chemother* 2016;60(5):3090–3095.

41. Kosaka M, Ushiki A, Ikuyama Y, et al. A four-center retrospective study of the efficacy and Toxicity of low-dose trimethoprim-sulfamethoxazole for the treatment of pneumocystis pneumonia in patients without HIV infection. *Antimicrob Agents Chemother* 2017;61(12):e01173–17.

42. Bahr NC, Rolfes MA, Musubire A, et al. Standardized electrolyte supplementation and fluid management improves survival during amphotericin therapy for cryptococcal meningitis in resource-limited settings. *Open Forum Infect Dis* 2014;1(2):ofu070.

43. Mayer J, Doubek M, Vorlicek J. Must we really fear toxicity of conventional amphotericin B in oncological patients? *Support Care Cancer* 1999;7(1):51–55.

44. Dimopoulos G, Falagas ME. Approach to the febrile patient in the ICU. *Infect Dis Clin North Am* 2009;23(3):471–484.

45. Patel RA, Gallagher JC. Drug fever. *Pharmacotherapy* 2010;30(1):57–69.

46. Cunha BA, Hage JE, Schoch PE, Cunha CB, Bottone EJ, Torres DC. Overview of antimicrobial therapy. In: Cunha CB, Cunha, BA eds. *Antibiotic Essentials* (15th ed.). New Delhi, India:Jaypee Brothers Medical Publishers Ltd, 2017:1–16.

47. McCloskey RV. Spontaneous reports of bleeding: Comparison of *N*-methylthiotetrazole side chain (MTT) and non-MTT cephalosporins. *J Infect Dis* 1988;158(6):1405.

48. Sattler FR, Weitekamp MR, Ballard JO. Potential for bleeding with the new beta-lactam antibiotics. *Ann Intern Med* 1986;105(6):924–931.

49. Fischer HD, Juurlink DN, Mamdani MM, Kopp A, Laupacis A. Hemorrhage during warfarin therapy associated with cotrimoxazole and other urinary tract anti-infective agents: A population-based study. *Arch Intern Med* 2010;170(7):617–621.

50. Saum LM, Balmat RP. Ceftriaxone potentiates warfarin activity greater than other antibiotics in the treatment of urinary tract infections. *J Pharm Pract* 2016;29(2):121–124.

51. Terasaki T, Nouda H, Tsuji A. Relationship between lipophilicity and binding affinity with human serum albumin for penicillin and cephem antibiotics. *J Pharmacobiodyn* 1992;15(3):99–106.

52. Wen X, Wang JS, Backman JT, Laitila J, Neuvonen PJ. Trimethoprim and sulfamethoxazole are selective inhibitors of CYP2C8 and CYP2C9, respectively. *Drug Metab Dispos* 2002;30(6):631–635.

53. Yamamoto H, Habu Y, Yano I, et al. Comparison of the effects of azole antifungal agents on the anticoagulant activity of warfarin. *Biol Pharm Bull* 2014;37(12):1990–1993.

54. Hashimoto H, Saito M, Kanda N, Yamamoto T, Mieno M, Hatakeyama S. Dose-dependent effect of daptomycin on the artificial prolongation of prothrombin time in coagulation abnormalities: In vitro verification. *BMC Pharmacol Toxicol* 2017;18(1):74.

55. Smith SE, Rumbaugh KA. False prolongation of international normalized ratio associated with daptomycin. *Am J Health Syst Pharm* 2018;75(5):269–274.

56. Pottegard A, Henriksen DP, Madsen KG, Hellfritzsch M, Damkier P, Stage TB. Change in international normalized ratio among patients treated with dicloxacillin and vitamin K antagonists. *JAMA* 2015;314(3):296–297.

57. Neftel KA, Hauser SP, Muller MR. Inhibition of granulopoiesis in vivo and in vitro by beta-lactam antibiotics. *J Infect Dis* 1985;152(1):90–98.

58. Andres E, Maloisel F. Antibiotic-induced agranulocytosis: A monocentric study of 21 cases. *Arch Intern Med* 2001;161(21):2619.

59. Olaison L, Belin L, Hogevik H, Alestig K. Incidence of beta-lactam-induced delayed hypersensitivity and neutropenia during treatment of infective endocarditis. *Arch Intern Med* 1999;159(6):607–615.

60. Singh N, Yu VL, Mieles LA, Wagener MM. Beta-lactam antibiotic-induced leukopenia in severe hepatic dysfunction: Risk factors and implications for dosing in patients with liver disease. *Am J Med* 1993;94(3):251–256.

61. LaVie KW, Anderson SW, O'Neal HR, Jr., Rice TW, Saavedra TC, O'Neal CS. Neutropenia associated with long-term ceftaroline use. *Antimicrob Agents Chemother* 2016;60(1):264–269.

62. Furtek KJ, Kubiak DW, Barra M, Varughese CA, Ashbaugh CD, Koo S. High incidence of neutropenia in patients with prolonged ceftaroline exposure. *J Antimicrob Chemother* 2016;71(7):2010–2013.

63. Brown RB, Levin J, Morris A. Adverse effects of antibiotics. *J Am Podiatr Med Assoc* 1989;79(10):500–504.

64. Vermes A, Guchelaar HJ, Dankert J. Flucytosine: A review of its pharmacology, clinical indications, pharmacokinetics, toxicity and drug interactions. *J Antimicrob Chemother* 2000;46(2):171–179.

65. Williamson DR, Lesur O, Tetrault JP, Pilon D. Drug-induced thrombocytopenia in the critically ill: A case-control study. *Ann Pharmacother* 2014;48(6):697–704.

66. Hui P, Cook DJ, Lim W, Fraser GA, Arnold DM. The frequency and clinical significance of thrombocytopenia complicating critical illness: A systematic review. *Chest* 2011;139(2):271–278.

67. Aster RH, Curtis BR, McFarland JG, Bougie DW. Drug-induced immune thrombocytopenia: Pathogenesis, diagnosis, and management. *J Thromb Haemost* 2009;7(6):911–918.

68. Attassi K, Hershberger E, Alam R, Zervos MJ. Thrombocytopenia associated with linezolid therapy. *Clin Infect Dis* 2002;34(5):695–698.

69. Lee EY, Caffrey AR. Thrombocytopenia with tedizolid and linezolid. *Antimicrob Agents Chemother* 2018;62(1):e01453–17.

70. Lodise TP, Fang E, Minassian SL, Prokocimer PG. Platelet profile in patients with acute bacterial skin and skin structure infections receiving tedizolid or linezolid: Findings from the phase 3 ESTABLISH clinical trials. *Antimicrob Agents Chemother* 2014;58(12):7198–7204.

71. Johansen ME, Jensen JU, Bestle MH, et al. The potential of antimicrobials to induce thrombocytopenia in critically ill patients: Data from a randomized controlled trial. *PLOS ONE* 2013;8(11):e81477.

72. Brown SJ, Desmond PV. Hepatotoxicity of antimicrobial agents. *Semin Liver Dis* 2002;22(2):157–167.

73. Navarro VJ, Senior JR. Drug-related hepatotoxicity. *N Engl J Med* 2006;354(7):731–739.

74. Andrade RJ, Tulkens PM. Hepatic safety of antibiotics used in primary care. *J Antimicrob Chemother* 2011;66(7):1431–1446.

75. Kullar R, Davis SL, Levine DP, et al. High-dose daptomycin for treatment of complicated gram-positive infections: A large, multicenter, retrospective study. *Pharmacotherapy* 2011;31(6):527–536.

76. Moise PA, Hershberger E, Amodio-Groton MI, Lamp KC. Safety and clinical outcomes when utilizing high-dose (> or =8 mg/kg) daptomycin therapy. *Ann Pharmacother* 2009;43(7):1211–1219.

77. Dare RK, Tewell C, Harris B, et al. Effect of statin coadministration on the risk of daptomycin-associated myopathy. *Clin Infect Dis* 2018;67(9):1356–1363.

78. N. C, Imhof A. Miscellaneous antibacterial drugs. In: Anderson JK ed. *Side Effects of Drugs Annual* (1st ed.). Oxford, UK: Elsevier, 2009;31:427–455.

79. Benattar YD, Omar M, Zusman O, et al. The effectiveness and safety of high-dose colistin: Prospective cohort study. *Clin Infect Dis* 2016;63(12):1605–1612.

80. Pogue JM, Ortwine JK, Kaye KS. Are there any ways around the exposure-limiting nephrotoxicity of the polymyxins? *Int J Antimicrob Agents* 2016;48(6):622–626.

81. Drusano GL, Ambrose PG, Bhavnani SM, Bertino JS, Nafziger AN, Louie A. Back to the future: Using aminoglycosides again and how to dose them optimally. *Clin Infect Dis* 2007;45(6):753–760.

82. Nicolau DP, Freeman CD, Belliveau PP, Nightingale CH, Ross JW, Quintiliani R. Experience with a once-daily aminoglycoside program administered to 2,184 adult patients. *Antimicrob Agents Chemother* 1995;39(3):650–655.

83. Wargo KA, Edwards JD. Aminoglycoside-induced nephrotoxicity. *J Pharm Pract* 2014;27(6):573–577.

84. Cunha BA. Vancomycin revisited: A reappraisal of clinical use. *Crit Care Clin* 2008;24:393–420.

85. Cunha BA, Mohan SS, Hamid N, McDermott BP, Daniels P. Cost-ineffectiveness of serum vancomycin levels. *Eur J clin Microbiol Dis* 2007;26:509–511.

86. Prybylski JP. Vancomycin trough concentration as a predictor of clinical outcomes in patients with *Staphylococcus aureus* bacteremia: A meta-analysis of observational studies. *Pharmacotherapy* 2015;35(10):889–898.

87. van Hal SJ, Paterson DL, Lodise TP. Systematic review and meta-analysis of vancomycin-induced nephrotoxicity associated with dosing schedules that maintain troughs between 15 and 20 milligrams per liter. *Antimicrob Agents Chemother* 2013;57(2):734–744.

88. Finch NA, Zasowski EJ, Murray KP, et al. A quasi-experiment to study the impact of vancomycin area under the concentration-time curve-guided dosing on vancomycin-associated nephrotoxicity. *Antimicrob Agents Chemother* 2017;61(12):e01293–17.

89. Heil EL, Claeys KC, Mynatt RP, et al. Making the change to area under the curve-based vancomycin dosing. *Am J Health Syst Pharm* 2018;75(24):1986–1995.

90. Gomes DM, Smotherman C, Birch A, et al. Comparison of acute kidney injury during treatment with vancomycin in combination with piperacillin-tazobactam or cefepime. *Pharmacotherapy* 2014;34(7):662–669.

91. Navalkele B, Pogue JM, Karino S, et al. Risk of acute kidney injury in patients on concomitant vancomycin and piperacillin-tazobactam compared to those on vancomycin and cefepime. *Clin Infect Dis* 2017;64(2):116–123.

92. Crass RL, Dunn R, Hong J, Krop LC, Pai MP. Dosing vancomycin in the super obese: Less is more. *J Antimicrob Chemother* 2018;73(11):3081–3086.

93. Mistro S, Maciel Ide M, de Menezes RG, Maia ZP, Schooley RT, Badaro R. Does lipid emulsion reduce amphotericin B nephrotoxicity? A systematic review and meta-analysis. *Clin Infect Dis* 2012;54(12):1774–1777.

94. Tseng AL, Dolovich L, Salit IE. Azithromycin-related ototoxicity in patients infected with human immunodeficiency virus. *Clin Infect Dis* 1997;24(1):76–77.

95. Wallace MR, Miller LK, Nguyen MT, Shields AR. Ototoxicity with azithromycin. *Lancet* 1994;343(8891):241.

96. Vasquez EM, Maddux MS, Sanchez J, Pollak R. Clinically significant hearing loss in renal allograft recipients treated with intravenous erythromycin. *Arch Intern Med* 1993;153(7):879–882.

97. Ariano RE, Zelenitsky SA, Kassum DA. Aminoglycoside-induced vestibular injury: Maintaining a sense of balance. *Ann Pharmacother* 2008;42(9):1282–1289.

98. Ahmed RM, Hannigan IP, MacDougall HG, Chan RC, Halmagyi GM. Gentamicin ototoxicity: A 23-year selected case series of 103 patients. *Med J Aust* 2012;196(11):701–704.

99. McGarity GJ, Ariano RE. Once-daily aminoglycosides. *Am J Health Syst Pharm* 2016;73(8):529.

100. Mo Y, Lorenzo M, Farghaly S, Kaur K, Housman ST. What's new in the treatment of multidrug-resistant gram-negative infections? *Diagn Microbiol Infect Dis* 2018;93(2):171–181.

101. Zahar JR, Rioux C, Girou E, et al. Inappropriate prescribing of aminoglycosides: Risk factors and impact of an antibiotic control team. *J Antimicrob Chemother* 2006;58(3):651–656.

102. Snavely SR, Hodges GR. The neurotoxicity of antibacterial agents. *Ann Intern Med* 1984;101(1):92–104.

103. Tanaka A, Takechi K, Watanabe S, Tanaka M, Suemaru K, Araki H. Comparison of the prevalence of convulsions associated with the use of cefepime and meropenem. *Int J Clin Pharm* 2013;35(5):683–687.

104. Fugate JE, Kalimullah EA, Hocker SE, Clark SL, Wijdicks EF, Rabinstein AA. Cefepime neurotoxicity in the intensive care unit: A cause of severe, underappreciated encephalopathy. *Crit Care* 2013;17(6):R264.

105. Cannon JP, Lee TA, Clark NM, Setlak P, Grim SA. The risk of seizures among the carbapenems: A meta-analysis. *J Antimicrob Chemother* 2014;69(8):2043–2055.

106. Chow KM, Hui AC, Szeto CC. Neurotoxicity induced by beta-lactam antibiotics: From bench to bedside. *Eur J Clin Microbiol Infect Dis* 2005;24(10):649–653.

107. Grill MF, Maganti RK. Neurotoxic effects associated with antibiotic use: Management considerations. *Br J Clin Pharmacol* 2011;72(3):381–393.

108. Owens RC, Jr., Ambrose PG. Antimicrobial safety: Focus on fluoroquinolones. *Clin Infect Dis* 2005;41(Suppl 2):S144–S157.

109. Gillman PK. Linezolid and serotonin toxicity. *Clin Infect Dis* 2003;37(9):1274–1275.

110. Lawrence KR, Adra M, Gillman PK. Serotonin toxicity associated with the use of linezolid: A review of postmarketing data. *Clin Infect Dis* 2006;42(11):1578–1583.

111. Taylor JJ, Wilson JW, Estes LL. Linezolid and serotonergic drug interactions: A retrospective survey. *Clin Infect Dis* 2006;43(2):180–187.

112. Narita M, Tsuji BT, Yu VL. Linezolid-associated peripheral and optic neuropathy, lactic acidosis, and serotonin syndrome. *Pharmacotherapy* 2007;27(8):1189–1197.

113. Woytowish MR, Maynor LM. Clinical relevance of linezolid-associated serotonin toxicity. *Ann Pharmacother* 2013;47(3):388–397.

114. Ramsey TD, Lau TT, Ensom MH. Serotonergic and adrenergic drug interactions associated with linezolid: A critical review and practical management approach. *Ann Pharmacother* 2013;47(4):543–560.

115. Ghannoum MA, Kuhn DM. Voriconazole—Better chances for patients with invasive mycoses. *Eur J Med Res* 2002;7(5):242–256.

37 Antibiotic Dosage Adjustment in Renal Insufficiency and Hemodialysis in the Critical Care Unit

Damary C. Torres, Kristina Bruno, and Danielle Maffei

CONTENTS

CLINICAL PERSPECTIVE

Acute kidney injury (AKI) is a common occurrence in critically ill patients with up to half of patients requiring some type of renal support. In patients with sepsis, AKI is associated with increased mortality and remains the leading cause of death in the critical care unit (CCU). Administering appropriate antibiotic doses to balance treating the infection while minimizing kidney injury is an important component of patient care in the CCU. The removal of antibiotics in critically ill patients is complex, influenced by factors such as the mode of renal support used, if any; drug characteristics such as solubility, molecular weight, and protein binding; and patient characteristics, including cardiovascular status and infection. The following table provides a guideline on treating patients with antimicrobials in the CCU, but as always, clinical judgement is necessary to ensure the best possible outcomes for patients.

ANTIMICROBIAL DOSING TABLE

Antibacterial Agents

Drug Name	Usual Dose	Dose Adjustments for Renal Insufficiency			Supplemental Dose Post-Dialysis		Dose in RRT
		>50	10–50	<10	Post-HD	Post-PD	CRRT
Amikacin	1 g (IV) or 15 mg/kg (IV) q24h	CrCl 50–80: 500 mg (IV) or 7.5 mg/kg (IV) q24h	500 mg (IV) or 7.5 mg/kg (IV) q48h	250 mg (IV) or 3.75 mg/kg (IV) q48h	500 mg (IV) or 7.5 mg/kg (IV)	500 mg (IV) or 7.5 mg/kg (IV)	500 mg (IV) or 7.5 mg/kg (IV) q48h
Ampicillin	1–2 g (IV/IM) q4–6h or 500 mg (PO) q6h	No change	1 g (IV) q8h / 250 mg (PO) q8h	1 g (IV) q12h / 250 mg (PO) q12h	1 g (IV) / 500 mg (PO)	1 g (IV) / 250 mg (PO)	1 g (IV) q12h / 250 mg (PO) q12h
Ampicillin-sulbactam	1.5–3 g (IV) q6h	CrCl >30: No Change	CrCl 15–30: 1.5–3 g (IV) Q12h	CrCl <15: 1.5–3 g (IV) q24h	1.5 g (IV)	None	1.5–3 g (IV) q24h
Azithromycin	500 mg (IV/PO) × 1 dose, then 250 mg (IV/PO) q24h	No change	No change	Use with caution	None	None	No change
Aztreonam	2 g (IV) q8h	No change	1 g (IV) q8h	500 mg (IV) q8h	500 mg (IV)	500 mg (IV)	1–2 g (IV) q12h
Cefamandole	2 g (IV) q6h	1 g (IV) q6h	1 g (IV) q6h	1 g (IV) q12h	1 g (IV)	1 g (IV)	1 g (IV) q12h
Cefazolin	1–1.5 g (IV/IM) q8h	CrCl 35–55: 1 g (IV) q12h	CrCl 10–35: 500 mg (IV) q12h	500 mg (IV) q24h	1 g (IV)	2 g (IV)	500 mg (IV) q12h
Cefepime	2 g (IV) q8–12h	CrCl 30–60: 2 g (IV) q12h	CrCl 10–30: 2 g (IV) q24h	1 g (IV) q24h	1 g (IV)	1 g (IV)	1 g (IV) q12h
Cefoperazone	2 g (IV) q12h	No change	No change	No change	No change	No change	No change
Cefotaxime	1–2 g (IV) q6h	No change	1 g (IV) q12h	1 g (IV) q24h	1 g (IV)	1 g (IV)	2 g (IV) q12h
Cefotetan	2 g (IM/IV) q12h	CrCl >30: No change	CrCl 10–30: 2 g (IV) q24h	2 g (IV) q48h	1 g (IV)	1 g (IV)	750 mg (IV) q12h
Cefoxitin	2 g (IV) q6h	CrCl 30–50: 2 g (IV) q12h	CrCl 10–30: 1 g (IV) q12h	1 g (IV) q24h	2 g (IV)	1 g (IV)	2 g (IV) q12h
Ceftaroline fosamil	600 mg (IV) q12h	No changes	CrCl 30–50: 400 mg (IV) q12h	CrCl 15–30: 300 mg (IV) q12h	200 mg (IV) q12h after HD	No data	300 mg (IV) q12h
Ceftazidime	2 g (IV) q8h	CrCl 30–80: 2 g (IV) q12h	CrCl 10–30: 2 g (IV) q24h	2 g (IV) q48h	500 mg (IV)	500 mg (IV)	2 g (IV) q12h
Ceftazidime/ Avibactam	2.5 g (IV) q8h	CrCl 31–50: 1.25 g (IV) q8h	CrCl 16–30: 0.94 g (IV) q12h / CrCl 5–15: 0.94 g (IV) q24h	CrCl <5: 0.94 g (IV) q48h	0.94 g (IV) given q48h	No data	No data
Ceftizoxime	2 g (IV) q8h	1 g (IV) q8h	1 g (IV) q12h	1 g (IV) q24h	1 g (IV)	1 g (IV)	1 g (IV) q12h
Ceftolozone/ Tazobactam	1.5 g (IV) q8h	No change	CrCl 30–50: 750 mg (IV) q8h	CrCl 15–29: 375 mg (IV) q8h	LD of 750 mg (IV) × 1 dose, 150 mg (IV) q8h after HD on HD days	No data	375 mg (IV) q8h
Ceftriaxone	1–2 g (IV/PO) q12–24h	No change	No change	No change	No change	No change	No change
Cefuroxime	1.5 g (IV) q8h or 500 mg (PO) q12h	No change	CrCl 10–20: 750 mg (IV) q12h / No change for PO	750 mg (IV) q24h / 250 mg (PO) q24h	750 mg (IV) / 250 mg (PO)	750 mg (IV) / 250 mg (PO)	1 g (IV) q12h / 500 mg (PO) q12h
Chloramphenicol	50–100 mg/kg/day (IV/PO) divided q6h	No change	No change	No change	500 mg (IV/PO)	None	No change
Ciprofloxacin	400 mg (IV) q12h or 500–750 mg (PO) q12h	No change	CrCl 30–50: 500 mg (PO) q12h	CrCl >30: 400 mg (IV) q24h / 500 mg (PO) q24h	200–400 mg (IV) / 250–500 mg (PO)	200–400 mg (IV) / 250–500 mg (PO)	400 mg (IV) q12h / 250 mg (IV) q12h
Clindamycin	600 mg (IV) q8h or 150–450 mg (PO) q6h	No change	No change	No change	None	None	No change
Colistin	2.5–5 mg/kg/day (IV/IM) in 2–4 divided doses	2.5–3.8 mg/kg/day (IV/IM) in 2 divided doses	CrCl 30–50: 2.5 mg/kg/day (IV/IM) in 1–2 divided doses	CrCl 10–29: 1.5 mg/kg (IV/IM) q48h	1.5 mg/kg (IV/IM) q24–48h, on HD, administer after HD	No data	2.5 mg/kg (IV/IM) q24–48h

(Continued)

Antibacterial Agents

Drug Name	Usual Dose	Dose Adjustments for Renal Insufficiency			Supplemental Dose Post-Dialysis		Dose in RRT
		>50	10–50	<10	Post-HD	Post-PD	CRRT
Dalbavancin	LD: 1 g (IV) × 1 dose MD: 500 mg (IV) 7 days later	No changes	CrCl <30: LD: 750 mg (IV) MD: 325 mg (IV) 7 days later	CrCl <30: LD: 750 mg (IV) MD: 325 mg (IV) 7 days later	None	None	No data
Daptomycin	Complicated skin infections: 4 mg/kg (IV) q24h; Bacteremia/endocarditis: 6 mg/kg (IV) q24h; Unresponsive to above dose: 12 mg/kg q24h	No changes	CrCl <30: 4 mg/kg (IV) q48h or 6 mg/kg (IV) q48h	CrCl <30: 4 mg/kg (IV) q48h or 6 mg/kg (IV) q48h	4 mg/kg (IV) or 6 mg/kg (IV) q48h, on HD days, administer after HD	4 mg/kg (IV) q48h or 6 mg/kg (IV) q48h, administer after PD	4 mg/kg (IV) q48h or 6 mg/kg (IV) q48h
Doripenem	1 g (IV) q8h	CrCl 30–50: 1 g (IV) q12h	CrCl 10–30: 500 mg (IV) q12h	500 mg (IV) q24h	250 mg (IV)	500 mg (IV)	500 mg (IV) q12h
Doxycycline	100 mg (IV/PO) q12h or 200 mg (IV/PO) q24h For serious infections can start with LD: 200 mg (IV/PO) q12h × 3d, then MD: 100 mg (IV/PO) q12h	No change	No change	No change	None	None	No change
Ertapenem	1 g (IV/IM) q24h	No change	CrCl <30: 500 mg (IV) q24h	CrCl <30: 500 mg (IV) q24h	if dosed less than 6 h prior to HD give 150 mg (IV)	No data	500 mg (IV) q24h
Erythromycin	1 g (IV) q6h or 500 mg (PO) q6h	No change	No change	No change	None	None	No change
Gentamicin	240 mg (IV) or 5–7 mg/kg (IV) q24h	120 mg (IV) or 2.5–3.5 mg/kg (IV) q24h	120 mg (IV) or 2.5–3.5 mg/kg (IV) q48h	80 mg (IV) or 1.25–1.75 mg/kg (IV) q48h	80 mg (IV) or 1 mg/kg (IV)	40 mg (IV) or 0.5 mg/kg (IV)	120 mg (IV) or 2.5–3.5 mg/kg (IV) q48h
Imipenem/Cilastatin	1 g (IV) q6h	CrCl 40–70: 500 mg (IV) q6h	CrCl 20–39: 250 mg (IV) q8h	CrCl <20: 250 mg (IV) q12h	250 mg (IV)	250 mg (IV)	500 mg (IV) q8h
Levofloxacin	500–750 mg (IV/PO) q24h	No change	CrCl 20–50: 750 mg (IV/PO) q48h or LD: 500 mg (IV/PO), then MD: 250 mg (IV/PO) q24h	CrCl <20: LD: 750 mg (IV/PO), then MD: 500 mg (IV/PO) q48h or LD: 500 mg (IV/PO), then MD: 250 mg (IV/PO) q48h	None	None	LD: 500–750 mg (IV/PO), then MD: 250–500 mg (IV/PO) q24h
Linezolid	600 mg (IV/PO) q12h	No change	No change	No change	None	None	No change
Meropenem	0.5–2 g (IV) q8h	No change	CrCl 26–50: 1 g (IV) or usual dose q12h CrCl 10–25: 500 mg (IV) or 50% dose q12h	CrCl <10: 500 mg (IV) or 50% usual dose q24h	500 mg (IV)	500 mg (IV)	LD: 1 g (IV), then MD: 500 mg (IV) q8h or 1 g (IV) q12h
Metronidazole	1 g (IV) q24h or 500 mg (IV/PO) q6–8h	No change	No change	500 mg (IV) q24h 250 mg (PO) q12h	1 g (IV) 500 mg (PO)	1 g (IV) 500 mg (PO)	No change
Mezlocillin	3–4 g (IV) q6h	No change	CrCl 10–30: 3 g (IV) q8h	CrCl <10: 2 g (IV) q8h	3 g (IV)	3 g (IV)	3 g (IV) q8h
Minocycline	100 mg (IV/PO) q12h or 200 mg (IV/PO) q24h	No change	No change	No change	None	None	No change
Moxifloxacin	400 mg (IV/PO) q24h	No change	No change	No change	None	None	No change
Nafcillin	2 g (IV) q4h	No change	No change	No change	None	None	No change
Nitazoxanide	500 mg (PO) q12h	No change	250 mg (PO) q12h	Use with caution	None	None	250 mg (PO) q12h

(Continued)

Antibacterial Agents

Drug Name	Usual Dose	Dose Adjustments for Renal Insufficiency			Supplemental Dose Post-Dialysis		Dose in RRT
		>50	10–50	<10	Post-HD	Post-PD	CRRT
Ofloxacin	300–400 mg (PO) q12h	No change	CrCl 20–50: 300–400 (PO) q24h	CrCl <20: 200 mg (PO) q24h	200 mg (PO)	200 mg (PO)	300 mg (PO) q24h
Oritavancin	1200 mg (IV) × 1 dose	No change	CrCl <30: no date	No data	No data	No data	No data
Oxacillin	1–2 g (IV) q4h	No change	No change	No change	None	None	No change
Penicillin G	2–4 mU (IV) q4–6h	No change	1–2 mU (IV) q4–6h	1 mU (IV) q8h	2 mU (IV)	0.5 mU (IV)	2 mU (IV) q6h
Piperacillin	3 g (IV) q4–6h	No change	CrCl 20–50: 3 g (IV) q8h	CrCl <20: 3 g (IV) q12h	1 g (IV)	2 g (IV)	3 g (IV) q8h
Piperacillin/ Tazobactam	3.375 g (IV) q6h or 4.5 g (IV) q8h	No changes	CrCl 20–40: 2.25 g (IV) q6h or 3.375 g (IV) q6h (nosocomial pneumonia) CrCl 11–20: 2.25 g (IV) q8h or 2.25 g (IV) q6h (nosocomial pneumonia)	2.25 g (IV) q8h	2.25 g (IV) q12h or 2.25 g (IV) q8h (nosocomial pneumonia); administer additional dose of 0.75 g (IV) after dialysis session if regular dose not due right after session	2.25 g (IV) q12h or 2.25 g (IV) q8h (nosocomial pneumonia); administer additional dose of 0.75 g (IV) after dialysis session if regular dose not due right after session	2.25–3.375 g (IV) q6h
Polymyxin B	1–1.25 mg/kg (IV) q12h 1 mg = 10,000 units	CrCl 20–50: 1 mg/kg (IV) q12h	CrCl 5–19: 0.5 mg/kg (IV) q12h	CrCl <5: 0.2 mg/kg (IV) q12h	No data	No data	0.5 mg/kg (IV) q12h
Quinupristin/ Dalfopristin	7.5 mg/kg (IV) q8h	No change	No change	No change	None	None	No change
Streptomycin	1–2 g (IM) q24h or 15–30 mg/kg (IM) q24h	No change	1 g (IM) q24h or 15 mg/kg (IM) q24h	1 g (IM) q96h or 15 mg/kg (IM) q72h	1 g (IM) or 15 mg/kg (IM) 2–3x/week	1 g (IM) or 15 mg/kg (IM) or 20–40 mg/mL in dialy q24h	1 g (IM) q96h or 15 mg/kg (IM) q72h
Tedizolid	200 mg (IV/PO) q24h × 6 days	No change	No change	No change	None	None	No change
Telavancin	10 mg/kg (IV) q24h	No change	CrCl 30–50: 7.5 mg/kg (IV) q24h CrCl 10–29: 10 mg/kg (IV) q48h	Avoid	None	None	7.5 mg/kg (IV) q24h
Ticarcillin/ Clavulanate	3.1 g (IV) q4–6h	CrCl 30–60: 3.1 g (IV) q8h	CrCl 10–30: 3.1 g (IV) q12h	2 g (IV) q12h	3.1 g (IV)	3.1 g (IV)	3.1 g (IV) q8h
Tigecycline	LD: 100 mg (IV) × 1 dose, then 50 mg (IV) q12h or High dose: LD: 200–400 mg (IV) × 1 dose, then 100–200 mg (IV) q24h	No change	No change	No change	None	None	No change
Tobramycin	240 mg (IV) or 5 mg/kg (IV) q24h	120 mg (IV) or 2.5 mg/kg (IV) q24h	120 mg (IV) or 2.5 mg/kg (IV) q48h	60 mg (IV) or 1.25 mg/kg (IV) q48h	80 mg or 1 mg/kg (IV)	40 mg or 0.5 mg/kg (IV) or 2–4 mg/L in dialysate q24h	120 mg or 2.5 mg/kg (IV) q48h
Vancomycin	15–20 mg/kg/dose q8–12h or 1 g (IV) q12h	Usual dose q12h	Usual dose q24h	1 g (IV) q week	None	None	1 g (IV) q24h

Abbreviations: CrCl, creatinine clearance; CRRT, continuous renal replacement therapy; HD, hemodialysis; IM, intramuscular; IV, intravenous; mU, million units; PD, peritoneal dialysis; PO, oral; q, every; RRT, renal replacement therapy.

Antifungal Agents

| Drug Name | Usual Dose | Dose Adjustments for Renal Insufficiency | | | Supplemental Dose Post-Dialysis | | Dose in RRT |
		>50	10–50	<10	Post-HD	Post-PD	CRRT
Amphotericin B	0.5–0.8 mg/kg (IV) q24h	No change	No change	No change	None	None	No change
Amphotericin B lipid complex (ABLC)	5 mg/kg (IV) q24h	No change	No change	No change	None	None	No change
Amphotericin B liposomal (L-amb)	3–6 mg/kg (IV) q24h	No change	No change	No change	None	None	No change
Amphotericin B cholesteryl sulfate complex (ABCD)	3–4 mg/kg (IV) q24h	No change	No change	No change	None	None	No change
Anidulafungin	Loading dose: 200 mg (IV) × 1, Maintenance dose: 100 mg (IV) q24h	No change	No change	No change	None	None	No change
Caspofungin	Loading dose: 70 mg (IV) × 1, Maintenance dose: 50 mg (IV) q24h	No change	No change	No change	None	None	No change
Fluconazole	Candidemia: loading dose: 800 mg (IV/PO) × 1, then maintenance dose: 400 mg (IV/PO) q24h Mucocutaneous candidiasis: loading dose: 400 mg (IV/PO) × 1, then maintenance dose: 200 mg (IV/PO) q24h Candida esophagitis or Candiduria: loading dose: 200 mg (IV/PO) × 1, then maintenance dose: 100 mg (IV/PO) q24h	No change	100 mg (IV/PO) q24h	100 mg (IV/PO) q24h	200 mg (IV/PO)	200 mg (IV/PO)	200–400 mg (IV/PO) q24h
Flucytosine	25 mg/kg (PO) q6h	No change	CrCl 20–40: 37.5 mg/kg (PO) q12h CrCl 10–20: 37.5 mg/kg (PO) q18h	37.5 mg/kg (PO) q24h	37.5 mg/kg (PO)	1 g (PO)	37.5 mg/kg (PO) q18h
Griseofulvin	Microsize: 500–1000 mg (PO) q24h Ultramicrosize: 330–375 mg (PO) q24h	No change	No change	No change	None	None	No change
Isavuconazole	Loading dose: 200 mg (IV) q8h × 48h Maintenance dose: 200 mg (IV/PO) q24h	No change	No change	No change	None	None	No change
Itraconazole	200 mg (PO) q12–24h If loading dose needed: 200 mg (IV) q12h × 2 days, then maintenance dose: 200 mg (IV) q24h or 200 mg (PO) q12h	No change	CrCl <30: No change for PO Avoid IV due to cyclodextrin	No change for PO Avoid IV due to cyclodextrin	100 mg (IV/PO)	None	No change for PO Avoid IV due to cyclodextrin
Ketoconazole	200 mg (PO) q24h	No change	No change	No change	None	None	No change
Micafungin	Candidemia: 100 mg (IV) q24h Esophageal candidiasis: 150 mg (IV) q24h Prophylaxis in stem cell transplant: 50 mg (IV) q24h	No change	No change	No change	None	None	No change

(Continued)

Antifungal Agents

Drug Name	Usual Dose	Dose Adjustments for Renal Insufficiency			Supplemental Dose Post-Dialysis		Dose in RRT
		>50	10–50	<10	Post-HD	Post-PD	CRRT
Posaconazole	*Aspergillus* and *Candida* prophylaxis: 200 mg (PO) q8h Oropharyngeal candidiasis: 100 mg (PO) q12h × 1, then 100 mg (PO) q24h × 13 days Fluconazole- or intraconzole-resistant strains: 400 mg (PO) q12h	No change	No change	No change	None, use with caution	None, use with caution	No change
Terbinafine	250 mg (PO) q24h	No change	Avoid	Avoid	Avoid	Avoid	Avoid
Voriconazole	IV loading dose: 6 mg/kg IV q12h × 1 day IV maintenance dose: 4 mg/kg (IV) q12h PO loading dose ≥40 kg: 400 mg (PO) q12h × 1 day PO maintenance dose ≥40 kg: 200 mg (PO) q12h, can increase to 300 mg (PO) q12h PO loading dose <40 kg: 200 mg (PO) q12h × 1 day PO loading dose <40 kg: 100 mg (PO) q12h, can increase to 200 mg (PO) q12h	No change	No change PO, avoid IV	No change PO, avoid IV	Usual dose PO, avoid IV	No data	4 mg/kg (PO) q12h, avoid IV

Abbreviations: CrCl, creatinine clearance; CRRT, continuous renal replacement therapy; HD, hemodialysis; IV, intravenous; PD, peritoneal dialysis; PO, oral; q, every; RRT, renal replacement therapy.

Antiviral Agents

Drug Name	Usual Dose	Dose Adjustments for Renal Insufficiency			Supplemental Dose Post-Dialysis		Dose in RRT
		>50	10–50	<10	Post-HD	Post-PD	CRRT
Adefovir dipivoxil	10 mg (PO) q24h	No change	CrCl 20–50: 10 mg (PO) q48h	CrCl <20: 10 mg (PO) q72h	10 mg (PO)	10 mg (PO)	10 mg (PO) q72h
Amantadine	200 mg (PO) q24h	No change	CrCl 15–30: 100 mg (PO) q24h	CrCl <15: 200 mg (PO) q week	None	None	100 mg (PO) q48h
Cidofovir	5 mg/kg (IV) weekly for 2 weeks, then 5 mg/kg q 2 weeks	CrCl >55: No change	CrCl <55: Avoid	Avoid	Avoid	Avoid	Avoid
Famciclovir	Meningitis/encephalitis: 500 mg (PO) q8h × 10 days Herpes zoster (dermatomal or disseminated shingles) or VZV pneumonia: 500 mg (PO) q8h × 7–10 days	CrCl 40–59: 500 mg (PO) q12h	CrCl 20–39: 500 mg (PO) q24h	CrCl <20: 250 mg (PO) q24h	250 mg	None	500 mg (PO) q24h
Foscarnet	HSV: 40 mg/kg (IV) q12h × 2–3 weeks CMV induction: 90 mg/kg (IV) q12h × 2 weeks CMV maintenance: 90–120 mg/kg (IV) q24h until cured CMV relapse/re-induction dose: 120 mg/kg (IV) q24h × 2 weeks	CrCl 50–80: Induction: 40–50 mg/kg (IV) q8h Maintenance: 60–70 mg/kg (IV) q24h	CrCl 20–50: Induction: 20–30 mg/kg (IV) q8h Maintenance: 65–80 mg/kg (IV) q48h	CrCl <20: Avoid	60 mg/kg (IV)	None	Induction: 20–30 mg/kg (IV) Maintenance: 65–80 mg/kg (IV) q48h
Leflunomide	100 mg/day (PO) × 3 days, then 20 mg (PO) q24h	No change	No change	No change	None	None	No change
Oseltamivir	Treatment: 75 mg (PO) q12h × 5 days Prophylaxis: 75 mg (PO) q24h × 10 days	No change	CrCl 30–60: Treatment: 30 mg (PO) q12h Prophylaxis: 30 mg (PO) q24h CrCl 10–30: 30 mg (PO) q24h	30 mg (PO) q24h	30 mg (PO)	30 mg (PO)	30 mg (PO) q24h
Pegylated interferon alfa-2a	180 mg (SQ) once weekly × 48 weeks	No change	180 mg (SQ) q week; avoid ribavirin	135 mg (SQ) q week; avoid ribavirin	135 mg (SQ) q week; avoid ribavirin	135 mg (SQ) q week; avoid ribavirin	135 mg (SQ) q week; avoid ribavirin
Pegylated interferon alfa-2b	Weight based dosing	No change	CrCl 30–50: reduce dose by 25%	CrCl 10–29: reduce dose by 50%	Avoid	Avoid	Avoid
Peramivir	600 mg (IV) × 1 dose	No change	CrCl 30–50: 200 mg (IV) × 1 CrCl 10–29: 100 mg (IV) × 1	No data	Give dose after HD	No data	100 mg (IV) × 1
Ribavirin	600 mg (PO) q12h	No change	Avoid	Avoid	Avoid	Avoid	Avoid
Rimantadine	100 mg (PO) q12h	No change	No change	100 mg (PO) q24h	None	None	No change

(Continued)

Antiviral Agents

Drug Name	Usual Dose	Dose Adjustments for Renal Insufficiency			Supplemental Dose Post-Dialysis		Dose in RRT
		>50	10–50	<10	Post-HD	Post-PD	CRRT
Valacyclovir	*Herpes labialis:* 2 g (PO) q12h × 1 day Genital herpes initial therapy: 1 g (PO) q12h × 3 days Genital herpes recurrent/intermittent therapy, <6 episodes/year, HIV-negative: 500 mg (PO) q24h × 5 days Genital herpes recurrent/intermittent, <6 episodes/year, HIV-positive: 1 g (PO) q12h × 7–10 days Genital herpes chronic suppressive therapy, >6 episodes/year, HIV-negative: 1 g (PO) q24h × 1 year Genital herpes chronic suppressive therapy >6 episodes/year, HIV-positive: 500 mg (PO) q12h × 1 year HSV-1 late-onset VAP: 1 g (PO) q8h × 10 days Meningitis encephalitis: 1 g (PO) q8h × 10 days Chickenpox: 1 g (PO) q8h × 5 days VZV pneumonia: 1–2 g (PO) q8h × 10 days Herpes zoster (shingles) dermatomal/disseminated: 1 g (PO) q8h × 7–10 days VZV meningitis/encephalitis: 1 g (PO) q6h	CrCl 30–50: 1 g (PO) q12h max	CrCl 10–30: 1 g (PO) q24h max	500 mg (PO) q24h max	1 g (PO)	500 mg (PO)	500 mg–1 g (PO) q24h max
Valganciclovir	Induction: 900 mg (PO) q12h × 21 days Maintenance dose: 900 mg (PO) q24h until cured for normal hosts and chronically for immune-compromised hosts	CrCl 40–60: Induction: 450 mg (PO) q12h Maintenance: 450 mg (PO) q24h	CrCl 25–40: Induction: 450 mg (PO) q24h Maintenance: 450 mg (PO) q48h	CrCl 10–25: Induction: 450 mg (PO) q48h Maintenance: 450 mg (PO) 2x/week	Avoid	Avoid	Induction: 450 mg (PO) q24h Maintenance: 450 mg (PO) q48h

Abbreviations: CrCl, creatinine clearance; CMV, cytomegalovirus; CRRT, continuous renal replacement therapy; HD, hemodialysis; HIV, human immunodeficiency virus; HSV, herpes simplex virus; IV, intravenous; IM, intramuscular; PD, peritoneal dialysis; PO, oral; q, every; RRT, renal replacement therapy; SQ, subcutaneous; VAP, ventilator associated pneumonia; VZV, varicella-zoster virus.

Miscellaneous Agents

Drug Name	Usual Dose	Dose Adjustments for Renal Insufficiency			Supplemental Dose Post-Dialysis		Dose in RRT
		>50	10–50	<10	Post-HD	Post-PD	CRRT
Atovaquone	PCP treatment: 750 mg (PO) q12h; PCP prophylaxis: 1500 mg (PO) q24h	No change	No change	No change	None	None	No change
Atovaquone/ proguanil	Malaria treatment: 4 tablets (1000/400 mg) (PO) q24 × 3 days; Malaria prophylaxis: 1 tablet (250/100 mg) (PO) q24 h for 2 days before entering endemic area, daily during exposure and for 1 week post-exposure	CrCl >30: No change	CrCl 10–30: No change for treatment; Avoid for prophylaxis	No change for treatment; Avoid for prophylaxis	Avoid	Avoid	Avoid
Capreomycin	1 g (IM) q24h	CrCl 50–80: 500 mg (IM) q24h	500 mg (IM) q48h	500 mg (IM) q72h	500 mg (IM)	None	500 mg (IM) q48h
Cycloserine	250 mg (PO) q12h	No change	250 mg (PO) q12-24h	150 mg (PO) q12h	None	250 mg (PO)	150 mg (PO) q12h
Dapsone	100 mg (PO) q24h	No change	No change	No change	None	None	No change
Ethambutol	15 mg/kg (PO) q24h	No change	CrCl	CrCl	None	None	15 mg/kg (PO) q36h
Ethionamide	500 mg (PO) q12h	No change	No change	No change	No data	No data	No data
Isoniazid	300 mg or 5 mg/kg (PO) q24h	No change	No change	No change	300 mg	300 mg	No change
Pentamidine	4 mg/kg (IV) q24h	No change	No change	No change	None	None	No change
Primaquine	Malaria treatment: 15 mg (PO) q24h; PCP treatment: 15–30 mg (PO) q24h (plus clindamycin)	No change	No change	No change	None	None	No change
Pyrazinamide	25 mg/kg (PO) q24h (max 2 g)	No change	CrCl <30: 25 mg/kg (PO) 3x/week	25 mg/kg (PO) 3x/week	25 mg/kg or 1 g (PO)	None	25 mg/kg (PO) 3x/week
Pyrimethamine	75 mg (PO) q24h	No change	No change	Use with caution	None	25 mg (PO)	No change
Quinine sulfate	650 mg (PO) q8h	No change	650 mg (PO) q12h	650 mg (PO) q24h	Administer dose after HD	650 mg (PO)	650 mg (PO) q24h
Rifabutin	300 mg or 5 mg/kg (PO) q24h	No change	CrCl <30: 150 mg (PO) q24h	150 mg (PO) q24h	None	None	No change
Rifampin	TB: 600 mg (PO) q24h; Antibiotic: 300 mg (PO) q12h	No change	No change	No change	None	None	No change
Spectinomycin	2 g (IM) × 1 dose	No change	No change	No change	None	None	No change

Abbreviations: CrCl, creatinine clearance, CRRT, continuous renal replacement therapy; HD, hemodialysis; IM, intramuscular; IV, intravenous; PD, peritoneal dialysis; PO, oral; q, every; RRT, renal replacement therapy.

BIBLIOGRAPHY

Bennett JE, Dolan R, Blaser MJ eds. *Mandell, Douglas and Bennetts Principles and Practice of Infectious Disease* (8th ed.). St. Louis, MO: WB Saunders, 2015.

Cunha CB, Cunha BA eds. *Antibiotic Essentials*. 15th ed. New Delhi. India: Jaypee Brothers Medical Publishers Pvt. Ltd. 2017.

Lexicomp Online®, Hudson, OH: Lexicomp, Inc. December 12, 2017.

Roberts JA, Lefrant J, Lipman J. What's new in pharmacokinetics of antimicrobials in AKI and RRT? *Intensive Care Med* 2017;43:904–906.

Zamoner W, de Freitas FM, Garms DS, et al. Pharmacokinetics and pharmacodynamics of antibiotics in critically ill acute kidney injury patients. *Pharmacol Res Perspect* 2017;4:1–7.

38 Antibiotic Failure: Apparent or Actual in the Critical Care Unit

Burke A. Cunha

CONTENTS

CLINICAL PERSPECTIVE

The clinical presentation is either that of persistent fever while on antimicrobial therapy or new fevers while in the critical care unit (CCU). Unfortunately, there are many causes of fevers in the CCU due to infectious as well as non-infectious causes (Table 38.1). For most physicians, continued fever suggests antibiotic treatment failure, and new fever suggests a new infectious process. Sustained or new fevers are often accompanied by leukocytosis [1–3]. Sometimes, consults are presented for leukocytosis without fever. As with fever, leukocytosis may be due to non-infectious or infectious causes and is not, per se, indicative of an infectious etiology, e.g., leukocytosis in patients on steroids. Since leukocytosis is reflective of stress due to any cause, most cases of leukocytosis with a left shift are due to non-infectious events/causes of fever [4,5].

TABLE 38.1

Differential Diagnosis of Fevers in the CCU: Unresponsive to Appropriate Antimicrobial Therapy

Infectious Causes	Non-infectious Causes
• CVC associated infections[a]	• Thrombophlebitis
• Nosocomial pneumonia	• Hemorrhage
• Nosocomial acute bacterial endocarditis	• Acute myocardial infarction
• Abscesses (undrained/inadequately drained)[a]	• Acute pulmonary embolism/infarction
• *C. difficile* diarrhea/colitis	• Acute pancreatitis
	• Drug fever
	• Gout flare
	• Acute adrenal insufficiency
	• Hematomas

Source: Cunha, C.B. and Cunha, B.A., *Antibiotic Essentials*, 17th ed., Jay Pee Medical Publishers, New Delhi, India, 2020.

[a] Require removal (infected devices) or drainage (abscesses).

DIAGNOSTIC APPROACH TO CONTINUED FEVERS ON ANTIBIOTIC THERAPY

UNDRAINED ABSCESSES

The approach is to first consider infectious causes that require non-antibiotic therapy/intervention, e.g., undrained/inadequately drained abscesses. Inadequate abscess drainage is usually accompanied by fever + leukocytosis. Persistent fever, in this setting, does not indicate an antibiotic failure. While antibiotics may penetrate into a phlegmon before the abscess is fully formed/walled off, few antibiotics are able to penetrate into the abscess and sterilize the abscess cavity. Therefore, antibiotics are adjunctive in the treatment of abscesses, and care requires adequate abscess drainage. This would seem obvious but is not in practice [6,7].

ANTIBIOTIC TREATMENT OF COLONIZATION VS. INFECTION

In general, colonization should not be treated with antibiotics. Colonization is not accompanied by fever, CCU patients often have fever from a variety of sources, but a positive culture forms respiratory secretions in a ventilated patient, a non-purulent wound drainage, a sacral decubitus ulcer culture with underlying chronic osteomyelitis, or a urine culture in a patient with an indwelling urinary catheter (CAB) (Tables 38.2 through 38.4).

Colonization should not be covered/treated for several reasons. First, colonization may rarely precede infection (the exception and not the rule), but nearly always, there is no progression from colonization to infection. Second, it is more difficult to eradicate colonization (no inflammatory component) than infection. Unnecessary prolonged treatment of colonization represents needless expense and prolonged length of stay (LOS) in the CCU and may predispose to multidrug-resistant (MDR) organisms or be complicated by *C. difficile* [8,9].

TABLE 38.2

Nosocomial Pneumonia: Colonization vs. Infection

- Colonization of respiratory secretions in ventilated patients is the rule and a function of time (days intubated).
- GNB from the CCU milieu colonize respiratory secretions.
- Common GNB colonizers include *Klebsiella, Enterobacter, Serratia, S. maltophilia, B. cepacian,* and *P. aeruginosa.*
- Most GNB colonizing organisms rarely, if ever, cause NP/VAP, e.g., *Enterobacter, S. maltophilia,* and *B. cepacia.*
- In ventilated patients with fever, leukocytosis, and infiltrates on CXR, unless accompanied by the characteristic clinical features of the pathogen, *organisms cultured from respiratory secretions should be considered as airway colonizers* and not the cause of NP/VAP.
- *Klebsiella* sp. pneumonia presents with fevers and cavitation (3–5 days after infiltrates) and *P. aeruginosa* pneumonia presents with high spiking fevers, elastin fibers in respiratory secretions, hemoptysis, and rapid cavitation (<3 days after infiltrates).

- Ventilated patients treated with antibiotics with minimal *S. aureus* activity, e.g., ciprofloxacin and ceftazidime, are often colonized with MSSA or MRSA but do not progress to *S. aureus* NP/VAP.
- *S. aureus* (MSSA or MRSA) CAP may complicate influenza pneumonia, but rarely, if ever, causes NP/VAP.
- Reports of *S. aureus* in ventilated patients with fever, leukocytosis, and infiltrates on CXR are based on respiratory secretion cultures and represent colonization and not the cause of NP.
- Without the distinctive clinical features of MSSA or MRSA CAP, e.g., high fevers, cyanosis, elastin fibers in respiratory secretions, hemoptysis, clinical deterioration, and rapid cavitation (<3 days) on CXR, patients should be considered as being colonized with MSSA or MRSA (or may have tracheobronchitis) but not MSSA/MRSA NP/VAP.

Source: Cunha, C.B. and Cunha, B.A., *Antibiotic Essentials*, 17th ed., Jay Pee Medical Publishers, New Delhi, India, 2020.

Abbreviations: GNB, gram-negative bacilli; NP, nosocomial pneumonia; VAP, ventilator associated pneumonia.

TABLE 38.3

Chronic Osteomyelitis: Colonization vs. Infection

Sacral Decubitus Ulcers (Stage III/IV) or Chronic/Deep Diabetic Foot Ulcers

- **Always treat the usual pathogens related to body site flora rather than "covering the cultured organism" from deep ulcers (since the culture specimen is not representative of the underlying pathogen in the infected bones).**
  - **Diabetic foot ulcers with chronic osteomyelitis:**
    Cover the usual osteomyelitis pathogens: GAS, GBS, common coliforms, *S. aureus,* and *B. fragilis* (not *P. aeruginosa*).
- **Do not cover surface ulcer colonizers cultured** *P. aeruginosa, Acinetobacter* sp., VSE/VRE, *Enterobacter* sp., *Burkholderia* sp., *Stenotrophomonas* sp.
  - Do not rely on deep ulcer/fistula cultures (which represent skin flora) and are not reflective of bone pathogens, i.e., osteomyelitis.
  - If *P. aeruginosa* is cultured from deep ulcer/fistula, do not cover for *P. aeruginosa.* Over 95% of diabetic foot ulcers/fistulas will be culture positive from *P. aeruginosa* (due to *P. aeruginosa* colonization from wet socks, wet dressings, whirlpool baths). In aseptically collected bone specimens in the OR.
  - *P. aeruginosa* is NOT a bone pathogen in diabetics with chronic osteomyelitis.
  - **Sacral decubitus ulcers (stage III/IV) = chronic osteomyelitis**
    Cover the usual chronic osteomyelitis pathogens:
    GAS, GBS, *S. aureus,* coliforms, and *B. fragilis.*
- **Do not cover ulcer surface colonizers cultured ("water organisms"):**
  - *Stenotrophomonas* sp., *Acinetobacter* sp., *Enterobacter* sp., *P. aeruginosa* sp., *Burkholderia* sp.

Source: Cunha, C.B. and Cunha, B.A., *Antibiotic Essentials*, 17th ed., Jay Pee Medical Publishers, New Delhi, India, 2020.

Abbreviations: GAS, group A streptococci; GBS, group B streptococci; VSE, vancomycin-susceptible enterococci; VRE, vancomycin-resistant enterococci.

TABLE 38.4

Urinary Tract: Infection Versus Colonization

Acute Uncomplicated Cystitis (AUC) = Infection	
Dysuria + Bacteriuria (cc: >100 K cfu/mL)	Treat with PO antibiotic[a]
Asymptomatic Bacteriuria (AB) = Colonization	
No rationale for UC if no dysuria	
AB = Bacteriuria (<100 K cfu/mL) + No dysuria	*Do not treat*
	(If treated, AB usually returns)
Catheter Associated Bacteriuria (CAB) = Infection versus Colonization	
Asymptomatic CAB (*bacteriuria without dysuria*) = **Colonization**	
Replace Foley and repeat UC (bacteriuria eliminated)	*Do not treat*
Symptomatic CAB (bacteriuria with dysuria) = **Infection** (if dysuria is not due to irritation)	Treat with PO antibiotic[a]

[a] Repeat UC/UA after 1–3 days on therapy to verify antibiotic response in AUC (urine colony counts rapidly decrease with effective therapy).

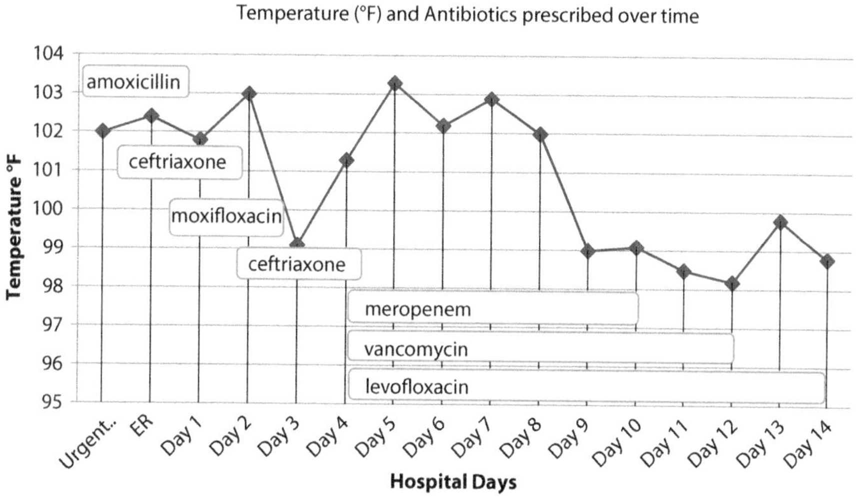

FIGURE 38.1 Apparent antibiotic failure (lack of response to prolonged multiple antibiotic therapy) with prolonged fevers due to Adenovirus pneumonia. (From Cunha, B.A. et al., *J. Clin. Med.*, 6, E42, 2017.)

NON-ANTIBIOTIC-RESPONSIVE INFECTIOUS DISEASES

Incredibly, all too often in the CCU, fevers persist on antibiotics if the underlying cause of fever is fungal or viral. The fever response to appropriate antimicrobial therapy has diagnostic importance, i.e., the lack of a decrease in temperature should suggest (after device-related infection and abscesses have been ruled out) a viral etiology of the fever, e.g., EBV and CMV, as well as non-infectious causes of fever, e.g., gout and SLE flare [1,10] (Figure 38.1).

ANTIBIOTIC-RELATED CAUSES OF ANTIBIOTIC FAILURE

First, the antibiotic being used should have a high degree of activity against the known or presumed pathogens. Once again, avoid "covering/chasing" isolates that have no clinical significance at the site that were cultured from, i.e., clinical correlation is required to assess the potential clinical significance (of the organism in this setting vs. its non-significance colonization of a body fluid).

Antibiotic underdosing is not uncommon. Dosing should be with the highest recommended dose while avoiding toxicity to minimize resistance potential. If the antibiotic selected has the appropriate spectrum (by body site) and is being dosed optimally, then consideration should be given to re-assessment of the interpretation of *in vitro* susceptibility data (organism/pathogen specific) vs. *in vivo* effectiveness [8,11] (Tables 38.5 and 38.6).

IN VITRO SUSCEPTIBILITY VS. IN VITRO EFFECTIVENESS

Some organisms, e.g., MRSA, are reported as "susceptible" to an antibiotic, but *in vivo*, they are ineffective, e.g., quinolones (excluding delafloxacin) and cephalosporins

TABLE 38.5

Antibiotic Failure: Apparent and Actual Causes—Persistent Fevers on Appropriate Antibiotic Therapy

Microbiologic Factors
- *In vitro* susceptibility but ineffective *in vivo*
- Treating colonization (no fever) vs. infection (fever)

Antibiotic Factors
- Inadequate antimicrobial spectrum (for site of infection)
- Inadequate antibiotic tissue levels (relative to serum levels)
- Decreased antibiotic activity (pH dependent)

Antibiotic Penetration Factors
- Undrained/inadequate abscess
- Device associated infections (no blood supply)
- Organ hypoperfusion/diminished blood supply, e.g., DM and PVD

Non-Infectious Diseases
- Disorders mimicking infections, e.g., SLE and malignancies
- Drug fever

Antibiotic Unresponsive Infectious Diseases
- Viral or fungal infections

Source: Cunha, C.B. and Cunha, B.A., *Antibiotic Essentials*, 17th ed., Jay Pee Medical Publishers, New Delhi, India, 2020.

(excluding ceftaroline) and should not be used to treat MRSA infections. Similarly, the type of MRSA matters; i.e., community-acquired MRSA (CA-MRSA) is reported susceptible to TMP-SMX, doxycycline, and clindamycin, but those drugs are relatively ineffective against community-onset MRSA (CO-MRSA) and hospital-acquired MRSA (HA-MRSA) strains [12–15].

Other common examples include TMP-SMX with *Klebsiella* sp. Although usually reported as TMP-SMX susceptible, TMP-SMX may not be effective in serious systemic *Klebsiella* sp. infections [8] (Tables 38.7 and 38.8).

Even though all streptococci are routinely reported as aminoglycoside "susceptible," aminoglycosides, e.g., gentamicin, have no inherent anti-streptococcal (groups A–D) activity. When penicillin or ampicillin is given with gentamicin, the synergistic combination is clinically effective [8].

INADEQUATE TISSUE PENETRATION

If the infection focus is in difficult-to-penetrate tissue/organ, there are two key factors that determine tissue potential penetration, i.e., the degree of local tissue inflammation and the lipid solubility of the antibiotic, as expressed by lipid solubility, i.e., V_d in L/kg.

TABLE 38.6

Presumed Antibiotic Failure: Differential Diagnosis Approach to Continued Fevers on Appropriate Antimicrobial Therapy

Infectious Causes

- **Treating colonization** (not infection)
- **Abscesses** (undrained/inadequately drained)
- **Viral infections**
- **Fungal infections**

Antibiotic Related
- **Inadequate tissue penetration**
  - Prostate: Cephalosporins, carbapenems (water, not lipid, soluble)
  - Synovial fluid: Vancomycin (↓ penetration, large molecule)
  - Device associated (no blood supply)
    – CVC
    – Prosthetic devices
- **Inadequate activity**
  - Urine: Low urine levels (~ CrCl)
  - Suboptimal urine pH for the antibiotic (↓ activity, not urine levels)
  - Lungs: Aminoglycosides (↓ activity, not low lung levels)
- **Suboptimal Dosing**
  - MDR GNB: Higher than usual doses may be needed for relative resistant strains (DD-S)
- **Inadequate tissue perfusion (DM, PVD)**
- **Susceptible *in vitro* but ineffective *in vivo***

Non-Infectious Causes

- **Drug fever**
- **Non-infectious disorders** (SLE flare)

Source: Cunha, C.B. and Cunha, B.A., *Antibiotic Essentials*, 17th ed., Jay Pee Medical Publishers, New Delhi, India, 2020.
Abbreviations: CVC, central venous catheter; PVD, peripheral vascular disease; MDR, multidrug resistant; GNB, gram-negative bacilli; DD-S, dose-dependent susceptibility.

TABLE 38.7
Limitations of Susceptibility Testing

Microbiology and Clinical Correlations

- *In vitro* data do not differentiate between colonizers and pathogens.
- *In vitro* data do not necessarily translate into *in vivo* efficacy.
- Antibiotic activity effectiveness depends on body site concentrations, local pH, degree of inflammation, cellular debris, local oxygen levels, blood supply, and penetrability.
- *In vitro* susceptibility testing is dependent on the microbe, methodology, pH, and antibiotic concentration.
- *In vitro* susceptibility testing assumes the isolate was recovered from blood, using serum concentrations of an antibiotic given in the usual dose.
- Some body sites, e.g., bladder urine, contain higher antibiotic concentrations than found in serum, while other body site levels may be lower than in serum, e.g., CSF. Therefore, *in vitro* susceptibility may be misleading for non-bloodstream infections.
- Antibiotics should be prescribed at the usual recommended doses; attempts to lower cost by reducing dosage may decrease antibiotic efficacy; e.g., cefoxitin 2 g IV inhibits ~85% of *B. fragilis*, whereas 1 g IV inhibits only ~20%.

Source: Cunha, C.B. and Cunha, B.A., *Antibiotic Essentials*, 17th ed., Jay Pee Medical Publishers, New Delhi, India, 2020.

TABLE 38.8
Discordance between *In Vitro* Susceptibility Testing and *In Vivo* Effectiveness

Antibiotic	"Susceptible" Organism
Penicillin	*H. influenzae, Yersinia pestis,* VSE[a]
TMP-SMX	*Klebsiella,* VSE, *Bartonella* sp.
Polymyxin B	*Proteus* sp., *Salmonella* sp.
Imipenem	*Stenotrophomonas maltophilia*
Vancomycin	*Erysipelothrix rhusiopathiae*
Gentamicin	*Mycobacterium tuberculosis*
Aminoglycosides	Streptococci, *Salmonella* sp., *Shigella* sp.
Clindamycin	*Fusobacteria* sp., *Clostridia* sp., *Listeria* sp.
Macrolides	*P. multocida*
First-, second-generation cephalosporins	*Salmonella* sp., *Shigella* sp., *Bartonella* sp.
Third-, fourth-generation cephalosporins	*Listeria* sp., *Bartonella* sp., MRSA[b]
Quinolones	MRSA

Source: Cunha, C.B. and Cunha, B.A., *Antibiotic Essentials*, 17th ed., Jay Pee Medical Publishers, New Delhi, India, 2020.

[a] Effective penicillin therapy for systemic enterococcal infections due to VSE requires an aminoglycoside, e.g., gentamicin (alone ineffective against enterococci).

[b] Although apparently testing susceptible against MRSA, *in vitro* susceptibility of antibiotics against MRSA is not reliable and may be misleading effective *in vivo* reliably are vancomycin, tigecycline, quinupristin/dalfopristin, linezolid, tedizolid, daptomycin, ceftaroline, telavancin, dalbavancin, oritavancin, delafloxacin, and minocycline.

The traditional "difficult to penetrate" uninflamed tissues are the CSF, sinuses/mastoid, and prostate. When any of these organ infections are chronic, e.g., chronic prostatitis, by definition, they have no acute inflammatory component and represent a penetration barrier to antibiotics. The other important determinant of tissue penetration is lipid solubility, as measured by the volume of distribution (V_d). The greater the V_d higher than the V_d of water = 0.7 L/kg, the better the tissue penetration [8].

ADEQUATE ANTIBIOTIC LEVELS SUBOPTIMAL AND ANTIBIOTIC ACTIVITY

There are two common clinical scenarios that demonstrate this concept. First, when treating pneumonia, virtually all antibiotics achieve therapeutic levels in the lungs. However, daptomycin lung levels are therapeutic, but the drug is inactivated by lung surfactant. It is a common misconception that aminoglycosides do not penetrate the lung well, but they do.

However, aminoglycoside activity is decreased by local acidosis, cellular debris, and local hypoxia, which are part of the pathology in pneumonia [8].

The effect of local pH on antimicrobial activity should be considered when no other explanation suffices to explain antibiotic failure, particularly in the treatment of cystitis and prostatitis. The activity of some antibiotics is enhanced in an acid urine (and decreased in an alkaline urine), while others are most active in an alkaline pH (and decreased in an acid urine). With some antibiotics, pH has no effect on activity but may affect urine levels by altering tubular reabsorption [16–18].

Inadequate urinary levels (with renal eliminate antibiotics) may result from decreased renal function. These points are well illustrated in healing chronic prostatitis. First, chronic prostatitis has no inflammatory component to facilitate antibiotic penetration. Second, the prostate is a multiseptate lipid gland laden, which prevents therapeutic levels of water-soluble antibiotic ($V_d \sim H_2O$). Third, the pH of infected prostate tissue is lower (acidic) than uninfected prostate [8,17–22].

DRUG FEVER

Drug fevers are hypersensitivity reactions (without rash) that usually occur after long exposure (years) to a sensitizing medication or, less commonly, after recent introduction of a new sensitizing medication. Drug fevers may present as new or prolonged fevers. Medications most often causing drug fevers are non-antibiotics, e.g., Colace and Lasix. The patient may be atopic but not always. Drug fever should be suspected when fever is accompanied by relative bradycardia and the patient looks "relatively well" (in light of underlying pathology). Leukocytosis with a left shift may lead the unwary away from considering the diagnosis of drug fever. Otherwise-unexplained relative bradycardia (provided patient is not on a β-blocker, verapamil, or diltiazem or has a pacemaker rhythm) is the cardinal clue to drug fever. Mild transaminitis is common. Eosinophils are often present, but eosinophilia is uncommon. Drug fever is a diagnosis of exclusion. The diagnostic test is to discontinue the most likely medication causing drug fever, and the temperature will decrease to normal after 3 days [1,8] (Tables 38.9 and 38.10).

TABLE 38.9

Clinical Features of Drug Fever

History
- Many, but not all patients are atopic
- Most patients have been on a "sensitizing medication" for years "without a problem"
- Less likely due to new or recent medications

Physical Exam
- Unexplained/persistent fevers with relative bradycardia
- Fevers usually between 102°F and 104°F but may exceed 106°F
- Patient appears "inappropriately well" for degree of fever

Laboratory Tests
- Elevated WBC count (usually with left shift) mimicking an infectious etiology
- Eosinophils almost always present, but eosinophilia is uncommon
- Elevated erythrocyte sedimentation rate over baseline
- Commonly transient, mild elevations of serum transaminases
- Negative blood cultures (excluding skin contaminants)

Commonest Sensitizing Medications Causing Drug Fever	
Common	**Less Common**
Amphotericin B	Allopurinol
Barbituates	Hydralazine
Methyldopa	Iodides
Penicillins	Isoniazid
Cephalosporins	Rifampin
Procainamide	Non-steroidal anti-inflammatory drugs
Quinidine	Anti-seizure medications
Sulfonamides	Sedatives
Opiates	Sleep medications
Colace	
Lasix	

Source: Cunha, C.B. and Cunha, B.A., *Antibiotic Essentials*, 17th ed., Jay Pee Medical
              Publishers, New Delhi, India, 2020.

TABLE 38.10

Relative Bradycardia: Pulse/Temperature-Pulse Relationships (Applies to Adult Patients with Temperatures >102°F)

Temperature	Appropriate Pulse Response (Beats/Min)	Relative Bradycardia Pulse with (with Beats/Min)[a]
106°F (41.1°C)	150/min	<140/min
105°F (40.6°C)	140/min	<130/min
104°F (47.7°C)	130/min	<120/min
103°F (39.4°C)	120/min	<110/min
102°F (38.9°C)	110/min	<100/min

Source: Cunha, C.B. and Cunha, B.A., *Antibiotic Essentials*, 17th ed., Jay Pee Medical Publishers, New Delhi, India, 2020.

Note: Relative bradycardia refers to heart rates that are inappropriately slow relative to body temperature (pulse must be taken simultaneously with temperature elevation).

[a] *Does not apply to patients with second/third degree heart block*, a pacemaker-induced pulse, or those on beta-blockers, diltiazem, or verapamil.

If more than one drug may be responsible for the drug fever, discontinue one at a time to identify the medication responsible.

DIAGNOSTIC APPROACH TO ANTIBIOTIC FAILURE

First, fever per se, should not be treated, unless harmful to the patient, e.g., extreme hyperpyrexia, severe cardiopulmonary disease, and brain trauma. Fever is an important host defense mechanism and provides diagnostic clues to the etiology of the fever. Fever is an indicator of effective antibiotic therapy. The usual approach to fever continues to be reflex pan culture of blood, wounds, respiratory secretions, and urine, without regard, for carefully considering clues indicating the likely source of the fever (infectious and non-infectious) [5,8].

In the CCU, in the absence of recent urologic procedures, urosepsis is rare. Catheter-associated bacteruria (CAB) alone does not produce fever or result in urosepsis in the normal host. Urosepsis may occur if the patient with an indwelling urinary catheter has obstruction, device (stent) urosepsis, or is a non-leukopenic compound host (DM, SLE, steroids, and cirrhosis).

Nosocomial pneumonias (NP) are difficult to diagnose, and respiratory secretion cultures are unhelpful and may be misleading. The diagnosis of NP is based on fever and new pulmonary infiltrates, but there are many mimics of NP, e.g., BOOP, ARDS (drug-induced pancreatitis), pulmonary hemorrhage, and heart failure. With NP, fever decreases with appropriately selected and dosed antibiotic therapy [23–25]. If no decrease in temperature, improvement of infiltrates on CXR, or resolution of leukocytosis after 2 weeks of therapy, the cause is not NP, and the patient needs a lung biopsy and not another or more antibiotics or a more prolonged course, e.g., HSV-1 NP [26,27].

REFERENCES

1. Cunha BA, Shea KW. Fever in the intensive care unit. *Inf Dis Clin North Am* 1996;10:185–209.
2. Cunha BA. Fever in the critical care unit. *Crit Care Clin* 1998;14:1–14.
3. Cunha BA. Fever in the intensive care unit. *Int Care Med* 1999;25:648–651.
4. Eljaaly K, Alshehri S, Aljabri A, et al. Clinical failure with and without empiric atypical bacteria coverage in hospitalized adults with community-acquired pneumonia: A systematic review and meta-analysis. *BMC Inf Dis* 2017;17:385.
5. Cunha BA, Ortega AM. Antibiotic failure. *Med Clin N Amer* 1995;79:663–672.
6. Garcia-Lamberechts EJ, Gonzalez-Del Castilo J, Hormigo Sanchez AL, et al. Factors predicting failure in empirical antibiotic treatment. *An Sist Sanit Navar* 2017;40:119–130.
7. Hassinger TE, Guidry CA, Rotstein OD, et al. Longer-duration antimicrobial therapy does not prevent treatment failure in high-risk patients with complicated intra-abdominal infections *Surg Inf* 2017;18:659–663.
8. Cunha CB, Cunha BA ed. *Antibiotic Essentials* (17th ed.). New Delhi, India: Jaypee Medical Publishers, 2020:1–15, 103–106, 596–599, 619–620, 657–658.
9. Cunha BA. Strategies to control antibiotic resistance. *Semin Respir Infect* 202;17:250–258.
10. Cunha BA. Intravenous line infections. *Crit Care Clin* 1998;14:339–346.
11. Ismail B, Shafei MN, Harun A, Ali S, Omar M, Deris ZZ. Predictors of polymyxin B treatment failure in gram-negative healthcare associated infections among critically ill patients. *J Micro Imm Inf* 2017;29:S1684.
12. McGuinness WA, Malachowa N, DeLeo FR. Vancomycin resistance in *Staphylococcus aureus*. *Yale J Biol Med* 2017;90:269–281.
13. Doern GV, Brecher SM. The clinical predictive value (or lack thereof) of the results of in vitro antimicrobial susceptibility tests. *J Clin Micro* 2011;49:S11–S14.

14. Tillotson GS, Zinner SH. Burden of antimicrobial resistance in an era of decreasing susceptibility. *Exp Rev Anti Inf Therapy* 2017;15:663–676.
15. Cunha BA. Predicting in vivo effectiveness from in vitro susceptibility: A step closer to performing testing of uropathogens in human urine. *Scand J Infect Dis* 2012;44: 714–715.
16. Musher DM, Minuth JN, Thorsteinsson SB, Holmes T. Effectivenes of achievable urinary concentrations of tetracyclines against "tetracycline-resistant" pathogenic bacteria. *J Infect Dis* 1975;131:S40–S44.
17. Stamey TA, Fair WR, Timothy MM, et al. Serum versus urinary antimicrobial concentration in cure of urinary tract infections. *N Engl J Med* 1974;291:1159.
18. Washington JA. Discrepancies between in vitro activity and in vivo response to antimicrobial agents. *Diagn Micro Inf Dis* 1983;1:25–31.
19. Yang L, Wang K, Li H, Denstedt JD, Cadieux PA. The influence of urinary pH on antibiotic efficacy against bacterial uropathogens. *Urology* 2014;84:713.e1–e7.
20. Ristuccia PA, Jonas M, Cunha BA. Antibiotic susceptibility of ampicillin resistant *E. coli* in urine to antibiotics at urinary concentration. *Adv Ther* 1986;3:163–167.

21. Cunha BA. Tigecycline dosing is critical in preventing tigecycline resistance because relative resistance is, in part, concentration dependent. *Clin Microbiol Infect* 2015;21:e39–e40.
22. Cunha BA, Cunha CB, Lam B, Giuga J, Chin J, Zafonte VF, Gerson S. Nitrofurantoin safety and effectiveness in treating acute uncomplicated cystitis in hospitalized adults with renal insufficiency: Antibiotic stewardship implications *Eur J Clin Micro Inf Dis* 2017;36:1213–1216.
23. Cunha BA. Slowly resolving and non-resolving pneumonias. *Drugs Today* 2000;36:829–834.
24. Cunha BA. Rash and fever in the critical care unit. *Crit Care Clin* 1998;141:35–53.
25. Cunha BA, Gian J, Klein NC. Severe adenoviral pneumonia in an immunocompetent host with persistent fevers treated with multiple empiric antibiotics for presumed bacterial co-infection: An antibiotic stewardship perspective of de-excalation derailed. *J Clin Med* 2017;6:E42.
26. Mohan S, Hamid NS, Cunha BA. A cluster of nosocomial herpes simplex virus type 1 pneumonia in a medical intensive care unit. *Inf Cont Hosp Epid* 2006;27:1255–1257.
27. Cunha BA, Eisenstein LE, Dillard T, Krol V. Herpes Simplex Virus (HSV) pneumonia in a heart transplant: Diagnosis and therapy. *Heart Lung* 2007;36:72–78.

Index

Note: Page numbers in bold and italics refer to tables and figures, respectively.

Printed and bound by CPI Group (UK) Ltd, Croydon, CR0 4YY

17/10/2024

01775663-0017